# GENERAL PSYCHOPATHOLOGY

# Volume One

# KARL JASPERS

# GENERAL PSYCHOPATHOLOGY

## Volume One

*Translated from the German by*

J. HOENIG

and

MARIAN W. HAMILTON

*With a new foreword by*

PAUL R. McHUGH, M.D.

THE JOHNS HOPKINS UNIVERSITY PRESS
Baltimore and London

Originally published in German as *Allgemeine Psychopathologie,* by Karl Jaspers
Copyright © Springer-Verlag Berlin Heidelberg 1959
Copyright © in the English translation 1963 Manchester University Press
Foreword, by Paul R. McHugh, M.D., © 1997 The Johns Hopkins University Press
Printed in the United States of America on acid-free paper

Johns Hopkins Paperbacks edition, 1997
9 8 7 6 5 4 3 2 1

The Johns Hopkins University Press
2715 North Charles Street
Baltimore, Maryland 21218-4319
The Johns Hopkins Press Ltd., London

Library of Congress Cataloging-in-Publication Data

Jaspers, Karl, 1883–1969.
   [Allgemeine Psychopathologie.   English]
   General psychopathology / Karl Jaspers ; translated from the German by J. Hoenig and
Marian W. Hamilton ; with a new foreword by Paul R. McHugh. — Johns Hopkins pbk. ed.
      p.     cm.
   Originally published: Chicago: University of Chicago Press, 1968.
   Includes bibliographical references and indexes.
   ISBN 0-8018-5775-9 (pbk. : v. 1 : alk. paper). — ISBN 0-8018-5815-1 (pbk. : v. 2 : alk.
paper)
   1. Psychiatry. 2. Psychology, Pathological. 3. Phenomenological psychology. I. Title.
   [DNLM: 1. Mental Disorders. 2. Psychology. WM 140 J39a 1968a]
RC454.J313   1997
616.89—dc21
DNLM/DLC
for Library of Congress                                                              97-18291
                                                                                      CIP

A catalog record for this book is available from the British Library.

# FOREWORD TO THE 1997 EDITION

## GENIUS IN A TIME, PLACE, AND PERSON

For those who would understand psychiatry, this book is indispensable. Although it draws from the clinical thought and practices of the late nineteenth and early twentieth centuries, its delineation of the methods for comprehending mental disorders remains unmatched to this day. It is, in fact, a product of a special time, place, and person.

### The Time

Consider first its time. The year *General Psychopathology* was published—1913—was pivotal in the history of psychiatry. It was the culmination of the most productive decade of this century. It was also the last year before the great German tradition of university-based empirical psychiatry was drowned by the chaos of war, economic depression, Nazi barbarism, and the Cold War's division of East and West Germany.

In the ten years from 1903 to 1913, the investment of fifty years of preparation and prior work bore fruit. In that decade, Emil Kraepelin published the eighth and definitive edition of his textbook (1909), Eugen Bleuler introduced the term *schizophrenia* (1906), and Alois Alzheimer described the condition that now bears his name (1907). These outstanding contributions to empirical psychiatry, though, were matched in the same decade by a maturing interpretive psychiatry. Sigmund Freud's fledgling movement, "psychoanalysis," gained international reputation through its spread among neurologists, private practitioners, and the sophisticated middle classes of Europe, through the interest of American physicians and society prompted by Freud's 1909 visit to Clark University, and through the revisionism and generation of alternative ideas provided by the breakaway in this decade of former students of Freud—Alfred Adler and Carl Gustav Jung. Freud, Jung, and Adler did more than propose explanations for psychiatric disorder; they generated a movement of thought about human mental life, well enough advanced by 1913 for any perspicacious student to predict its eventual power and claims.

As is obvious from this mere sketch, the initial collision between empirical and interpretive psychiatry occurred in this decade and originated in two linear Teutonic thinkers (Kraepelin and Freud). Their contention demanded resolution, but—with the exception of this great book—no such effort was made, in part because of the social chaos that enveloped the original champions and their followers. Enervating as it is to teaching and practice, this psychiatric conflict festers to the present day, with empiric and interpretive psychiatry retitled "biologic" and "dynamic." The monolithic tyrannies of the originators persist.

## The Place

If 1913 was a propitious year for someone to identify and resolve the warring concepts of psychiatry, then the place where this book was written was itself ideal. The Psychiatric Clinic of the University of Heidelberg, the preeminent German university and academic center, was under the direction of Franz Nissl, he of the Nissl stain in neurohistology. Nissl was an intense, hardworking, odd character who started on the wrong side in the battle of the neuron theory and learned from his mistakes. He was the perfect chief for such a clinical research institution: a methodical scientist himself who had learned about the difficulties of discovery.

A man of integrity without envy, Nissl could get others to join him in the enterprise of clinical and investigative psychiatry. He emphasized his colleagues' strengths rather than harping on their weaknesses. With these traits, combined with a passionate interest in scientific effort and achievement, he created an atmosphere of vigorous and free discussion among his faculty. For all that his own creativity was modest, his choices of colleagues, his enthusiasm for new enterprises, and his lack of autocratic tyrannies helped to create an environment in which inventiveness of all kinds flourished.

Nissl was not initially enthusiastic about this work of Karl Jaspers, wondering whether it was merely philosophical hairsplitting or "monkey business," as he called abstract treatises. Once he had read it, however (carrying the galley sheets around in the pocket of his white coat for weeks), he became its champion. Jaspers noted that Franz Nissl in Heidelberg in 1913 was just the right leader to produce a "genius of place."

## The Person

The time and place inspired a special person to write this book. Karl Jaspers came to Heidelberg right from medical school in 1908. He brought with him a unique set of qualities. Although initially interested in philosophy, he had turned to study medicine, which, he believed, best illuminated life itself and the challenges of human existence. However, he was chronically ill with bronchiectasis and could not assume heavy clinical duties. Jaspers won Nissl's begrudging permission to work in the library rather than the clinic or laboratory. His skills as an open-minded, critical, indeed often skeptical, thinker about psychiatric opinions and practices came to the fore. Jaspers soon realized, and as promptly said, that the library volumes (and the psychiatric periodical literature) were filled with "unfounded chatter." This "chatter" derived from the mushrooming of independent self-referential schools of thought about patients—each with its own terminology. Jaspers discerned that there was no commonly accepted, science-based, logical approach to psychiatry, not even a common observational method for identifying the manifestations of psychiatric disorders.

The problem was not just in the library. In the clinics as well, psychiatrists on one day seemed to work to a Kraepelinian diagnostic formula, but on the next proposed some theoretical explanation that took nothing from the previous day's ideas. It seemed to Jaspers that psychiatrists struggled to make sense of their discipline. They were aware of concepts and facts, but were unsure of when particular explanations for disorder might apply, and adopted treatments and research programs almost on impulse. Coincidentally Jaspers also appreciated why many of his more gifted contemporaries restricted their work to brain studies. At least they could get their hands around the brain, even if the problem of importance to the patient lay somewhere else.

"To make real progress psychiatrists must learn to think," he said during one discussion with colleagues. "Jaspers ought to be spanked," replied his contemporaries.

Jaspers sensed that psychiatry inhabited a middle ground between science, where laws of nature are discerned, and history, where fateful events are conceived as emerging from human choices and actions. That is, Jaspers knew that some mental disorders derive from brain diseases, and therefore psychiatrists should be close allies with neurologists. But he also knew that mental distress could emerge as consequences of some conflict between an individual's wishes and actual life circumstances, so psychiatrists should naturally share interests with students in the social and cultural disciplines. In fact, Jaspers saw more coherence and conceptual development among neurologists and social scientists than among most psychiatrists. The students in the disciplines surrounding psychiatry tended to reflect on the methods behind their opinions and thus learned to judge them.

Jaspers turned to three prominent social scientists to organize his thought: the philosopher Edmund Husserl, the historian Wilhelm Dilthey, and the political scientist Max Weber. Husserl comes first because Jaspers took from Husserl an approach to examining patients. Husserl taught that the contents of the conscious mind of others could be accessed and described by what he called at first "descriptive psychology" and later "phenomenology." Jaspers followed Husserl's lead and, with modifications for the clinical setting, defined a phenomenological approach to interviewing and examining psychiatric patients.

The phenomenological method hinges on the human capacity for self-expression—a means of communicating one's experiences to another. This capacity makes it possible for patients to describe the contents of their minds and for psychiatrists listening to these descriptions to enter the mental life of such patients. Through this process psychiatrists can empathically penetrate (almost co-experience) their patients' thoughts, perceptions, and feelings and note the similarities and differences among the "phenomena" they find.

The phenomenologically inspired interaction between psychiatrists and patients calls for efforts that go beyond the definition and cataloging of disordered mental events such as delusions and hallucinations. The psychiatrist attempts to grasp these events as experiences within the consciousness of the patient—a kind of "living with" the events as the patient recounts them.

Jaspers, following Husserl, proposed that psychiatrists could achieve such an understanding of their patients' mental life if they approached the task of inquiry without prejudice of theory but rather by attempting to gain from a patient a full description of his or her mental experience. The process is not some secret seeking but rather a true "meeting of minds." In this book Jaspers lays out a treasury of characteristic disruptive experiences within human consciousness accessible to psychiatrists prepared to take up such a "walk in your shoes" stance with their patients.

Once he clarified the "phenomenologic" approach and described the characteristic features of disordered thoughts, perceptions, and emotions, Jaspers's next issue was to differentiate the several prevailing explanations for mental disorders. Again he had little help from the psychiatric literature, where he found a muddle of conflicting schools of thought. Here he turned to Dilthey and Weber. These social scientists taught that drawing explanatory "connections" between events—as, for example, concluding that the loss of a parent in childhood produced a revengeful character in the adult—was a hazardous business if not done methodically and systematically.

The social scientists had two methods at hand. An empirical, statistical demonstration of the regular co-occurrences of certain events in a population might provide evidence for the "connection" between them, but an empathic assertion that a particular experience had special meaning in the life story of an individual might suggest even more powerfully the link between an experience and a later behavior. Jaspers's goal became the appropriation and practical differentiation of these two social science methods of explanation so as to make them available to psychiatric teaching, investigation, and practice.

Thus, he could support Kraepelin's opinions on heredity and mental illness based on the statistical study of hundreds of patients and their families. And, as well, he could identify what Freud and Adler were claiming for "connections" between early life experience and the development of a disorder such as hysteria or anxiety. Jaspers, taking the terminology from Dilthey, distinguished these two modes of work by speaking of Kraepelin's method as "explanation" (*erklären*). "Explanation," Jaspers noted, was the attempt to discern nature's laws acting impersonally, through "causal connections," to produce a mental disorder.

Jaspers identified Freud's method as "understanding" (*verstehen*). "Understanding," Jaspers taught, grasped for "meaningful connections" in an attempt to demonstrate that disorder emerged because of a conflict between experience and a specific individual's hopes and desires—a conflict and its emotional consequences that could be empathically appreciated for the person even though not statistically demonstrable.

By differentiating "explanation" and "understanding," Jaspers emphasized that there was a critical epistemological divide within the field of psychiatry and that psychiatrists could bridge this divide only by appreciating these different methods at their disposal. But woe to the psychiatrist who confused "understanding" with "explanation" (as Jaspers believed Freud to have done), because then false claims and misdirected hypotheses would once again muddle this field.

Thus, from each method Jaspers identified contributions to psychiatry. But he emphasized those contributions as having limits implicit in the method itself. For example, he noted that Kraepelinian labels might slight the personal suffering of an individual, whereas Freudian interpretations might overlook a neurobiologic process.

Jaspers also emphasized those limits because he held that neither provided full views of human mental life and its potentials. He believed and emphasized in his phenomenological studies that the individual human being—even afflicted by mental disorder—was always more than we can know. In essence, Jaspers's object was to show psychiatrists exactly what they know, how they know it, and what they do not know and cannot claim. He wrote this book with these aims in mind.

*Aftermath*

*General Psychopathology* was a splendid achievement for anyone but amazing for a man of barely thirty years of age. A fascinating fact, though, is that it culminated the psychiatric productivity of its author, who, with the exception of revising the text (with some expansion) for subsequent editions (this is the seventh), left psychiatric work forever. He became a distinguished leader in twentieth-century existential philosophy. He was also a voice of reason in the catastrophic events that overcame his university and his country. He was a prodigy in many ways, but as a physician, who led a philosophical movement and denounced tyranny when others were silent, he was most special.

Jaspers always claimed that the work in *General Psychopathology* was his avenue to understanding human nature. An open, unblinkered view of mental illness gave him a comprehension of mental health. As well, his dedication to identifying limits to imperious claims about human beings protected him from the huge ideological errors of this century. His emphasis on the phenomena of human consciousness helped him grasp an essential characteristic of human mental life—its promise. His commitment to this promise provoked his enmity to the totalitarian systems that sprang up in the West (Fascism, National Socialism, Marxism/Leninism).

From the same allegiance to promise he also opposed physician/scientists who, emphasizing a fragmentary knowledge of human biology, slighted the value and grounds for hope in the lives of their patients. Thus, right from 1913, Jaspers attacked the growing power of the eugenics movement, which engaged psychiatrists around the world seeking "racial hygiene." His strong and persisting enmity toward racism in all its forms came from the same source and was based on his recognition of the fundamental unity of human mental experiences played out in individual lives and purposes.

His quarrels with psychoanalysis grew over time and increased with each edition of *General Psychopathology*. (They can also be reviewed in his philosophical works, such as *Man in the Modern Age*.) The quarrel began in the first edition, in which he challenged the views of Freud and his followers that they had a scientific—that is, "causal" or "explanatory" rather than a "meaningful"—approach to mental disorders. Later, when the requirement for a training analysis became psychoanalytic policy, Jaspers attacked the movement both for its indoctrinating methods toward its students and for its fundamental nihilism (deriving even what is best in a person from base origins that only psychoanalysis can unveil).

At the very heart of all his teaching is Jaspers's radical commitment to two great themes, freedom and responsibility. These two themes must interrelate either for a person to reach his or her innate promise or for all of us to build a society worthy of mankind. The first of the two themes declares that the essence of human beings is freedom. Unlike all other creatures, men and women face an unpredictable future and have unlimited opportunities for progress. Jaspers's sense of human freedom aroused his hatred for simplistic notions about our nature and for coercive forces that would restrict our development to certain paths. He foresaw situations in which thinking about human beings as animals would eventually lead to treating them as such—culling them as if they were a flock or a herd.

The second theme—responsibility—reflects his appreciation that the way things are formed—families forged, societies built, cities sustained, and the future realized—depends in the last analysis on the decisions and deeds of individuals. "Each individual—by his way of life, his daily small deeds, by his great decisions, testifies to himself as to what is possible. By this, his present actuality, he contributes unknowingly toward the future." This idea—that there is no law of nature or law of history which determines what is and what will be, but rather it is the many and repeated choices of free individuals which make or break this world—was fundamental to Jaspers's thought as a psychiatrist and as a philosopher. It made him inspect the choices suggested to and imposed on people by authorities of all kinds—scientific authorities as much as political authorities—and ultimately set him at odds with tyrannies—both the tyrannies of governments and the tyrannies of the crowd.

The central problem of modernity is how to tie freedom to self-government. In *General Psychopathology*, Jaspers addresses this issue as he describes the conceptual foundations of psychotherapy. He discloses that order in mental life is a consequence of enlightened freedom, not an imposition on it. Here Jaspers voices opinions that he derives from that quintessential modern source, psychotherapy, but that have had earlier advocates and other derivations (Thucydides from war, Augustine from the ruins of an imperial civilization, Jefferson from revolution). The main point of these advocates—and the essence of Jaspers's thought—is that people are free but can learn that they are responsible for the consequences of their actions.

These ideas, the promise in human nature and its realization through the interplay of freedom and responsibility, with all their implications for both psychiatric practice and a democratic society, are not found in the clinical writings of Jaspers's contemporaries, Kraepelin or Freud. This is another seldom-noted, distinguishing feature of his work in both psychiatry and philosophy. Thus Jaspers *alone* advances the wisdom about patients needed to dispel the contemporary agitations around psychiatry that characteristically clamor for rights and disregard implications. These include the antipsychiatry of Michel Foucault and Thomas Szasz, the demand for physician-assisted suicide in the Netherlands, and the subtle forms of eugenics that the Human Genome Project has in store.

*Conclusion*

I call this book indispensable even though it was written eighty-four years ago—before the discovery of the EEG, DNA, or norepinephrine. I hold this view because, despite these many scientific advances, most of the problems that Jaspers noted in 1913 remain as problems to psychiatry today. We have more information than Jaspers found crowding the shelves in Heidelberg, but we still disagree about how best to order this information so as to encourage its steady progress and to read its fundamental messages.

Jaspers noted that psychiatrists must "develop and order knowledge guided by the methods through which it is gained—to learn the process of knowing and thereby to clarify the material." The twentieth century brought more facts to us. But a systematic appreciation of the methods of observation and interpretation that psychiatrists employ is essential to transform these facts into knowledge and its ultimate implications. No one since Jaspers has done it better.

PAUL R. McHUGH, M.D.
Henry Phipps Professor and Director
Department of Psychiatry and Behavioral Sciences
Johns Hopkins Medical Institutions

REFERENCES

Jaspers, K. The Phenomenological Approach in Psychopathology. *British Journal of Psychiatry* 114:1313–1323, 1968.
Jaspers, K. Philosophical Autobiography. In Paul A. Schilpp (ed.), *The Philosophy of Karl Jaspers*. La Salle: Open Court Publishing Company, 1981.
Shepherd, M. Karl Jaspers: General Psychopathology. *British Journal of Psychiatry* 141:310–312, 1982.

Shepherd, M. The Sciences and General Psychopathology. In M. Shepherd and O. L. Zangwill (eds.), *Handbook of Psychiatry*, Vol. 1. Cambridge: Cambridge University Press, 1982.

Slavney, P. R., and McHugh, P. R. *Psychiatric Polarities* (Chapter 3, Explanation and Understanding). Baltimore: Johns Hopkins University Press, 1987.

Wiggins, O. P., and Schwartz, M. A. Chris Walker's Interpretation of Karl Jaspers' Phenomenology: A Critique. *Philosophy, Psychiatry, and Psychology* 2:319–343, 1996.

Wiggins, O. P., and Schwartz, M. A. Edmund Husserl's Influence on Karl Jaspers' Phenomenology. *Philosophy, Psychiatry, and Psychology* 4:15–36, 1997.

# FOREWORD

I am honoured that the task of writing a foreword to the English translation of the seventh and latest edition of this great psychiatric classic should devolve upon me. An English translation is long overdue. It is a source of satisfaction to me also that this translation should emerge from the Manchester University Department of Psychiatry. Karl Jaspers has worldwide eminence as a philosopher; his outstanding contribution to psychiatric thought is less well-known, at least amongst psychiatrists in England and America. The first edition of the *Allgemeine Psychopathologie* appeared nearly fifty years ago, in 1913, when the author was barely thirty years of age. Before this, in 1910, Jaspers had created a stir in the world of German psychiatry by the publication of his seminal article on morbid jealousy in which he first brought to the light of day his method and fundamental principles. As one of his biographers has remarked, Jaspers showed in this momentous contribution his sure eye for psychopathological detail and it was in this article that he first introduced his concept of 'process' versus 'personality development'. This laid the basis of so-called psychopathological phenomenology which, through the work of Jaspers and a brilliant group of colleagues, amongst whom may be mentioned Hans Gruhle, Kurt Schneider, the late Professor Mayer-Gross, well-known to us in this country, and several others, became the particular decoration of the Heidelberg school of psychiatry. The importance of this development in psychiatric thought has been on the whole insufficiently recognised, even in the land of its origin. In recent years, however, there has been an evident increase of interest in and attention to the teachings of this school. The Heidelberg school, until recently under the leadership of Professor Kurt Schneider, whose own contributions over the last fifty years have been outstanding, has stimulated a large number of younger men who have broken fresh ground. It may, I think, be fairly said that the school of phenomenology with its developmental offshoots is at the moment the most significant school in present-day German psychiatry. That this school should have been insufficiently recognised in England is perhaps hardly suprising. Many reasons can be adduced for this, first and foremost of which is the linguistic barrier. Secondly, even for those familiar with the German language, Jaspers' thought and style are difficult, due no doubt to his training as a philosopher, and his consequent use at times of terms specially devised to express some nuance of meaning not easily, if at all, to be translated intelligibly. To the English with their ingrained empiricism such an approach might well repel at first sight as academic and theoretical. Yet this would be a superficial valuation. In fact, the whole basis of Jaspers' work is strongly empirical and, as he is at pains to affirm, strictly within the framework of the inductive method of the natural sciences as far as the often intangible subject matter of this difficult field allows. By a remarkable paradox, however, our supposedly empirical countrymen have accepted readily enough, and on the whole with an astonishing lack of criticism, the often unproved and unprovable assertions of the so-called psychodynamic schools. To those to whom such teachings form an acceptable psychopathology, the work of Jaspers might well appear static and arid. Static it is certainly not, arid it may be to those for whom the still sparse and inconvenient facts of mental illness must be circumvented by romantic fancies. This statement implies no facile derision of psychoanalytic teaching, it reflects rather an unvoiced Utopian regret that, due no doubt to the nature of the subject, psychoanalytic teaching, often enough characterised by profound insight into human behaviour, could not have been limited to the thoughtful and critical few. On the other hand the phenomenological approach involves painstaking, detailed and laborious study of facts observed in the individual patient at the conscious level. It is the method which forms the basis of the clinical practice and teaching of the Manchester Department of Psychiatry and one which I believe is fundamental to sound clinical work. Moreover, I believe that whatever other paths the young clinical psychiatrist may come ultimately to tread, whatever particular orientation he may come later to adopt, a knowledge of the principles stated in this book is indispensable to him. For whilst one of the great merits of the book lies in its tentative formulations and the resolute determination of the author to go no further than the facts, and whilst some of Jaspers' interpretations and analyses of morbid phenomena have been subjected to searching criticism, and some are now not widely accepted, the principles remain and with these the continuing influence of the work.

As long as psychiatric diagnosis and treatment rest on psychopathological investigation, the continuing improvement and sharpening of this tool of investigation must remain a prime concern to psychiatrists. This book is a guide to that technique, still irreplaceable, much of it is still as fresh as the day it was written and still a lively stimulus to others yet to come.

The world of English-speaking psychiatry stands in debt to the translators, my two colleagues Dr. J. Hoenig and Miss M. W. Hamilton. It had been for long my earnest desire that this key work should be translated into English. When Dr. Hoenig joined my staff I was gratified to learn that he had already contemplated doing so. Miss Hamilton, who had had already some considerable experience in translating from the German other works of this particular school, seemed an obvious collaborator. I wish therefore to thank them particularly for having undertaken this immensely difficult task. If here and there the translation may seem to have faltered, this can, I am sure, be charged for the most part to the difficulty and at times impossibility of rendering the author's subtle thought into concise and comprehensible English.

E. W. ANDERSON

# TRANSLATORS' PREFACE

Being concerned with the teaching of psychiatry, we have felt as keenly as others the lack of a fundamental textbook in psychopathology. The existing difficulties of psychiatry as a subject are many but they seem rooted in two major shortcomings:

1. Although modern clinical psychiatry is still largely based on the achievements of continental psychiatrists, particularly of those French and German workers, who wrote in the first quarter of this century, much of what has been written remains inaccessible to the English-speaking psychiatrist who is unfamiliar with these languages. This often results in a very superficial understanding of the concepts, which are either used out of their proper context or put into a wrong one. The confusion which follows is suffocating.

2. As a consequence of this confusion, but also going beyond it, there is an absence of common terminology. Identical expressions tend to be used for entirely different entities, and one and the same entity is often given two, three or more different names as if it were so many different things.

It is said that the development of psychiatry has at present reached a stage where a unification of viewpoints is impossible. This is true; more than that, a unification is not even desirable. Thought and research must be free to explore in many directions and within many different theoretical frameworks. But conceptual confusion and the lack of a common, basic terminology far from safeguarding this freedom constitute a major threat to it. It is precisely because there are now so many different interpretations of the few known facts that the need for improved communication within the profession has become paramount. We need to know better what psychiatry has already achieved and discipline ourselves more, to use a shared terminology within clearly defined theoretical frameworks.

Though none, perhaps, are better placed to further such an aim than the editors of the psychiatric journals themselves, professional education remains the function of the University Departments. With this in mind we decided to translate Karl Jaspers' *General Psychopathology*. To make the book available in English had been a firm objective with one of us (J.H.) since 1951, but hitherto the scale of the work had failed to attract a publisher. However the University Department in Manchester seemed to offer an excellent opportunity for a fresh endeavour since the climate of this Department under Professor Anderson's teaching was very favourable to the Heidelberg School and one of us (M.W.H.) had already had experience in translating other psychiatric texts from the German.[1] No other work better meets the need for

---

[1] K. Schneider, *Psychopathic Personalities* (Cassell, 1958); *Clinical Psychopathology* (Grune & Stratton, 1959).

a critical introduction to continental psychiatry and for the creation of a terminology which would be commonly acceptable. The translation therefore was begun in 1958 but, as we were only able to work in our own time, it was not completed until 1962. The task has proved exacting but very instructive and always enjoyable.

One of Jaspers' explicit aims was to systematise the main methods of approach in psychopathology and thus facilitate the building of a common terminology. To do justice to this latter has presented us with some formidable difficulties. We have tackled these in several different ways:

1. We retain the original German or French term (e.g. 'Gestalt', 'Anlage', 'Querulant', 'Milieu', 'Absences'), where the words have already become part of English usage. Where a possible translation has suggested itself, but we have felt doubtful, we have given the German term in brackets with a cross-reference in the index, e.g. Thought-resonance (Gedankenlautwerden), Thrust (Schub) of the schizophrenic process, Talking past the point (Vorbeireden), Inhibition on becoming (Werdenshemmung), etc.

2. Where the obvious English translation is already in technical usage but represents quite a different concept from its German step-brother, e.g. 'Psychopathy' for 'Psychopathie', we have avoided it, since its use would give rise to confusion. We have, therefore, translated 'Psychopathie' as 'personality disorder', which is a term relatively free from any other specific meaning and appears to express quite adequately what is meant by the term 'Psychopathie' in continental psychiatry. But we have retained 'neurosis' for 'Neurose' since here the term has retained the same sense in both languages, namely, a psychogenic disorder of behaviour and thought.

3. The term 'paranoid' presented us with special difficulties. We have used it in keeping with the Oxford Dictionary definition of Paranoia (n. Mental derangement, esp. when marked by delusions, of grandeur, etc. [Gk. -noia f. para (noos—mind), distracted]. The German usage is also in line with this definition and implies a 'wrong notion', synonymous with 'delusional'. In English, however, 'paranoid' is often used to mean 'persecutory' both in technical psychiatry and in general usage. This has led to a good deal of confusion with such expressions as 'paranoid schizophrenia' (i.e. a schizophrenic picture in which delusions predominate), since the content of the delusions can have other than persecutory content, e.g. messianic, hypochondriacal, magical, etc. Thus the expression 'paranoid features' does not properly mean 'ideas of persecution' but merely the 'presence of delusions'. As there does not seem any philological justification for the use of this word in the narrower sense of 'persecutory', we have retained the broader meaning in accordance with the dictionary definition.

4. We have translated the philosophical terms as best we could. We were not able to get much help from translations of Jaspers' philosophical works nor from other writings. These translations have not been consistent nor particularly happy, and, on advice from our colleagues in the University Depart-

ment of Philosophy, we decided to go our own way, keeping the other translations in mind as much as possible. Terms such as 'Existenz' (Existence itself), 'Dasein' (Existence as such; existence in a world; human existence), 'Sein' (Being), 'So-Sein' (Being-Thus), 'Das Umgreifende' (that which encompasses, the Encompassing) or 'Geist' presented some of our greatest difficulties. The latter we found impossible to render by any single English word. It appears as 'mind', 'spirit', 'culture', according to the context.

5. Certain words in common German usage have been 'coined' by Jaspers and given specific meanings. The two most important 'Verstehen' (understanding) and 'Erklären' (explanation) run through the whole book and are related to his central theme, the dichotomy of psychic phenomena into 'psychogenic development' versus 'organic process'. Both these orders of psychic phenomena occur in all the conditions encountered in psychiatric practice, are usually inextricably intertwined and must be separated out for complete comprehension of the mental state. Jaspers uses 'Verstehen• and 'Erklären' to describe the methods of their respective exploration. Words which would fully convey his exact meaning do not exist in either German or English and even for the German reader lengthy comment was needed (p. 301, footnote). We therefore thought it best to retain the literal translation throughout the book, wherever possible. However, for clarity's sake we have been forced to 'coin' certain phrases, especially in respect of 'Verstehen' and its adjectival use 'verstehende' (e.g. 'verstehende Psychologie'—'the psychology of meaningful connections, meaningful psychology, psychology of meaning'), Where 'understanding' is non-specific in Jaspers' sense, the term 'comprehend'. —'Begreifen' has been used.

Finally, we are aware that in trying to be faithful to the text and preserve in some measure the author's style, our translation may at times leave the reader, as it has us, dissatisfied, but we hope that in all major matters the intention of this great work has been served truly by its English rendering.

We were greatly helped by many; we would like to acknowledge the sympathetic support accorded by Professor E. W. Anderson and the unceasing encouragement offered us in particular by Sir Aubrey Lewis and the late Professor Mayer-Gross. A number of colleagues have helped in preparing the scripts and proofs in their various stages. We wish to thank particularly Mr. J. C. Kenna and Dr. N. L. Gittleson. We are also indebted to colleagues and friends who have helped in the compilation and paging of the index, in particular Mr. Harold Smith, Dr. Uma Sreenivasan and Mrs Meti Abraham.

Last but not least we wish to thank Mr. T. L. Jones, Secretary of the Manchester University Press, for his constant help and the patience he has brought to bear on the many problems involved.

*Manchester, 1962*                                                                          J.H.
                                                                                                      M.W.H.

# AUTHOR'S PREFACES

*To the first edition* (1913)

This book sets out to survey the entire field of general psychopathology and the facts and viewpoints of this science. It also sets out to be a guide to the literature for all those who are interested.

Instead of presenting dogmatic statements of results, it prefers to introduce the reader to problems, approaches and methods, and instead of a system based on a theory, it would like to achieve some kind of order based on a deliberate methodology.

There are in psychopathology a number of viewpoints, a number of parallel approaches which in themselves are quite justifiable and complement rather than oppose each other. My efforts have been directed towards sorting these approaches out, separating them clearly and at the same time demonstrating the many-sided nature of our science. An attempt has been made to include every empirically-based approach and every field of psychopathological interest, so that as far as possible the reader may gain a really comprehensive view of psychopathology as a whole and not merely be presented with a personal opinion, a particular school or a set of ideas that happens to be in vogue.

In many parts of the book we have had simply to record and enumerate facts so far available, data still lacking in context and experiments that are as yet tentative. But in psychopathology it is dangerous merely to learn the matter, our task is not to 'learn psychopathology' but to learn to observe, ask questions, analyse and think in psychopathological terms. I would like to help the student to acquire a well-ordered body of knowledge, which will offer a point of departure for new observations and enable him to set freshly acquired knowledge in its proper place.

*To the second and third editions* (*extracts*, 1919 *and* 1922)

. . . We trail around with us a great number of vague generalities. I have tried to clarify them as far as possible. But the deep intentions, which sometimes find expression through them, should not simply be put aside and let fall, because full clarification has not been attained. . . . The opinion has been expressed in medical quarters that this book is too hard for students, because it attempts to tackle extremely difficult and ultimate problems. As far as that is concerned, I am convinced that either one grasps a science entirely, that means in its central problems, or not at all. I consider it fatal simply to adjust at a low level. One should be guided by the better students who are interested in the subject for its own sake, even though they may be in a minority. Those who teach should compel their students to rise to a scientific level. But this is made impossible if 'compendia' are used, which give students fragmentary, superficial pseudo-knowledge 'for practical purposes', and which sometimes is more subversive for practice than total ignorance. One should not show a façade of science. There is a decline in culture and intellectual effort in our days and it is the duty of everyone not to compromise. This book has, as a matter of fact, found its way to students; I feel justified in hoping that it will remain in the hands of students.

. . . In general, the methodological climate of the book remains important. In the midst of all the psychopathological talk, we have to learn to know what we know and do not know, to know how and in what sense and within what limits we know something, by what means that knowledge was gained and on what it was founded. This is so because knowledge is not a smooth expanse of uniform and equivalent truths but an ordered structure of quite diverse kinds of validity, importance and essence.

## To the fourth edition (1942)

The intention of this book has remained unchanged. Its working-out however has called for a complete re-writing. This was so because of the extensive research done in psychopathology during the last two decades and because of the deepening of my own basic knowledge.

The book aims very high. It would like, as far as the subject matter is concerned, to satisfy the universal demand for knowledge. It wishes to be of service to physicians and all those who make mankind their theme.

I have attempted to get to know all the material provided by research, obtain an over-all picture and present it vividly. Everything, which has been contributed to the knowledge of the sick human psyche by psychiatrists in the main, but also by general physicians, psychologists, psychotherapists, biologists and philosophers, has needed to be analysed in respect of its basic features and also found a place within a realistic classification. The illumination brought by analysis of methods has provided me with the means. Such a task, in all its width, can only be achieved for the time being and then only incompletely. I hope that now I have succeeded better than in my previous attempt.

I want to thank *Professor Kurt Schneider*[1] of Munich. Not only has he stimulated me with penetrating criticism and valuable suggestions but he has greatly encouraged my work through his positive and exacting attitudes.

I am also grateful to *Professor Oehlkers* of Freiburg for information on biological questions and for clarifying them in discussion. He read through the chapter on Heredity and made improvements.

[1] Now (1946) in Heidelberg.

I wish to thank my publisher *Dr. Ferdinand Springer*. My impulse to re-write was aroused through his expressed wish in the spring of 1941 that I should again work over the book which Springer and Wilmanns stimulated me to write thirty years before, and through the generosity with which he left it entirely to me to determine the scope and time in which to write it. After the first hesitation I became wholly absorbed by the task and instead of making minor adjustments set myself once more to reconstruct the whole.

*Professor Carl Schneider* made my work much easier by admitting me to the free use of the Library at the Heidelberg Clinic for Neuro-psychiatry and by being always ready, even at the cost of considerable trouble, to obtain books for me, for which I am most grateful.


## To the seventh edition (1959)

A long time ago this book came into being in the Heidelberg Clinic. Under Nissl's leadership, Wilmanns, Gruhle, Wetzel, Homburger, Mayer-Gross and others created a community of living research. (See my brief description in *Philosophie und Welt*, 1958, pp. 286–92. Regarding Franz Nissl, there is an excellent essay by Hugo Spatz in the *Grosse Nervenärzte*, vol. 2, 1959, ed. K. Kolle). Within the framework of Wundt's brain-research and accompanied by much fierce discussion, phenomenology and the psychology of meaningful connections came into being. At the same time as they appeared, they were established methodologically. The psychology of meaningful connection has become an undisputed part of psychiatry, drawing today from other sources, some of which are productive, others highly confused. When my book has been on occasion described as representative of the phenomenological trend, or of the trend of meaningful psychology, this has been only partly correct. It reaches into a far wider sphere: the clarification of psychiatric methods in general, modes of comprehension and ways of research. The aim has been to work through all the available empirical knowledge critically, by reflecting on the methods whereby it was gained, and then give it a general presenta-tion.

To bring the book up to date on the basis of the psychiatric research of the last two decades, would have necessitated my living for a while as an observer in a clinic in order to refresh and extend my own experience. Even if this had been possible, nowadays I would not be able to manage it. The book however rouses a steady interest and does not seem to be out of date. Considerable extensions in its material might be necessary, particularly as regards researches into the brain and somatic research in general, but the methodological principles remain largely unaffected by the increased material. It would certainly be possible nowadays to write a better book even on the methodological side. Such a task must fall to a younger scientist who might well succeed if he would appropriate the methodological clarification of this book, expand it and put it perhaps into a different context. I would gladly welcome such a book. Until it appears this present old one is well suited to help the physician who wants to learn how to 'think' in psychopathological terms.

KARL JASPERS

# SUMMARY OF CONTENTS

## Volume One

# Volume Two

### Part One: Individual Psychic Phenomena

### CHAPTER I

### SUBJECTIVE PHENOMENA OF MORBID PSYCHIC LIFE (PHENOMENOLOGY)

#### SECTION ONE: ABNORMAL PSYCHIC PHENOMENA

## CHAPTER II

### OBJECTIVE PERFORMANCES OF PSYCHIC LIFE— (PERFORMANCE PSYCHOLOGY—LEISTUNGSPSYCHOLOGIE)

## CHAPTER V

## MEANINGFUL CONNECTIONS

## CHAPTER VI

## MEANINGFUL CONNECTIONS AND THEIR SPECIFIC MECHANISMS

### SECTION ONE: NORMAL MECHANISMS

CHAPTER VII

THE PATIENT'S ATTITUDE TO HIS ILLNESS

CHAPTER VIII

THE TOTALITY OF THE MEANINGFUL CONNECTIONS
(CHARACTEROLOGY)

# VOLUME TWO

## Part Three: The Causal Connections of Psychic Life
### (Explanatory Psychology—Erklärende Psychologie)

# CHAPTER IX

## EFFECTS OF ENVIRONMENT AND OF THE BODY ON PSYCHIC LIFE

# CHAPTER X

## HEREDITY

CHAPTER XI

EXPLANATORY THEORIES—THEIR MEANING AND VALUE

Part Four: The Conception of the Psychic Life as a Whole

CHAPTER XII

THE SYNTHESIS OF DISEASE ENTITIES (NOSOLOGY)

## CHAPTER XIII

## THE HUMAN SPECIES (EIDOLOGY)

## CHAPTER XIV

## BIOGRAPHICAL STUDY (BIOGRAPHIK)

## Appendix

# GENERAL PSYCHOPATHOLOGY

# Volume One

# INTRODUCTION

The aim of this introduction is to remind the reader of the wide, unrestricted field in which the science of psychopathology has to make its way. Since each chapter provides the necessary basis for its subject-matter there is no need to lay any general foundation in these opening remarks. We shall simply centre discussion on the modes of human experience and the meaning of psychopathology. Patients' actual experiences will be reported on later.

## § 1. THE BOUNDARIES OF GENERAL PSYCHOPATHOLOGY

### (a) *Psychiatry as clinical practice and psychopathology as a science*

The psychiatrist as a practitioner deals with individuals, with the human being as a whole. These individuals may be patients in his care or under treatment, he may give testimony on their behalf in a Court of Law or to other authorities, or a personal opinion on them to historians, or may just see them in his consulting-room. Every case is entirely 'unique' but to deal with it competently the psychiatrist has to look to psychopathology to provide him with certain general concepts and laws. Psychiatrists function primarily as living, comprehending and acting persons, to whom science is only one resource among many; for psychopathologists, however, science is the sole and ultimate aim of their work. Their interest is not the individual human being. Their aim is to know, recognise, describe and analyse general principles rather than particular individuals. Their major concern is not the usefulness of science (this comes automatically as progress is made) but what the real, distinguishable phenomena are, what truths can be discovered about them and how they can be tested and demonstrated. Empathy and observation bring complex material, indispensable for study, but psychopathologists want more than this; they want communicable concepts for this material which can then be formulated into laws and principles and demonstrable relationships. This being so, they have to accept certain limitations so as not to transgress but on the other hand they gain freedom and power to explore the wide field which is left to them.

*Psychopathology is limited* in that there can be no final analysis of human beings as such, since the more we reduce them to what is typical and normative the more we realise there is something hidden in every human individual which defies recognition. We have to be content with partial knowledge of an infinity which we cannot exhaust. As a person, not as a psychopathologist, one may well see more; and, if others see more which is exceptional and unique, we should refrain from letting this interfere with our psychopathology. Ethical, aesthetic and metaphysical values are established independently from psychopathological assessment and analysis.

I

Apart from this field of values, which has nothing to do with psychiatry, instinctive attitudes and personal intuitions, which are usually quite incommunicable, are essential nevertheless for clinical practice. It has often been emphasised that psychiatry is still an 'expertise' and has not yet reached the status of a science. Science calls for systematic, conceptual thinking which can be communicated to others. Only in so far as psychopathology does this can it claim to be regarded as a science. What in psychiatry is just expertise and art can never be accurately formulated and can at best be mutually sensed by another colleague. It is therefore hardly a matter for textbooks and we should not expect to find it there. Training students in psychiatry is always more than a communication of concepts, more than mere scientific teaching. A textbook of psychopathology, however, must be scientific and is valuable only for this reason, so that we are deliberately confining ourselves in this book to what can be understood in scientific terms, while we fully recognise the practical importance of clinical art in the examination of the individual case.

*Psychopathology is concerned* with every psychic reality which we can render intelligible by a concept of constant significance. The phenomenon studied may also be a matter of aesthetic, ethical or historical interest, but we can still examine it psychopathologically. Different frames of reference are involved. Further, there is no sharp line of demarcation between the art and science of psychiatry. Science is continually extending into the field of clinical art but the latter always remains indispensable in its own right and reaches out on its own into ever new territory, but scientific practice is to be preferred in principle, even if it is not always possible. When it is attainable, we should always deprecate the use of our own personal intuitions which by their very nature are unreliable.

Psychopathology has, *as its subject-matter*, actual conscious psychic events. Although the main concern is with pathological phenomena, it is also necessary to know what people experience in general and how they experience it; in short, to take the full range of psychic reality. It is necessary not only to examine the actual experience but also the causes and conditions at work, as well as the relationships and the modes in which the experience comes to expression. We can make an analogy with somatic medicine, where in individual cases physiology and pathology seem equally concerned. We find the two are really interdependent. They work with the same principles and there is no clear, dividing line between the two disciplines. In the same way psychology and psychopathology belong to each other and learn from one another. There is no sharp division and many mutual problems are tackled by psychologists and psychopathologists alike. There is no unitary concept of what is morbid, but rather a number of concepts which in principle can all be differentiated but in practice have to allow for borderline cases and transitional states. We are not insisting here on any precise definition of mental illness, and our selection of material will be seen to follow conventional lines. We do not think it so important if in somebody's view this or that material should be included as morbid or some other material excluded as not morbid. A full discussion on the concept of illness has been left to the last part of this book. We must admit that we have demarcated our field of psychopathology from the larger field of psychology in what may seem rather an arbitrary manner, and it should be remembered that they really belong together, just as physiology and pathology belong to each other.

### (b) Psychopathology and psychology

Psychology studies what has been called normal psychic life. Theoretically psychology is as necessary for the psychopathologist as physiology for the pathologist,[1] but in fact we find many instances to the contrary. This is due to the fact that psychopathologists are concerned with much material of which the normal counterpart has not yet been studied by psychologists and they often have to provide their own psychology, since the psychologist can give no counsel. Academic psychology seems to be too preoccupied with those primary processes that are affected by neurological disorders and organic lesions but rarely suffer any disturbance in psychic illnesses proper. Psychiatrists, therefore, need some wider psychology which will give them better provision from the thousand-year-old stores of psychological thinking. Such a psychology seems to be finding a place for itself in academic circles recently.

### (c) Psychopathology and physical medicine

We said earlier that psychic events, their conditioning factors, causes and consequences all provide the subject-matter for psychopathology. Any enquiry into the connections between them must bring us to the theory of extra-conscious mechanisms and ultimately in many cases to definite, somatic events as the remote causes of psychic phenomena.

In every individual event soma and psyche form an inseparable unity. The two stand in a mutual reciprocity which shows itself much more directly in psychopathology than it does in normal psychology. There are somatic phenomena, universally accepted as such, which are in part dependent on

[1] We cannot quote any one text on psychology which would serve as a complement to the study of psychopathology. Psychology is divided into as many different camps as psychopathology. We have to get to know the schools and their teachings one by one if we are to learn anything about psychology. The *Physiologische Psychologie* of Wundt is the main text on psychic problems connected with the physiology of the senses and somatic phenomena but in many respects it is out of date. Ebbinghaus, *Lehrbuch* in Buhler's new edition is preferable so far as it goes. No new principle but a new thoroughness in the old method is offered by Husserl in his phenomenological basis for psychological enquiry. Contributions from the school of Külpe follow the same line. Messer provides a short popular exposition of this type of enquiry in *Empfindung u. Kenken*. As an introduction to certain sections of modern psychology, there is the well-written and realistic text by Bumke, *Psychologische Verlesungen* (Wiesbaden: Bergmann, 1919). More recent texts can only be recommended with some reserve. For an overall picture of the literature we might mention S. J. Fröbes, *Lehrbuch der experimentellen Psychologie* (Freiburg, 1917, vol. 1; 1920, vol. 2). A. Messer, *Psychologie*, 7 bis 9 Tausend (Stuttgart, 1922). Th. Elsenhaus, *Lehrbuch der Psychologie*, 3rd edn. (Giese, Gruhle and Dorsch, Tübingen, 1937).

psychic events: for example, duration of menstrual flow, the nutritional state and perhaps in certain circumstances any one of the somatic functions. On the other hand, the most complex psychic events originate in part from somatic sources. These relationships are responsible for the close connection between psychopathology and medicine. Quite apart from the fact that the actual treatment of human beings calls for thorough medical training, insight into the aetiology of psychic events cannot be achieved at all without some knowledge of somatic function, more particularly the physiology of the nervous system. Thus psychopathology finds in neurology, internal medicine and physiology its most valuable auxiliary sciences.

Investigation of somatic function, including the most complex cortical activity, is bound up with investigation of psychic function, and the unity of soma and psyche seems indisputable. Yet we must remember that neither line of enquiry encounters the other so directly that we can speak of some specific psychic event as directly associated with some specific somatic event or of an actual parallelism. The situation is analogous with the exploration of an unknown continent from opposite directions, where the explorers never meet because of impenetrable country that intervenes. We only know the end links in the chain of causation from soma to psyche and vice versa and from both these terminal points we endeavour to advance. *Neurology* has discovered that the cortex with the brain-stem provides the organ most closely associated with psychic function and its researches have reached their highest peak so far in the theory of aphasia, agnosia and apraxia. It seems, however, as if the further neurology advances, the further the psyche recedes; *psychopathology* on the other hand explores the psyche to the limits of consciousness but finds at these limits no somatic process directly associated with such phenomena as delusional ideas, spontaneous affects and hallucinations. In many cases, which increase in number as we gain in knowledge, the primary source of psychic change is found to lie in some cerebral disorder. Yet we always find that no one specific psychic change is characteristic for any one of these disorders. The facts seem to be that cerebral disorders may be responsible for almost all possible psychic changes though the frequency with which they appear may vary in different disorders (for example, in General Paralysis of the Insane).

From these observations we may conclude that it is vital for us when investigating somatic changes to bear possible psychic causation in mind and vice versa. Since every psychopathologist has to study neurology and internal medicine independently, we shall not try to deal here with matters of neurology and internal medicine best learned from the many textbooks available (such as neurological methods of examination, pupillary changes, abnormal reflexes, sensory or motor disturbances). Furthermore, the principle of this book is to present a psychopathology which, in its concept-building, its methods of investigation and general outlook, is not enslaved to neurology and medicine on the dogmatic grounds that 'psychic disorder is cerebral disorder'. Our particular scientific contribution is not to imitate neurology and construct a system with constant cross-reference to the brain—this always seems unreal and super-ficial—but to develop a standpoint from which to investigate the various problems, concepts and relationships within the framework of the psycho-pathological phenomena themselves. This is the special task of psycho-pathology, but time and again and at many points we shall of course find ourselves close to associated problems of neurology (e.g. the dependence of particular defects of psychic function on focal brain injury as in aphasia, etc.; the finding that some mental disorders are based upon cerebral disorders as with General Paralysis, arteriosclerosis, etc.; the conjecture that this is also the case with a number of others such as dementia praecox).

### (d) Methodology—the contribution of philosophy

Psychology and medicine are the scientific disciplines most closely linked with psychopathology but the latter, of course, like any other science, has re-moter connections with all other branches of human enquiry, one of which should have a special mention here—the discipline of philosophy with its accent on methodology.

In psychology as in psychopathology there are very few, perhaps no, assertions which are not somewhere and at some time under dispute. If we wish to raise our statements and discoveries to firm ground, above the daily flood of psychological notions, we shall almost always be forced to reflect on our methodology. Not only assertions but methods themselves come under dispute and it is quite an achievement if two investigators will agree upon method and only argue over their actual findings. Compared with this situation in psychopathology, somatic investigations in psychiatry at present pursue a relatively firm and smooth traditional path. There is, for instance, a wide community of aim in such fields of research as the histology of the central nervous system, serology, etc., whereas even the mere possibility of a scientific psychopathology will be questioned. Voices are raised asserting that no pro-gress has been made in this field for a long time, nor could any be made since psychopathology, it is said, is involved with that 'popular psychology' familiar to psychiatrists of an earlier date, which has already provided all that is really needed for psychiatric purposes. We also find a tendency to cling to newly discovered somatic phenomena as a means of gaining better knowledge of the psyche. Salvation is thought to lie in experiments where results are either expressed in figures or are objectively demonstrated or plotted as a curve. The upholders of such views are guilty of one omission. They fail to train themselves in psychological methods and therefore may be charged with uncritical thinking. Observation is not enough. If we are to obtain some clear, communicable concepts and if we are to reach an adequate differentiation of our field, valid thinking in addition is essential, otherwise no advance in our knowledge will take place.

It is not surprising, therefore, that every psychopathologist is driven to concern himself *with his methods*. For the same reasons some discussion of

methodology is necessary in this book. In the face of outside criticism we are
forced to defend ourselves and clarify our own position. A science in dispute
must first of all show its merits by factual results but, particularly when these
are not so readily accessible, we must anticipate some criticism of the methods
we employ.[1]

So far as concrete research is concerned, a thorough study of *philosophy* is
not of any positive value to psychopathologists, apart from the importance
of methodology. There is nothing that we can, so to speak, take over 'ready-
made', but philosophical studies undoubtedly exercise a certain restraining
influence of their own. They can protect us from putting the wrong question,
indulging in irrelevant discussions and deploying our prejudices, all of which
activities appear only too often in the psychopathological field among individual workers bereft of any such training. In the second place the study of
philosophy makes a positive contribution to the human quality of the psychopathologist himself and with its help he can clarify his motives.

## § 2. SOME BASIC CONCEPTS

Psychopathology is concerned with the ill person as a whole, in so far as
he suffers from a psychic illness or one that is psychically determined.

If we knew the elements that constituted the human psyche and all the
forces at work we could begin with a broad outline of the psyche and leave
details to be filled in later. But we need no such blue-print, since we conceive
the psyche as an unending effort at comprehension, an effort which can never be
concluded wholly, though we are always advancing through the many methods
of research. We have no basic concept in terms of which we could define man
nor any theory that would wholly cover his actual, objective existence. We
must, therefore, as scientists, keep an open mind for all the empirical possibilities and guard against the temptation to reduce human existence to one
common denominator. We have no psychic master-plan, but we shall simply
discuss a number of horizons within which our psychic realities present
themselves.

1. We are going to discuss *Man*. Does the fact that man is not an animal
have any bearing on human illness?

2. We are going to discuss the human *psyche*. How is this actually objectified?

3. The psyche is *consciousness*. What do 'conscious' and 'unconscious'
mean?

[1] Among psychiatrists writing on methodology, we would recommend Gaupp, 'Über die
Grenzen psychiatrischer Erkenntnis', *Zbl. Nervenkh.*, etc. (1903). Wege and Ziele, *Psychiatrischer
Forschung* (Tübingen, 1907). Professional philosophers who generalise have less to offer than
papers on methodology written by research workers who have in their possession a wealth of
concrete observations. Max Weber's book, for instance, *Gesammelte Beiträge zur Wissenschaftslehre* (Tübingen, Mohr, 1922), is of value, dealing in part with problems closely touching on
psychopathology.

4. The psyche is not a thing but *'being in one's own world'*. What do 'inner' and 'outer' world mean?

5. The psyche is not an end state but becoming, developing, unfolding. What does psychic *differentiation* mean?

## (a) Man and animal

Medicine draws little distinction somatically between man and animal. Both are studied in anatomy, physiology, pharmacology, pathology and somatic therapeutics. In psychopathology, however, human existence is, so to speak, a constant problem since the human mind and spirit are involved in every psychic illness.

It is altogether doubtful whether animals suffer from psychic illness. They can it is true suffer from diseases of the brain and nerves. We may, for instance, study the heredity of syringomyelia in rabbits. Then there are such phenomena as restiveness in horses, so-called hypnosis in animals (a different matter from the hypnosis of humans) and panic reactions. Animals can also suffer 'symptomatic psychoses' due to organic brain diseases. They show disorders of sense-perception, of stance, movement and changes in their 'personality', such as running in circles, biting, apathy and so on.

The following illustrates this: Dogs and cats in a state of experimental hypo-parathyroidism sometimes behave in such a way that Blum,[1] who has reported on such observations, speaks of a borderland between motor and psychic symptoms. He noticed attacks of savagery in which a cat rushed round its pen as if possessed, tried to jump up the smooth walls, attacked another friendly cat and bit it, until it finally collapsed with exhaustion. With dogs and cats he also noticed the adoption of unusual and uncomfortable postures, sudden jerky movements or a gait never seen with normal animals, such as parading or prancing like a show-horse. The head might be held consistently low as with an attacking bull, or the animal might stagger to the extent of falling or run or try to creep backwards in spite of a wall behind it, which it was bound to feel. A dog in a state of hallucination and delusion would sniff around and stare when there was nothing to see, and without the slightest apparent cause. He would scratch on the tin floor of his cage or try to burrow with his muzzle in an empty corner. From time to time he would bark but pay no attention to the environment. The cats obviously saw visions, striking out into emptiness and slowly retracting their paws.

'Functional psychoses proper' in animals have not been described (hysteria in animals is far from proven). Schizophrenia and the cyclic psychoses are found in every human race but not in animals. 'There is indeed no evidence for any specific animal psychoses and certainly none for any hereditary ones,'

---

[1] F. Blum, *Arch. Psychiatr.* (D), vol. 96 (1932), p. 215. Covering the whole subject: Dexler, 'Über die psychotischen Erkrankungen der Tiere', *Mschr. Psychiatr.*, vol. 16, Erg. H.99. Dexler, 'Die Erkrankungen des Zentralnervensystems der Tiere'. *Hdbuch. der normalen u. pathologischen Physiologie* von Bethe, Bergmann, etc. (1927), vol. X, p. 1232. R. Sommer, *Tierpsychologie* (Leipzig, 1925). K. Lorenz, 'Durch Domestikation verursachte Störungen arteigenen Verhaltens', *Z. angew. Psychol.*, vol. 59 (1940).

states Luxenburger, who quite rightly attacks anthropomorphic attitudes which tend to attribute human motives to animal behaviour. There is a striking contrast here between somatic medicine and psychopathology. Our quest for the particular human factor in psychic illness constrains us to view the latter as a specific human, rather than a universal natural, phenomenon. In so far as man exhibits his specific *human* nature, there can be no analogy with animals.

Man holds a unique position. He brought into the world an element alien to the animals but what this is still remains a problem. Although man can be classified somatically with the zoological species even his body remains unique, not only because of its erect gait and other characteristics but because his specific constitution sets him apart since, if we take the whole range of living forms into account, the human form preserves within itself more possibilities and less specialisation than any other. In addition man differs from all the animals in the expressive use he makes of his body. Psychologically there is a complete break. Animals do not laugh or cry as men do nor is the intelligence of apes mind or genuine thought but a sharp attentiveness which in man is a pre-condition of thought and not thinking itself. Freedom of action, conscious reflection and qualities of intellect and spirit have been considered the fundamentals of our humanity from time immemorial. The animal is bound to a natural fate which automatically fulfils itself in accordance with natural laws. Man is likewise bound but in addition he has a destiny the fulfilment of which lies in his own hands. Nowhere, however, do we find man as a completely rational being; he is borne along by natural necessity, which reaches into the furthest ramifications of his reason. In earlier centuries the imagination of men conceived of angels as pure intelligences. Man, however, is himself neither animal nor angel; he shares the condition of both but the existence of neither.

A further question is how man's special position influences the nature of human illness. In physical illness we so resemble the animals that experiments on the latter can be used to reach an understanding of vital bodily function in humans, though the application may be neither simple or direct. But the concept of human psychic illness introduces a completely new dimension. Here the incompleteness and vulnerability of human beings and their freedom and infinite possibilities are themselves a cause of illness. In contrast with animals, man lacks an inborn, perfected pattern of adaptation. He has to acquire a way of life as he goes along. Man is not merely pattern, he patterns himself. In so far as he is merely pattern, he is nearer to the animals.

In psychopathology the human being has himself become the object of scientific study and thus observations on animals do not contribute anything essential and there is a qualification of another kind. Not everything that happens in a psychic illness can be explained by using the criteria of science. Human beings are creators of culture, they develop beliefs and moral standards and constantly transcend their own empirical human self which is the only self that scientific research can recognise and grasp.

Animal psychology and psychopathology—so far as they can be said to exist—are not without some interest for our study. Firstly, we learn from them the basic phenomena of life, which may be discerned in humans also, but can be evaluated more objectively in this wider context—phenomena such as habits, learning abilities, conditioned reflexes, automatisms, trial-and-error behaviour and specific kinds of intelligent behaviour (e.g. W. Kohler, *Intelligenzpruefungen an Anthropoiden*). Secondly we learn what are the idiosyncracies of animal life itself, and we see that none of the animal forms were the predecessors of man but are all like him branches of the great tree of life. From such contrasts we learn to understand the exact implications of specific human existence.

### (b) Objective manifestations of psychic life

We can grasp and investigate only what has become an object to us. Psychic life as such is not an object. It becomes an object to us through that which makes it perceptible in the world, the accompanying somatic phenomena, meaningful gestures, behaviour and actions. It is further manifested through communication in the form of speech. It says what it means and thinks and it produces works. These demonstrable phenomena present us with the effects of the psyche. We either perceive it in these phenomena directly or at least deduce its existence from them; *the psyche* itself does *not* become *an object*. We are aware of it as conscious experience in ourselves and we represent the experience of others to ourselves as similar, whether the related phenomena are objectively observed by us or reported by others. But this experience too is a phenomenon. We can try to objectify the psychic life through symbol and analogy but it remains simply *the encompassing of existence*; a comprehension which in itself *can never be comprehended as an object*, yet it remains the framework of all the individual objective phenomena which we encounter.

We must emphasise once again that the psyche is not a thing. Even talking of 'the psyche' as an object is misleading. (1) Psyche means *consciousness*, but just as much and from certain points of view it can even, in particular, mean 'the unconscious'. (2) Psyche is not to be regarded as an object with given qualities but as *'being in one's own world'*, the integrating of an inner and outer world. (3) Psyche is a becoming, an unfolding and a differentiating, it is nothing final nor is it ever fully accomplished.

### (c) Consciousness and the unconscious

The term 'consciousness' has acquired a threefold significance: it implies *awareness of experience* and as such is distinct from loss of consciousness and from what is extra-conscious; secondly, it implies *awareness of an object*, knowing something, and as such is distinct from unconscious subjective experience, in which 'I' and 'object' are as yet undifferentiated; thirdly, it implies *self-reflection*, awareness of one's self and as such is distinct from the unconscious experience where I experience the self and the object as separate entities but am not explicitly aware of this differentiation.

Consciousness is indispensable for the manifestation of the psyche, provided by consciousness we mean every mode of inner experience, even where
there is no differentiation into 'I' and 'object' and even where all that takes place
is simply a feeling, devoid of object or any discrete self. There is no psyche
where there is no consciousness of this order.

Psychic life, however, cannot be fully understood in terms of consciousness,
nor is it to be grasped by consciousness alone. To reach a full and satisfactory
explanation we must add to the actual psychic experience *a theoretical extra-
conscious construct that goes beyond it*. Phenomenology and objective observation are founded in the actual phenomena of psychic experience and need no
theory. They are only concerned with what is given, but once we look for
explanation, this requires a theoretical framework and the assumption of
certain extra-conscious mechanisms and apparatuses. Direct, accessible psychic
experiences are like the foam on the sea's surface. The depths are inaccessible
and can only be explored in an indirect and theoretical way. But the test of
theoretical assumptions is in their effects. Their value never lies solely in their
self-consistency but rather in how well they explain the actual experience and
how capable they are of refining our observation. In order to explain psychic
life we have to work with extra-conscious mechanisms and unconscious
events, which of course can never be visualised as such but can only be
conceived in simile and symbol, whether physical or psychic.

In contrast to century-old tradition a dislike for speculative theory has
been asserting itself for some time. This seems a move in the right direction
since theories are so easily thought up and lead to irreparable confusion,
particularly when they are mingled with facts. We shall make it a principle to
be as economical as possible with our theoretical concepts and use them in the
full consciousness of their hypothetical character and consequent limitations.

It has often been debated whether *unconscious* psychic events exist. First,
we must differentiate between psychic events which though they have been
actually experienced go unnoticed by the individual and those events which
are in fact extra-conscious and have never actually been experienced. The
unnoticed psychic events can be brought to notice given certain favourable
circumstances, and their reality can thus be established. Extra-conscious events,
however, can by definition never be brought to notice.

Psychology and psychopathology have the important task of extending
knowledge into wide areas of the unnoticed psychic life and they illuminate
this life for consciousness (= knowledge). To do this within one's self is a
necessary pre-condition in the quest for truth and in the achievement of
individual development; to enhance this latter is one type of psychotherapy.

Extra-conscious events can never be directly demonstrated unless they
happen to appear as perceivable somatic events. It is undeniable, however, that
conscious psychic phenomena can be explained very plausibly and usefully
in this way by adding extra-consious events as cause and effect. They are
therefore theoretical constructs and their aptness and consistency are debatable,

but we cannot establish their actual reality, nor need we. The extra-conscious factors appear in many different forms, such as acquired memory patterns, acquired habits and attitudes and one's intellectual and temperamental endowment. It is not uncommon for a person to be aware that he is faced or even perhaps being overwhelmed by an experience which has emerged from extra-conscious depths within him.

The *numerous meanings* which have become attached to the term '*unconscious*' are shown by the following:

(*a*) The 'unconscious' is thought to be a *derivative of consciousness*. As such it may be (1) *automatic behaviour* (e.g. a past conscious activity is now carried out automatically and hence unconsciously), e.g. walking, writing, riding a bicycle; (2) *forgotten experience* that is *still effective*, e.g. the so-called complexes, after-affects of previous experience; (3) *memories* in reach of recall.

(*b*) The 'unconscious' is thought of in relation to *inattentiveness*. As such it is (1) *unnoticed*, yet lived through; (2) *unwilled*, unintended yet performed; (3) *unremembered* (it has been in consciousness but was straightway forgotten; seniles, for instance, often no longer know what was their clear intention a moment before —'I go into another room—what did I want there?'); (4) something that *has never become objective* and is not definable in speech.

(*c*) The 'unconscious' is thought of as *a power*, an *original source*. As such it is (1) the *creative, vital* element; (2) haven, shelter, *first cause* and *final end*. That is, everything essential comes to us from the unconscious, our passionate aspirations and inspirations, every impulse, every idea, every shape and form of our creative imagination, all the grandeur and the desolation of life. Fulfilment becomes the unconscious into which we return.

(*d*) The 'unconscious' is thought of as 'Being'—the very sense of being. As such it is thought to be (1) *psychic reality* (but we can no more explain consciousness as something mechanically and accidentally added to psychic reality than we can equate what is psychic with mere consciousness, rooted as the psyche is in the unconscious, influenced by it and influencing it in turn). Psychic reality has been variously conceived: as the spontaneous *play of basic elements* (Herbart), of which conscious psychic life is the manifestation; as a *series of deepening unconscious levels* (Kohnstamm, Freud); as that *personal unconscious* which every individual gathers to himself in the course of his life; as the *collective unconscious* (Jung) which operates in each individual as a substratum of universal human experience. In all these instances the unconscious is conceived as 'being for its own sake', the reality which gives us our existence. (2) 'Absolute being.' (This is a *metaphysical concept*: the 'unconscious'—like Being, Non-Being, Becoming, Substance, Form and almost all categories—is used as an analogy for this in an effort to make the unthinkable, thinkable; 'absolute being' is not however a concept that belongs to psychology.)

(*d*) *Inner and outer world*

There are certain categories of thought valid for the apprehension of all

living things, even of the psyche in its highest flights, though we have then
to exchange exact meaning for analogy. Among these categories is that of life
as 'an existence in its own world' since all life reveals itself as a continuous interchange between an inner and an outer world (v. Uexküll). To live in its own
world is a fundamental phenomenon of life. Even physical existence cannot be
adequately explored as if it were merely a matter of anatomical structure and
physiological function, arbitrarily located in space. It has to be regarded as a
living engagement with the world around it, whereby it achieves form and
reality through constant adaptation to stimuli, which it receives in part and in
part creates. This primal, integrative process of life as an existence in and along
with its own world is exemplified in human life too, but human beings take
the process even further *through conscious discrimination and an active influence on their own world* and then through their *generalised knowledge of it*. By
such means life transcends itself and moves on into other possible worlds and
beyond the concept of World itself. Empirical research must turn to certain
particular manifestations of this basic inter-relatedness and thereby to certain
isolated aspects of the relation between inner and outer world. For instance:

(1) In physiological thinking we find *stimulus* related to *response*; in
phenomenological thinking we find the 'intentional' relationship of the 'I' to
'*what confronts it*' ('subject' v. 'object').

(2) Individual life develops out of *constitution* (Anlage) and *environment*
(milieu); it springs from innate potentialities which may be stimulated and
moulded by the environment or left dormant to wither away. Constitution
and environment operate at first through biological events that lie outside
consciousness and we try to understand causal relationships at this level. Next,
in our conscious life they function in a psychologically comprehensible way,
when environmental factors, our birth, for instance, and changing life-situation,
pattern our existence and are in turn challenged and patterned by us. Because
of a natural self-development, the individual with his constitution confronts
the environment and enters into effective exchange with it. From this springs
all experience of human destiny, deed, effort and pain.

(3) Above all, environment fosters *situations*.[1] These provide the individual
with opportunities which he may make use of or waste or in which he may
reach decisions. He can contrive situations himself, letting them arise or not
arise in some meaningful pattern. He submits to the ordered regularity and
conventions of a world and at the same time he can convert them into means
of escape. In the end, however, he comes upon *frontier-situations*, the final
frontiers of existence—death, chance, suffering, guilt. These may awaken in
him something we have called Existence itself—a reality of selfhood.

(4) Everyone has his own *private world*[2] but an objective world also exists

[1] The concept of 'the situation' is discussed in my *Geistige Situation der Zeit* (Berlin, 1931),
pp. 19 ff.
[2] See my book *Philosophie* (Berlin, 1932), vol. 1, pp. 61 ff., on concepts of the world. Also
my *Psychologie der Weltanschauungen* (Berlin), pp. 122 ff.; 3rd edn. (Berlin, 1919), pp. 141 ff.

—a *general world common to all*. This general world exists for 'common consciousness' (or 'consciousness-as-such') and participation in this ensures a criterion for accuracy of thinking and its objective validity. Individual consciousness is but a portion of what is universal and generally possible, for which it provides *a concrete historical framework*, and so sets the stage for misapprehension and mistake.

(5) The psyche *discovers itself in its own world* and with that *creates a world*. In the world it becomes intelligible to others and the world brings it to creativity.

Thus the meaning of the fundamental relation between inner and outer is so often transposed that we may suddenly find ourselves confronted with what seem to be completely heterogeneous entities. But the general analogy holds good; there is a basic relatedness between what is within and what is without; we are in a world common to all living things and to all psychic life and to every human being in his separate reality.

## (e) *The differentiation of psychic life*

Psychic reality enlightens our understanding best when it is most highly developed. The furthest evolved and the most complex illumines the simple and the primitive, not vice versa. For research purposes, therefore, we look to those who have the best cultural endowment and a rich psychic life, but the very highly differentiated is something rare. Yet it is just the rare case which gives orientation to knowledge, in so far as it is not a freak but the full development of a classical extreme. Exceptional not ordinary cases are the psychologically illuminating ones and through them we gain a firmer grasp of the great company of more commonplace instances. The degree of psychic differentiation is a fundamental factor which exerts a constant influence on all phenomena.

To be able to distinguish the unusual is very important from a clinical point of view. What happens most often is most often reported on or complained of, but the mere fact of frequency does not mean that the phenomenon is fully understood nor that it is more akin to natural law, nor that somehow it has more reality. We may ask why one thing occurs rarely and another frequently. Why are the paranoics as defined by Kraepelin so rare, yet when they do occur they are so typical? Why should the classic types of hysteria be so common in the environment of Charcot's world but so rare nowadays?

Psychic life offers us enormous variety right up to the elaborate developments of genius. Hashish will produce in one person a dull, animal glow, uproariousness in another, in another a rich fabulous bliss. The same illness, dementia praecox for example, may be characterised in one individual by simple delusions of jealousy and persecution, while in another, Strindberg for instance, the same ideas can develop to an extraordinary degree of richness and the changed experience of life turn into a fountain of originality and poetic creativity. The symptomatology of every psychic disturbance will correspond with the degree of psychic development attained by the patient.

Psychic phenomena are generally only possible where there is some psychic differentiation. This applies both to the complexity of content and to the actual form the psychic event takes. For instance, compulsive ideas and the phenomena of depersonalisation only appear when there is a relatively advanced degree of differentiation; compulsive ideas, which call for a high degree of self-awareness, are not observed in young children, but are common in generally well-differentiated persons. The same applies to that large group of subjective inhibitions, specific to vulnerable people who are given to self-scrutiny.

The *concept of differentiation* can be further analysed: *in the first place*, it means a numerical increase in qualitative modes of experience. *Secondly*, it means the breaking up of vague experiences into several well-defined ones, thus giving richness and depth to the total experience. Low-level individual phenomena differentiate into higher ones; the vague instinctive life gains in content. Increased differentiation brings increased clarity and awareness. Undefined intuitions and feelings give place to clear, definite ideas. From an undifferentiated state of innocence emerge the innumerable contradictions and conflicts of our psychic life. *Thirdly*, it implies analysis and synthesis of object-consciousness, whereby we increase the possibilities for thought, comprehension, attitude, discrimination and comparison. *Fourthly*, it means a growing consciousness of self through the process of self-reflection. We have to distinguish here differentiation as a subjective experience which need not be conscious from conscious differentiation which takes the form of self-observation. Someone may have a compulsive idea without attempting to understand what he is undergoing. Usually, however, differentiation and self-awareness go together. Sometimes the mere registering of all kinds of unimportant feelings may create the false impression of a growth in differentiation. *Fifthly*, we should know at what level of development the differentiation takes place; this is decisive for understanding the personality. The whole force and vigour of the individual need to be taken into account besides the actual degree of differentiation, so that we come across different levels of the personality as a whole (Klages' concept of levels of development—'Formniveau'). Here we are at one of the limits of what we can conceive. Yet if we wish to understand personality we must try to find our way confidently beyond this point. Individuals can really be compared only when they have the same degree of differentiation and are at the same level of development (have the same 'Formniveau'), and this applies as much to the comparison of personal bearing and conduct as to comparison in the narrower field of handwriting, etc.

These distinctions are not really enough to give us any clear definitive point of view on the psyche as a whole. At present, so far as psychopathological phenomena are concerned, we have no satisfactory basis for estimating *degrees* of differentiation nor of the *direction* taken, and the same applies to degrees of disintegration and the direction they take. The general point of view which we have outlined will therefore have to suffice.

We can, however, distinguish two fundamental *causes* of differentiation. One is rooted in the *individual disposition* (Veranlagung); the other springs from the *cultural milieu*.

In *mental defectives*[1] psychosis exhibits a relatively poor symptomatology, the disturbances seem fewer in number and more primitive; delusions are hardly systematised and below a certain level of intelligence certain types of delusion (such as delusions of profound guilt) are never encountered. Excitement manifests itself invariably as loud, monotonous shouting or screaming; apathy appears as general, dull torpidity.

The *cultural milieu* in which a human being grows up and lives merely furthers or retards the unfolding of the individual constitution (Anlage). Man lives by participating in the collective cultural achievements of history and only reaches his own individual development through them. Untaught deaf-mutes remain at the level of idiots. What from the external social point of view seems to emerge by stages is actually already there in the totality of the psyche. Manifestations of mental illness obviously attain far more richness and variety when they occur at higher cultural levels. For this reason the advance of psychopathology gains nothing from the study of animals and is largely dependent on the study of people who come from the higher levels of culture. Doctors in private clinics possess incomparably valuable case-material in their educated patients, whereas public clinics know only too well the monotony of hysteria in the simpler type of patient.

Both differentiated and undifferentiated psychic phenomena, however, call for our attention. Analysis of highly differentiated psychic life throws light on the lower levels of development so that typically our interest finds itself swinging to and fro in both directions. For the natural sciences the proper object of investigation is the average phenomenon or that which most commonly appears. Other studies, equally partisan, maintain that the only proper object for examination is the rare and highly differentiated psyche. In the realm of 'belles lettres', we may find an analogy in the early French novel of manners and morals and the psychological novel of modern times.[2]

## (f) Recapitulation

From the above selected points of view we have visualised a number of horizons within which psychic phenomena appear. The only common factor is the shift in meaning, so that any contrast takes on manifold form. But discussion of the above five points of view should give us some preliminary feeling for the extent of the realities with which we have to deal, and make it quite

---

[1] Luther, *Z. Neur.*, vol. 16, p. 386. Plaskuda, *Z. Neur*, vol. 19, p. 596.

[2] Bourget, commenting on the 'psychological novel' in contrast to the novel of manners and morals, says 'il devra choisir les personnages chez lesquelles cette vie interieure soit le plus ample' (i.e. choice needs to be made of characters whose inner life is rich and ample).

clear how little can be said in general terms. When it comes to individual application, we need a firm grasp of the particular meaning in relation to the concrete issue. Discussion in general terms is usually meaningless in view of their indefinite nature.

## § 3. Prejudice and Presupposition

Whenever we apperceive, we have already brought into the situation that which renders apperception possible and gives it form. If what we bring falsifies our view we call it 'prejudice' but if on the contrary our apperception has been enabled and enhanced, we speak of 'presupposition'.

### (a) Prejudice

It is an enlightening process of self-criticism to make ourselves realise how much we have taken unconsciously for granted. There are many reasons for this, e.g. the urge to get some unified picture of the whole, or the wish to arrive at a few primary concepts that are simple and definitive. As a result we tend to generalise isolated points of view, specific methods and categories. Or, what happens more commonly, we confuse what is definitely knowable with what we believe.

Prejudices of this sort weigh on us unconsciously but with paralysing effect and we shall have to try and free ourselves from them in every chapter of this book. At this point we will only look at one or two very pronounced examples, and if we can recognise them in these extreme forms we shall be ready for the disguises which they more often assume.

(1) *Philosophical prejudice.* There have been periods in which great value has been placed on speculative and *deductive thinking*, based on principles that sought to comprehend and explain everything without the test of experience. Such thinking was more highly valued then than the irksome examination of particulars. These were periods in which philosophy tried to create from 'above' what only experience could bring from 'below'. Nowadays we seem to have abandoned this orientation but it reappears here and there in the form of abstruse theories. Behind our accepted systems of general psychopathology the old spirit hovers and can be identified. Our rejection of purely deductive and barren philosophical theorising is justified but it is often linked regrettably with the opposite misconception, that the only useful approach is to go on with the collection of particular experiences. It is thought better to amass data blindly than sit down and think. From this follows a contempt for the activity of thinking, which alone gives a place to facts, a plan to work to, a standpoint for observation and the passionate drive for rewarding scientific goals.

Deductive philosophies were generally associated with value-judgments and displayed *moralistic and theological tendencies*. Sins and passions were ascribed as the causes of mental illness and human qualities divided categorically into bad and good. Maximilian Jakobi, writing in the first half of the nineteenth century, completely annihilated such 'philosophising in the wrong place'. Science indeed has no room for philosophies of this sort, however important they may be as expressions of human attitudes to the world. Philosophies in conflict are commonly a mere battle for power, but in an exchange of scientific views there is always some chance for sensible discussion and a rational conclusion. All the same, it is difficult to keep psychology and psychopathology wholly free from value-judgments, which often prove to be an expression of some background philosophy. The simple *separation of observation and value-judgment* is something that must be required from every psychopathologist in his work, not so that all human values must be relinquished but that, on the contrary, we shall possess truer, clearer and profounder values the more we observe before we judge. What is needed is a quiet absorption into the facts of psychic life without the adoption of any specific attitude to them. Human beings have to be approached in an unbiased fashion with lively interest and without any kind of appraisal. This principle of keeping simple observation and value-judgment apart is easy to accept in theory but in practice it calls for such a high degree of self-discipline and real objectivity that we can never take it for granted at any time.

(2) *Theoretical prejudice.* The natural sciences rest on *comprehensive* and well-founded theories which provide us with a uniform background for individual observations. The atom-theory and the cell-theory are cases in point. We find nothing similar in psychology or psychopathology, where no *uniform theoretical framework* is attainable, except perhaps as the speculative construct of an individual. Our methods do not lead us to discover any ultimate elements, mechanisms or laws, in terms of which psychic life becomes explicable or will eventually do so; they merely introduce us by certain paths to various aspects of it. In our view psychic life is an infinite whole, a totality that resists any consistent attempt to systematise it; much like the sea, we may coast along the shore, go far out into the deeps but still only traverse the surface waters.

If we try to reduce psychic life to a few universal principles and seek comprehensive laws, we beg a question that cannot be answered. Where our theories may seem to have some kinship with the natural sciences, it is in the forming of tentative hypotheses, which we make for limited research ends only and which have no application to the psyche as a whole. Wherever we prejudge because of a theory, the appreciation of facts is curtailed. Findings are viewed from the angle of that particular theory; anything that supports it or seems relevant is found interesting; anything that has no relevance is ignored; anything that contradicts the theory is blanketed or misinterpreted. Reality is constantly seen through the spectacles of one theory or another. We have, therefore, to make a continual effort to *discount* the theoretical prejudices ever present in our minds and train ourselves to *pure appreciation of the facts*. We can only appreciate these latter in terms of category and method, and we have therefore to be fully aware of the presuppositions lying in every discovery according to the nature of its subject-matter—'theory lurks in every fact'. We can thus learn to look at reality in the clear knowledge that what we see is never reality itself nor ever the whole reality.

(3) *Somatic prejudice.* Tacit assumptions are made that, like everything else biological, the actual reality of human existence is a somatic event. Man is only comprehensible when he is understood in somatic terms; should the psyche be mentioned, this is in the nature of a theoretical stop-gap of no real scientific value. A tendency arises to discuss all psychic events as if their essence were something somatic, already in one's grasp, or as if such a concept merely pointed the way to discoveries of a somatic nature. Genuine research provides hypotheses which stimulate investigation, verification or refutation of ex-periential facts through somatic findings, but where this somatic prejudice is operative an imaginary 'soma' receives great emphasis as a heuristic pre-supposition, when in fact it is nothing but the unconscious expression of an unscientific prejudice. The attitudes of resignation sometimes shown when psychological matters are under consideration reflect the same prejudice; we can see it, for instance, in the statement that all psychological interest in schizophrenia will vanish when once the morbid somatic process that underlies it is discovered.

This somatic prejudice comes up again and again in the disguise of physi-ology, anatomy or vague biology. At the beginning of the century we would find it expressed as follows: there is no need to investigate the psyche as such; it is purely subjective. If it is to be discussed scientifically, it must be presented anatomically, somatically—as a physical function. Even provisional anatomical constructs are preferable to mere psychological investigation. These ana-tomical constructions, however, became quite fantastic (e.g. Meynert, Wer-nicke) and have rightly been called 'Brain Mythologies'. Unrelated things were forcibly related, e.g. cortical cells were related to memory, nerve fibres to association of ideas. Such somatic constructions have no real basis. Not one specific cerebral process is known which parallels a specific psychic phen-omenon. Localisation of various sensory areas in the cerebral cortex and of the aphasias in the left hemisphere only means that these organs must be intact for a specific psychic event to be possible. There is no difference in principle here from the equal necessity of having intact function of the eye or of the motor mechanism, etc., which are also essential 'tools'. With regard to the neuro-logical mechanisms, the position is more advanced, but we are still infinitely far removed from finding exact parallels to psychic events. It was entirely erroneous to suppose that the discovery of the aphasias and apraxias would lead us into psychic territory, and empirically we cannot decide whether psychic and somatic phenomena are parallel or interacting. There is not a single instance where we could demonstrate this. Psychic and somatic phen-omena, in so far as we can have some scientific understanding of them, appear separated by a measureless expanse of intermediary events, of which at present we are ignorant. In practice we can speak of parallelism or of interaction— usually of the latter. We can do this all the more easily in that it is always possible to convert the one set of terms into the other. As regards this tendency to translate psychic into somatic terms (imaginary or real), we may refer to Janet who said: 'if we are always to think anatomically where psychiatry is concerned, we might as well resign ourselves to think nothing'.

(4) *'Psychologising'* and *'intellectualising'*. Empathy is often itself responsible for 'psychologising'. There is a desire to 'understand' everything and all critical awareness of the limits of psychological understanding is lost. This happens whenever 'psychological understanding' is turned into 'causal explanation' under the misconception that in every case there is a meaningful determinant of experience to be found. People ignorant of psychology and with a somatic orientation are most prone to fall into this trap. Too much is attributed to ill-will or malingering but this is due perhaps not so much to actual psychologising as to moralising. Some physicians have a definite dislike for hysterics and they suffer profound irritation if they cannot find any of the physical signs with which they are familiar. In their heart of hearts they think it all plain naughtiness, and when the situation is out of hand, only then do they pass the case on to the psychiatrist. Crude, naïve psychologising is found precisely in those medical men who do not want to have anything to do with psychology, nor to know anything about it.

Psychic life provides many contexts where people seem to act purposefully and out of rational motives, and there is a very widespread inclination to assume 'conscious reasons' behind all human activity. In actual fact rational behaviour plays a very small part in human affairs. Irrational drives and emotional states usually prevail, even when the individual wishes to convince himself that he is acting on purely logical grounds. Exaggerated search for rational connections gives rise to intellectualising, which obstructs any hope of reaching a true and penetrating understanding of human behaviour. Reasoning is then over-rated as against the forces of suggestion. When the patient appears irrational, there is a hasty resort to a diagnosis of 'dementia' and all the complex richness of human experience is ignored.

(5) *Use of False Analogy.* Psychic life is objectified through expression and through creative impact, through behaviour and through action, through somatic events and speech. But the psyche itself cannot be observed; we can only see it through *metaphor and simile*. It is something we experience and implement, something we realise in ourselves but never actually see. In discussing the psyche we always have to fall back on imagery, usually of a three-dimensional kind, and in psychological thinking analogies for the psyche abound, e.g. the psyche is a stream of consciousness; consciousness is like a space where individual psychic phenomena come and go as figures on a stage; it is a space that recedes infinitely into the unconscious; the psyche is constituted of layers—layers of consciousness, of experience, function and personality; the psyche is made up of elements in various combinations; it is moved by fundamental forces, the factors and components of which we can analyse; it has attributes that can be described as with any other thing. Such

three-dimensional analogies are invaluable to us. We could not do without them and they do no harm as long as we do not try to prove anything by them, but merely use them descriptively. It is not uncommon, however, for the original analogy to be taken as a valid construct and become established as one of our prejudices. Vivid and comprehensible analogies readily dominate our minds so that from time to time we no longer see them as analogies but as valid concepts of the thing itself. For instance, the psyche is broken down into atom-like elements or psychic events are seen as mechanical movements (mechanistic theory) or psychic connections as a series of combinations analogous to a chemical compound (psychic chemistry). In any case there is a constant human tendency to let imagery and metaphor become the preferred mode of thought and work in our minds prejudicially.

(6) *Medical prejudice relating to quantitative assessment, objectivity and diagnostics*. The prejudice in favour of *quantitative* findings derives from the exact sciences. Examination of qualitative changes is regarded as arbitrary, subjective and not scientific. Statistical and experimental methods, which by their use of measurement, calculation and graphs seem so valuable for the investigation of certain problems, are held to be the one and only scientific method. Even when this sort of investigation is no longer possible, quantitative concepts are often still applied, though in the context they are meaningless. Sometimes we find it put forward quite seriously that the 'intensity' of ideas is the primary cause of compulsive thinking, hysterical phenomena, delusions and hallucinations—ideas are projected outward simply because of their intensity.

The only suitable object for investigation then becomes *that which can be perceived through the senses*. The examination of physical phenomena, of performance and productivity is indeed very valuable but all the same we can only penetrate to what is psychic if we let the psyche confront us directly and the psyche, as we shall find, is always qualitatively singular. Psychic events can never be directly perceived, only indirectly in the way they express themselves. This self-evident point explains why a psychopathology which simply confines itself to what can be directly perceived through the senses becomes inevitably a psychopathology without a psyche.

In the psychiatric assessment of a case, diagnosis is left to the last but in practice, except in the case of well-known cerebral changes, diagnosis is the least relevant factor. If it is made the main issue, it will prejudge what ideally should emerge from the investigation. What matters is the process of analysis. The chaos of phenomena should not be blotted out with some diagnostic label but bring illumination through the way it is systematically ordered and related. Psychiatric diagnosis is too often a sterile running round in circles so that only a few phenomena are brought into the orbit of conscious knowledge.

## (b) Presupposition

The opposite of prejudging our investigations is to try and make every possible approach to psychic reality, using all the means in our power. In the empirical sciences every investigator is driven on to find reality, so that as regards the somatic aspects of psychiatry the psychiatrist will ask for histological, serological and neurological facts and will discard anatomical constructs and speculations. In psychopathology the basic reality for research is psychic life as it is presented to us through observed behaviour and through what can be understood from the patient's remarks. We have to feel, grasp and contemplate all that is really happening in the human psyche. The reality we are driven to look for is the reality of psychic life and we want to know it in a context that to some extent is open to scientific observation. It is the understanding of psychic reality which alone gives body and richness to our concepts, and we refuse to have this reality dissolved away in empty theoretical prejudice and anatomical or other constructs taking its place. Indeed, we cannot practise psychopathology at all if we lack the capacity and the desire to bring the psyche home to ourselves in all its rich complexity.

The investigator, however, is more than a vessel into which knowledge can be poured. He is a living being and as such an indispensable instrument of his own research. The *presuppositions* without which his enquiry will remain sterile are contained within his own person. Clarification may free us from prejudice, but presuppositions are a necessary part of understanding. They appear as tentative ideas which we then take as experimental hypotheses; they are certain basic attitudes in ourselves, derivations of our own being, without which we cannot comprehend the essence of anything. Presuppositions provide guiding ideas, and form the mental life of those engaged in research; they need to be strengthened and cultivated and they should be acknowledged. They do not prove the correctness of an insight but are the source of any truth or relevance it attains.

*Prejudices* (*that are false*) are rigid, circumscribed presuppositions which are wrongly taken as absolutes. They are hardly realised by those who hold them; they do not reach consciousness and when clarified can be dissolved. *Presuppositions* (*that are true*) are rooted in the investigator himself and are the ground of his ability to see and understand. Once elucidated, they will be well and truly grasped.

The most vital part of the psychopathologist's knowledge is drawn from his *contact* with people. What he gains from this depends upon the particular way he gives himself and as therapist partakes in events, whether he illuminates himself as well as his patients. The process is not only one of simple observation, like reading off a measurement, but the exercise of a self-involving vision in which the psyche itself is glimpsed.

It is possible to partake in the inner life of another person through a tentative exchange of roles; a certain dramatic play, as it were, which nevertheless is no play but real. There is a natural way of empathic listening to others in which we simultaneously keep touch with ourselves. Every psychopathologist depends on his power to see and experience and on the range, receptivity and complexity of such power. There is an immense difference between those who blunder about among the sick and those who take an unhesitating course in the light of their sensitive perceptions.

This sympathetic tremulation of one psyche with the experiences of another means that, if we are to be scientific, we must objectify such experience critically. Sympathy is not the same as knowledge, but from it springs that vision of things which provides knowledge with indispensable material. Completely dispassionate observation misses the essence of things. Detachment and sympathy belong together and should not be seen in opposition. If we are to gain in scientific knowledge, the interplay of both is needed. The psychopathologist with this genuine vision has a psychic life vibrant with experiences which he is constantly subduing to a rational order.

The critique of his own basic reason, when confronted with objects, forces him to ask: what state of mind is governing my perception of these objects? Have I got their correct relevance and importance as an observed reality? What construction am I putting on them? How do they affect my own conscious reality? In order to appreciate facts properly we must always work on ourselves as well as on our material. Only that knowledge is a full knowledge which leads to growth of the self and as such it can move into new dimensions beyond the level of mere confirmatory practice.

Research workers and clinicians should create in themselves a universe of different approaches. Memories of things seen, concrete clinical pictures, biological insights, important encounters—in brief, all their personal past experience should be readily available for constant comparison. They also need a set of well-differentiated concepts, so that the interpretation of what they perceive can be made clear to others.

## § 4. METHODS

In psychiatric literature there is much discussion of mere possibilities and a great deal of subjective and speculative comment that lacks the substance of authentic experience. In studying the contributions of others as well as in our own researches, therefore, we should always ask: 'What are the facts?'—'What am I being shown?'—'What are the original findings and what are the present ones?'—'What interpretation has been put upon them?'—'How much is pure speculation?'—'What experience do I need to follow these ideas up properly?' When the ideas presented are not based on experience, we should ask whether we might not discard them as immaterial. Ideas should lead to new findings or enrich those findings that already exist by making them more tangible or giving them a fuller context. It is a pity to waste time on tortuous, meaningless argument or on imaginary models, however much they clamour for attention. If we are to apperceive essentials with certainty, our guide should be a clearly grasped methodology. This helps us to draw a line between genuine, empirical research, pointless experiment and compilations that are uninformative, poorly designed and repetitive.

Every advance in factual knowledge means an advance in method. The latter is often adopted consciously, but by no means always so. Not all great scientific advances begin with complete methodological insight, though when this is present it always clarifies and establishes the factual knowledge gained.

Research methods define their objects by the method chosen. The object is therefore never reality as a whole but always something in particular, an aspect or a perspective, never the happening in its totality.

### (a) Techniques

Psychopathology finds its objects for study in clinics, consulting rooms, institutions, in collected papers, reports, in research laboratories, etc. We are dependent in the beginning on such facts as can be found, and on the way they have been tackled. Discovery often enough consists in simply drawing attention to observed facts. The first person to count suicides and list other comparable figures (population-statistics, seasons of the year) discovered something, even if only in the first instance a routine technique. The important thing is to see the significance of something hitherto ignored and to watch the chance of winning fresh facts through the use of a number of techniques.

1. *Case-study*. Research in psychopathology is based on verbal exploration of the patient and on an intimate acquaintance with his behaviour, gestures and attempts at communication. We also try to get material information on his present condition and on his earlier personal history, so far as it can be obtained. We use the patient's own description of himself, the history as given by him or his relatives, official documents when he has been in the hands of authority, personal papers, information from acquaintances, superiors, etc.

The individual case remains the basic source for all that counts as experience in psychopathology. The description of cases and case-histories—which may range from a description of individual phenomena to a comprehensive biography—is called case-study. This method provides the foundation for our particular science and orientates our approach.

Besides this commonly used and readily grasped method, psychopathology has also developed certain special methods which are not so well suited for routine enquiries, but are appropriate for the exploration of correlates. These are the statistical and experimental methods.

2. *Statistics*. Statistics[1] first appeared in psychopathology as a method of social research, e.g. criminal statistics, suicide rates, etc. Then came the statistical handling of certain specific psychiatric problems: duration of paralysis, interval between luetic infection and onset of paralysis, ages of patients and onset of their respective psychoses; annual distribution curve of admissions, etc. Finally, statistics gained a prominent place in genetics, in correlation-finding in personality studies, in intelligence testing and in somatotyping. The pull towards precision, so characteristic of the natural sciences, operates

---

[1] F. W. Hagen, *Statistische Untersuchungen über Geisteskrankheiten* (Erlangen, 1876). Also later works such as Roemer, *Allg. Z. Psychiatr.*, vol. 70, p. 804.

no less in the field of psychopathology and spurs us on to try to measure and enumerate everything we can.

Statistical methods present a particular problem of their own. We would comment briefly as follows:

(*aa*) Statistical findings never show anything conclusive, when applied to *the individual case*. They can only work with probabilities (usually to the most modest degree). Individual cases can never be subsumed under a statistical finding. For instance, if I know the percentage mortality for an operation, I still do not know what will happen in the individual case. Or if I know the correlation between somato-type and psychosis, I cannot assess the significance of the somatotype in the individual. Any one case may be totally unaffected by the statistical findings.

(*bb*) A clear definition of *the original data* is of decisive importance. If it is not unequivocally defined and identifiable by any other research worker at any time, calculation becomes meaningless. Exact method based on inexact data can lead to the most remarkable mistakes.

(*cc*) Whenever simple enumeration gives place to *mathematical manipulation* a high degree of mathematical and critical ability is required in evaluating results. All the different steps must be kept in mind as well as the sense of the findings; it is only too easy to get lost in a nightmare world of pseudo-mathematical abstractions.

(*dd*) Statistical findings lead to *correlations* but not to *causal connections*. They hint at possibilities and stimulate us to interpret. Causal interpretation demands hypotheses which we can test out. This leads to the danger of numerous *ad hoc* hypotheses multiplying in support. The limits of interpretation must be realised. We should be aware when the point has been reached of artificial hypotheses explaining every correlation. No one case can be contradictory because the supposed factors in all their possible combinations have become all-inclusive and by the application of mathematics every finding can be turned into a confirmation. Friess' theory of the periodicity of biographical events provides an instance. But even with relatively simple numerical comparisons, misinterpretation is quite a risk and often not easily perceived as such. Figures are convincing and we must see they do not smother the useful overstatement 'figures can prove anything'.

3. *Experiments.* Experiment has occupied a prominent position in psycho-pathology. *Experimental psychopathology*, as it was called, was separated off from the rest of the subject and regarded as a special field, i.e. scientific psycho-pathology proper. Such a division seems to us a mistake. Under certain circumstances experiments can be most valuable auxiliaries but the ultimate goal of a science cannot be merely to obtain experimental results. Valid experiment in this field can only be carried out by a psychopathologist who has psychological training, and who knows what questions to ask and how to evaluate the answers. Practice in experiment may give technical skill but it does not in itself constitute the ability for psychological work. Hence the many pseudo-scientific experiments carried out by experimental psychopathologists. Complicated experiments are performed and figures produced but they tell us nothing. There is no supporting theory at the back of them nor any guiding

point of view. The brilliant investigations of Kraepelin in regard to the work-curve, his measurements of memory, his association experiments, etc., constitute a most valuable contribution but comparing the results of psycho-pathological enquiry in general with the results of experimental psychology, Möbius[1] seems to state the truth when he writes of the latter 'they are, to put it crudely, very small beer'.

The main problem is to find those methods that will extract some definite realities from the endless and confusing flood of life; methods that will help us to construct models, find measurable data, draw graphs, schemata and likenesses—in brief create the configurations whereby reality can be properly structured and comprehended. Discovery of a way to make certain facts comprehensible, so that they can be re-identified by others, is the beginning of all research.

Technical methods, such as experiments, calculations, measurements, very often result in accidental observations on the patient which may be extremely useful, though within their own term of reference these methods may yield little. Intelligence tests, for instance, can produce situations in which the patient offers an interesting piece of behaviour which the objective clinical examination did not bring to light. Somatotyping induces a scrutiny of the body from all possible angles, although the actual measurements may be without significance. Thus it is easy to make false evaluations, once we confuse a method's objective findings with what comes to light incidentally in the course of its application.

## (b) The practical logic of research

In the actual course of acquiring knowledge we find ourselves using several methods simultaneously. For theoretical purposes we can discriminate between them and along with them the main types of material gained from their use. There are three major groups: the collection of *individual phenomena*, the enquiry into *the connections* and the grasping of *complex unities*.

1. *Collection of individual phenomena.* Individual facts emerge out of the living flow of psychic reality. Their infinite number fall into various groupings determined by the method of their collection.

(*aa*) The first step towards a scientific knowledge of the psyche is the selection, delimitation, differentiation and description of particular *phenomena of experience* which then, through the use of the allotted term, become defined and capable of identification time and again. Thus we shall presently describe the different kinds of hallucinations, delusions, compulsive phenomena and the different modes of personal awareness, drives, etc. So far there is no concern with the sources of such phenomena nor with the emergence of one psychic phenomenon from another, nor yet with any theories about underlying causes. The only concern is with the actual experience. This representation of psychic experiences and psychic states, this delimitation and definition

[1] P. J. Möbius, *Die Hoffnungslosigkeit aller Psychologie*, 2nd edn. (Halle, 1907).

of them, so that we can be sure the same term means the same thing, is the express function of *phenomenology*.

(*bb*) The descriptions of phenomenology only help us to get to know our material indirectly. We depend on patients' self-descriptions, which we can only grasp by analogy with our own modes of experience. Phenomena of this sort may be called *subjective* as opposed to those *objective* phenomena which can be directly demonstrated as they occur, which they do in a number of fundamentally different ways, e.g. as somatic accompaniments (the pulse rate during excitement, dilatation of pupils during fear), or as expression (facial expressions of happiness or gloom), as measurable performance (work-output, memory performance), or in the shape of actions, behaviour or literary or artistic creation. All such objective phenomena help to elucidate the question —what are the basic types of objective psychic facts?

Differentiation is very often made between *subjective* (the patient's immediate experience, which can only be indirectly grasped by the observer) and *objective* (that which can be directly demonstrated in the external world). But such differentiation is not unequivocal. 'Objective' has various meanings; it is not identical in the case of pulse rate, memory performance or meaningful gesture. The following shows the different meanings which this dichotomy into 'subjective' and 'objective' can produce :

1. *Objective* means everything that can be *perceived by the senses*: reflexes, recordable movements, actions, conduct, etc.; every measurable performance, work-output, memory-span. *Subjective* then means everything that can be comprehended by *empathy* into psychic events, or by some realisation of psychic content.

2. Rational content, e.g. of delusions, can be called *objective*, in so far as this can be understood in a *purely intellectual* way, i.e. without empathy. *Subjective* then is applied to the actual events in the psyche which can only be grasped by *sympathetic insight*, i.e. the original delusional experience.

3. *Objective* can be used ultimately for a part of what was up to then subjective, for the *outward sign* of some psychic content directly understood by empathy, e.g. the fear shown by a patient. In this context, *subjective* becomes what we get to know indirectly *through the patient's own statements*, e.g. when a patient with no outward signs of fear tells us he is afraid.

4. It is a remarkable fact that one can have psychic experience without knowing the exact manner of it. For instance, patients may be retarded, which we can either note objectively in the slowing down of their reactions or detect as an objective fact through the exercise of our own empathy. They themselves, however, need not be subjectively aware of this at all. The less psychic differentiation there is, the less is the subjective awareness. In this context, therefore, we can find *objective retardation* as opposed to *subjective retardation* or an objective flight of ideas as opposed to a subjectively experienced 'pressure of thought' (the feeling of a disjointed, restless and shifting flow of ideas).

5. So far all the phenomena, whether objective or subjective, provide matter for scientific investigation but there is one last aspect of the dichotomy into subjective and objective under which *objective* phenomena become those *which can*

*be tested* and discussed, while *subjective* phenomena are those that remain vague matters, *untestable*, cannot be discussed, seeming to rest on inexplicable impressions and purely personal judgments.

2. *Enquiry into connections* ('Understanding' or 'perception of meaning'— Verstehen; 'Explanation' or 'perception of causal connection'—Erklären). Phenomenology presents us with a series of isolated fragments broken out from a person's total psychic *experience*. Other studies present us with data of a different order, e.g. psychological performances, somato-psychic events, expressive gestures, psychotic actions and inner worlds. How are all these various data to be related? In some cases the meaning is clear and we understand directly *how one psychic event emerges from another*. This mode of understanding is only possible with psychic events. In this way we can be said to understand the anger of someone attacked, the jealousy of the man made cuckold, the acts and decisions that spring from motive. In phenomenology we scrutinise a number of qualities or states and the understanding that accompanies this has a *static* quality. But in this question of connectedness, we grasp a psychic perturbation, a psyche in motion, a psychic connection, the actual emergence of one thing from another. Here our understanding has a *genetic* quality. (A psychopathology of meaningful phenomena.) Not only do we understand subjectively-experienced phenomena in this way, but all the other phenomena which are directly visible to us in their objective manifestations, e.g. actual performances and the works and personal worlds of our patients, which may all have provided us with the material for our static observation.

Broadly speaking, however, 'understanding' has two different meanings, according to whether it is termed *static* or *genetic*. The *static mode* denotes the presentation to oneself of psychic states, the objectifying to oneself of psychic qualities, and we shall exercise this kind of understanding when we come to the chapters on phenomenology and the psychology of expression, etc. In the second part of the book we shall occupy ourselves with the *genetic mode*, that of empathy, of perceiving the meaning of psychic connections and the emergence of one psychic phenomenon from another. The qualification of 'static' or 'genetic' will only be added to 'understanding' (Verstehen) where there might be some confusion. Otherwise we shall use the term 'understanding' according to context, implying in one chapter the static mode, in another the genetic.

In psychopathology our genetic understanding (or perception of meaningful connection) soon reaches its *limits*. (We can call this process 'psychological explanation' if we like, but then we must keep it clearly distinct, as of a different order from objective causal explanation, which is the perception of causal connection in the strict sense.) In psychopathology psychic phenomena appear suddenly as something entirely new, in a way we cannot understand at all. One psychic event follows another quite incomprehensibly; it seems to follow arbitrarily rather than emerge. Stages of psychic development in normal people, psychic phases and episodes in abnormal people are all incomprehensible events and appear as purely temporal sequences. It is equally difficult to understand the whole range of a person's psychic development and its full meaning in genetic terms. We can only resort to *causal explanation*, as with phenomena in the natural sciences, which, as distinct from psychological phenomena, are never seen 'from within' but 'from the outside' only.

In order to be clear we shall keep the expression '*understanding*' (Verstehen) solely for the understanding of psychic events 'from within'. The expression will never be used for the appreciation of objective causal connections, which as we have said can only be seen 'from without'. For these we shall reserve the expression '*explanation*' (Erklären). These two different expressions denote something very specific which will grow clearer as the reader proceeds and the number of examples increases. In questionable cases where one or the other expression could be used interchangeably we shall use the term '*comprehend*' (Begreifen). The very possibility of any systematic study or clear-sighted research in psychopathology depends on grasping the fact that we are dealing here with polar opposites, static understanding as opposed to external sense-perception and genetic understanding as opposed to causal explanation of objective connections. These represent totally different, ultimate sources of knowledge.

Some scientists tend to deny the validity of any psychological source of scientific knowledge. They only accept what can be perceived objectively by the senses, not what can be meaningfully understood through the senses. Their viewpoint cannot be refuted since there is no proof of the validity of any ultimate source of knowledge. But at least we might look for consistency. Such scientists should abstain from talking of the psyche or even thinking in terms of psychic events. They should give up psychopathology and confine themselves to the study of cerebral processes and general physiology. They should not appear as expert witnesses in Court, since on their own showing they know nothing about the subject-matter; they can give no expert opinion on the psyche, only on the brain. They can only help expertly with reference to physical phenomena and they should give up any pretence to history-taking. Such consistency would gain one's respect and we might think it worthy of the name of science. More commonly we find, however, denials and doubts expressed in interjections such as 'this is only subjective', etc. This seems a sterile nihilism shown by people who would persuade themselves that their incompetence is due to their subject-matter, not to themselves.

3. *Grasp of complex unities*. All research differentiates, separates and studies individual particulars in which it tries to discover certain general laws. Yet all these individual particulars are taken out from what is in reality a complex unity. In grasping particulars we make a mistake if we forget the comprehensive whole in which and through which they exist. This never becomes the direct object of our study but only does so via the particulars. It is never examined

in itself but only in the form of some schema of its essence. In itself it remains an idea.

We can state the following in relation to it: the whole comes before its parts; the whole is not the sum of its parts, it is more than them; it is an independent and original source; it is form; the whole cannot therefore be grasped from its elements alone. The whole can persist in its totality even when its parts are lost or changed. It is impossible to derive the whole from its parts (mechanistic philosophy) nor can the parts be derived from the whole (Hegelianism). We have rather to conceive a polarity. The whole must be seen through its parts and the parts from the aspect of the whole; there can be no comprehensive synthesis of the whole from its parts nor any deduction of the parts from the whole; there is only something that encompasses. The infinite whole comprises a mutual interplay of parts and wholes. We have to enter upon an infinite analysis and relate everything analysed to its appropriate whole. In biology, for instance, all the particular causal connections obtain their coherence through mutual interaction within a living whole. Genetic understanding (the perception of psychic connection) enlarges the 'hermeneutic round'; we have to understand the whole from the particular facts and this whole in turn preconditions our understanding of the facts.

The same question arises in *somatic medicine*. In the old days when illnesses were thought to be demons in possession, a man was held to be either sick or not; he had a devil in him or he had not. He was thought to be wholly possessed, sick as a person. Then came one of the greatest advances in scientific knowledge, when it was found that the body was not sick as a whole at all, but that the trouble could be localised in certain anatomical organs or biological processes, from which point it exercised more or less far-reaching effects on other organs, functions or even on the whole body. Reactive and compensatory processes were observed between the morbid development and the body as a whole, which was seen as a life-process making for health. It was now possible to distinguish purely local and limited diseases, which had no effect on the rest of the body and were of slight importance—what we might, using other criteria, call a blemish—from those other disorders which became vitally important because of their effect on the body as a whole, which then began to react to these effects. Instead of the numerous ills which had been supposed rather vaguely to affect the whole body, it was now possible to describe a number of well-defined diseases which could be the cause of widespread symptoms but did not spring from the living body as a whole. There remained a by no means unimportant group of somatic disorders which seemed to be grounded in the total constitution of the body. In the last resort, however, we find that with all individual disturbances once they have been identified there is always some relation to the 'constitution', that complex unity of the living individual.

The same polarity of whole and part will be found to exist in our study of *the psyche*. But in this case from the point of view of methodology everything is much less clear scientifically, with many more dimensions and much more complex. The relationship between part and whole enters into every chapter of this book. At critical points the meaning of wholeness will be explored in some detail, but it becomes the main theme in the fourth part, as the empirical whole, and in the sixth part as that all-encompassing whole which is beyond empirical investigation. The following are a few general preliminary remarks:

Though we speak of 'a human being as a whole' we mean something infinite and as a whole unrealisable. A vast number of individual psychic functions go to its construction. Let us take for example some extremely circumscribed particular, such as colour-blindness, tone-deafness or outstanding memory for digits; these are so to speak deviant parts of the psyche which may eventually—sometimes during a lifetime—exert an influence on the total personality. Similarly we can think of many other particulars as isolated functions of the psyche which provide the varied equipment of personality and we can contrast abnormalities arising in these functions, in memory for instance, with abnormalities of a quite different kind, which are rooted in the whole individual right from the start and do not seem to originate in any individual part of the psyche. For instance, there are patients in whom brain injury has produced severe memory defects, speech disorders and motor paralyses which seem destructive to the total personality. If we observe closely, however, under certain favourable conditions, the original unchanged personality becomes apparent; it is only 'put out of action' for a time or made incapable of expressing itself. It remains potentially intact. In contrast with this we find patients whose 'equipment' seems all in order but who appear deviant in their personality as a whole, sometimes in a way which defies definition. It was this which led the older psychiatrists to call mental illnesses 'illness of personality'.

This general polarity of the human being as a whole and his individual psychic parts does not provide the sole dimension for our analysis. There are many kinds of wholes and parts in psychological research. Phenomenological elements are contrasted with the totality of the momentary state of consciousness; an individual's particular performance with his over-all performance; the individual symptom with the typical syndrome. As to more comprehensive and complex unities, we find these in the constitution, in the disease entity and in the person's whole history. Yet even these ultimate empirical wholes remain relative and cannot be taken as the whole of the human being as such. This encompasses all these things and springs from an unconfined freedom which lies beyond the reach of empirical enquiry into Man.

Scientific endeavour makes progress only by analysis and by relating one particular to another, but if it does no more than this, it dies in failing to discern the essential; it simply slips into the comfort of bare enumeration. Science must always be carried along by the idea of some unifying whole, without being seduced by facile anticipation into tackling any such whole directly. When this happens we tend to get drunk with phrases and narrow our horizons through a presumed mastery of the whole and through an apparent elucidation of the psychic forces which encompass us all. In our research we need to keep as our farthest horizon the consciousness of this encompassing quality of the human being, which reduces every object of our enquiry to a part or an aspect, to something relative, however comprehensive it may seem in its empirical wholeness.

What Man actually is remains the great question that stands at the margins of all our knowledge.

*(c) Inevitable mistakes in formal logic that have to be constantly overcome*

1. *The slide into endlessness.* Facts and thinking are 'correct' but yet do not bring knowledge. Every research worker has the experience of being on the wrong track and baffled, without knowing why. We have to learn to meet this hazard consciously, having grasped wherein it lies. I now try to point out a number of these hazards.

*(aa)* If I write my *case-histories* on the principle that I must lay judgment aside and describe everything, put down all that the patient says, collect everything that can be known, my case-histories will soon become nothing but endless description and if I am too conscientious, they will grow into fat tomes which nobody reads. The mass of irrelevant data cannot be justified by saying that later research workers may look at it from some fresh point of view. Very few facts can be well described without there being some intuitive awareness of their possible meaning. We can only avoid pointless activity of this sort if we start with a vision of what is essential and if we formulate some ideas to govern the collection of our data and its presentation. It is no help to cut the process short with some schema of popular appeal.

*(bb)* One of the surest ways to establish facts is *to count what can be counted.* But we can count ad infinitum. Figures may now and then command interest, particularly for a beginner, but they make sense only when such figures can be compared from different points of view. Yet even that lacks point. The important thing is to make the whole counting operation into an instrument for some exploratory idea which will penetrate reality and not merely re-present itself in a string of endless figures. Thus we find complex investigations which produce certain figures but teach us nothing; there is no basic idea to check diffusiveness and give the work methodical shape.

*(cc)* It has become popular to calculate the *correlation* between two sets of facts, and this may vary from certainty (coefficient = 1) to complete independence (co-efficient = 0). Personality traits, individual abilities, genetic factors, test-results, are all examined statistically for degrees of correlation. Such correlations appear very satisfying; there seems to have been a conclusive demonstration of real connections. If however such correlations are multiplied endlessly and are only of moderate significance in any case, they begin to lose their value. Correlations are after all only superficial facts, an end effect which cannot inform us of the real relationships obscured by such mass statistics. In this world almost everything is related to everything else. The facts will attain to meaning and the endless correlation stop only if we can introduce some standpoint to give significance. This should derive from a theory based upon other sciences and be itself illumined with a fresh idea. As with everything else, the mere beauty of the presentation must not blind one. Diffusiveness of this

sort can be checked only with the help of some methodological principle to which we must adhere.

(*dd*) Another protracted, yet sterile, undertaking is the enumeration of all the parts of a reality and the explanation of it by the *combination and permutation* of these same parts. Even if, judging by methods of pure logic, this were quite correct, our knowledge of fresh, essential matters is advanced not at all. The important thing is to possess the formula whereby all the real possibilities may be deduced as required, not to make ad hoc use of the play of permutations without any over-riding notion of what it is all about.

(*ee*) In studying the *physiology of reflexes*, because the reality of mutual conditioning of elementary reflexes is so complicated, we may quickly get caught in an endless maze, while trying to establish all the possible combinations of certain conditioned reflexes. But knowledge of the integration of reflexes will overcome this endless interchange by helping us to grasp the principle of such an integration, which we can test by a number of well-designed experiments. Such knowledge illuminates for us the endless process and informs it with a principle.

(*ff*) Generally speaking in all fields of research we find the same enumerative process at work. Clinical syndromes are described and combined endlessly, phenomenological descriptions accumulate and tests of performance multiply.

In research we have to go through the same experiences again and again. We first have to commit ourselves and then embark on a long journey. After countless attempts we have so to feel the impact of our efforts that—saturated with what we have gathered on the way—we at last gain the idea which will bring order, create categories and differentiate between what matters and what does not. Every true discovery is a conquest over endlessness. It is a prime mistake for a scientist, however industrious, to lose sight of this and work away in sterile repetition. We should retain the capacity to be startled and to stop, to feel the challenge of our work and discover in this experience of endlessness the beginning of new possibilities. For a time, it is true, the slide into endlessness is always necessary. Every piece of original work is followed by analogous studies, by repetition of the same experiments on other material, by work which serves the purpose of confirming or enlarging upon the previous findings, until the unending nature of the repetition becomes obvious. But the forward march, the beat in the real rhythm of research, springs from the periodic fertilisation of our consciousness with a new idea which solves the endless riddle that has baffled us so far. In putting the clear question, we already have our reply.

This discussion on the danger of diffuse effort rests on the principle that all concrete reality is infinite. Knowledge lies in discovering concepts whereby we can *master this unendingness* and bring it *under the control of discerning insights* which, though limited, are nonetheless well fitted to help us grasp the essence of their matter, in so far as they grow organically out of it and are not forcibly imposed upon it.

There are many ways in which we can lose the point of our efforts, and we will now describe a few that are typical:

*Unlimited 'ad hoc' hypotheses.* We need working hypotheses for the interpretation of our facts. They have no value per se but only as a means of widening experience, so that we can pose the right questions and develop a line of research. It is usual to endow these working hypotheses with a certain significance, often quite unconsciously. We keep on making more and more far-reaching concepts, develop our theoretical constructions and employ one concept after another simply for the sake of concept-building. We need only to consider the psychiatric literature attentively to see how much writing consists of unobjective thinking without foundation in experience. We can see how easily this happens. Theoretical possibilities are endless in themselves. To develop them is an intellectual game, differing, according to taste, in line and pattern and in persuasive power. But for thought to have meaning, this endless game has to be controlled. We can set a limit by requiring every concept so to justify itself in the reality of experience that our experience is furthered. This cannot be done by unproductive play with the experiences already available. Thought that leads us away from living experience without again returning to it builds a fable. We must, therefore, ask of every method whether it increases our knowledge and gives it depth and shape, and whether it makes it more possible to identify phenomena as they arise. Does it widen our experience and increase skill? Or does it lead to a void of abstractions and so entangle us with ideas and paper-schemes that we suddenly find ourselves in a world remote from what we see and do, and ourselves moving from one vacuum into another?

*Acceptance of endless possibility.* If our theoretical explanations are such that a combination and variation of the available facts will explain every possible instance in such a way that no case remains to contradict the theory, we have fallen into the trap of another endless activity—one that tries to explain everything and therefore explains nothing. An initially clarifying theory will encounter contradiction at some time or other. There will be realities which will oppose it. 'Ad hoc' theories may then be formed to explain these new facts and finally a point is reached where so many premises have been made that all thinkable eventualities are provided for. Probably all successful theories that have held sway from time to time have fallen into the practice of this magical, confusing play. Such theories 'explain everything' and thereby nothing and can offer the faithful only an unending application of the theory and the all-embracing possibilities of combination. Every time explanation becomes too complex, scientists should be on their guard against being drawn into an acceptance of endless possibilities, which at one stroke turns them into omniscient individuals, whose only means of progression in fact is to revolve in tautologous circles.

*Unlimited use of references.* Anyone who does research wants to know what has been discovered previously. In describing a given field of knowledge, one must know the literature referring to it, but too exacting a thoroughness in this comprehensive occupation may go on for ever. We may then consider important only the collection of ideas, opinions and individual differences as such, the matching and selecting of them. This activity will grow endless once we fail to recognise certain areas of agreement because different terms and phrases have been employed. It will be equally endless if we do not see the indefiniteness of certain aspects because we believe that the whole has already been explained; or if, for lack of proper scrutiny, the author's ideas have overgrown the actual argument; or if the literature has not been extracted on relevant lines and according to the factual value of its contents, there being instead a wholesale collection of it, as if everything described were of equal importance. In the face of the enormous psychiatric literature that has accumulated, we have to acquire a power of discrimination which will protect us from confusing what are only 'efforts of Sisyphus' with the accumulation of knowledge.

(2) *The impasse created by absolutes.* Almost all the methods and material of research come to be regarded as necessary, of central importance and absolute. Once we feel we are on the right course, we are eager to subordinate all our findings to the one point of view which now is no longer seen simply as our method of working, but takes on an ontological value in itself. We believe we have now grasped reality, instead of remembering that we are in fact using a large variety of methods and our enquiry must be kept in a proper perspective. We have come to regard what is only partial knowledge as if it were an absolute, whereas all knowledge is partial and of the particular. To safeguard against this pitfall, we should have a clear idea of the different methods and points of view and weigh them one against the other, those of biology, for instance, as against those of the social sciences, or vice versa; or the psyche against the brain, or nosology against phenomenology. By regarding our own point of view as an absolute we create nothing but prejudice.

In psychopathology and in psychology, theories have grown up from a far too readily satisfied urge to explain the whole in some one particular way by means of a limited number of elements. This has resulted in the construction of 'systems', certain all-embracing frameworks, broad classifications and apparently final, totally comprehensive structures, which need only further perfecting in their details. In all these efforts, theories of the nervous system have always been the model. We, on the contrary, are asking for a systematic grasp of all the existing methods and viewpoints and insist that there should be no confusion of them, and no generalisation beyond certain well-defined limits, and within these limits methods should be systematically used and carefully applied.

From its inception this book has been averse from every kind of fanatical teaching, which creates absolutes so readily out of the human desire for attention. In the course of an enquiry and in following up all its consequences, absolutes may be necessary and even meaningful to an enthusiastic investigator, caught up in some phase of his work. When however we are trying to construct some comprehensive picture, such practices should be discarded. The first requisite is to fight fanaticism—and who is there without it? Only so will theory spring from an appreciation of the whole rather

than from some partial truth that has been raised arbitrarily to the status of an absolute. The unifying whole which we look for is always incomplete. In contrast to the
totality of closed and would-be universal systems, my own over-all point of view
starts, not from an apparently known, factually demonstrable principle of things, but
rather points down many perspectives and in many directions. It suggests movement in various planes and constrains us to remain alert and look far afield, while at
the same time we try to keep a firm grasp on all the systematised knowledge we have
won so far.

But it is a delicate matter to unify the manifold findings of research. Every investigator is apt to consider the facts in his own field misrepresented by others. He
will resent that anybody who has not worked in this same field should interfere with
his judgments and he will lightly dispose of arguments which arise from an objective
interpretation of the whole field, treating them as purely theoretical. Any such
unification would indeed be a distortion, if it were built on ontological principles,
but, as it is, our attempt does not take the form of a universal theory bent on explaining everything. It takes the form only of a comprehensive methodology, in which all
possible knowledge can be accommodated. Such a methodology must be so constructed that it is an open one which constantly allows for new methods.

The basic attitude expressed in this book is that of fighting against all attempts to
create absolutes, of exposing the various forms of endlessness and of doing away
with obscurities, but we hope at the same time to recognise every genuine experience
and comprehend it in its own way. We want to understand and accommodate all
the knowledge that is possible and find a natural place for it within the framework
of our method.

(3) *Pseudo-insight through terminology.* Precise knowledge always lends
itself to clear formulation. Happy or unhappy formulations have exceptional
importance for the effective dissemination and general intelligibility of our discoveries. But only where the knowledge gained is itself clear will the resulting
terminology be both factual and of intrinsic value. There is a recurrent demand
for some unified terminology in psychology and psychopathology and the
difficulty lies not in the words so much as in the actual concepts themselves. If
only our concepts were clear, there would be no problem of terminology. As
it is, to create a scientific terminology at this juncture by setting up some com-
mittee or other appears quite impracticable. We have not yet arrived at any
universal acceptance of the necessary concepts. We can expect only that everyone who publishes any work in psychopathology will be familiar with the
concepts which outstanding investigators have associated with certain terms
and that he himself will deliberately associate precise concepts with the words
he himself uses. At present people do not hesitate to introduce new words into
scientific publications and discussions, words which carry manifold meanings
in general usage. Frequently, too, fruitless attempts are made to suggest a
whole number of new words rather than do any real research.

(d) *The relatedness of psychopathological methods to other scientific studies*

Medicine is only one of the roots of psychopathology. Psychopathological phenomena may also be reinterpreted as *biological events* against a general ground of biological theory, e.g. genetics, where human existence and mental illness can be studied from this point of view. Only when the biological aspects have been clearly distinguished can we proceed to discuss what essentially belongs to Man.

Whenever the object studied is Man and not man as a species of animal, we find that psychopathology comes to be not only a kind of biology but also one of the Humanities. With psychiatry the doctor enters a world which lies outside the other disciplines with which he is already familiar. The fundamentals of his education generally consist of chemistry, physics and physiology, but here he is in need of a different basic training. This situation is responsible for the fact that psychiatry, in so far as it is practised by doctors without training in the Humanities, lacks any consistency in its scientific standing. Young doctors study their psychiatry more or less haphazardly and some psychiatrists can show little more than a dilettante learning.

Psychopathology requires us to study specially, not only to understand the work of others, but to do so methodically and with a reasonable certainty, as well as to make further progress ourselves.[1] The literature is pervaded by inadequate contributions in this respect. The average psychiatrist is officially recognised as an expert only in so far as cerebral pathology, somatic, forensic, nursing and administrative problems are concerned.

According to Kant[2] expert opinion in the Courts on mental states should fall within the competence of the philosophical faculty. From a purely logical point of view perhaps this is correct but in practice of course it will not do. No one but a doctor can treat mental patients because somatic medicine is indispensable for this. Consequently only a doctor should be concerned with the collection of factual data necessary for the Court. Kant's dictum stands, however, in that the psychiatrist's competence is really commensurate with how far his education and knowledge would qualify him to belong to the philosophic faculty. This goal is not served where (as has occurred in the history of psychiatry) he learns a certain philosophical system by heart and applies it automatically. This is worse than if he had learnt nothing at all. But he should acquire some of the viewpoints and methods that belong to the world of the Humanities and Social Studies.

In fact the methods of almost all the Arts and Sciences converge on psychopathology. Biology and morphology, mensuration, calculation, statistics, mathematics, the Humanities, sociology, all have their application. This dependence on other branches of learning and the proper taking over of their methods and concepts are both matters of some importance to the psychopathologist, who is concerned with the human being as a whole and more especially the human being in times of sickness. The essence of psychopathology as a study can only emerge clearly from a composite framework. It

---

[1] Külpe, 'Medizin u. Psychologie.', *Z. Pathopsych.*, vol. 1 (1912).
[2] Kant, *Anthropologie*, 51.

is true that methods taken over from elsewhere may lose thereby and are often misapplied, thus producing a pseudo-methodology, and this is a weakness. Yet psychopathology is impelled to make use of methods that have been perfected elsewhere in order to improve the status of its subject-matter, which is unique and irreplaceable for our apprehension of the world and humanity, and to bring it to a level where it can be properly grasped and its significance fully comprehended.

The channels provided by society for psychopathological enquiry are the hospital practice, the outpatient departments, the institutions, the medical and psychotherapeutic consulting-rooms. Scientific knowledge emerges first as the consequence of 'practical necessity' and most often remains within these confines. More rarely, but then all the more effectively, the thirst for fundamental knowledge has led great personalities within these fields to break new grounds.

### (e) *The demands of a satisfactory methodology: a critique of methods in contrast to methods that mislead*

What can we expect from our methods? They should help us to gain new ground and enrich our knowledge in depth while they widen our experience. They should enable us to understand cause and effect and they should indicate to us comprehensible relationships, the verification of which is tied to our presuppositions. They should not involve us with what are mere logical possibilities divorced from observation and experience, and their value should show itself in the extent to which we can assess and influence events that arise from our contact with persons.

Criticism of methods is of value in testing the foundations of our knowledge from time to time. We can then detect pseudo-knowledge due to wrong method. Such a critique also helps us to grasp the inner organisation of our knowledge. It refines our methods of enquiry, making them more practicable and better understood.

Every scientific approach has its pitfalls and methodology is no exception. It can degenerate into an empty, logistic checking and rechecking. Such superficial juggling with figures or shuffling of concepts is merely destructive. The true source of all our knowledge is always the contemplative gaze. It may well happen that a writer who has seen something new cannot formulate what he has seen into an unexceptionable theory; although he is right, formal logic may apparently demonstrate contradiction and error. Constructive criticism, however, will grasp the essential and valuable part of what he wants to say and only improve formulation and clarify method. This necessary, if only formal, correction will be dangerous only if the real significance of the new insight is overlooked. We may find also that clear, correct concepts have been fatal for a particular problem at a certain time, inasmuch as they were premature and as yet unsubstantiated.

Discussion of method makes sense only when there is a concrete case to consider and when the particular effects can be shown. Discussion of method in the abstract is painful. Only a concrete logic is valid in the empirical sciences. Without factual investigations and concrete material, arguments become suspended in mid-air. There is little point in thinking up methods which are not put into practice and perhaps can never be.

Finally there is a type of methodological approach which works quite categorically and negates 'de facto' every positive attempt at fresh knowledge. It works on purely logical grounds and the result is entirely unproductive. For example, there is the typical objection against any attempt at precise differentiation, which is said to be 'breaking down' what is properly a 'unit' (e.g. body and soul, knowing and living, personality development and morbid process, perceiving and conceiving, etc.). Another such argument is that 'transitions' between the separated elements make differentiation illusory. However broadly true this 'unit' thesis may be, its application to the processes of research is generally untrue. Knowledge can be gained only by differentiation. True unity precedes knowledge in the form of an unconscious comprehension that pervades in the form of Idea, creating clear perspectives that once more unify what has been separated. Knowledge itself cannot anticipate this unity, which can be achieved only through actual practice, through the reality of the live human being. To know is to differentiate; knowledge is always concrete and structured, pregnant with opposites and unlimited in its movement towards unity. The discussion over 'transitions' is usually nothing but a retreat from observation and thinking. It is a negative quibbling and such pseudo-methodology does nothing to strengthen genuine unity; it only makes for greater confusion. An amorphous enthusiasm for unity produces chaos and obscurity instead of knowledge which should have a wide mastery over its means.

Certain standards should be expected from publications in psychopathology. Arguing until domesday should be impermissible. Before communicating any research, writers should live themselves into the major observations of the past, familiarise themselves with the essential differences and be clear about their methods. This is the only way to ensure that ancient matter is not being presented again as something new and perhaps even in inferior form. It is the only way to avoid abstract theorising, a lapse into endlessness and the charge that a great deal of hard-won knowledge has got lost in surmise.

## § 5. What a General Psychopathology has to do: a Survey of this Book

General psychopathology is not called upon to collect individual discoveries but to create a context for them. Its achievement should be to clarify, systematise and shape. It should *clarify* our knowledge of the fundamental facts and the numerous methods used; it should *systematise* this knowledge into comprehensible form and finally shape it so that it *enriches the self-*

*understanding of mankind.* It thus specifically assumes the function of furthering knowledge, a function which far exceeds the simple process of fact-finding. A mere didactic classification that can be of practical use and committed to memory is not enough; only that didactic matter suffices which coincides with a grasp of the essential facts.

General psychopathology takes its place within a stream of earlier attempts to comprehend the whole. It takes its orientation from them and in turn becomes the starting-point for fresh attempts which contradict, elaborate or advance them yet further. Let us turn to some of these earlier contributions:

When my *Psychopathology* appeared for the first time (1913) there were books by *Emminghaus* and *Störring*; later we had those by *Kretschmer* and *Gruhle*.[1] All these works were written with different intentions and it would not be fair to class them all on the same level as to aim and value. Each, however, was the expression of a comprehensive theory, an attempt to mould material of unlimited extent.

General psychopathology is far from being a didactic presentation of available facts; it tries consciously to fit the whole together. Every psychiatrist is characterised by the way he formulates his complex material into some over-all pattern, flexible or rigid as the case may be. Every book on psychopathology wants to contribute to this total picture and find some mode of thinking which will give meaning and definition to the individual methods used. Books which aim at a total presentation gain relative importance from the way in which they take a comprehensive view and represent this throughout the whole of their methodology and line of reasoning. In comparing and characterising the following works I hope to draw an illuminating contrast with what I have tried to do in my own *General Psychopathology.*

*Emminghaus. (1878).* He chose a medical classification, analogous to other clinical specialities. His book treats 'seriatim' nosology (symptomatology, diagnostic criteria, course, duration and outcome of psychiatric illness), aetiology (predisposition, precipitating factors, etc.) and lastly, pathological anatomy and physiology. His method is purely descriptive and displays the untested general attitudes of medicine based on the natural sciences of his day. In his detailed psychology he makes use of very diverse points of view and there is little conscious criticism or development of ideas. The standard is little more than that of everyday psychology which is obscured by an apparently scientific terminology and the contemporary interest in externals. The advantage of the book is its orderly comprehensive character, but its very comprehensiveness obscures the gulf which always exists between psychiatry and other clinical specialities. (We can make a real synthesis only after a conscious effort to clarify the partly heterogeneous principles and methods involved.) Presentation is attractive and vivid throughout and the extensive bibliography makes the book an excellent reference book even today, for the older literature in particular. A wide perspective (the interest, for instance, in ethnic psychology), which is maintained along with the general medical interest, derives from the psychiatric education of earlier times. The medical classification of earlier times, which Emminghaus employed, continues in use in the general psychiatric textbooks.

---

[1] Emminghaus, *Allgemeine Psychopathologie zur Einführung in das Studium des Geistesstörungen* (Leipzig, 1878). Störring, *Vorlesungen über Psychopathologie* (Leipzig, 1900): Kretschmer, *Medizinische Psychologie* (Leipzig, 1922, 5th edn., 1949). Gruhle, 'Psychologie des Abnormen', *Hdbuch der vergleichenden Psychologie*, Kafka, vol. 3, sect. 1 (München, 1922).

*Störring (1900):* aimed at a different target. He wanted to discuss the importance of psychopathology for normal psychology and stressed the theoretical issues from the beginning, taking Wundt's theories as a standard. He devotes much space to discussions on the genesis of phenomena, using Wundt's methods, which nowadays strike us as rather out of date. Classification follows the old schema: cognition, emotion and volition. He uses 400 pages for cognition, 35 pages for emotion and only 15 pages for volitional phenomena. The trend of thought is consistent throughout and this lends a particular value to the book. Interesting points emerge but the net contribution is so meagre that though the title is attractive one puts the book down with some disappointment. The theoretical approach brings much more shape into the material than the traditional medical classifications used by Emminghaus, but in view of the enormous range of psychic reality, Störring's work offers very limited solutions.

*Kretschmer (1922).* This book cannot be compared with the other two. Its aim is didactic and it deals with that part of psychology which is supposed to be of real importance to the doctor, but without—as we think quite justifiably—differentiating in principle between normal and pathological. Kretschmer also constructs his over-all picture with the help of a theory and this gives his thought a particular configuration. He conceives a number of psychic levels, which appear as stages of development in history, phylogeny and ontogeny and are simultaneously present in the mature individual. To this he adds a second idea which concerns types of personality and modes of reaction. Both notions are then rigidly schematised. He stresses the value of simplification into a small number of formulae and he refers to the natural sciences which have found this method fruitful in gaining control over subject-matter. He wants to show how, using exact methods, he can reduce the multifarious richness of real life to a few basic biological mechanisms, universally recurrent. In doing this, however, he meets his own confusion. In the natural sciences there is a constant interplay between theory and observation, which then either confirms or disproves the theory so that exact hypotheses emerge which can get exact answers. Science progresses in a generally connected way, step by step, or with the leap of a new formulation. But in psychiatry, and this applies to Kretschmer, theory always has to have the character of a tentative approach which will allow for varied classifications and further observations.

Kretschmer supplies us with an original example of the 'psychology of meaningful phenomena' disguising it as one of the natural sciences to suit the climate of the medical faculty, but in fact he manages to do this only by misusing the logic of the natural sciences and their exact methods. His simplifications were 'to bring life into dry bones'. 'Sometimes I have tried to startle people with the barest of formulae', he says. So much compression of his material, however, and so much theoretical simplification produce an air of omniscience, with which we are only too familiar in the history of psychological medicine. His omniscience rushes to classify and pigeon-hole such phenomena as 'expressionism' or 'historical personality' and the book is pervaded by that incredible delusion adhered to by many psychiatrists that the 'psychology of the neuroses is nothing else but the psychology of the human heart'—'to understand neurosis is, "eo ipso", to understand human nature'. It is perhaps typical that the book should be written in a literary style. It has little respect for the infinite possibilities of the human individual, or for the eternal problem of the psyche. There is no sense of wonder. Instead we are offered a number of clichés, the use of which gives us a satisfactory feeling of penetrating human understanding. But

Kretschmer creates no real concept of the totality of psychic life. He gets as far as an initial selection of problems. His language is figuratively telling rather than conceptually sharp and we are more impressed by the slickness of the expression than by the genuine force of his ideas.

*Gruhle (1922):* This work seems in perfect contrast to Kretschmer's. The externals of careful work and dry style already point to this. Gruhle tries to find an unbiased classification. He does not theorise schematically but deals with his material as to the whole. He distinguishes quantitative, qualitative and functional abnormalities, the latter to include intentional acts and motivated behaviour. He comments on abnormal relationships between physical and psychic events and on abnormal psychic development. By using broad concepts, such as quality and quantity, he is able to classify all his material and find accommodation for all observed phenomena. No underlying concept or fresh idea is developed. There is no systematic exploration of the inner organisation of phenomena. As he said, he simply sets up a number of boundary-stones, to contain everything that seems of psychopathological importance. His superficially wide-reaching system gives us a number of broad concepts but no creative picture of the whole. He has a passion for formal clarity and this forces him to avoid everything in the way of creative construction. In the end he is left surrounded by his innumerable facts but unable to differentiate the important from the unimportant. This indeed is something which formal classifications cannot achieve; it can be done only by the use of ideas and Gruhle therefore misses the substance of the problem. He does not try to impress and one has the feeling that there is not one inaccurate sentence in the whole book. Yet the writing has a certain charm in spite of the dryness of style. The author is a man of culture and keeps a certain distance from the things he writes about. He would have had no difficulty in cultivating a literary style but he feared nothing more than the confusion of 'belles lettres' with science. If we accept the book for what it purports to be, a careful collection of existing material, we shall find it most useful. A wide literature is referred to, and old, forgotten work has been put to much good use.

My own book (1913) intends something quite different from all the publications both before Gruhle and after. As the author I cannot of course characterise this intention unfavourably. But I want to make it clear from the start that what I intend to do in no way invalidates what others have attempted so far. On the contrary I would recommend everybody who wants to penetrate into the problems of psychopathology to read all these texts and compare them. Only by correcting the one by the other can we hope to gain a proper grasp of this complex subject.

The following are some observations on the purpose and format of this book:

## (a) *Conscious critique of methods in place of dogmatism*

In 1913 I described my methodology as follows: 'Instead of forcing the subject-matter into a strait-jacket of systematic theory, I try to discriminate between the different research methods, points of view and various approaches, so as to bring them into clearer focus and show the diversity of psychopathological studies. No theory or viewpoint is ignored. I try to grasp each different view of the whole and give it place according to its significance and limitations. The all-embracing factor will be the mental search. Every theory that aims at completeness will be taken as valid for that particular standpoint only. I then try to master the sum of all such views in their entirety. But in the end no more can be done than to order them according to the methods and categories by which they have been individually constructed. I indicate how we come to perceive the various aspects of the psyche and each chapter presents one such aspect. There is no system of elements and functions to be applied generally in psychopathological analysis (as one might apply knowledge of atoms and the laws of chemical combination); we must simply be satisfied with a number of different methods of approach. The data are ordered not in terms of any one consistent theory, but simply in terms of the methods used.'

The above statement reflects a common conflict of scientific opinion that cannot be overestimated in its importance. Either we think every piece of knowledge gives us the thing itself, *reality as such*, Being in its totality, or we think that there can be no more than an *approximate appreciation of context*, which implies that our knowledge is rooted in our methods and limited by them. We may thus rest content with a knowledge of 'what is' or know ourselves constantly *on the move against expanding horizons*; we may simply emphasise some *theory of reality* as sufficiently explanatory or prefer the *systematic approach to methods used*, hoping this will throw light on what is after all an unlimited obscurity. We may discard our methods as *temporary* but *necessary tools*, to be dropped when we supposedly grasp at the thing itself, or *things in themselves* may become *temporary* though *necessary myths* attending our incessant efforts to know; they are theoretical realities which we discard as incomplete, but which keep the doors open for further experience and research.

A *conscious critique of methods* will keep us prepared in the face of enigmatic reality. *Dogmatic theories* of reality shut us up in a kind of knowledge that muffles against all fresh experience. Our methodological approach, therefore, is in full opposition to the attitude that would establish absolutes. We represent searching in opposition to finding.

We have to remember that methods become creative only when we use them, not when we theorise about them. Early investigators who widened knowledge by their methods sometimes did not understand what was happening. (They paid for their lack of understanding by becoming dogmatic about their discoveries.) The conscious study of methods as such is not creative; it only clarifies, but in doing so it creates the conditions under which discoveries can arise, whereas all forms of dogmatism inhibit fresh findings.

In a naïve thirst for knowledge people want to grasp the whole at once and grope after seductive theories which seem to point in this direction. Critical enquiry, however, would rather know the limitations and possibilities. It wants a clear understanding of the *boundaries* and implications of each viewpoint and fact, as well as a *continuous exploration* of hard-won, ever-expanding possibilities.

It seems to me that only through the use of some systematic methodology can we obtain the widest extension of our limits and the greatest clarity about what it is possible to know.

### (b) Classification according to methods

By reducing our methods to some order we become fully aware of the differing modes of apprehension, the various kinds of observation, forms of thought, ways of research and basic scientific attitudes, which we can then test out on appropriate objects of investigation. In this way differentiation between individual entities becomes sharper and our organs of apprehension and enquiry are refined. On each several occasion limits can be clearly drawn and we can test out possible concepts of the whole and put them in some kind of perspective. This training in methodological order provides a reliable critique of the meaning and limits in every piece of knowledge, and enhances our unprejudiced apprehension of facts.

To the psychopathologist, reality displays itself as an individual whole, in the form of a living human being. As we get to know, we analyse, and by one method or another we secure our facts. It follows that (1) all our knowledge is of particulars; we have never seen the whole before our analysis starts; we have already made analysis in the act of seeing. (2) the observable facts and our methods of observation are closely related. We obtain our facts only by using a particular method. Between fact and method no sharp line can be drawn. The one exists through the other. Therefore a classification *according to the method used* is also *a factual classification* of that which is, as it is for us. It is the ever-moving function of knowledge through which empirical being reveals itself to us. By classification of method and the indication of what is revealed thereby, we gradually come to see the basic varieties of existing fact. Only so can we arrive at any well-defined statement about observed facts and grasp the possible range of definable fact. Classification of method introduces an order into observed facts which is in accordance with the order of these same facts.

Where work develops successfully, object and method coincide. A classification according to the one is at the same time in accord with the other. This may seem to contradict the statement that *'every object should be examined by a number of different methods'*. This maxim is correct but means that what is only superficially one single objective fact (what we call an individual person) has to be investigated by a number of different methods, as an illness, an alteration in consciousness, as memory etc. The bject obecomes in this sense something ill-defined and inexhaustible, a crude fact, indefinable in its totality. What it really is as an object reveals itself only through the methods we use. Whether and to what extent the object which we tackle by so many methods really is a single object and what kind of entity this may finally prove to be can be determined only by methods specific to it.

If on the other hand we have some *theory of reality* to go by, the classification of our knowledge appears much easier. A few principles and basic factors will then afford us a comprehensible whole—'we grasp reality itself'. Hence the often transitory success of attractive theoretical systems in which the thing in itself seems to be completely comprehended, and every newcomer gets a grasp of the whole very quickly, feeling that he has reached the heart of reality straightaway. All he need do is repeat, confirm, apply and elaborate. A more difficult process, but a truer one, is this process of *classifying by method*. This is neither attractive nor particularly comfortable; it cannot be done quickly and there is no immediate grasp of the whole; it is however a scientific exercise. It will stimulate research and further one's abilities. We can see clearly how far we have got, and what certain methods will tell us, but the total human being is left as an open question.

Classification by method is therefore a task which never finishes. There is no construction of a complete science but a constant endeavour to bring out the structure of idea from the observed facts, in the course of defining them and demonstrating them in their various relationships.

### (c) The idea of the whole

Classification of methods provides a scaffolding but by itself this is not enough. We use it only to look for something that lies beyond our reach, namely the whole. But any comprehensive formulation has to be diverse in character. Out of all the diversity therefore we have to select just those basic varieties of fact, those fruitful viewpoints and orientations which will open up for us broad expanses of experience. Superficial connections have to be analysed, true affinities united. In each case the essential unifying agent needs to be clarified. In this way we shall discover basic structures that give meaningful form to the individual parts as they are presented.

Some concentration of basic principles is necessary because we can so easily lose sight of them when presentations ramify. Simple lines of orientation are wanted and we need to confine ourselves to essentials, to the most universal and fundamental considerations only. There is something creative in finding these basic classifications, even if there is no new discovery. Every classification which has been established becomes by its own inconsistencies a stimulus for further research and we make specific experiments to test our views of the whole, since the problematical part of knowledge appears only when we are actually exploring some current concept of the whole.

We try to take the attitude of unprejudiced reason, which is critical of its limits and by a process of classification tries to reach deeper and truer insight into its own activities.

### (d) The objective validity of the classifications

If the basic classifications found in the book are objective, arise out of realities and are not mere theoretical speculations, they will lead on to form an over-all picture which cannot but impress the reader more and more convincingly as the exposition proceeds.

The truth of aesthetically satisfying and didactically convenient classifications can be tested only in the actual application of them. The criterion of their validity lies in their power to increase our insight. A classification that is not merely a loose grouping of events contains objective judgment; it already implies the taking up of a definite attitude.

Classification should bring out basic principles and, where the subject is seen from a number of points of view, show us which are the main points and which are secondary. By defining positions in this way it can lend weight to findings which up to then had not perhaps been considered of importance. At the same time it can show the relativity of all such emphases by again re-defining the position gained. The arrangement should be such that every possible experience can be accommodated therein.

Each chapter is presented within the framework of its specific method and illustrates the phenomena obtained by this method. The basic modes of apprehension and enquiry, the various presentations of the subject, Man, follow one another steadily throughout the book. In actual practice, however, this involves some forcing of the situation. When related phenomena appear to fit together readily, classification has succeeded but when the phenomena seem constricted into a forced order, we have a hint that classification is at fault. To note this and use the occasion as a stimulus for further enquiry is a constant challenge. Each of us can reach only as far as his limit, that point where energies run out because inspiration fails, but our successors may well make use of our work to supersede us in their turn.

The arrangement of the book as a whole and in detail is not accidental but most carefully considered. I beg my readers to think hard about the meaning of the classifications used and to study critically the way the chapters follow one another. I would like them to appraise the basic ideas continually right through to the last part. Only if they set themselves to grasp the book as a single whole will they see the total expanse properly, from which the in-dividual chapters with their own particular perspectives have emerged.

*(e) The plan of the book*

The following is a rough outline of the six main parts: The first part presents the *empirical psychic phenomena*. These are presented serially: sub-jective experiences, somatic findings, concrete performances, meaningful phenomena, i.e. patients' expressions, productions, and personal worlds. The whole of Part I tries to sharpen the perceptiveness of the psychopathologist and demonstrate what are the immediate data.

The second and third parts are concerned with *psychic connections,* that is, the second part with '*meaningful connections*' and the third part with '*causal connections*'. We cannot discover either of these directly from a simple col-lection of facts but only through a process of enquiry which will verify one set of facts against another. These two parts, so to speak, train the *research capacity* of the psychopathologist. Man is part mind, part nature, and at the same time both. The whole of our learning therefore is needed for his proper understanding. In the second part our enquiry calls for some knowledge of the Humanities; in the third part, we need a knowledge of biology.

In the fourth part, the predominantly analytical procedures of the previous sections are followed by what is in chief an effort at synthesis. We are now concerned with the way in which we can apprehend the *individual psychic life as a whole*. We present the *comprehensive approach of the clinician*, who has before him the individual man as a whole and thinks, in diagnosis, in terms of a *personal history*, which in its entirety provides the essential setting for every individual life.

The fifth part considers *abnormal psychic life* in its *social setting* and *in history*. Psychiatry differs from the rest of medicine amongst other things because its subject-matter, the human psyche, is not only a product of nature but also of culture. Morbid psychic events depend in their content and in their form on the cultural milieu which is affected by them in turn. The fifth part trains *the appreciation of the scientist for the historical aspects* of human reality.

In the sixth part we finally discuss *human life as a whole*. We are no longer making empirical observations but present a philosophical reflection. The specific frames of reference, which as complex unities contributed a guiding principle to every previous chapter, are in the end all relative. Even the comprehensive approach of the clinician cannot grasp empirically the human life as a whole. The individual is always more than what is known of him. The final discussion, therefore, no longer adds to our knowledge but tries to clarify *our philosophical position*, into which we can gather all that we know and understand of Man.

The book, therefore, sets out to show us what we know. Practical questions of clinical work are outlined in *the appendix* and there is a short survey of the history of psychopathology as a science.

### (f) Comments on the plan of the book

1. *Empiricism and Philosophy.* In the first five parts I hope I am a thorough-going empiricist and that I am successful in my fight against platitudinous speculation, dogmatic theorising and absolutism in every form. But in the sixth part, and here in this introduction, I have discussed philosophical questions, where these seem to me essential, if as psychopathologists we are to achieve any real degree of clarity. Not only does unprejudiced empiricism bring us to the real boundary where philosophy begins but conversely only philosophical clarity can make reliable, empirical research possible. Philosophy is not so related to science that philosophic studies can find application in the sciences and it has always been a fruitless, though often repeated, undertaking to recast empirical findings into some philosophical terminology. Philosophy can only help towards an inner attitude of mind, which will enhance science by delineating its boundaries, giving it inner direction and stimulating an insatiable thirst for knowledge. Philosophical logic has to grow indirectly into a concrete logic by the conceptual organisation of facts. Psychopathology

does not need philosophy because the latter can teach it anything about its own field, but because philosophy can help the psychopathologist so to organise his thought that he can perceive the true possibilities of his knowledge.

2. *Overlapping of chapters.* In describing the phenomena of experience we sometimes hint at their causal and meaningful connections and vice-versa. So in most of the other chapters we shall encounter phenomenology in one way or another. Thus we review delusional ideas, phenomenologically, as a psychological performance and in their meaningful connections. So with suicide—outwardly it is a straightforward fact the incidence of which can be counted; it can also be investigated by a number of methods, directed towards motive, or in accordance with age, sex and time of year, or with regard to its connection with psychosis, or with social conditions, etc. Thus we shall find the same facts appearing in different chapters and it will become progressively apparent what it is that remains 'the same'. Different schools of thought (psychoanalysis, for instance, or Kretschmer's 'theory of body-build') also appear in several places, wherever they happen to include different methodological aspects (be it consistently or otherwise). The different chapters therefore do overlap but it should be understood that this is necessary and we should be clear in what sense it is permissible.

In each chapter there is only one method that is paramount, and the reader's gaze is directed to all that it reveals. But each of these methods is already using other methods and allows an echo to be heard of what is the master-principle of another chapter, though not yet, or no longer, the prevailing principle (for instance, the phenomenology of some memory-failure can be rendered precise only if the facts are also comprehended from the point of view of the psychological performance, while functional defects of memory can be analysed only along with the phenomenology of the experience in question). Or, to express this differently, every method is related to its own subject-matter, but what becomes apparent through it has at the same time some relation to other subject-matter which is duly comprehended by other methods that point towards it. What we therefore regard as the same set of facts has to appear in several chapters which are in fact complementing each other; yet seen severally from these different perspectives the facts are not the same. One method in isolation can always go only so far and no farther. No one method can allow its subject-matter to segregate itself aloofly within it. It is therefore quite natural that in writing one chapter we should relate it, either with facts or references, to one of the others. All divisions are un-natural at some point. The coherence of things themselves demands that the various methods should remain tangible in their relatedness.

There is also the basic fact that every human being is in some sense one, and this brings a universality into all the possible relationships between the facts that can be found out about him. We need the viewpoints of all the different chapters in order to apprehend one man. No single chapter by itself gives us sufficient understanding.

Division into chapters is necessary for clarity but to reach truth and comprehension they must all be reunited. The themes of the different chapters are related to each other and do not lie mechanically side by side. In every chapter however a specific method of approach will be seen to prevail, a particular mode of observation of presentation and explanation.

3. *Specific methods and the total picture.* In every chapter—to put it rather grandly—the whole field of psychopathology is touched upon, but only from one, single point of view. There is no complete set of facts, ready-made, which are being considered merely from diverse points of view. Through the application of each method, something becomes apparent that belongs only to it, as well as something rather vaguely defined which does not belong. Similarly, the totality that becomes apparent through all our methods is not any consistent total reality nor is there any one universal method which will reveal everything that is. All we can do is to try and apprehend individual realities clearly and unequivocally with the help of individual methods.

Hence enquiry will always be limited by the fact that only one way can be traversed at any given time. Yet there are still many other ways to tread, essential conditions for critical knowledge. In so far as the total picture can remain only a collection of methods and categories, it must stay for ever unfinished; the circle is never closed. The question remains open, not only what will emerge as future additional data, but also what at a later time will appear as new methods of thinking and new perspectives. Therefore the book is probably lacking in that individual chapters may still be insufficiently clarified, with something hiding there that derives from some different principle of which we are not yet aware and which at a later date will have to be extracted. Each chapter tries to give a complete viewpoint but there is no guaranteed completeness; other chapters are possible and to this extent the whole book is incomplete. There is a challenge to develop further chapters, not as simple additions but as part of the connected series of methods. Only so would we keep that total picture of infinite extent which cannot be attained as a concrete reality but only as a system of methods.

It is wrong to call this book 'the principal text of phenomenology'. The phenomenological attitude is one point of view and one chapter has been devoted to it in some detail as the viewpoint is a new one. But the whole book is directed to showing that it is only one point of view among many and holds a subordinate position at that.

## (g) Technical lay-out

1. *Illustration by example.* Experience must in the last resort remain a personal matter. A book can enhance our experience but cannot be a substitute for it. What is seen at a glance, the actual experience of human intercourse and conversation, the confirmation that comes from factual investigation, none of this can be transmitted by a text, even with the most circumstantial presentation. If we have had our own personal experiences we can understand those of

others better, imagine them and use them for our own understanding. Written descriptions cannot substitute for the actual experience, but some account of concrete examples helps us to grasp further possibilities. My book offers many such examples. All my own experience is here and I have added certain striking and characteristic examples from the work of other investigators.

These should help the reader to build up a store of experiences. Though this can be properly achieved only through experiences of his own, he will find good preparation and confirmation in the reports and interpretations set out in the literature.

The essential requirement stands that every speculation should find fulfilment in experience. No experience should be without its theoretical explanation nor should we find theories unsupported by experience. We need plastic views on life, clearly structured and containing neither too much nor too little. They should be the 'fixed lights' to give our thoughts inner direction when the way is uncharted. So it becomes possible for us while we observe and theorise always to know and say what it is we mean.

2. *The form of presentation.* A comprehensive presentation needs to be readable. It should not be simply a reference book. This involves us in maintaining a line of thought throughout and in concentrating on what is essential. Concise definition is desirable even to the point of what might seem a legalistic brevity.

But every idea we formulate has to be lifted out of an endless host of facts and accidental events. Enumeration of these ought to be minimal but they have to be mentioned and their presence felt. The danger of making endless enquiry is always with us but in presenting our material we have always to remember those ever-present, as yet unmastered elements which are important and must be given a place. Interesting accidentals are among our data also, though perhaps as yet nothing much more can come of them than the evocation of a surprised 'well, that is how it is . . .'. We must not forget that undetermined, unmastered elements and surprising happenings are always marks of failing comprehension; we recognise these things but as yet we do not know them.

Every chapter has a prevailing point of view. The reader would do well to familiarise himself with the whole series. In the individual chapters however he may want to leave out this or that, depending on his own particular interests and he will then find the table of contents a useful guide.

3. *References to the literature.* It is always a problem to know how to cope with the continuous stream of publication. The extent of the literature is vast even if we discount all the many repetitions, the muddle of happy ideas, the noisy arguments and indifferent reporting. To get at the factors of value, we must go for the following: first and foremost, the facts themselves, cases, personal histories, self-portrayals, reports and every other kind of *material evidence*; secondly, any really *new insight*; thirdly, the concrete observations made, the images, forms and types adopted, the *pregnant formulations*: fourthly, the

*basic attitude* behind the new discoveries, their 'atmosphere', shown in the style of the work and the kind of criteria used. There may be an unconscious grasp of the whole, some hidden philosophy, or an attitude determined by the worker's social status, calling or occupation, or it may be a practical attitude founded in the need for action and the wish to help. What publications should be mentioned? It is impossible to give them all. Recently reference books have grown to an unwieldy size,[1] and our aim is something different. We are not after the compilation of facts but what characterises them, so our use of the literature must be selective: First we include epoch-making contributions which have led to the foundation of new schools of research, the classic original papers. Secondly, we mention the most recent summaries, where the bibliographies introduce us to a particular field. Thirdly, we take representative samples from various lines of research, which can stand for much other analogous work. Selection in this case is haphazard and does not imply any value-judgment.

The immense task of a real survey of the literature has hardly begun. In the individual sciences the problem is the same as in the great libraries. A hierarchy of importance is sorely needed, so that really valuable material can be recognised and not tend to get lost among the rabble. Inessentials could well be dispensed with, yet they have to be categorised somehow, for the use of specialists. At present there seems no hope of any final evaluation nor of any formal purge by some scientific court. At a later date investigators may well find something of value among the discards; so far as psychopathology goes, we have at present only an unselective set of references.

## (h) Psychopathology and culture

A comprehensive presentation aims at more than mere knowing; it tries to cultivate. It would like to see psychopathologists exercise their thinking, differentiate their knowledge, discipline their observations and introduce method into their experiences. While preserving a great tradition, we also wish to serve it by re-shaping it. Knowledge as such is only relevant when it contributes to the further cultivation of sight and thought.

I would like my book to give the reader a wide education in psychopathology. It is indeed much simpler to learn up formulae and technical terms and appear to have the answer to everything. An educated attitude has to grow slowly from a grasp of limits within a framework of well-differentiated knowledge. It lies in the ability to think objectively in any direction. An educated attitude in psychiatry depends on our own experiences and on the constant use of our powers of observation—no book can give us that—but it also depends on the clarity of the concepts we use and the width and subtlety of our comprehension, and it is these which I hope my book will enhance.

[1] The following texts cover the literature: the specialist journals and original contributions: Aschaffenburg, *Handbuch der Psychiatrie*. Bumke, *Handbuch der Geisteskrankheiten*, Zentralblatt für Neurologie u. Psychiatrie (Berlin, 1910, onwards); Fortschritte der Neurologie (Leipzig, 1929, onwards); the reference section of many journals.

# PART I

## INDIVIDUAL PSYCHIC PHENOMENA

# PART I

# INDIVIDUAL PSYCHIC PHENOMENA

*Introduction*

Phenomena form the groundwork of our knowledge. Empirical research depends on our seeking out as many phenomena as possible, since it is through them alone that our ideas receive verification.

The collection of phenomena always means collection of *individual* phenomena. These are far from uniform and the need for clarification forces us to group them according to certain *basic types*. Such classification is sometimes of a superficial character only, that is according to the source material, e.g. case histories, Court records, patients' own writings, photographs, departmental files, school reports, statistics, experimental test results. But a real classification must work on the principle that its basic phenomena are of an observable nature. We shall, therefore, classify our phenomena into four main groups: the patients' subjective experiences, objective performances, somatic accompaniments and meaningful objective phenomena (i.e. expression, actions and productions).

*Group 1.* The psyche *experiences* life—and experience is a psychic phenomenon. Metaphorically we call it the stream of consciousness, a unique flow of indivisible occurrences which, however many people we take, never seems to flow in quite the same way. How then is it best apprehended? Experiences crystallise out for us in their course into a number of objective phenomena and take relatively fixed forms. We can speak of an hallucination, an affect, a thought, as if we were dealing with some definite object; it at least maintains a certain span of existence in our mind. *Phenomenology* is the study which describes patients' subjective experiences and everything else that exists or comes to be within the field of their awareness. These *subjective* data of experience are in contrast with other *objective* phenomena, obtained by methods of performance-testing, observation of the somatic state or assessment of what the patients' expressions, actions and various productions may mean.

*Group 2. Psychic performances* (for instance, those of apperception, memory, work-capacity, or intelligence) provide the material for what we call the *study of psychological performance* (Leistungspsychologie). Performance can be measured as to quality and quantity. The common factor is the use of set tasks in an attempt to answer specific enquiries or meet the accidental problems posed by some given situation.

*Group 3. Somatic accompaniments of psychic events* provide the material for what we call somatopsychology, the *study of bodily events* (Somato psychologie). Here somatic events are observed which are not psychological in character and in no way express the psyche nor are they meaningful. Psychologically they are incomprehensible and have only a factual relationship with psychic events or happen to coincide with them.

*Group 4. Meaningful objective phenomena* are perceivable phenomena that show their psychic origin only because we understand their meaning. They fall into three categories: bodily appearance and movements that we directly understand (giving rise to a psychology of expression—Ausdruckspsychologie); personal worlds of meaningful activity and behaviour (giving rise to a psychology of the personal environment—Weltpsychologie); and meaningful literary, artistic and technical productions (giving rise to a psychology of creativity—Werkpsychologie).

These four main groups of phenomena will be set out in the four following chapters. From these we shall see that (*a*) every datum described raises the immediate question—*why* is it as it is, *how* is it so and *to what end?* The answer to these questions will be discussed in the latter part of this book. We continually experience dissatisfaction in the face of mere facts, though we also experience a very special satisfaction in establishing facts as such, 'This is a fact!' 'We have found something!', but in the end we find this field of pure fact is infinitely wider than the field where such facts stand properly related and fully understood. (*b*) *Apparently identical* phenomena can be *aetiologically different* from each other; so that the realisation of meaningful relationships can throw light on the facts themselves and show differences between them which at first sight had gone unobserved. External facts, such as murder, suicide, hallucination, delusion etc., mask a heterogeneous reality. Therefore even during the stage of fact-finding we are always going beyond the facts themselves. (*c*) All individual phenomena derive their specific quality from *a whole to which they currently belong*: for instance, the phenomena of experience arise within a consciousness; somatic symptoms arise within a body–mind unit; individual performances within a unified intelligence and expression, actions and productions within what is sometimes called the level of development (Formniveau), the psychic totality or some such name.

# CHAPTER I

# SUBJECTIVE PHENOMENA OF MORBID PSYCHIC LIFE

## (PHENOMENOLOGY—PHENOMENOLOGIE)

*Introduction*

Phenomenology[1] sets out on a number of tasks: it *gives a concrete description* of the psychic states which patients actually experience and *presents* them *for observation*. It reviews the inter-relations of these, *delineates* them as sharply as possible, differentiates them and creates a suitable terminology. Since we never can perceive the psychic experiences of others in any direct fashion, as with physical phenomena, we can only make some kind of representation of them. There has to be an act of empathy, of understanding, to which may be added as the case demands an enumeration of the external characteristics of the psychic state or of the conditions under which the phenomena occur, or we may make sharp comparisons or resort to the use of symbols or fall back on a kind of suggestive handling of the data. Our chief help in all this comes from the patients' own *self-descriptions*, which can be evoked and tested out in the course of personal conversation. From this we get out best-defined and clearest data. Written descriptions by the patient may have a richer content but in this form we can do nothing else but accept them. An experience is best described by the person who has undergone it. Detached psychiatric observation with its own formulation of what the patient is suffering is not any substitute for this.

So we always have to fall back on the 'psychological judgment' of the patient himself. It is only in this way that we get to know the most vital and graphic pathological phenomena. The patients themselves are the observers and we can only test their credibility and judgment. At times we have accepted patients' communications too readily and at times on the contrary we have doubted them too radically. Psychotics' self-descriptions are not only unique but yield reliable results and through

[1] Cf. my paper, 'Die phänomenologische Forschungsrichtung in der Psychopathologie', *Z. Neur.*, vol. 9 (1912), p. 391. *The term phenomenology* was used by Hegel for the whole field of mental phenomena as revealed in consciousness, history and conceptual thought. We use it only for the much narrower field of *individual psychic experience*. Husserl used the term initially in the sense of 'a descriptive psychology' in connection with the phenomenon of consciousness; in this sense it holds for our own investigations also, but later on he used it in the sense of 'the appearance of things' (Wesensschau) which is not a term we use in this book. Phenomenology is for us purely an *empirical method of enquiry* maintained solely by the fact of *patients' communications*. It is obvious that in these psychological investigations descriptive efforts are quite different from those in the natural sciences. The object of study is non-existent for the senses and we can experience only a representation of it. Yet the same logical principles are in operation. Description demands the creation of systematic categories, as well as a demonstration of relationships and orderly sequences on the one hand and of sporadic appearances, unheralded and unforeseen, on the other.

them we have discovered many of our basic concepts. If we compare what patients say we find much that is similar. Some individuals are very reliable and also very gifted. On the other hand with hysterical patients and psychopaths (those suffering from personality disorder) there is very little one can trust. Most of their extensive self-description has to be taken very critically. Patients will report on experiences in order to oblige and please. They will say what is expected of them and often if they realise that they have aroused our interest, they will more than rise to the occasion.

The first step, then, is to make some representation of what is really happening in our patients, what they are actually going through, how it strikes them, how they feel. We are not concerned at this stage with connections nor with the patients' experience as a whole and certainly not with any subsidiary speculations, fundamental theory or basic postulates. We confine description solely to the things that are present to the patients' consciousness. Anything which is not a conscious datum is for the present non-existent. Conventional theories, psychological constructions, interpretations and evaluations must be left aside. We simply attend to what exists before us, in so far as we can apprehend, discriminate and describe it. Experience shows us that this is by no means easy to do. We refuse to prejudge when studying our phenomena, and this openmindedness, so characteristic of phenomenology, is not something which one just has, but it has to be acquired painfully through much critical effort and frequent failure. When we were children we drew things not as we saw them but as we imagined them, so, as psychopathologists, we go through a phase in which we have our own notions about the psyche and only gradually emerge into a direct, unprejudiced apprehension of psychic phenomena as they are. Phenomenological orientation is something we have to attain to again and again and involves a continual onslaught on our prejudices.

Close contemplation of *an individual case* often teaches us of phenomena common to countless others. What we have once grasped in this way is usually encountered again. It is not so much the number of cases seen that matters in phenomenology but the extent of the inner exploration of the individual case, which needs to be carried to the furthest possible limit.

In histology, when we examine the cerebral cortex, we expect to account for every fibre and every cell. So in phenomenology we *expect to account for every psychic phenomenon*, every experience met with in our investigation of the patient and in his own self-description. In no circumstances should we rest satisfied with a general impression or a set of details collected ad hoc, but we should know how to appreciate every single particular. If we persevere in this way we shall cease to marvel at the phenomena we see so frequently but which those who are satisfied with general impressions either miss or find extraordinary according to how they feel at the time and how impressionable they are. On the other hand this method draws attention to what is really out of the ordinary and therefore justifies our wonder. There is no danger that wonder will ever be exhausted.

In phenomenology, therefore, the main thing is to train ourselves in a fruitful scrutiny of what the patient's immediate experiences are, so that we come to recognise what is identical in all the manifold manifestations. We need to collect a rich store of observed phenomena in the form of concrete examples and in this way provide ourselves with some measuring-rod and frame of reference when we come to the examination of any new case.[1]

There is value too in the description of unusual and unexpected phenomena and the ability to recognise them for what they are, i.e. fundamental phenomena of conscious existence. Normal phenomena are also often better understood following some study of the abnormal, but there is little point in a purely logical differentiation without concrete examples.

We shall now proceed to deal with (1) *individual phenomena*, isolated for purposes of study, e.g. hallucinations, emotional states, instinctual drives, and (2) a clarification of the properties of *the conscious state*, which in its own way influences the phenomena studied and lends them different meanings according to the different psychic contexts in which they appear.[2]

## SECTION ONE

## ABNORMAL PSYCHIC PHENOMENA

(a) *The dissection of the total relational context of the phenomena*

In all developed psychic life we find the confrontation of a subject with an object and the orientation of a self towards a content as an absolutely basic phenomenon. In this respect *awareness of an object* may be contrasted with *self-awareness*. This first distinction enables us to give an independent description of objective abnormalities (e.g. altered perceptions, hallucinations) and then ask in what ways awareness of the self may have changed. But the state

---

[1] The following are good self-descriptions: Baudelaire, *Paradis artificiels*. Beringer and Mayer-Gross, *Z. Neur.*, vol. 96 (1925), p. 209. J. J. David, 'Halluzinationen', *Die neue Rundschau*, vol. 17. p. 874. Engelken, *Allg. Z. Psychiatr.*, vol. 6, p. 586. Fehrlin, *Die Schizophrenie* (Selbstverlag, 1910) Fr. Fischer, *Z. Neur.*, vol. 121, p. 544; vol. 124, p. 241. Forel, *Allg. Z. Psychiatr.*, vol. 34, p. 960. Fraenkel and Joel, *Z. Neur.*, vol. 111, p. 84. Gruhle, *Z. Neur.*, vol. 28 (1915), p. 148. Ideler, *Der Wahnsinn* (Bremen, 1848), pp. 322 ff., 365 ff. *Religiöser Wahnsinn* (Halle, 1848), vol. 1, p. 392 ff. Jakobi, *Annalen der Irrenanstalt zu Siegburg* (Köln, 1837), p. 256 James, *Die religiöse Erfahrung in ihrer Mannigfaltigkeit* (Leipzig, 1907). Janet, *Les obsessions et la psychasthenie.* Jaspers, *Z. Neur.*, vol. 14, pp. 158 ff. Kandinsky, *Arch. Psychiatr.* (D), vol. 11, p. 453. *Kritische u. klinische Betrachtungen im Gebiet der Sinnestäuschungen* (Berlin, 1885). Kieser, *Allg. Z. Psychiatr.*, vol. 10, p. 423. Klinke, *J. Psychiatr.*, vol. 9. Kronfeld, *Mschr. Psychiatr.*, vol. 35 (1914), p. 275. Mayer-Gross, *Z. Neur.*, vol. 62, p. 222. Mayer-Gross and Steiner, *Z. Neur.*, vol. 73, p. 283. Meinert, *Alkoholwahnsinn* (Dresden, 1907). Nerval, *Aurelia* (München, 1910). Quincey, *Bekenntnisse eines Opiumessers* (Stuttgart, 1886). Rychlinski, *Arch. Psychiatr.* (D), vol. 28, p. 625. Gerhard Schmidt, *Z. Neur.*, vol. 141, p. 570. Kurt Schneider, 'Pathopsychologie im Grundriss', *Handwörterbuch der psychischen Hygiene* (Berlin, 1931). Schreber, *Denkwürdigkeiten eines Nervenkranken* (Leipzig, 1903). Schwab, *Z. Neur.*, vol. 44. Serko, *J. Psychiatr.*, vol. 34 (1913), p. 355. *Z. Neur.*, vol. 44, p. 21. Staudenmaier, *Die Magie als experimentelle Naturwissenschaft* (Leipzig, 1912). Wollny, *Erklärungen der Tollheit von Haslam* (Leipzig, 1889).

[2] Regular annual reports on phenomenological research appear in *Fortschritte der Neurologie, Psychiatrie u. ihrer Grenzgebiete* (Leipzig, 1929 ff.). Initial reports by Kurt Schneider; since 1934 by K. F. Scheid; since 1939 by Weitbrecht.

of self-awareness and the objective aspects of that 'other', to which the self directs itself, interlock in a mutual movement whereby the 'self' is caught up by what is given externally and is at the same time driven internally to grasp at what is there. Description of what is objective leads on to the meaning of this for the self and a description of the states of the self (emotional states, moods, drives) turns into a description of the objective aspects under which these states become apparent.

Subjective orientation towards an object is certainly a constant and basic factor in all meaningful psychic life but we cannot achieve differentiation of the phenomena by this alone. Immediate experience is always *within a total relational context* which we have to dissect if the phenomena are to be described.

This total relational context is founded in the way we *experience space and time*, in the mode of *body-awareness* and the *awareness of reality*; it is moreover self-divided through the opposition of *feeling-states* and *drives*, and these create further self-divisions in their turn.

The division of phenomena into *direct* and *indirect* cuts across all these other divisions. Every phenomenon has the character of direct experience but for analytical and purposive thought it is essential for the psyche to stand outside this immediate experience. The basic phenomenon that renders such thinking and purpose possible may be called *reflection*, the turning-back of experience on itself and on its content. Hence indirect phenomena come into being and indeed all human psychic life shows the pervasiveness of this reflective activity. Conscious psychic life is not just an agglomeration of separable and isolated phenomena, but presents a total relational context which is in constant flux and from it we isolate our particular data in the very act of describing them. This total relational context changes with the *conscious state* in which the psyche may be at the time. All differentiations that we make are transient and must grow obsolete at some point, if we do not discard them altogether.

According to this broad principle of a total relational context it follows that (1) phenomena can only be partially *delimited and defined*, simply to the extent that they can again be identified. Isolation of phenomena makes them clearer and sharper than they really are. However, we have to accept this limitation if we are to aim at any fruitful points of view, precise observation or accurate presentation of the facts. (2) Phenomena can *reappear* in our descriptions *repeatedly* according to the particular aspect stressed (e.g. qualitative phenomena of perception may appear in respect of object-awareness or in respect of feelings).

*(b) Form and content of phenomena*

The following points are of general application for all the phenomena to be described: Form must be kept distinct from content which may change from time to time, e.g. the fact of a hallucination is to be distinguished from its content, whether this is a man or a tree, threatening figures or peaceful landscapes. Perceptions, ideas, judgments, feelings, drives, self-awareness, are all forms of psychic phenomena; they denote the particular mode of existence in which content is presented to us. It is true in describing concrete psychic events we take into account the particular contents of the individual psyche, but from the phenomenological point of view it is only the form that interests us. According to whether we have the content or the form of the phenomenon in mind, we can disregard for the time being the one or the other—the phenomenological investigation or the examination of content. For patients content is usually the one important thing. Often they are quite unaware of the manner in which they experience it and they muddle up hallucinations, pseudo-hallucinations, delusional awarenesses, etc., because they have never had to differentiate what seems to them so unimportant a matter.

Content, however, modifies the mode in which the phenomena are experienced; it gives them their weight in relation to the total psychic life and points to the way in which they are conceived and interpreted.

*Excursus into form and content.* All knowledge involves a distinction between form and content, and throughout psychopathology from the simplest of psychic events right up to the most complex wholes this distinction is in constant use. For example:

1. In all psychic experience there is a *subject* and *object*. This objective element conceived in its widest sense we call psychic content and the mode in which the subject is presented with the object (be it as a perception, a mental image or thought) we call the form. Thus, hypochondriacal contents, whether provided by voices, compulsive ideas, overvalued ideas or delusional ideas, remain identifiable as content. In the same way we can talk of the content of anxiety and other such emotional states.

2. *The form of the psychoses* is contrasted with their *particular content*: e.g. periodic phases of dysphoria are to be contrasted as a form of illness with the particular type of behaviour that furnishes the content (e.g. dipsomania, wandering, suicide).

3. Certain very *general psychic changes*, which can only carry a psychological interpretation, may also be formally conceived, e.g. the schizophrenic or hysteric experience. Every variety of human drive and desire, every variety of thought and phantasy, can appear as content in such forms and find a mode of realisation (schizophrenic, for instance, or hysteric) in them.

Phenomenology finds its major interest in form; content seems to have a more accidental character, but the psychologist who looks for meaning will find content essential and the form at times unimportant.

## (c) *Transitions between phenomena*

Many patients seem mentally able to view the same content in quick succession in a number of widely varied phenomenological forms. Thus in an acute psychosis the same jealous content may come up in the most diverse shapes (as an emotional state, a hallucination or as a delusion). We might well talk of 'transition' between these several different forms but this would be a mistake. 'Transition' as a general term is simply a cloak for insufficient analysis. The truth is that the fabric of the individual momentary experience is woven from a number of phenomena which we can separately discern by description. For instance, a hallucinatory experience is pervaded by delusional conviction; the perceptual elements gradually disappear, and in a given case we can often be no longer sure whether they ever existed or, if so, in what form. There are, therefore, clear differences between phenomena, real phenomenological gulfs (as for instance between physical and imaginary events) which remain in contrast to phenomenological transitions (from awarenesses, for example, to hallucinations). Psychopathology should reach a clear understanding of these differences and should deepen, extend and classify them since only this will help us in the analysis of our cases.

## (d) Classification of groups of phenomena

The following paragraphs give a description *seriatim* of abnormal phenomena. We proceed from concrete experiences to the experience of space and time, then to body-awareness, to the awareness of reality and to delusion. Next we deal with emotional states, drives and will and so on to the awareness of self. Finally we present the phenomena of self-reflection. The paragraphs are determined by the distinctness and singularity of the relative phenomena. They are not arranged according to any preconceived scheme, since at present it is not possible to classify our phenomenological data in any satisfactory manner. Phenomenology, though one of the foundation-stones of psychopathology, is still very crude. Our present effort at description does not hide this fact, but we have to classify somehow, even if tentatively. This is best done by a classification which gives some plastic impression of what the facts will naturally yield. The inevitable discrepancies will at the same time stimulate us to try and grasp the full significance of the phenomena, not on the basis of some purely theoretical order but by trying to master them repeatedly from more comprehensive and profounder points of view.

## § 1. AWARENESS OF OBJECTS

*Psychological preface.* We give the name 'object' in its widest sense to anything which confronts us; anything which we look at, apprehend, think about or recognise with our inner eye or with our sense-organs. In short anything to which we give our inner attention, whether it be real or unreal, concrete or abstract, dim or distinct. Objects exist for us in the form of *perceptions* or *ideas*. As perceptions the objects stand *bodily* before us (as 'tangibly present', 'vividly felt' and 'apperceived' or 'with a quality of objectivity'). As ideas they stand before us imaginatively (as 'not actually there', 'with a quality of subjectivity'). In any of our perceptions or ideas we can discern three elements: the *qualitative aspect of sensation* (red, blue, pitch of sound, etc.), the *spatial and temporal arrangement* and the *purposeful act of perception* (apperception and objectification). The purely sensory factors are, so to speak, brought to life by the purposeful act and only gain objective meaning through it. We can term this act 'thought' or 'awareness of meaning'. There is the further phenomenological fact that these purposeful acts need not always be founded in sense-data. For instance, we can be abstractly aware of something, there can be a mere knowing of it (e.g. in rapid reading). We are clearly aware of the meaning of the words without actually conjuring up the precise image of what is alluded to. This abstract representation of content is termed *an awareness*. Depending on the type of perception this awareness may be *physical*, e.g. awareness of 'someone's presence' without actually seeing him and with no mental image of him (colloquially a 'feeling that someone is there'), or it may be a purely *ideational* awareness, which is by far the most common.

The following are certain first-hand accounts of how objects may be experienced in an abnormal way:

(*a*) *Anomalies of perception*

(1) *Changes in intensity.* Sounds are heard louder, colours seem brighter, a red roof is like a flame, a closing door thunders like a cannonade, crackling in the bushes sounds like a shot, wind like a storm (in deliria, in the initial stages of narcosis, in poisoning, before epileptic seizures, in acute psychoses).

A patient who had suffered for some years from a non-penetrating shot-wound in the head wrote: 'Since my head-injury I feel from time to time that my hearing has become extraordinarily sharp. This is so at intervals of 4–8 weeks, not in the day but at night when I am in bed. The change is sudden and surprising. Noises which, when I am normal, are almost inaudible strike me with a shattering intensity and are un-cannily clear and loud. I am forced to try and lie perfectly still as even the slight crackling of sheets and pillows causes me a lot of discomfort. The watch on the bed-side-table seems to have become a church clock; the noise of passing cars and trains to which I am accustomed and which normally never bothers me now roars over me like an avalanche. I lie drenched in sweat and instinctively assume a rigid posture until I suddenly find normal conditions have returned. It lasts about 5 minutes but it seems absolutely interminable' (Kurt Schneider).

On the other hand a diminution of intensity may also occur. The environment seems dimmed, taste is flat or everything tastes almost the same (melancholia). A schizophrenic gave the following description:

'The sunshine pales when I face it directly and talk loudly. I can then look quietly into the sun and am only dazzled moderately. On the days when I am well looking into the sun for several minutes would be quite impossible for me as it must be for anyone else' (Schreber).

Absence or reduction of pain (analgesia and hypalgesia) may occur in local or generalised form. The local kind is usually neurological in origin, sometimes psychogenic (Hysteria). The generalised form occurs as a hysterical or hypnotic phenomenon or as the result of strong affect (soldiers in battle). It also occurs as the sign of a particular constitution (hypalgesia only). Hyperalgesia shows the same diversity of conditions.

(2) *Shifts in quality.* While one is reading, the white paper suddenly appears red and the letters green. The faces of others take on a peculiar brown tint, people look like Chinese or Red Indians.

Serko observed himself in the early stages of mescalin intoxication and noted that everything he perceived took on an infinite richness of colouring so that he was actually *intoxicated with colours*: 'The most inconspicuous objects outside one's normal attention suddenly lit up in a host of brilliant colours difficult to describe. Objects like cigarette-ends, and half-burned matches on the ash-trays, coloured glass on a distant rubbish heap, ink-blots on the desk, monotonous rows of books, etc. In particular, certain indirectly viewed objects attracted my attention almost irresistibly through their vivid colouring—even the fine shadows on the ceiling and on the walls and the dim shadows which the furniture cast on the floor had a rare and delicate colour which gave the room a fairy-tale magic.'

(3) *Abnormal concomitant perceptions*. A schizophrenic gives the following description:

'With every word spoken to me or near me, with every slight noise, I feel a blow on my head, producing a certain pain. The pain-sensation feels like an intermittent pulling in my head, probably linked with a rending of part of the skull-bone' (Schreber).

In such cases, which are fairly common in schizophrenia but which may also appear quite independently of it, we are dealing with genuine concomitant perceptions and not with the well-known association of sound and colour images. (Audition colorée, synopsia.)[1]

## (b) Abnormal characteristics of perception

Perception has a number of characteristics, it may seem familiar or strange, or have an emotional quality or seem imbued with a certain atmosphere. The following appear to be abnormal characteristics:

### (1) Alienation from the perceptual world[2]—Derealisation

'Everything appears as through a veil; as if I heard everything through a wall' . . . 'The voices of people seem to come from far away. Things do not look as before, they are somehow altered, they seem strange, two-dimensional. My own voice sounds strange. Everything seems extraordinarily new as if I had not seen it for a long time' . . . 'I feel as if I had a fur over me . . . I touch myself to convince myself that I exist.'

These are complaints of patients who have this disturbance in a relatively mild form. Such patients are never tired of describing how strangely their perceptions have altered. Their experience is so odd, peculiar, eerie. Description always proceeds by metaphor as it is impossible to express the experiences directly. Patients do not think that the world has really changed but only feel as if everything were different to them. We should always remember that in

---

[1] On the theory of synaethesia cp. Bleuler, *Z. Psychol.*, vol. 65 (1913), p. 1. Wehofer, *Z. angew. Psychol.*, vol. 7 (1913), p. 1. Hennig, *Z. Psychother.*, vol. 4 (1912), p. 22. Georg Anschuetz, *Das Farbe-Ton-Problem in psychischen Gesamtbereich* (Halle, 1929). (*Deutsche Psychologie*, Bd. V, vol. 5) (careful investigation of a rare and interesting case).

[2] Oesterreich, *J. Psychiatr.*, vol. 8. Janet, *Les Obsessions et la psychasthenie*, 2nd edn. (Paris, 1908).

reality they can see, hear and feel sharply and distinctly. We are dealing, there-fore, with a disturbance in the actual process of perception, not in its material elements nor in the apprehension of meaning nor in judgment. Thus in every normal perception there must be yet another factor which would elude us had these patients not presented us with these peculiar complaints. Where there is a severer degree of disturbance the descriptions become more noteworthy:

'All objects appear so new and startling I say their names over to myself and touch them several times to convince myself they are real. I stamp on the floor and still have a feeling of unreality' . . . Patients will feel lost and think they cannot find their way about though they can do this as well as ever. In really unknown surroundings this feeling of strangeness will increase. 'I held on to my friend's arm in panic; I felt I was lost if he left me for one moment'—'All objects seemed to retreat into infinity.' (This is not to be confused with physical illusions of distance.) 'One's own voice seems to die away into infinity.' Patients often think they can no longer be heard any more; they feel as if they have floated away from reality, away into outer space in a frightening isolation—'Everything is like a dream. Space is infinite, time no longer exists; the moment endures for ever, infinite expanses of time roll by'—'I am en-tombed, totally isolated, no human is by me. I only see black; even when the sun is shining, it is still all black'. Yet we find such patients see everything and have no disturbance in the sensory part of their perception.

With these more severe grades of disturbance (if we explore the patients carefully) actual judgment does not seem disturbed at first but the feelings are so forceful that they cannot entirely be suppressed. Patients have to handle things to make sure they are really still there, have to convince themselves of the existence of the ground by stamping on it. In the end, however, the psychic disturbance becomes so serious that we can no longer speak of patients having any judgment at all. Other severe disturbances usually appear as well. Terrified and restless, the patients begin to experience their feelings as the reality itself and are then inaccessible to reason. Now the world has escaped them. Nothing remains. They are alone in terrible isolation, suspended between infinities. They have to live for ever because time no longer exists. They themselves no longer exist; their body is dead. Only this fake-existence remains as their horrible fate.

(2) Just as the perceptual world may be experienced as something strange or dead, so it can be experienced as something *entirely fresh* and of *overpowering beauty*:

'Everything looked different—I saw in everything the touch of a divine magni-ficence'—'It was as if I had come into a new world, a new existence. Every object wore a bright halo, my inner vision was so enhanced I saw the beauty of the universe in everything. The woods rang with celestial music.' (James.)

(3) These descriptions have shown that objects are not only perceived in a purely sensory manner but are accompanied by an emotional atmosphere. *Empathy into other people* is an important instance of this, in that we no longer have pure sense-perception but the latter has now become an occasion for psychic understanding. The pathological phenomena consist either in a *failure*

*of empathy*—other people seem dead, patients feel they only see the outside and are no longer conscious of the psychic life of others, or in an *unpleasantly forceful empathy*—the psychic life of others impinges with a fierce vividness on the defenceless victim, or finally in a *fantastically mistaken empathy*—where this is entirely unwarranted:

A patient with encephalitis lethargica reported: 'During that time I had an incredibly fine feeling for imponderables, atmospheres etc. For instance I would feel immediately the minutest misunderstanding among two of my student friends'. The patient also reported that he did not really share in these feelings, he only registered them. 'It was not a natural participation' (Mayer-Gross and Steiner).

Increased empathy into highly differentiated psychic states is found among other signs at the beginning of process-disorders. A patient many years before the onset of an acute psychosis experienced an increased sharpening of his feeling-sensitivity, which he himself regarded as abnormal. Works of art appeared to him profound, rich, impressive, like ravishing music. People appeared much more complex than before and he felt that he had a much more intricate understanding of women. Reading gave him sleepless nights.

There is one particular mode of misunderstanding the psychic life of others which may be found in the initial stages of process-disorders. Other people appear so curious and baffling to the patient that he considers these healthy people as mentally ill rather than himself (Wernicke—Transitivismus).

## (c) *Splitting of perception*

This term covers phenomena described by schizophrenic patients and patients in toxic states:

'A bird chirrups in the garden. I hear it and know that it is chirruping but that it is a bird and that it is chirruping are two things which are poles apart. There is a gulf between them and I am afraid I shall not be able to bring them together. It is as if the bird and the chirruping have nothing at all to do with each other' (Fr. Fischer).

In mescalin intoxication: 'When I opened my eyes I looked towards the window without actually appreciating it as a window and I saw a number of colours or green and light blue blotches; I knew they were the leaves of a tree and the sky which could be seen through them, but it was impossible to relate these perceptions of different things with any definite location in space.' (Mayer-Gross and Steiner).

## (d) *False perceptions*

We have now described all abnormal perceptions in which no fresh set of unreal objects is perceived, but only a set of real objects which somehow appear to be different. Now we turn to false perceptions as such, in which fresh, unreal objects seem to be perceived.[1] Since the time of Esquirol a discrimination has been made between illusions and hallucinations. *Illusion* is the term for perceptions which in fact are transpositions (or distortions) of real per-

[1] Johannes Müller, *Über die phantastischen Gesichtserscheinungen* (Koblenz, 1826). Hagen, *Allg. Z. Psychiatr.*, vol. 25, p. 1. Kahlbaum, *Allg. Z. Psychiatr.*, vol. 23. Kandinsky, *Kritische u. klinische Betrachtungen im Gebiete der Sinnestäuschungen* (Berlin, 1885). I myself have written a detailed account of false perception in *Z. Neur.* (Referaten-teil), vol. 4 (1911), p. 289. See my further work

ceptions; here external sensory stimuli unite with certain transposing (or distorting) elements so that in the end we cannot differentiate the one from the other. *Hallucinations* are perceptions that spring into being in a primary way and are not transpositions or distortions, of any genuine perception.

(*aa*) There are three types of illusions (*illusions due to inattentiveness, illusions due to affect* and *pareidolia*):

1. *Illusions due to inattentiveness.* Experimental investigation into perception shows that almost every perception collects some elements of reproduction that tend to transpose or distort it. When attention is scanty and therefore external sensory stimuli are meagre, the latter are nearly always filled out in some way or other. For instance, in listening to a lecture we constantly piece out the meaning and only notice we are doing this when occasionally we make a mistake. We overlook misprints in a book and complete the meaning correctly according to the context. Illusions of this sort can be corrected immediately once our attention is drawn to them. Errors in identification and inexact, faulty perceptions that arise in General Paralysis and deliria, etc., belong to some extent to this category. Illusions of this sort (failure to identify) play a part in these patients' mistakes in reading and hearing and in the way they recast their visual impressions.

2. *Illusions due to affect.* When walking alone in the woods at night we may become frightened and mistake a tree-trunk or a rock for a human figure. A melancholic patient beset by fears of being killed may take the clothes hanging on the wall for a corpse, or some trivial noise may strike him as the clang of prison chains. Illusions of this sort are mostly rather fleeting and always comprehensible in terms of the affect prevailing at the time.

3. *Pareidolia.* Imagination can create illusionary forms from ill-defined sense-impressions, such as clouds, old patchy walls, etc. No particular affect is involved nor any reality-judgment, but the imaginary creation need not disappear when attention is directed upon it. Johann Mueller gives us the following description:

'As a child I was often teased by this vivid gift of imagination. I remember one fantasy particularly. From the living-room I could see a house opposite, old and shabby with blackened plaster and patches of various shape through which the colours of older plaster could be seen. As I looked through the window at this dark, dilapidated wall I made out a number of faces in the contours of the peeling plaster. As time went on they became more and more expressive. When I tried to draw other people's attention to these faces in the dilapidated plaster no one would agree with me. All the same I saw them distinctly. In later years I could still remember them clearly though I could not recreate them again in the contours which had given them birth.'

Similar illusions can be observed in patients. They appear to the onlooker as something alien; only the patients observe them and see them constantly

'Zur Analyse der Trugwahrnehmungen', *Z. Neur.*, vol. 6, p. 460. More recent works are W. Mayer-Gross and Johannes Stein, 'Pathologie der Wahrnehmung' in Bumke's *Handbuch der Geisteskrankheiten* (Berlin, 1928), vol. 1.

coming and going, whereas with the other two types of illusion they either vanish when attention is drawn to them or when the affect from which they sprang undergoes a change.

A patient in the clinic at Heidelberg, while fully collected, saw animal and human heads 'as if embroidered' on the counterpane and on the wall. She also saw grimacing faces in the spots of sunlight on the wall. She knew they were deceptions and said: 'My eye evokes faces in the unevenness of the wall'. Another patient reported with surprise: 'Things shape themselves; the round holes in the window-frames [the fastenings] become heads and seem to be biting at me'.

Another patient described the following illusions while he was out hunting: 'On all the trees and bushes I saw, instead of the usual crows, dim outlines of panto-mime figures, pot-bellied fellows with thin bow-legs and long thick noses, or at another time elephants with long trunks swinging. The ground seemed to swarm with lizards, frogs and toads; sometimes of portentous size. All kinds of animal forms and evil shapes seemed to surround me. Trees and bushes took on wild, provoking shapes. At other times a girl's figure rode on every bush, and on the trees and reeds. Girls' faces smiled from the clouds, enticing me and when the wind moved the branches, they waved at me. The rustle of the wind was their whispering' (Staud-maier).

Illusions which are a matter of sensory experience must be clearly differ-entiated from *misinterpretations*, or wrong deductions. If shining metal is mistaken for gold or a doctor for a public prosecutor, this does not imply any alteration in the actual sense-perception. The perceived object remains exactly the same but a wrong interpretation has been put upon it. Illusions must also be differentiated from the so-called *functional hallucinations*; a patient, for instance, hears voices while the water is running but they stop when the tap is turned off. He hears the running water and the voices simultaneously. While illusions contain an element of genuine perception with functional hallucina-tion we have simultaneous hallucinations running alongside with a constant element of genuine sense-perception and disappearing at the same time as the sense-perception.

(*bb*) *Hallucinations proper* are actual false perceptions which are not in any way distortions of real perceptions but spring up on their own as something quite new and occur simultaneously with and alongside real perceptions. This latter characteristic makes them a different phenomenon from dream-hallucination. There are a number of normal phenomena *comparable* to halluci-nations proper. For instance, the after-images which arise in the retina, the rarer phenomenon of *sense-memory* (the subsequent, deceptive yet real hearing of words already heard, and the seeing of microscopic objects at the end of a heavy day of microscope work, all phenomena particularly common when one is tired). Lastly there are the *fantastic visual phenomena* classically described by Johannes Mueller and the now well-known phenomenon, *the subjective eidetic image*.

An example of *sense-memory* has been given me personally by Geheimrat

Tuzcek of Marburg: 'I had been gathering apples for the greater part of the day without a break. I had been standing on a ladder to work the apple-picker and had been gazing continuously up into the branches as I pulled away at the long stick of the 'picker'. As I walked back through the dark streets to the station, I was painfully hindered by the fact that I kept on seeing apple-hung branches before my eyes. The image was so powerful that I could not stop myself from waving my stick in front of me as I walked. The state persisted for several hours until at last I went to bed and fell asleep.'

The following is an extract from the self-observations made by Johannes Mueller on *fantastic visual phenomena*:

'I would shorten my sleepless nights by wandering as it were among my own visual creations. If I want to watch these bright images, I relax my eye-muscles, close my eyes and look into the darkness of the visual field. With a feeling of complete relaxation in my eye-muscles I let myself down into the sensuous stillness of my eyes or into the darkness of the visual field. I ward off any thought or judgment . . . at first the dark field shows patches of light here and there, hazy clouds, shifting and moving colours; these are soon replaced by well defined pictures of all sorts of objects, at first dim, then increasingly clear. There is no doubt that they are really luminous and sometimes coloured as well. They move and change. Sometimes they arise at the margin of the visual field with a vividness and distinctness which ordinarily never occurs in that area. With the slightest movement of the eye they are usually gone. Reflection too will chase them away. They rarely represent known figures; usually they are strange people and animals I have never seen, or an illuminated room in which I have never been . . . I can conjure up these visions not only at night but at any time during the day. At night I have spent many sleepless hours watching them with my eyes closed. I have only to sit down, shut my eyes, abstract myself from everything and watch the automatic arrival of these images which I have known and loved from my childhood . . . Bright pictures frequently appear in the dark visual field but equally often the dark field brightens into a kind of mild, inner daylight before the actual picture appears, which it then does immediately. The gradual brightening of the visual field seems to me as remarkable as the actual appearance of the luminous images. It is astonishing to sit as a spectator, in the daytime, with eyes closed and see the 'daylight' entering gradually from inside and in the daylight of one's eyes to witness luminous moving figures, produced apparently by the private life of the senses, and all this happening in a waking state, a state of quiet reflection, with nothing magical about it nor any sentimental fancy. I can determine with the greatest precision the exact moment when the images will become luminous. I sit with my eyes closed for a long time. If I try to imagine anything deliberately it remains a mere idea, which does not shine or move within the dark visual field; but suddenly there is a congruence between the fantasy and the light-nerve, suddenly there appear luminous forms, quite apart from the train of ideas. These are sudden apparitions not forms imagined in the first place and then growing luminous. I do not see what I make up my mind to see. I simply have to accept what lights up in front of me without any effort on my part. The short-sighted objection that these are the same as luminous dream-images or 'merely fancied' can certainly be discarded. I can weave fancies for hours but what I imagine never becomes living and vivid in this way. There must be a disposition to experience these luminous phenomena. Something bright suddenly appears which has not previously been imagined, is unwilled and has no recognisable associations. This phenomenon which I see in my waking state shines as brightly as the flashes which we can create in the visual field by pressing on the eyeballs'.

*Subjective eidetic images* are sensory phenomena found in 50 per cent of all adolescents and among a certain number of adults (the so-called eidetics). If pictures of flowers, fruit or other objects are laid on grey paper and then removed, these people will see the objects again in full detail on the paper, sometimes in front or behind the plane of the paper. Such images are distinct from after-images since they are not complementary. They can also shift and change and they are not exact copies but modifiable by reflection. They can be recalled even after some considerable time. According to Jaensch, before an examination an eidetic person could read out extensive texts from such a visual image alone.[1]

(*cc*) A certain class of phenomena were for a long time confused with hallucinations. Looked at closely these proved to be not really perceptions but a special kind of imagery. *Kandinsky* has described these phenomena very fully under the title of *Pseudo-hallucinations*. The following is an example:

'During the evening of August 18th, 1882, Dolinin took 25 drops of tincture opii simplicis and went on working at his desk. One hour later he observed great facilitation in the way his imagination worked. He stopped what he was doing and still conscious and with no inclination for sleep he noticed in the course of one hour while his eyes were closed a number of faces and figures seen during the day, faces of old friends not seen for a long time and faces of unknown people. Now and then there appeared white pages with different kinds of writing; then repeatedly a yellow rose and finally—pictures of people in various costumes standing in all sorts of positions but quite motionless. These pictures appeared for a moment then vanished. They were followed at once by a fresh set, not logically connected. They were projected outward distinctly and seemed to stand there in front of his eyes. They were in *no relation whatever with the dark visual field* of his closed eyes. It was necessary to divert his gaze away from this field if he was to see the pictures. Fixing on the visual field interrupted the visual phenomena. In spite of many attempts he failed to make the subjective picture part of the dark background. In spite of the sharp outlines and vivid colours and the fact that the pictures seemed to stand out in front of the subject's gaze they *lacked the character of objectivity*. Dolinin felt that though he saw these things with his eyes, they were not his outward, physical eyes, which only saw a black visual field flecked with patches of foggy light; they were "*inner eyes*" located somewhere behind the outer ones. The distance of the pictures from these "inner eyes" varied from 0·4–6·0 metres. Usually it was that of clearest vision which in his case was very small, because of his short-sightedness . . . The human figures varied in size from normal to that of a photograph. Optimal conditions for the pictures to appear were as follows: "An attempt must be made to make the mind blank as far as possible and direct one's attention idly to the sense-activity concerned [in Dolinin's

[1] Urbantschitsch, *Über subjektive optische Anschauungsbilder* (Vienna, 1907). Silberer, 'Bericht über eine Methode gewisse symbolische Halluzinationserscheinungen hervorzurufen', *Jb. Psychoanal.*, vol. 1 (1909), p. 513. E. R. Jaensch, *Über den Aufbau der Wahrnehmungswelt u. ihre Struktur im Jugendalter.*

case, the visual sense]. Where the spontaneous pseudo-hallucination is actively appreciated, it is possible to retain this for a little in the focus of awareness and longer than one could do without such active effort. Direction of attention to another sense-activity (for instance from vision to hearing) whether in part or wholly will interrupt the pseudo-hallucination that first appeared. Interruption also will take place when attention is focused on the black visual field of the closed eyes or on real objects in the environment when the eyes are open; also when there is any onset of spontaneous or deliberate abstract thinking." ' (Kandinsky).

The first thing one notices about this description is that the phenomena in question are seen by an 'inner eye'; they are not within the black visual field, like the previous fantastic visual phenomena nor do they possess the reality of perception (the character of objectivity—Kandinsky). If we are to get our orientation among these many phenomena of our imagination, of which Dolinin furnishes only one example, it would be as well to arrange the varying characteristics in some order whereby normal perception and normal imagery can be phenomenologically distinguished. Thus:

| Sense-perception (Wahrnehmung) | Image or Idea (Vorstellung) |
|---|---|
| 1. Perceptions are of concrete reality. They have a character of objectivity. | Images are figurative. They have a character of subjectivity. |
| 2. Perceptions appear in external objective space. | Images appear in inner subjective space. |
| 3. Perceptions are clearly delineated and stand before us in a detailed fashion. | Images are not clearly delineated, and come before us incomplete, only individual details evident. |
| 4. The sensory elements are full, fresh. Colours, for instance, are bright. | Though occasionally sensory elements are individually the equal of those in perception, most are relatively insufficient. The majority of people's visual images are neutral-toned. |
| 5. Perceptions are constant and can easily be retained unaltered. | Images dissipate and have always to be recreated. |
| 6. Perceptions are independent of our will. They cannot be voluntarily recalled or changed, and are accepted with a feeling of passivity. | Images are dependent on our will. They can be conjured up or deliberately altered. They are produced with a feeling of activity. |

With regard to point 2, we must add that objective space and subjective space can appear to coincide, for instance, when I form the visual image of something behind me. I can also imagine something standing between certain objects in front of me but I do not see it there (in that case it would be a hallucination). Both spaces only seem to coincide; there is always a jump from the one to the other and they are widely separated in fact.

From the above table we may now be able to derive the specific characteristics of pseudo-hallucinations. The only absolute difference from sense-perception appears in points 1 and 2 (i.e. pseudo-hallucinations are figurative, not concretely real and occur in inner subjective space, not in external objective space). These two opposing characteristics divide perception sharply from imagery, as by a gulf, and there are no transitions. With the other characteristics, as shown in points 3 and 4, the differences are not so clear-cut. Images which always remain configurations of our inner space may progressively assume certain characteristics ascribed to perceptions. Thus we find an infinite variety of image-phenomena ranging from normal imagery to fully developed pseudo-hallucinations. We may now characterise these as follows: pseudo-hallucinations lack concrete reality and appear in inner subjective space. To the 'inner eye' however they seem to have definite contours and are fully detailed (point 3); in their sensory elements they have all the sufficiency of normal perception (point 4). We may be fully conscious and find ourselves suddenly confronted with them, sharply articulated and with a wealth of vivid detail. They do not dissipate at once but may be retained as constant phenomena until they abruptly take their departure (point 5). Lastly, they cannot be deliberately altered or evoked. The subject is receptive and passive (point 6) in regard to them.

Such fully developed phenomena are, however, by no means the most common. The phenomena are generally rather more imprecise and show only one or two of the above characteristics. We may get pale, vague images which appear involuntarily, or detailed, constant phenomena that have been deliberately invoked. Thus a patient recovering from an acute psychosis could imagine things most vividly for a time. He inwardly visualised a chessboard with all the men on it but he soon lost this capacity. Pseudo-hallucinations have so far been found only in the visual and auditory field in the form of inner pictures and voices.

In describing sense-experience in false perception, we distinguished illusions from hallucinations and similarly we draw a clear distinction between sense-phenomena and the phenomena of imagery (i.e. between hallucination and pseudo-hallucination). This does not prevent us from finding actual 'transitions' in that pseudo-hallucination can *change over* into hallucination and there may be a florid sensory pathology in which all the phenomena *combine*. We cannot reach any analysis, however, unless we attempt sharp distinctions of this sort which provide us with some kind of standard.

Illusions, hallucinations and pseudo-hallucinations are extremely varied and range from elementary phenomena, such as sparks, flames, rushing sounds, bangs and cracks, to the perception of shapes and forms, heard voices, and visions of figures and landscapes. If we review the different sense-fields we will get a certain over-all picture:

*Vision:*[1] Real objects are seen enlarged or diminished or distorted or in motion. Pictures jump about on the walls, the furniture comes to life. Optical hallucinations in alcoholic delirium are myriad and changing, in epilepsy their colouring is vivid (red, blue) and they tend to be overpowering. In acute psychoses hallucinations have

---

[1] For illustrations of visual hallucinations see Serko, *Z. Neur.*, vol. 44, and Morgenthalre, *Z. Neur.*, vol. 45.

been observed that take the form of whole scenic panoramas. Here are some examples:

(*aa*) *In inner subjective space:* A schizophrenic patient, while awake, saw ghastly pictures, she did not know how. They were inner pictures; she knew they were really nothing. But the pictures crowded in on her. She saw a graveyard with half-open graves; figures walking about without heads; the pictures were agonising. By diverting her attention to external objects, she could make them go.

(*bb*) *With open eyes:* Figures appear in the whole visual field, but there is no integration with objective space: 'The figures grouped themselves round me 3–6 metres away. Grotesque human figures, who made some kind of noise like a jumble of voices. The figures were there in space, but as if they had their own private space, peculiar to themselves. The more my senses were diverted from their usual objects, the more distinct grew this new space with its inhabitants. I could give the exact distance but the figures were never dependent on the objects in the room nor were they hidden by them; they could never be perceived simultaneously with the wall or the window etc.'

'I could not accept the objection that I had only imagined these things; I could not find anything in common between these perceptions and my own imagination nor can I do so to this day. I feel the figures of my imagination are not in space but remain faint pictures in my brain or behind my eyes while with these phenomena I experienced a world which had nothing to do with the world of the senses. Everything was "real", the forms were full of life. Later on the ordinary world still contained this other one with its own separate space and my consciousness was gliding between the two as it chose. The two worlds and their perceptions are utterly dissimilar' (Schwab).

Serko described false-perceptions during mescalin intoxication as follows:

'They appear in the one constant, disc-like and microscopic visual field and are greatly diminished in size; they are not integrated with the real surroundings but form a miniature theatre of their own; they do not touch on the immediate content of consciousness and are always subjective . . . they are chiselled to the finest particular, and vividly coloured. They appear in sharp relief and change constantly . . . when my eye moves, they do not change position in space.' The content of these false perceptions is 'in continuous movement' . . . 'Patterns dissolve into bouquets, whirls, domes, Gothic doorways . . . and so on; there is an everlasting coming and going and this restless moving to and fro seems to be their hallmark'.

(*cc*) *With eyes closed.* A schizophrenic counterpart to Johann Mueller's description is as follows:

'With closed eyes I would perceive a diffused, milky-white light out of which appeared exotic forms of plants and animals in relief and often in shining colours. I thought the pale light lay in the eye itself but the shapes were like an experience and seemed to come from another world. The perception of light was not always the same. When my mental state was better the light was brighter but after some trivial social set-back (annoyance, excitement) or some physical discomfort (e.g. after overeating) it would get darker and sometimes it was pitch-black night. Light appeared about 1–2 minutes after my eyes were shut. When I travelled by train through a tunnel and shut my eyes it would become bright and I thought wrongly that the train was in the open again but when I opened my eyes suddenly there was nothing but the pitch black of the tunnel. The light vanished not only because I opened my eyes but because I tried to look and see. As soon as I stopped looking fixedly I could see the light with my eyes open even during the day, but less clear. The shapes did not appear every time. The plants were beyond imagination; I was astounded by their loveliness and grace; there was something magnificent about them as if the plants I ordinarily know were only their degenerate descendants. The animals were pre-historic; they had something benign about them. Occasionally some one part became extremely prominent, but I was surprised how harmoniously the rest of the form was adapted to these peculiarities so that a certain type emerged. There was no movement among them, they seemed three-dimensional and after a few minutes disappeared' (Schwab).

(*dd*) *Integration with outer objective space:* Kandinsky described his own psychotic experiences thus: 'Some of my hallucinations were relatively pale and indistinct. Others were bright with all sorts of colours, like real objects. They obscured real objects. For a whole week I saw on one and the same wall, which was covered with a smooth, plain wallpaper, a series of gilt-framed frescoes, landscapes, seascapes, and sometimes portraits.'

Uhthoff[1] described the following:

'The patient suffered from an old chorioiditis. Central positive scotoma. Had it for 20 years without particular symptoms; one day, a dull feeling in the head and tiredness. The patient looked out of the window and suddenly noticed a "vine" moving and growing in size on the pavement of the courtyard. The appearance of leaves persisted for six days and then it became a tree with buds. Walking along the street she saw the tree as in a fog between the real bushes. On closer observation real leaves could be distinguished from the fictitious ones; the latter were 'as if painted'— the colour was bluer and greyer "as if shaded"; the "fantasy leaves" were as if "pasted on" while the natural ones "stand out from the wall". After a time the patient also saw "exquisite flowers, of every possible colour, little stars, sprays, bouquets". On closer scrutiny this intelligent patient gave the following description: "The leaves, bushes, etc., seemed localised in the positive, central visual field defect and the size changed with distance. At 10 cm. the phenomena had a diameter of 2 cm." If projected on to a house across the street they were so big as to cover the whole window. When the eyes were moved, the phenomena moved too. This was the criterion by which the patient realised that they were not real objects. When the eyes were closed, the phenomena disappeared and gave way to patterns (golden star on a black background—and round it often a concentric blue and red ring). The hallucinatory objects hid the background and were opaque.'

A patient suffering from a schizophrenic process gave the following description:

'Once I was visited for a few days by a pretty young woman. A few days later I was lying in bed at night and turning over on to the other side I saw to my great surprise on the right beside me the girl's head protruding from the bedclothes as if she was lying by me. It looked magical, beautiful, ethereally transparent and softly gleaming in the dark room. I was completely dumbfounded for a moment but the next moment I knew what I was dealing with, all the more as at the same time a rough, unkind voice whispered sarcastically inside me. I turned crossly on to the left side and swore without paying any more attention to the phantom. Later a friendly inner voice said—The girl has gone' (Staudenmaier).

[1] Uhthoff, 'Beiträge zu den Gesichtstaeuschungen bei Erkrankungen des Sehorgans', *Mschr. Psychiatr.*, vol. 5, pp. 241, 370.

A schizophrenic girl reported:

'At first I was very busy catching the "Holy Ghost" with my eyes; by this I mean those little white transparent flecks which jump in the air or out of the eyes of those around me and look like dead, cold light. I also saw people's skins emitting fine black and yellow rays; the air too became pervaded with other strange rays and layers . . . All day I have been afraid of wild animals which race through the closed doors; they steal, slow and black, along the wall to hide under the couch and watch me from there, with bright eyes. I have been frightened by headless men who walk about the passages and by soul-less bodies of murdered people that lie in the middle of the parquet floor; when I look at them they vanish at once; I "catch them away" with my eyes' (Gruhle).

*Hearing:* In acute psychoses patients hear tunes, confused noises, whistling and the rattling of machines, a racket which appears to them louder than guns. Here as in the chronic states we often find 'voices' as well, the 'invisible' people who shout all kinds of things at the patient, ask him questions and abuse him or order him about. As to content, this may consist of single words or whole sentences; there may be a single voice or a whole jumble of voices; it may be an orderly conversation between the voices themselves or between them and the patient. They may be women's, children's or men's voices, the voices of acquaintances or unknown people, or quite indefinable human voices. Curses may be uttered, actions of the patient may be commented on or there may be meaningless words, empty repetitions. Sometimes the patient hears his own thoughts spoken aloud. (*Voiced thoughts*—Gedankenlautwerden.)

Here is a self-description (Kieser):

'It is amazing, horrible and for me humiliating, to think what acoustic exercises and experiments—musical ones too—have been conducted with my ears and body for nearly 20 years. Sometimes I could hear one and the same word repeated without interruption for two to three hours. I had to listen to long continuous speeches about me; frequently the content was insulting and there was often an imitation of well-known persons. These lectures, however, had little truth about them, usually they were infamous lies and slanders about my person, sometimes also of others. . . . it was often proclaimed that "I" said all these things . . . the scoundrels wanted to pass the time with onomatopoeia, paronomasia and other figures of speech and kept up a perpetuum mobile of speech. Sometimes one could only just hear these incessant, uninterrupted sounds but sometimes one could hear them a half or full mile away. They were being catapulted out of my body and the most varied sounds and noises got slung about, especially when I entered some house or village or town. This is the reason I have been living like a hermit for the last few years. All the time my ears keep ringing and sometimes so loudly that it can be heard far and wide. When I am among woods or bushes and the weather is stormy, some horrible, demoniacal poltergeist is aroused; when it is quiet, each tree starts rustling and uttering words and phrases when I approach. So with water—all the elements are being used to torture me.'

Another patient had been hearing voices for months, on the street, in the shops, in trains and restaurants. The voices talked and called out quietly but clearly and distinctly. 'Do you know him, he is crazy Hagemann'. 'He is looking at his hands again.' 'Lie down, now, your spinal cord is diseased.' 'He is a man without character', etc.

Schreber gives a description of those *functional hallucinations* that are heard at the same time as a real noise. They can be heard only then, not when it is quiet:

'I should remark on the circumstance that all the noises I hear, specially those that last rather long, like the rattle of trains, the throbbing of a steamer, the music at concerts, all seem to speak. It is a subjective feeling, of course, not like the speech of the sun or of the miraculous birds. The sound of words spoken or developed by me links up with my sense-impressions of train, steamer, squeaking boots etc. I would not think of saying that the train, steamer etc. are really speaking as in the case of the sun and the birds'.—Schizophrenic patients often hear the voices localised inside, in the body-trunk, head, eyes, etc.

We have to differentiate 'inner voices' ('voices of the mind') that is 'pseudo-hallucinations' from 'voices proper':

Perewalow, a chronic paranoic, distinguished voices that talked directly from the outside, through walls and pipes, from those voices brought by a current which his persecutors used to *force him sometimes to hear inwardly*. These inward voices were neither localised outside nor were they physical; he distinguished them from 'made thoughts' unaccompanied by any inner hearing and directly conducted into his head. (Kandinsky). Mrs. K. reported she had two memories; with one she could recall at will like anyone else; with the other, voices and inner pictures would appear before her involuntarily.

'Voices' are of particular importance with schizophrenic patients. Many different names and interpretations are given to them; for instance (Gruhle), communications, rapport, magical talk, secret language, voices in uproar etc.

*Taste and smell:* These senses have no objective pattern. In principle and sometimes in practice we can differentiate spontaneous hallucinations from those false perceptions in which objective smells and tastes are sensed as smelling and tasting somehow differently: A patient gives the following description—'It is odd about taste . . . food may taste just anyhow; sprouts like honey or the soup so unsalty I want to salt it heavily but, just before I do, it seems to me over-salted' (Koppe). Other patients complain about coal-dust, sulphur, air that stinks, etc.

*Simultaneous activity of several senses.* In actual sense-perception we deal ultimately not with one single sense, but with an object. This object seems to us as one and the same through the operation of several senses. So with hallucination, one sense supplements the other.

But there is a melêe of the senses, a different matter altogether, which makes clarity impossible. Experiences have been observed where the object is never exhibited to the patient in any clearly defined way by any one sense but is mixed up in a whirling confusion of shifting sense-data in which consciousness vainly tries to establish some meaning. We are not dealing here with a co-ordinated hallucination of several senses but with real synaesthesias that have become the dominant mode of perception. Genuine perceptions are now one with hallucinatory and illusory ones. Bleuler describes how he 'tasted' juice on his finger-tips. Under mescalin intoxication it is reported:

'One thinks one hears noises and sees faces and yet everything is still one and the same . . . what I see, I hear; what I smell, I think . . . I am music, a grating, everything is one and the same . . . then there are the auditory hallucinations which are also visual perceptions, zig-zag, angular, like oriental ornamentation . . . all this is not only thought by me, but felt, smelt, seen by me and seem to be my own movements as well . . . all is clear and definite . . . in the face of this actual experience of the impossible, criticism becomes nonsensical' (Beringer).

### (e) Abnormal Imagery—False Memory

The phenomena of abnormal perception have now been described and our account of pseudo-hallucinations brings us to the phenomenology of abnormal imagery.

Abnormal imagery has some correspondence with alienation from the perceptual world. The anomaly is not so much of the image itself but only of certain aspects which we might call the 'character of the image'. Some patients complain they are quite unable to imagine anything; such images as they can summon up are pale, shadowy, dead and do not seem to appear in consciousness.

One of Foerster's patients complained: 'I cannot even imagine how I look, how my husband and children look . . . when I look at an object, I know what it is but as soon as I close my eyes afterwards it has gone completely. It is as if one tried to imagine what air looked like. Surely, doctor, you can hold an object in your mind, but I can't keep an idea of it at all. I feel as if my thought had gone black.' Foerster found on examination that this patient could describe things perfectly from memory and that she was in fact extremely sensitive to colours, etc.

We are not dealing, therefore, with real inability to imagine but rather with something like derealisation in perception. The sensory elements and the mere direction of attention to an object are not all there is to a perception nor to an image. There are certain accessory characters which are of even greater importance for imagery than for perception, as with imagery the sensory elements tend in any case to be few, slight and fleeting. As a result we seem far more dependent upon these 'accessory' characters. If they are in abeyance we can well understand the patient when he says that he cannot imagine anything at all.

In the discussion of imagery a special place must be assigned to memories, that is the images which occur with the conscious knowledge that they constitute a previous perception of ours, that we have experienced their content before and that the object they represent is or was real. False perceptions mislead our judgment and false memories can do the same. Later on, when we discuss theories of memory, we shall see how nearly all memories are slightly falsified and become a mixture of truth and fantasy. It is necessary to differentiate Kahlbaum's hallucinatory memory from simple falsification of memory. For example:

A patient suffering from a process schizophrenia reports during the final stage of an acute phase of paranoid anxiety: 'For the past few weeks so many things have suddenly occurred to me over what happened with Emil [her lover] . . . just as if someone had told me'. She had completely forgotten these things. Later she even talked of the time 'when I suddenly remembered so many things'. The things she remembered were of this sort: 'Emil had, I'm sure, hypnotised me, because I was sometimes in such a state that I surprised myself; I had to kneel down on the floor of the kitchen and eat out of the pig-bucket. Afterwards he told it all triumphantly to his wife . . . I once had to go into the pig's sty. How long I was there and how I got there I don't know; I only came to as I was coming out of the sty on my hands and feet . . . Emil also nailed a couple of boards together and I had to say I wanted to be crucified after which I had to lie face downwards . . . once it seemed to me as if I had been riding a broomstick . . . once I felt as if Emil had me in his arms and there was a terrible wind . . . once I stood in the muck and was being pulled out . . .' Sometime before she had to go for a walk with Emil, and she knew exactly what happened under the lamp but did not know how she got home again.

Three criteria distinguish these cases which have often been observed.[1] The patients know for certain that *what comes to their mind is something they have forgotten.* They have the feeling that at the time they were in *an abnormal state of consciousness.* They talk of doped states, attacks of faintness, being half-asleep or half-awake, being in some peculiar state, a state of hypnosis, etc. Lastly there are indications that the patients feel that they must have been the *passive tools* of someone or something at the time and could not do anything about it. They were just made to do things. The mode of description in such cases is suggestive of false memory but in certain individual cases it has been shown (Oetiker) that the behaviour of the patient was actually disturbed during the period to which the false memory referred.

With the phenomena of false memories the patient gets a sudden image of a previous experience that has all the vivid feeling of a memory, but in actual fact nothing, not even a slender basis for it, is really remembered. Everything is *freshly created.* There are however apparently similar phenomena where everything is not freshly created but there is a *distortion* of *actual scenes,* for instance an innocuous scene in a public-house is distorted into an experience of being poisoned or hypnotised. There are, lastly, false memories that seem to have a neutral content: the patient announces that an hour ago he had a visitor when actually he was alone in bed. The only feature left here sometimes to differentiate such phenomena subjectively from normal falsifications of memory is the 'sudden coming to mind', which gives us an impression of primary phenomena.

This 'sudden coming to mind' of supposed 'forgotten' experiences can be difficult to distinguish from a progressive illumination of memory regarding real experiences which have been undergone during a twilight state.[2] Alter described the case of a high-ranking civil servant, who recalled step by step the details of a sexual murder he thought he had committed some time previously. Some circumstantial evidence indicated this. After his death, a detailed self-accusation was found among his papers, but neither the patient's other psychopathic symptoms nor the objective data were

---

[1] Oetiker, *Allg. Psychiatr. Z.,* vol. 54. Cp. Schneider's case, *Z. Neur.,* vol. 28, p. 90. Cp. Blume, *Z. Neur.,* vol. 42, p. 206, regarding a possible relation between falsification of memory and dreams.

[2] Alter, 'Ein Fall von Selbstbeschuldigung', *Z. Neur.,* vol. 15, p. 470.

definite enough to support any conclusion. However the phenomena as described by Alter suggest that he really went through this experience. There was a gradual illumination of memory through the help of a number of individual facts which could have aroused associations, and there was no sign that he felt he had been a passive tool, or subject to alien influences, etc.

Another false-memory phenomenon looks rather like *a déjà vu*, but here the patient consciously *accepts* everything *as real*. For example:

A dementia praecox patient reported that she couldn't help noticing that she saw faces in the clinic which she had seen at home a few weeks before; a witch-like form, for instance, that walked through the ward during the night as an attendant; she said that she had also seen the Matron some time ago in Pforzheim dressed in black. 'There was my recent experience in the garden when Dr. G. asked why didn't I work . . . I had already told this to my landlady four weeks ago. It struck me as very funny and I asked him with surprise what he had in mind.' When conversing in the clinic, she thought it had been like this before; she believed in any case that she had been in a mental hospital before.[1]

The patients accept these phenomena as real and because of this they should be distinguished from déjà-vu experiences proper, which are never thought to be real. Moreoever, the total experience itself leaves one with a different impression. This certainty of having seen or experienced something before may only refer to certain aspects of the present, sometimes it may refer to the whole situation; sometimes it occurs for only a brief period, a few minutes at the most, and sometimes it accompanies psychic events for weeks on end. It is not an uncommon phenomenon in schizophrenia.

The above examples of hallucinatory memory and this latter special form of déjà vu are phenomenologically all of the same character. The following group of falsifications of the past are not strictly speaking false memories and *do not have this same phenomenological character:*

(a) *Pathological lying.* Stories about the past which are pure fantasy are eventually believed by their inventor himself. Such falsifications range from harmless tall stories to a complete falsification of the whole past.

(b) *Reinterpretation of the past.* Insignificant past scenes suddenly acquire new meaning as the patient looks back at them. 'A meeting with an officer of high rank means the patient was of noble origin etc.'

(c) *Confabulations.* We use this term for a shifting series of false memories, briefly retained or immediately lost. They can appear in a number of forms: Confabulation out of embarrassment, which involves filling in the gaps of a severely impaired memory, e.g. in senile patients. With these and in cases with severe head injuries we find productive confabulations as part of the Korsakow syndrome. Patients will tell long stories about accidents they have had, a walk they have taken and other activities when they have been quietly in bed all the time. Lastly we have the well-characterised phenomena of the fantastic confabulations common in paranoid processes: A patient had lived through the Great War when he was about 7

[1] Other instances are given by Pick, *Fschr. Psychol.,* vol. 2 (1914), pp. 204 ff.

years old; in Mannheim he had seen large armies fighting; he had a special decoration because of his noble descent; he made a journey to Berlin with a big entourage to visit his father, the Kaiser; all that happened a long time ago; he was changed into a lion and so it goes on, endlessly. One patient called his whole fantastic world 'the novel'. The content of these confabulations can be influenced by the investigator. One can sometimes bring completely new stories to light. On the other hand, we can observe individual cases, for instance after head injury, where one of the confabulatory contents is tenaciously and continuously held.

### (f) Vivid physical awarenesses

In discussing false perception, false memory and pseudo-hallucinations, etc., emphasis was laid on the concrete vividness. We can now add to these phenomena one which is not vivid in the concrete sense but is for all that an equally forcible deception. This is the phenomenon of a false awareness.[1]

A patient felt someone was always walking next to him or rather obliquely behind him. When the patient got up, this one got up too; when he went, the other went with him; when he turned round, the other kept behind him so that the patient could never see him. He always remained in the same position though sometimes he came a little nearer or moved a little further away. The patient had never seen or heard him and had never felt him nor touched him and yet he experienced with an extraordinary certainty the feeling that somebody was there. In spite of the keenness of the experience and though he sometimes let himself be deceived, he concluded in the end that in reality no one was there.

If we compare phenomena such as this with normal experiences of a similar character, the following points emerge: For instance, we know when we are at a concert that someone is sitting behind us; we have just seen him; while walking in a dark room we suddenly stop because we think a wall is in front of us, etc. In such cases we are *aware that something is present* which at that moment is not based on any obvious sensory sign. Nevertheless these normal phenomena are either based on previous perceptions or on fine momentary ones which can be demonstrated if one will examine the situation more carefully (such as changes in sound, or density of atmosphere as in the case of the awareness of a wall), but with pathologically vivid awarenesses, the experience appears as a completely primary phenomenon and has the character of *urgency, certainty and vividness*. We have termed phenomena of this sort vivid physical awarenesses in contrast to other vaguer awarenesses which bring something abstract or fantastic before the psyche (e.g. awarenesses of thoughts or delusional awarenesses).

There are transitions from vivid physical awareness to hallucination proper:

'One thing is always with me. I feel and see a wall around me about 3–4 metres away; it is made of some wavy and hostile substance and under certain conditions devils keep on breaking out from it' (Schwab).

[1] Cp. my article on 'Concrete Awareness', *Z. Pathopsychol.*, vol. 2 (1913).

There are transitions to primary delusions as well: patients feel they are 'being observed' or 'watched' without anyone near them. A patient said, 'I did not feel free any longer, *that* wall in particular kept me.'

## § 2. Experience of Space and Time

*Psychological preface.* Space and Time are *always present* in sensory processes. They are not primary objects themselves but they invest all objectivity. Kant calls them 'forms of intuition'. They are *universal.* No sensation, no sensible object, no image is exempt from them. Everything in the world that is presented to us comes to us in space and time and we experience it only in these terms. Our senses cannot transcend the space–time experience of existence nor can we escape from it but are always confined within it. We do not perceive space and time as such, as we do other objects, but we perceive them along with these objects, and even in experience barren of any object we are still within time. Space and time do not exist on their own account; even where they are empty, we have them only in conjunction with objects that inform and define them.

Space and Time, underivative and primary, are always present in abnormal as well as in normal life. They can *never vanish.* Only the way in which they are present, how they appear to us, our mode of experiencing them, our estimate of their extent and duration, only these may be modified.

Space and Time are real for us only through their content. It is true we conceive them as a void, although we try to picture this emptiness to ourselves in vain. As *voids*, they share a *basic characteristic* of a quantitative kind: we find dimensions, homogeneity, continuity, infinity. The parts so constituted are not, however, instances of a universal called space or time, but parts of a perceptual whole. *Informed with content*, they immediately become qualitative. Although space and time are inseparable, they are radically different from each other; space being a homogeneous manifold and time a spaceless occurrence. If we want to bring these primary things home to ourselves in some neat phraseology we may say that they both represent the sundered existence of Being, separated from itself. Space is extended being (the side-by-side) and time is sequential being (the-one-after-the-other).

We can sometimes *do without* space and enjoy a kind of inner objectless experience, but time is always there. Or can we also break through time? The mystics say we can. In breaking through time, eternity is experienced as time standing still, an everlasting now, a 'nunc stans'. Past and future become one lucid present.

If space and time only become real for us through the objects that give them content the question arises what can we regard as the *essence* of space and time? Their universality has misled us in the past to take them as the very basis of Being. But it is a mistake to consider space and time as absolutes of Being itself and the experience of them as an absolutely basic one. Although everything that exists for us is spatial and temporal, whether real or symbolic, we should not impute to space and time that which gives them their content and intrinsic value. Though we all fulfil our fate in space and time in such a way that both gain substance for us in the all-embracing present, they are both nothing but the outer covering of events, with no significance but that which comes from our attitude towards them. It is the significance, not the specific experience, which turns them both into a psychic language, a psychic form, which should be kept out of the discussion when space and time are themselves the theme. In this chapter we are concerned only with *space and time as they are actually experienced*. It is altogether another matter that this experience, if it suffers any change, will modify all the psychic contents and be itself altered by the psychic contents—that is, the awareness of the significance of space and time may be changed.

Both space and time exist for us in a *number of basic configurations*, though what they have in common is not always immediately clear. In regard to *space* we have to distinguish: (1) the space I perceive as a qualitative structure, when I view it from my present orientation within the centre of my body, e.g. left to right, up and down, far and near. This is the space I contact around me as I live and move, which my eye grasps, the place where I am. (2) objective three-dimensional space, the space through which I move, which I constantly have with me as my immediate space of orientation. (3) theoretical space, including the non-euclidean space of mathematics—the space which is simply a theoretical construct. What *significance* I feel may lie in the configurations of space, in the spatial experience itself and in spatial change is another matter. As to *Time*, we have to distinguish: the time-experience, clock-time, chronological and historical time and time as the historical aspect of the individual's Existence.

For phenomenological purposes there is no point in psychopathology taking these philosophical problems as a starting-point, however relevant they may be for philosophy itself. It will be better to work out the actual abnormal phenomena and, as the case may be, see whether this theorising about space and time may not contribute something towards a clearer comprehension of the phenomena.

### (a) Space[1]

Appreciation of space can be assessed quantitatively as a performance, but there may be a very poor performance and yet the experience of space may still be normal. On the other hand space as a phenomenon may be being experienced quite differently. Where this experience is unconscious, we can only see it through its effects, i.e. through faulty performance. Where it is conscious, the patient can himself compare his present changed experience of space with what he remembers of his normal experience or with what normal spatial perception still remains to him.

1. Objects may seem smaller (*micropsia*) or larger (*macropsia*) or aslant, larger on one side than the other (*dysmegalopsia*). We also know of double vision or multiple vision up to a sevenfold vision. (All these phenomena may occur in deliria, epilepsy, and in acute schizophrenic psychoses, but we can also find them in psychasthenic conditions.)

*Exhaustion neuroses.* An overworked student sometimes saw letters and music, sometimes the wall and door as small and distant. The room became a long corridor. At other times his movements appeared to take on enormous dimensions and a mad speed. He thought he made enormous strides.[2]

Lubarsch (quoted by Binswanger) reported fatigue experiences when in bed in

---

[1] L. Binswanger, 'Das Raumproblem in der Psychopathologie', *Z. Neur.*, vol. 145 (1933), p. 598.

[2] Veraguth, 'Über Mikropsie u. Makropsie', *Dtsch. J. Nervenheilk.*, vol. 24 (1903).

the evening at the age of 11–13 years. 'My bed became longer, wider and so did the room, stretching into infinity. The ticking of the clock and my heartbeats thudded like huge hammers. A passing fly seemed like a sparrow.'

A presumably schizophrenic patient reported: 'There were times when everything I saw around me assumed enormous proportions. Men seemed gigantic, everything near and far seemed to me as if seen through the end of a telescope. I always seem when looking outside, for instance, to see everything through fieldglasses; so much perspective, depth and clearness in everything' (Ruemke).

2. *Experience of infinite space.* This occurs as an alteration of the whole spatial experience:

A schizophrenic reported: 'I still saw the room. Space seemed to stretch and go on into infinity, completely empty. I felt lost, abandoned to the infinities of space, which in spite of my insignificance somehow threatened me. It seemed the complement of my own emptiness . . . the old physical space seemed to be apart from this other space, like a phantom' (Fr. Fischer).

Serko described the feeling of infinite space under mescalin. The depth dimension of space seemed to enlarge. The wall moved away and space diffused itself everywhere.'

3. As with the contents of perception, so it is with the appreciation of space, which also takes on *an affective character.* L. Binswanger called it '*space with an atmosphere*' (or *emotionally-coloured space*). Space can have something of a psychic character so that it can exist as a threatening or a pleasing reality. Even in the previous examples it is difficult to distinguish sharply what are the actual changes in perception and what are merely alterations in the affective components of perception, although conceptually it is important to keep these two situations apart.

A schizophrenic patient of Carl Schneider said: 'I see everything as through a telescope, smaller and at a very great distance, yet not smaller in reality but more in the mind . . . less related to each other and to myself as it were . . . colours are dimmer and so is the significance . . . everything is far away . . . it is more a mental remoteness . . .'

Here the described alterations in perception are clearly already in essence affective changes. In the following example of schizophrenic experience, the fact of a reality experience seems to be in the foreground, although perception itself seems altered:

A schizophrenic reported: 'Suddenly the landscape was removed from me by a strange power. In my mind's eye I thought I saw below the pale blue evening sky a black sky of horrible intensity. Everything became limitless, engulfing . . . I knew that the autumn landscape was pervaded by a second space, so fine, so invisible, though it was dark, empty and ghastly. Sometimes one space seemed to move, sometimes both got mixed up. . . . It is wrong to speak only of space because something took place in myself; it was a continuous questioning of myself' (Fr. Fischer).

Another schizophrenic reported: 'when he looked at objects, things often seemed so empty, sometimes there, sometimes here. The air was still there between things, but the things themselves were not there.'

Another patient said: He only saw the space between things; the things were there in a fashion but not so clear; the completely empty space was what struck him. (Fr. Fischer).

## (b) Time

*Preliminary remarks.* We have to make three distinctions:

1. *Knowledge of time.* This relates to objective time and the performance of judging time-intervals rightly or wrongly. It also relates to wrong or delusional ideas on the nature of time (e.g. a patient says his head is a clock, that he is making time; or another patient says: 'new time is being produced so they must be turning the black–white knob' (Fr. Fischer).

2. *Experience of time.* The subjective experience of time is not the estimation of any particular span of time but a total awareness of time, in respect of which the ability to assess the time-span is only one of many other characteristics.

3. *Handling of time.* Everyone has to handle the basic fact of time. We may or may not be able to wait, to allow something to mature; we have to make decisions; we have to handle time in the context of our over-all awareness of our past life and our whole existence.

*Knowledge of time* concerns the study of psychological performance; *handling of time* is a matter for the psychology of meaningful phenomena (Verstehende Psychologie); in the following paragraphs we shall deal with the *experience of time* only. We are merely describing phenomena and there is no need to explain or grasp the meaning of these immediately.

In addition to the three above lines of enquiry, we are left finally with the biological problem of *the time-bound nature of life*, including psychic life. Every life has its own time, peculiar to it, whether it be the mayfly or man; each has its own life-span, its own life-curve and periodicity. This vital time is an objective, biological and qualitatively differentiated time. Time always plays a part in physiological events. (For instance, the beginning of the hormonal impulse which brings about a timely puberty.) It also plays a part in all forms of regulation; not only those which are merely chemical, varying in rate according to the temperature, for instance, but also those which show a rhythmic build-up, as interplay of stimuli, harmoniously ordered in their time-relationships. Finally, time plays a part in that extraordinary 'inner time-keeping' which can accurately determine any time interval (for instance, during sleep after a resolve to wake at a certain hour or after hypnotic suggestion).[1]

The reality of this vital time raises *certain questions*: Do time-events, if they differ for different species, also vary within the species in power, impetus, increase or decrease of tempo? Can time-events be disturbed as a whole, not only in one or other of their constituent factors? Is our experience of time, experience of events as such and therefore disturbed by any disturbance of these events? What kind of perception is implied in our experience of time? Do we perceive some kind of objective, every-day event, such as the objects of ordinary sense-perception or is it the vital bodily event

---

[1] Ehrenwald (*Z. Neur.*, vol. 134, p. 512) reports two cases of Korsakow syndrome; the time-sense was severely disturbed and he induced the patients by hypnosis to wake at certain times with some accuracy; conscious awareness was lost but a primitive, unconscious time-sense seemed there.

which we perceive? Do we perceive something concrete or are we experiencing something that is basically ourselves, or do both these things happen? We can ask all these questions but so far we are left without answer. Carrell is still circling round the riddle when he writes: 'Time is told in the tissues of our body. Possibly when this reaches the threshold of consciousness, it explains our deep-rooted, indefinable feeling of the flow of silent waters on which our conscious states waver like searchlights on some great, dark river. We realise we are changing and are no longer one with our previous self and yet we realise our identity.' We cannot explain the experience of time nor can we derive it from anything else; we can only describe it. We cannot avoid asking what are the causes of abnormal experience of time but so far demonstrable answers do not exist.

The following points are material when we come to discuss the phenomena of the experience of time: *Knowledge of time* (and actual orientation in time) takes place on the basis of our experience of time but it is not the experience of time itself. Our *experience of time* involves a basic awareness of the constancy of our existence; without this constancy in time there can be no consciousness of time passing. Consciousness of time passing is an *experience of basic continuity* (Bergson's durée, Minkowski's temps vécu). Experience of time is also an experience of *having a direction*, a growing forward, in which the awareness of the present stands as a reality between the past as memory and the future as planned. Finally there is *the experience in time of timelessness*, of Being as the eternal present, as the transcendence of all becoming.[1]

(1) *Momentary awareness of time*. Normal experience of the momentary passage of time varies understandably. Interesting and changing occupation makes us aware how rapidly time passes; idleness, lack of events and waiting, all make us feel how slowly the time goes and generally bring about a state of boredom, though not always. Mental patients do nothing for years on end without suffering from boredom. Exhausted and tired people can have the feeling of vacuity without boredom. These are all understandable variations, but there is an abnormal experience of the time-lapse found in seizures, psychoses and poisoning. The manner of the experience is altogether different and rooted in the vital events themselves:

(aa) *Time hurrying or slowed*. Klien[2] reports a boy who had attacks during which he would be frightened and run to his mother, saying:

'It's starting again, mother, what is it? Everything starts going so quickly again. Am I talking faster or are you?' He also thought the people on the street were walking faster.

In mescalin intoxication, Serko had the feeling that the immediate future was rushing on at chaotic speed:

'At first you have the peculiar feeling that you have lost control over time, as if it were slipping through your fingers; as if you were no longer capable of holding on

---

[1] Re abnormal experience of time see E. Straus, *Mschr. Psychiatr.*, vol. 68, p. 240. v. Gebsattel, *Nervenarzt*, vol. 1, p. 275. Also Roggenbau, *Die Störungen des Werdens u. Zeiterlebens* (Stuttgart, 1939). Fr. Fischer, *Z. Neur.*, vol. 121, p. 544; vol. 132, p. 241. G. Kloos, *Nervenarzt*, vol. 11 (1938), p. 225 (Störungen des Zeiterlebens in der endogen Depression).

[2] Klien, *Z. Psychopath.*, vol. 3 (1917), p. 307.

to the present in order to live it out; you try to cling on to it but it escapes you and streams away . . .'

(*bb*) *Lost awareness of time.* As long as there is some awareness the feeling of time cannot be lost altogether but it can be reduced to a minimum. Patients, for instance, if severely exhausted, may say that they do not feel time any more at all. If activity is lost, there is also a corresponding loss in the awareness of the passage of time:

In mescalin intoxication, when the chaotically racing moments of time are streaming away, when the intoxication is at its height, time vanishes altogether. Serko: 'Particularly when there is a wealth of hallucination, you have the feeling of swimming in a boundless stream of time, somewhere, somehow . . . you have to pull yourself up repeatedly and make a real effort to appreciate the time situation actively so as to escape from the chaotic flight of time, if only for a moment; only for a moment, however, since as soon as you relax, boundless time returns.' As Beringer commented, it is life 'for the moment only, no past or future'.

(*cc*) *Loss of reality in the time-experience.* Consciousness of time is primarily linked with feelings of immediacy, of something being present or absent, feelings of reality. With the disappearance of a time-sense, the present disappears and with it reality. Reality is felt purely as a temporal immediacy; or, to put it another way, we feel as if nothing were timelessly there. Some psychasthenic or depressive patients describe this experience as follows: 'It feels as if it is always the same moment, it is like a timeless void.' They do not live their time any more, although in some way they know it.

A depressed patient feels as if time did not want to go on. This experience has not got the elementary character of the previous cases but there is something of an elementary character in this particular feeling, which symbolises self and time locked together . . . 'The hands of the clock move blankly, the clock ticks emptily . . . they are the lost hours of the years when I could not work' . . . Time goes backwards. The patient sees that the hands move forward but, for her, actual time is not going on with them but is standing still. 'The world is all of a piece and cannot go forward or backward; this is my great anxiety. I have lost time, the hands of the clock are so light . . .' On looking back, on recovery, the patient said: 'It seems to me that January and February passed just like a blank, all of a piece, at a standstill; I couldn't believe time really went on. As I kept working and working and nothing came of it, I had the feeling that everything was going backwards and I would never be done' (Kloos).

(*dd*) *The experience of time standing still.* A schizophrenic patient reported:

'I was suddenly caught up in a peculiar state; my arms and legs seemed to swell. A frightful pain shot through my head and time stood still. At the same time it was forced on me in an almost superhuman way how vitally important this moment was. Then time resumed its previous course, but the time which stood still stayed there like a gate'. (Fr. Fischer).

2. *Awareness of the time-span of the immediate past.* After a hard day and

many experiences we are understandably conscious of having had a long day, while an empty, slowly passing day is felt in retrospect to have been short. The livelier our memory of past events, the shorter seems the time-span that has passed, but the more experiences intervene, the longer does this time-span appear. There is, however, a mode of recalling the time-span which is of a different order and has something new and primary at its root:

Following an acute and florid psychosis a paranoid patient reported: 'My own memory gives me the impression that this time-span, 3–4 months by ordinary reckoning, was an immensely long time for me, as if every night had the length of centuries.'

Serko experienced an enormous subjective over-estimation of the length of time during mescalin intoxication. 'Time seemed stretched out', 'Recent experiences seemed far away'.

Frequent reports are made of an overwhelming richness of experience packed into seconds, for instance during a crash or in a dream. A French investigator of dreams (quoting from Winterstein) reported as follows: 'He dreamed of the terror régime of the Revolution, of scenes of death, tribunals, condemnation, of a journey to the guillotine, of the guillotine itself; he felt his head severed from his trunk and then he woke up; the head of the bed had collapsed and hit him on the back of the neck.' 'The end of the dream was its source.'

The authenticity of similar reports cannot be doubted. But in one second of time we do not experience as a sequence what has become a series in our memory. There has to be some concerted act of intense momentary representation which gathers up together all those things that our memory has interpreted as a sequence in time.

Psychasthenic and schizophrenic patients report ecstatic experiences lasting in fact a few minutes as if they might have lasted for ever.

With the epileptic aura, a second in time is experienced as timeless or as eternity itself (Dostoievski).

3. *Awareness of time-present in relation to time-past and future.* A number of remarkable but very varied phenomena have been described:

(*aa*) *Déjà vu and jamais vu.* Patients are seized at moments by an awareness that everything they see has been seen before in exactly the same way. The moment has been clearly experienced before, down to the last detail. Objects, persons, postures and movements, words, even the tone of the voice, are all surprisingly the same, everything has been like this before. Conversely the 'jamais vu' experience consists in the awareness that everything is seen for the very first time, everything strikes as unfamiliar, fresh and incomprehensible.

(*bb*) *Discontinuity of time.* Individual schizophrenic patients report, for example, that one has fallen from heaven between one moment and the next: that time appears void, that awareness of the flow of time is lost (Minkowski); a patient of Bouman's (Korsakow) suddenly felt (during transfer from one institution to another) as if he were abruptly transplanted from one place to another; the two moments stood side by side; no time-span intervened.

(*cc*) Months and years fly by with *excessive speed.* 'The world races on and when it is autumn, spring is here already. It never used to be as fast as that in the old days' (A schizophrenic woman—Fr. Fischer).

(*dd*) *The shrinking of the past:* Bouman's patient felt a past of twenty-nine years had lasted only four years at most and the smaller time-spans within this period were correspondingly shortened.

4. *Awareness of the future.* The future vanishes:

A depressed patient, suffering from 'terrible emptiness' and a feeling of 'having lost all feeling' reported—'I cannot see the future, just as if there were none. I think everything is going to stop now and tomorrow there will be nothing at all'. Patients know there is another day tomorrow but this awareness has changed from what it was like before. Even the next five minutes do not lie ahead as they used to do. Such patients have no decisions, no worries, no hopes for the future. They have also lost the feeling for past stretches of time. 'I know the exact number of years, but I have no real appreciation of how long it was' (Kloos).

This is not an elementary experience of time. Changes in the emotional atmosphere of the patient's perception and in his awareness of things also make themselves noticeable in the experience of time. What is lost is the feeling of immediate content. Things are there but the patient can only know them, not feel them, so the future disappears like everything else. The concept of time is there and the correct knowledge of time but not the actual time-experience.

5. *Schizophrenic experience of time standing still, flowing together, and stopping.* Schizophrenic patients report that sometimes during transient, brief attacks, they have remarkable, elementary yet somehow significant experiences, sensorily keen but of a supernatural strangeness. They report these experiences as some kind of transformation of their time-experience:

A schizophrenic described one attack thus: 'Yesterday I looked at the clock . . . I felt as if I was put back, as if something past was coming to me . . . I felt as if at 11.30 a.m. it was 11.0 a.m. again but not only the time went back but what had happened to me during it. Suddenly it was not just 11.0 o'clock but a time long past was there too . . . midway in time I came towards myself out of the past. It was terrible. I thought perhaps the clock was put back; the attendants had played a stupid trick . . . then I had a feeling of frightful expectation that I could be drawn into the past . . . the play with time was so uncanny . . . *an alien time* seemed to dawn. Everything blended with everything else and I said in a strained way to myself: I must hold on to everything . . . then lunch came and everything was as usual . . .' (Fr. Fischer).

A schizophrenic woman said: 'There is no more present, only a backward reference to the past; the future goes on shrinking—*the past* is so intrusive, it envelops me, it *pulls me back*. I am like a machine which stands in one place and works by itself. It is worked to breaking-point but it still stands . . . I am living much faster than before . . . It is the contact with old things. I feel this sustains me. I let myself be carried away, so that at least one can reach an end and be at peace . . . if I were to hang on to all this speed I would get swept away with it . . . time chases me and ravenously eats itself away and I am in the middle of it all' (Fr. Fischer).

Another schizophrenic woman described the painful admixture she suffered of emptiness, non-existence, time standing still and the return of the past: 'Life is now a running conveyor-belt with nothing on it. It runs on but is still the same . . . I did not know death looked like this . . . I am now living in eternity . . . outside everything carries on . . . leaves move, others go through the ward but for me time does not pass . . . when they run around in the garden and the leaves fly about in the wind, *I wish I could run too so that time might again be on the move* but then I stay stuck . . . time stands still . . . one swings between past and future . . . it is a boring, endless time. It would be fine to start again from the beginning and *find myself swinging along with the proper time,* but I can't . . . *I get pulled back,* where to ? . . . there where it comes from, where it has been before . . . it goes into the past—that is what is so elusive . . . time slips into the past . . . the walls which used to stand firm have all fallen down . . . do I know where I am, oh yes—but the elusive thing is there is no time and how can one get hold of it? Time is in collapse' (Fr. Fischer).

Another schizophrenic described his attack: 'One evening during a walk in a busy street, I had a sudden feeling of nausea . . . afterwards a small patch before my eyes, no bigger than a hand. The patch glimmered inwardly and there was a to and fro of dark threads . . . the web grew more pronounced . . . I felt drawn into it. It was really *an interplay of movements* which had replaced my own person. *Time had failed* and stood still—no, it was rather that time re-appeared just as it disappeared. *This new time* was infinitely manifold and intricate and could hardly be compared with what we ordinarily call time. Suddenly the idea shot through my head that time did not lie before or after me but in every direction. It came to me from looking at the play of colours . . . but the disturbance was soon forgotten'.

This patient also reported: Thinking stood still; everything stood still *as if there were no more time.* I seemed to myself as a timeless creature, clear and transparent, as if I could see right down into myself . . . at the same time I heard quiet music far away and saw dimly lit sculptures . . . it all seemed a never-ceasing flow of movement very different from my own state. These distant movements were, it seemed, a "folie" of my condition.'

Yet another experience of the same patient was as follows: 'I was *cut off from my own past,* as if it had never been like that, so full of shadows . . . as if life had started just now . . . then the past turned round . . . *everything got intermingled* but in no comprehensible way; everything shrank, fell together, packed up, like a wooden shack which has collapsed, or as if a well-perspectived painting became two-dimensional and everything flicked together' (Fr. Fischer).

## (c) *Movement*

Perception of movement involves space and time simultaneously. Disturbances in the perception of movement are principally reported as disturbances of function following neurological lesions. So far as abnormal experiences go, our description of the time-experience has already covered movement, thus, there is discontinuity; movement is not perceived, but the object or person is now here, now there, without any time intervening. There is also the speeding up or slowing down of visible movements etc.

Perceptions of movement in an object have been noted even though this has made no actual change of position:

Under the influence of scopolamine: 'I suddenly saw how the pen—apparently surrounded by a kind of fog—crawled towards me like a caterpillar with fine wavy movements. It seemed to get nearer. At the same time I realised that the distance between the end nearest me and the line of the cover on the desk never got any smaller' (Mannheim—quoted from C. Schneider), (*Z. Neur.*, vol. 131).

## § 3. Awareness of the Body

*Psychological preface.* I am aware of my body as my existence. I also see it and touch it. The body is the only part of the world that is both felt from within and—so far as its surface goes—at the same time perceived. The body provides me with an object and I am also that body. There is a difference, it is true, between what I feel about myself as a body and how I perceive myself as an object, yet the two are inextricably interwoven. Bodily sensations whereby a certain object builds itself up for me and sensations which remain as a feeling of my bodily state are the same and indivisible, though one can differentiate between them: *Sensations that give rise to feelings* blend into *an awareness of our physical state*. Awareness of our body's existence, normally an unnoticed, neutral background for consciousness—neither a disturbing nor an influential factor, may undergo a number of exceptional changes as a whole: states of sexual excitement, anxiety or pain may involve the body profoundly, absorbing the individual and compelling him to further effort or destroying him completely.

Our body becomes *an object* to us because we are aware of our own body, which follows our every movement not as a clear-cut, isolated object but as an intuition of our three-dimensional self. *Head* and *Schilder*[1] have clarified this phenomenon. According to Head the impressions relating to space—kinaesthetic, tactile, optical— build up organised models of ourselves which may be termed *body-schemata*. What we make of our bodily sensations and how we execute our movements are both maintained through the relationship these sensations and movements have with previous bodily impressions that have found their way unconsciously into the body-schema.

The awareness of our physical state and the three-dimensional body-schema combine as a whole to form what Wernicke called the *somato-psyche*. *Awareness of the physical state* has to be analysed physiologically according to the specific sense-perceptions which go to build it up. All the senses play some part in this, those of the eye and ear to the smallest degree, only reaching such a level if the external content is accompanied by intensive stimuli which give rise to a bodily sensation. Taste and smell play a larger part and the bodily sensations continuously so. These latter can be classified into three groups: those of the body-surface (thermic, haptic, hygric etc.); those belonging to movement and posture (kinaesthetic, vestibular); and those belonging to the organs (which intimate the condition of the inner organs). The physiological basis for these sensations lies in the histologically well-known nerve-endings. Whether this list exhausts all the sensations we receive may be questioned.

Awareness of the body has to be clarified *phenomenologically* by relating it to our experience of the body as a whole. *The close relationship* of *the body to awareness of self* is best exemplified in the experience of muscular activity and movement, rather

---

[1] Paul Schilder, *Das Körperschema. Ein Beitrag zur Lehre vom Bewusstsein des eigenen Körpers* (Berlin, 1923).

less well in the sensations contributed by the heart and circulatory system and least of all in the vegetative changes. Specific feelings of one's bodily existence arise from the following: movement and posture, the style, ease and grace of our motor-activity or its heavy and clumsy nature, the impression we think our physical presence makes on others, our general weakness or strength and any alteration in our normal feeling-state. All the above are factors of our *vital self.* There are wide variations in the extent to which we feel *our oneness* as well as in the amount of *distance* we establish between ourselves and our body. This may reach a maximal distance in medical self-observation when we see our pains only as symptoms and consider the body as some alien object, consisting of anatomical findings, or as a kind of garment, something in the last resort quite different from ourselves and in no way identical, though our unity with it in fact is inseparable.

*Awareness of our body* need not *be confined* to the actual *boundaries of our body.* We may still feel at the end of the stick which guides us in the dark. Our proper space, the space of our anatomical body, may be extended by the feeling of something at one with ourselves. So the car I drive, if I am a good driver, becomes part of my body-schema or image and is like an extended body which I invest fully with my own senses. External space begins where my senses and I come up against objects that emerge from it.

My bodily awareness is able to detach itself from objective, organised space, that is from the realities of space, in two directions: either negatively, in giddiness (as loss of vital feeling and certainty) or positively, in dancing (as an access of vital feeling and sense of freedom).[1]

The experience of one's body as one's own is phenomenologically closely linked with the experience of feeling, drive and awareness of self.

We should distinguish between phenomenological description of *actual bodily experiences* and any discussion of the *significance* for the individual of his own body, in terms of the effective meaningful connections, where there are hypochondriacal, narcissistic or symbol-forming tendencies influencing the self-awareness.

### (a) *Amputated limbs*

It is remarkable how amputated limbs may be sensed as a result of habituation to the body-schema, which remains a reality after the amputation has taken place. The body-schema is not a mere free-floating concept of one's own body but a mode of apprehending oneself that has been deeply imprinted throughout all one's life, a mode in which at any one time all the body sensations are unified into a whole. Just as we think we can see within the normal blind spot in the visual field, so we still sense the lost limb as real and fill out the gap that has been rent in the body-schema. These sensations must be localised in the cerebral cortex. Head saw such a phantom limb disappear following a focal cortical lesion.

Riese[2] describes a healthy leg-amputee thus: in all his body movements the lost leg was still sensed. When he got up, the knee extended; it bent again when he sat

---

[1] E. Straus, 'Die Formen des Räumlichen', *Nervenarzt.*, vol. 3 (1930).
[2] Riese, 'Neue Beobachtungen am Phantomglied', *Dtsch. Z. Nerevnkh.* (1932), p. 127. D. Katz, *Zur Psychologie der Amputierten* (Leipzig, 1921).

down; he could stretch the leg luxuriously along with all the other limbs; when asked whether he really believed all this, the patient knew the leg was no longer there, but it somehow still kept its own peculiar reality for him.

### (b) Neurological disturbances

With localised cerebral lesions orientation in relation to one's own body is disturbed in a number of ways. For instance (taking psychological performance) the ability to recognise an irritable place on the body-surface or the position of a limb is partially or wholly absent. Patients can no longer touch nose, mouth or eyes or the orientation for the left and right side of the body may be disturbed. Patients can no longer say on which side of their body the stimulus is applied etc. In these states we do not know how the bodily awareness itself is altered phenomenologically.[1]

*Giddiness* may be either (1) vertigo (2) a sensation of falling (3) general unsystematised dizziness, experienced as an uncertain awareness, without rotation of objects or any sensation of falling. Here we are dealing with three heterogeneous phenomena. They have in common a total uncertainty as to posture and position.

This uncertainty normally occurs at the critical point of transition from one state to another, whether due to one's physical surroundings or some psychological reason. It arises neurologically from somatic causes, particularly in the vestibular apparatus. It may arise neurotically in connection with the upset of psychic conflict. Giddiness is the experience of an existence which as a whole has lost its ground; as such it is a symbol for everything that is on the verge but not yet brought within the orderly clarity of immediate being. This is the reason why philosophers could adopt the expression 'giddiness' for the original experience from which their basic insights into Being as a whole derived.

### (c) Bodily sensations, perception of bodily shape, hallucinations of the bodily senses, etc.

These may be classified and grouped as follows:

(1) *Hallucinations of the bodily senses.* We may distinguish between *thermic* hallucinations (the floor is burning hot, unbearable feelings of heat) and *haptic* ones (cold wind blows on the patient, insects creep under the skin, the patient is being stung all over). Within the latter category, *hygric* hallucinations have been further differentiated (perceptions of wetness and fluids). The hallucinations of *muscle sense* (Cramer)[2] are interesting. The floor rises and sinks, the bed is raised, patients sink, fly, feel they are light as a feather, an object in the hands feels very light or heavy, patients feel they are making movements, although motionless themselves; they think they are speaking, when actually they are silent (hallucinations of the speech apparatus). 'Voices'

---

[1] Cf. Schilder, *Das Körperschema. Ein Beitrag zur Lehre vom Bewusstsein des eigenen Körpers* (Berlin, 1923).

[2] Craner, *Die Halluzinationen im Muskelsinn* (Freiburg, 1889).

can be in part conceived as hallucinations of this sort but some of them must be interpreted as hallucinations of the vestibular apparatus.

2. *Vital sensations.* These give rise to feelings which make us aware of our vital bodily state. Reports from patients about their bodily sensations are inexhaustible. They feel turned into stone, dried up, shrunk, tired, empty, hollow or blocked. Sensations such as these cannot but alter the feeling of bodily existence. The patient feels he is a soap-bubble, or that his limbs are made of glass or describes himself in one or other of the countless ways in which patients try to depict their feelings. We have a host of reports on these puzzling sensations, particularly from schizophrenic patients. It is difficult to separate the actual sense experience from the delusion-like interpretation and in the latter case to clarify the underlying sensory events.

3. *Passivity experiences in the form of bodily sensation.* Bodily sensations may be accompanied by the vivid experience that they have been contrived from outside. In such cases the patients are not merely interpreting various abnormal organic sensations in one way or another but have an immediate perception of this 'coming from outside'. We observe that patients will correctly perceive pain and other sensations such as may be caused by physical illness (angina, rheumatoid arthritis), but they will experience these specific sensations as something externally contrived. Schizophrenic patients know the experience of being made to be sexually excited, of being raped and of being made to have sexual intercourse without any person being present. They may feel that wires are pulling at their hair and their toes.

4. *Experience of bodily distortion.* The body enlarges, gets stronger, becomes coarse and heavy and along with this the pillows and bed grow bigger and bigger.[1] Head and limbs get thick and swollen, parts are twisted, limbs become alternatively larger or smaller.

Serko describes himself during mescalin intoxication (the picture presents us with a vivid analogy to some psychotic experiences): 'I feel my body is exceptionally three-dimensional and highly detailed . . . I suddenly have a sensation that my foot has left my leg; I feel it lying apart from my body below the truncated leg. (N.B.— it is not just the sensation that the foot is missing but rather that there are two positive sensations—that of the foot and that of the truncated leg with the hallucinatory sensation of a lateral shift in position) . . . then I have the sensation that my head is being turned right round, 180°, that my abdomen is becoming a soft fluid mass, my face growing to gigantic dimensions, my lips swelling, my arms becoming peculiarly wooden and serrated in outline, like the Nurnberg puppets, or growing long and ape-like, while the lower jaw hangs down heavily. Among many other things I have the hallucination that my head has become separated from my body and is floating free in the air half a mile behind me. I really feel it floating and yet still belonging to me. To control myself I say a few words aloud and even the voice seems to come from a certain distance behind me. More peculiar still are the transformations; for instance,

[1] R. Klein, 'Über Halluzinationen der Körpervergrösserung', *Mschr. Psychiatr.*, vol. 67 (1928), p. 78 (cases of head-injury and encephalitis).

my feet become key-shaped and turn into spirals, while my lower jaw twists into the curls of a section-mark; my chest seems to melt away . . .'

In states of altered consciousness, the integration of bodily awareness with the space in which the body senses its objects may take on grotesque forms. A patient feels 'he is the water-mark on the paper which is being written upon'. Serko again describes his mescalin intoxication:

'Haptic hallucinations sometimes fuse with visual ones in an odd way difficult to describe. In a vaguely illuminated visual field there form certain strips of light with a lively movement, turning into spirals which move to and fro in the visual field while rapidly rotating. There is at the same time a transformation in the haptic field whereby my leg assumes a spiral form too. The light spirals and the haptic spirals fuse together in consciousness so that the same spiral that is visually hallucinated is also perceived haptically . . . one feels a complete bodily and visual unity . . .'

Under hashish intoxication the proband states: 'my body feels like a husk, a coffin in which the soul is suspended, as something delicate, transparent, like spun-glass and floating free within the confines of the shell. Arms and legs can see, all the senses are one; the shell is heavy and immobile; but the kernel thinks, feels, and ex-periences.' All this was not just imagined but actually felt to be real. The proband was afraid of being damaged by others (Fraenkel and Joel).

A schizophrenic patient said: 'I saw my new "self" like a new-born baby; power came from it but it could not fully pervade my body; it was too big and I wanted them to take a leg or an arm off so that it could be filled completely. Things got better later and at last I felt my "self" sticking out of my body into space.' (Schwab).

The phenomena recounted above show a good deal of variety but it is difficult to sort them out any more clearly than this. For the most part these abnormal experiences of the body-schema have no analogy with normal ex-perience of the body. Vital sensations, experience of symbolic meanings, neurological disturbances, all merge into each other. Awareness of self permits each to represent itself in the other.

## (d) The 'Double' or Heautoscopy

Heautoscopy is the term used for the phenomenon when someone vividly perceives his own body as a double in the outer world, whether as an actual perception or as an imaginary form, as a delusion or as a vivid physical aware-ness. There have been patients who will actually speak with their doubles. The phenomenon is not at all uniform.[1]

1. Goethe (in *Drang und Verwirrung*) had seen Frederika for the last time and was riding to Drusenheim when the following happened: 'In my mind's eye, not with my physical eyes, I saw myself distinctly on the same road riding towards myself. I was dressed as I had never been before in grey and gold. Immediately I shook myself out of this dream, the figure went' . . . 'The strange phantom gave me a certain peace of mind at that moment of parting.' What is noteworthy in the episode is the dreamy

---

[1] Menninger-Lerchenthal, 'Eine Halluzination Goethes', *Z. Neur.*, vol. 140 (1932), p. 486.

state, the mind's eye and the satisfaction derived from the meaning of the apparition—he was riding in the opposite direction back to Sesenheim—he will return.

2. A schizophrenic patient of Menninger-Lerchenthal complained that 'she sees herself from behind, naked; she has the feeling that she is not dressed and sees herself naked and feels cold too; it is her mind's eye that sees'.

3. A schizophrenic patient (Staudenmaier) said: 'During the night while I walked up and down in the garden I imagined as vividly as possible that there were three other people present besides me. Gradually the corresponding visual hallucination took shape. There appeared before me three identically clothed Staudenmaiers who walked along in step with me; they stopped when I did and stretched out their hands when I stretched out mine.'

4. A patient of Poetzl with a hemiplegia and diminished self-perception felt the hemiplegic side did not belong to him. While looking at his paralysed left hand he explained it by saying that it probably belonged to the patient in the next bed; during nocturnal delirium he affirmed that another person lay on his left side in the same bed and wanted to push him out.

We can see that we are dealing with phenomena that are really not the same although they are superficially similar. They may occur in organic brain lesions, in deliria, in schizophrenia and in dream-like states, never at least without a mild alteration in consciousness; day-dreaming, intoxication, dream-sleep or delirium. The similarity consists in the fact that the body-schema gains an actuality of its own out in external space.

## § 4. DELUSION AND AWARENESS OF REALITY

Since time immemorial delusion has been taken as the basic characteristic of madness. To be mad was to be deluded and indeed what constitutes a delusion is one of the basic problems of psychopathology. To say simply that a delusion is a mistaken idea which is firmly held by the patient and which cannot be corrected gives only a superficial and incorrect answer to the problem. Definition will not dispose of the matter. Delusion is a primary phenomenon and the first thing we have to do is to get it into a proper focus. The experience within which delusion takes place is that of experiencing and thinking that something is real.

*Awareness of reality—logical and psychological comment.* Things that are for the moment most self-evident are also the most enigmatic. Thus it is with Time, the Self and Reality. If we have to say what we think reality is we find ourselves answering something like this: it means *things in themselves* as compared with how they appear to us; it means *what is objective* in the sense of something generally valid as opposed to subjective error; it means *underlying essence* as distinct from masking effects. Or we may call reality *that which is in time and space*, if we want to differentiate it from the theoretically valid objectivity of ideal Being—that for instance of mathematics.

These are the answers of our reason and through them we define to ourselves a concept of reality. But we need something more than this purely logical concept of reality; there is also *the reality we experience*. Conceptual reality carries conviction only if a kind of presence is experienced, provided by reality itself. As Kant says, 100 imaginary dollars cannot be distinguished from a 100 real dollars so far as the actual concept goes; the difference is only noted in practice.

What the *experience of reality* is in itself can hardly be deduced nor can we compare it as a phenomenon with other related phenomena. We have to regard it as a primary phenomenon which can be conveyed only indirectly. Our attention gets drawn to it because it can be disturbed pathologically and so we appreciate that it exists. If we want to describe it as a phenomenon, we shall have to take the following points into account:

1. What is real is what we *concretely perceive*. In contrast with our imaginings, perception has a quality not determined by the particular sense-organ, e.g. the eye or ear, but rooted in the actual mode of what is sensed, which is something absolutely primary and constitutes sensory reality (normally connected with external stimuli). We can talk about this primary event, name and rename it, but we cannot reduce it any further.[1]

2. Reality lies in the simple *awareness of Being*. Awareness of reality may fail us, even when we concretely perceive. For instance it is lost in 'derealisation' and 'depersonalisation'. Awareness of reality must therefore be a primary experience of existence and as such Janet called it a 'fonction de réel'. Descartes' 'cogito ergo sum' holds even for the person in a state of derealisation who says paradoxically: 'I am not but have to go on being nothing for ever'. Descartes' phrase therefore cannot convince us by logic alone; in addition it requires the primary awareness of Being and the awareness of one's own existence in particular. 'I exist and thereby the things in the world outside me are experienced as equally existent.'

3. What is real is *what resists us*. Whatever may inhibit our bodily movements or prevent the immediate realisation of our aims and wishes is a resistance. The achievement of a goal against resistance or defeat thereby brings with it an experience of reality; all experience of reality, therefore, has a root in the practice of living. But the reality itself which we meet in practice is always an *interpretations*, a meaning, the meaning of things, events or situations. When I grasp the meaning, I grasp reality. The resistance we meet in the world gives us the wide field of the real which extends from the concreteness of tangible objects to perceived meanings in things, behaviour and human reaction. This brings to us awareness of the reality with which in practice we have to reckon and deal, to which we have to accommodate every moment, which fills us with expectation and which we believe in as something which is. Awareness of this reality pervades us all more or less clearly as a knowledge of the reality with which we are individually most concerned. This individual reality is embedded in a more general reality that has been structured and amplified for us through the traditional culture in which we have grown up and been educated. What is real for us in all this has many grades of certainty and usually we are not completely clear about it. We only need to test how much we would risk in our ordinary judgments of what is real or not for us to see the measure of this certainty.

We have to distinguish between *immediate certainty of reality* and *reality-judgment*. A vivid false perception may be recognised as a deception and judged as such

---

[1] Gerhard Kloos, *Das Realitätsbewusstsein in der Wahrnehmung und Trugwahrnehmung* (Leipzig, 1938). This is an excellent survey of all the efforts made at definition hitherto and makes its own fresh contribution, but an unsuccessful one in my opinion, though it helps us to appreciate the primary nature of the phenomenon.

and yet continue to be what it is, as happens with simple after-images and sometimes in the case of hallucinated mental patients. Even when the deception is recognised the patient may still act unawares as if the content were real. For instance, an amputee has a phantom limb, steps on it and falls; or there was the case of the famous botanist Naegeli who wanted to put a glass of water on a hallucinated table. Reality-judgment is the result of a thoughtful digestion of direct experiences. These are tested out against each other; only that which stands the test and is confirmed in this way is accepted as real; and hence only that is real which is commonly identifiable and accessible to others and not merely a private and subjective matter. A judgment of reality can itself be transformed into a new direct experience. We live continuously with a knowledge of reality acquired in this way but not always made fully explicit in the form of a judgment. The characteristics of this reality as evinced by our judgments (implicit or explicit) are: that reality is not a single experience 'per se' but only as it is there *in the context* of the experience and ultimately in the experience as a whole; reality is *relative* in so far as it is recognised only up to the point at which it has disclosed itself; it can alter; reality *discloses* itself; it rests on insight and how certain this is; it does not depend on concreteness nor on an immediate experience of reality as such; the latter are only supporting features for the whole, they are indispensable but have constantly to be checked. Hence, the reality of our reality-judgments is a flexible reality—a movement of our reason.

If now we want to characterise the field of *delusion*, we shall have to make some distinctions. There is first *diminished awareness of Being and of one's own existence*, which were discussed under derealisation of perception and which we shall meet again among the disturbances of self-awareness. Then there is *hallucinatory vividness*, which was discussed under false perceptions. Delusion proper, however, implies *a transformation in our total awareness of reality* (including that secondary awareness which appears in the form of reality-judgments). This builds itself up on judgmental experiences as well as on the world of practical activity, resistance and meanings, in which, however, hallucinatory vividness plays only an accidental and relatively minor part beside the transformation of basic experience which we have such great difficulty in grasping.[1]

## (a) The concept of delusion

Delusion manifests itself *in judgments*; delusion can only arise in the process of thinking and judging. To this extent pathologically falsified judgments are termed delusions. The content of such judgments may be rudimentary but take a no less effective form as mere awareness. This is usually spoken of as a 'feeling' that is also an obscure certainty.

The term delusion is *vaguely* applied to all false judgments that share the following external characteristics to a marked, though undefined, degree: (1) they are held with an *extraordinary conviction*, with an incomparable, *subjective certainty*; (2) there is an *imperviousness* to other experiences and to compelling

[1] Gerhard Schmidt, 'Der Wahn im deutschsprachigen Schrifttum der letzten 25 Jahre' (1914–29), *Zbl. Neur.*, vol. 97, p. 115.

counter-argument; (3) their content is *impossible*. If we want to get behind these mere external characteristics into the psychological nature of delusion, we must distinguish the original *experience* from the *judgment* based on it, i.e. the delusional contents as presented data from the fixed judgment which is then merely reproduced, disputed, dissimulated as occasion demands. We can then distinguish two large groups of delusion according to their *origin*: one group *emerges understandably* from preceding affects, from shattering, mortifying, guilt-provoking or other such experiences, from false-perception or from the experience of derealisation in states of altered consciousness etc. The other group is for us *psychologically irreducible;* phenomenologically it is something final. We give the term '*delusion-like ideas*' to the first group; the latter we term '*delusions proper*'. In their case we must now try and get closer to the facts of the delusional experience itself, even though a clear presentation is hardly possible with so alien a happening.

With every hallucination proper, a need is experienced to regard the hallucinated object as real. The need remains even when the false judgment of reality has been corrected in the light of the total context of perception and subsequent knowledge. But should the patient, although such a correction is feasible, retain his false judgment of reality in spite of the known objections, in spite of reflection and with absolute certainty—overcoming indeed any initial doubts he may have had—then we are dealing with delusion proper: such a belief is no longer understandable in terms of hallucination alone. With delusion-like ideas that originate from hallucinations we only find a tendency towards false judgment of reality (or a quite transient certainty) but with delusion proper all doubt has ceased. Some other psychic factors than mere hallucinations must be at work and these we will now try to explore.

The content of the delusions which the patient may disclose to us in the course of an interview is always a secondary product. We are faced with a customary formulation of a judgment, which simply differs from other judgments perhaps in having a different content. When investigating, therefore, we are always confronted with the question—what is the primary experience traceable to the illness and what in the formulation of the judgment is secondary and understandable in terms of that experience? There are *three existing points of view*: the *first* denies that there is any experience at all of delusion proper; all delusions are understandable in themselves and secondary. The *second* believes that lack of critical capacity due to poor intelligence allows delusion to emerge from any kind of experience; the *third* requires the singular phenomenon of delusional experience, which it regards as the essential pathological element. The first point of view is represented by Westphal.[1] According to him the first step is an awareness of change in one's personality, much as one might feel, for instance, if one had put on a uniform for the first time and felt conspicuous. So paranoics think that the change in themselves, which they alone appreciate, is also noticed by their environment. From this delusion that one has become noticeable arises the delusion that one is watched and from that the delusion

---

[1] Westphal, *Allg. Z. Psychiatr.*, vol. 34, pp. 252 ff.

that one is being persecuted. It is true such understandable connections do play a part, particularly in paranoid developments of personality, and in psychoses so far as content is concerned. We can thus understand over-valued ideas and secondary delusions in general, but we are still without an explanation of the essential nature of delusion. The same may be said for the attempt to derive delusion from preceding affects, the affect of distrust, for instance. There is no clear delineation here of the specific phenomenon, the actual delusional experience; we are only offered an understandable context for the emergence of certain stubborn misconceptions. If these misconceptions turn into delusion, something new has to arrive, which as an experience can also be grasped phenomenologically. The *second* point of view holds that the cause—or perhaps more modestly the precondition—for delusion lies in *weakness of intelligence.* We always tend to look for the logical errors and blunders in the paranoid patient's thought in order to prove some such weakness. Sandberg,[1] however, pointed out quite rightly that paranoics have by no means a poorer intelligence quotient than healthy persons and in any case the mentally ill person surely has as much right to be illogical as the healthy one. It is wrong to consider the failure in reasoning a morbid symptom in one case but normal in the other. Actually we find every degree of mental defect without delusions of any kind and the most fantastic and incredible delusions in the case of people of superior intelligence. The critical faculty is not obliterated but *put into the service of the delusion.* The patient thinks, tests arguments and counter-arguments in the same way as if he were well. A highly critical attitude is as rare in paranoics as in healthy people, but if it does occur it naturally colours the formal expression of the delusional content. For any true grasp of delusion, it is most important to free ourselves from this prejudice that there has to be some poverty of intelligence at the root of it. Any dependence on the latter is purely formal. We have to assume some *specific alteration in psychic function,* not a failure of intelligence, if after some delusional experience an individual, who is fully conscious and—as occasionally happens—quite free from any other morbid symptom, maintains a delusion that everyone else recognises as such, and if he simply declares: 'Well, that is how it is; I have no doubts about it, I know it is so'. With delusion proper there is material falsification while formal thinking remains intact. Where there is formal thought disturbance, then misapprehensions, confused association and (in acute conditions) the wildest notions may follow, which as such do not have the character of delusion proper. The *third* point of view, that there is some phenomenologically peculiar delusional experience, sets out to find what this basic primary delusional experience may be.

*Methodologically* delusion can be viewed from a number of standpoints: *phenomenologically* it is an experience; from the point of view of *psychological performance* it is a disturbance of thinking; as a psychological product, it is a *mental creation*: from the

[1] Sandberg, *Allg. Z. Psychiatr.,* vol. 52.

point of view of *meaningful connections*, it is motivated, dynamic content; and in the framework of *nosological-biographical* study we may ask whether we are to comprehend it as a break in the normal life-curve or simply as a part of the continuum of personality development.

### (b) Primary delusions

If we try to get some closer understanding of these primary experiences of delusion, we soon find we cannot really appreciate these quite alien modes of experience. They remain largely incomprehensible, unreal and beyond our understanding. Yet some attempts have been made.[1] We find that there arise in the patient certain primary sensations, vital feelings, moods, awarenesses: 'Something is going on; do tell me what on earth is going on', as one patient of Sandberg said to her husband. When he asked what she thought was going on, the patient said, 'How do I know, but I'm certain *something is going on.*' Patients feel uncanny and that there is something suspicious afoot. Everything gets a *new meaning*. The environment is somehow different—not to a gross degree—perception is unaltered in itself but there is some change which envelops everything with a subtle, pervasive and strangely uncertain light. A living-room which formerly was felt as neutral or friendly now becomes dominated by some indefinable atmosphere. Something seems in the air which the patient cannot account for, a distrustful, uncomfortable, uncanny tension invades him (Sandberg). The use of the word 'atmosphere' might suggest psychasthenic moods and feelings perhaps and be a source of confusion; but with this *delusional atmosphere* we always find an 'objective something' there, even though quite vague, a something which lays the seed of objective validity and meaning. This general delusional atmosphere with all its vagueness of content must be unbearable. Patients obviously suffer terribly under it and to reach some definite idea at last is like being relieved from some enormous burden. Patients feel 'as if they have lost grip on things, they feel gross uncertainty which drives them instinctively to look for some fixed point to which they can cling. The achievement of this brings strength and comfort, and it is brought about only by forming an idea, as happens with healthy people in analogous circumstances. Whenever we find ourselves depressed, fearful or at a loss, the sudden clear consciousness of something, whether false or true, immediately has a soothing effect. As judgment gains in clarity, the feelings loosed by the situation will (ceteris paribus) dwindle in their force. Conversely no dread is worse than that of danger unknown' (Hagen). Experiences such as these give rise to convictions of persecution, of having committed crime, of being accused or, by contrast, of some golden age, transfiguration, sanctification, etc.

It is doubtful whether the foregoing analysis will hold in all cases. Content sometimes seems immediately present, vividly clear. In the former instances,

---

[1] Hagen, *Fixe Ideen in: Studien auf dem Gebiete der ärztlichen Seelenkunde* (Erlangen, 1870). Sandberg, *Allg. Z. Psychiatr.*, vol. 52.

however, it is certainly possible to wonder whether the patients have found any content adequate for their actual experience. We will try therefore to explore the original experience further, with its feelings and sensations rather than the content itself, though it is true our exploration can only be a limited one. The content in these cases is perhaps accidental; it is certainly not meant literally and is quite differently experienced from similar content in the case of a person whom we can fully understand.

Let us now try to imagine what the psychological significance is of this delusional experience of reality in which the environment offers a *world of new meanings*. All thinking is a thinking about meanings. If the meaning is perceived directly with the senses, if it is directly present in imagination and memory, the meaning has the character of reality. Perceptions are never mechanical responses to sense-stimuli; there is always at the same time a perception of meaning. A house is there for people to inhabit; people in the streets are following their own pursuits. If I see a knife, I see a tool for cutting. If I look at an unfamiliar tool from another culture, I may not see its precise meaning but I can appreciate it as a meaningfully shaped object. We may not be explicitly conscious of the interpretations we make when we perceive but nevertheless they are always present. Now, the *experiences of primary delusion are analogous to this seeing of meaning*, but the awareness of meaning undergoes a radical transformation. There is an immediate, intrusive knowledge of the meaning and it is this which is itself the delusional experience. If we distinguish the different sense-data in which meaning of this sort can be experienced, we can speak of delusional perception, delusional ideas, delusional memories, delusional awarenesses etc. In fact there is no kind of experience with a known object which we could not link with the word 'delusion' provided that at the level of meaning, awareness of meaning has become this experience of primary delusion (Kurt Schneider, G. Schmidt).[1]

We will now look more closely at delusional perceptions, delusional ideas, and delusional awarenesses:

(*aa*) *Delusional perceptions*. These may range from an experience of some vague meaning to clear, delusional observation and express delusions of reference.

Suddenly things seem to mean something quite different. The patient sees people in uniform in the street; they are Spanish soldiers. There are other uniforms; they are Turkish soldiers. Soldiers of all kinds are being concentrated here. There is a world war (this was before 1914). Then a man in a brown jacket is seen a few steps away. He is the dead Archduke who has resurrected. Two people in raincoats are Schiller and Goethe. There are scaffoldings up on some houses; the whole town is going to be demolished. Another patient sees a man in the street; she knows at once he is an old lover of hers; he looks quite different it is true; he has disguised himself with a

[1] Kurt Schneider, 'Eine Schwierigkeit im Wahnproblem', *Nervenarzt.*, vol. 11 (1938), p. 462. He recognises only delusional perception as a two-stage phenomenon and specifically distinguishes this from other sources of delusion, the 'delusional notions'.

wig and there are other changes. It is all a bit queer. A male patient says of such experiences—'everything is so dead certain that no amount of seeing to the contrary will make it doubtful'.

These are not considered interpretations but direct experiences of meaning while perception itself remains normal and unchanged. In other cases, particularly at the beginning of process disorders, no clear, definite meaning accompanies the perceptions. Objects, persons and events are simply eerie, horrifying, peculiar, or they seem remarkable, mystifying, transcendental. Objects and events signify something but nothing definite. *Delusional significance* of this sort appears in the folowing examples:

A patient noticed the waiter in the coffee-house; he skipped past him so quickly and uncannily. He noticed odd behaviour in an acquaintance which made him feel strange; everything in the street was so different, something was bound to be happening. A passer-by gave such a penetrating glance, he could be a detective. Then there was a dog who seemed hypnotised, a kind of mechanical dog made of rubber. There were such a lot of people walking about, something must surely be starting up against the patient. All the umbrellas were rattling as if some apparatus was hidden inside them.

In other cases patients have noticed transfigured faces, unusual beauty of landscape, brilliant golden hair, overpowering glory of the sunlight. Something must be going on; the world is changing, a new era is starting. Lights are bewitched and will not burn; something is behind it. A child is like a monkey; people are mixed up, they are imposters all, they all look unnatural. The house-signs are crooked, the streets look suspicious; everything happens so quickly. The dog scratches oddly at the door. 'I noticed particularly' is the constant remark these patients make, though they cannot say why they take such particular note of things nor what it is they suspect. First they want to get it clear to themselves.

The patients arrive at defining the meaning more clearly when there are *delusions of reference*. Here the objects and events perceived are experienced as having some obvious relation to the patient himself:

Gestures, ambiguous words provide 'tacit intimations'. All sorts of things are being conveyed to the patient. People imply quite different things in such harmless remarks as 'the carnations are lovely' or 'the blouse fits all right' and understand these meanings very well among themselves. People look at the patient as if they had something special to say to him.—'It was as if everything was being done to spite me; everything that happened in Mannheim happened in order to take it out of me.' People in the street are obviously discussing the patient. Odd words picked up in passing refer to him. In the papers, books, everywhere there are things which are specially meant for the patient, concern his own personal life and carry warnings or insults. Patients resist any attempt to explain these things as coincidence. These 'devilish incidents' are most certainly not coincidences. Collisions in the street are obviously intentional. The fact that the soap is now on the table and was not there before is obviously an insult.

The following is an account extracted from the report of a patient who went on working, while finding throughout the day all sorts of imaginary connections among otherwise quite real perceptions:

'I was hardly out of the house when somebody prowled round me, stared at me and tried to put a cyclist in the way. A few steps on, a schoolgirl smiled at me encouragingly.' He then arrived at his office and noticed leg-pulling and ragging by his colleagues . . . 'at 12 o'clock there were further insults, the time when the girls came from school; I tried hard to confine myself to just looking at them; I simply wanted to see a bevy of girls, not to make any gesture . . . but the lads wanted to make out I was after something immoral and they wanted to distort the facts against me but nothing could be further from my mind than to be a nuisance staring and frightening . . . in the middle of the street they imitated me and laughed straight in my face and in a hateful way they pushed humorous drawings my way. I was supposed to read likenesses to third persons from the faces . . . the lads talked about me afterwards at the police station . . . they fraternised with the workers . . . the nuisance of being stared at and pointed at went on during meals . . . before I entered my flat somebody always had to annoy me with some meaningless glance but the names of the police and the private people involved I did not know . . .' The patient objected to 'eye-language' used even by the judge who examined him. In the street 'the police tried to stalk me several times but I drove them away by my looks . . . they became a kind of hostile militia . . . all I could do was to stay on the defensive and never take the offensive with anybody.'

A fine example of delusional reference is provided by a 17-year-old patient reported by G. Schmidt.[1] She was suffering from a schizophrenic psychosis and recovered after a few months. There is a mass of detailed self-reference:

'My illness first showed itself in loss of appetite and a disgust for "serum". My periods stopped and there came a kind of sullenness. I didn't speak freely any more; I had lost interest; I felt sad, distraught and was startled when anyone spoke to me.

My father, who owned a restaurant, said to me the cookery examination (which was to take place next day) was only a trifle; he laughed in such an odd tone that I felt he was laughing at me. The customers were looking oddly at me too as if they had guessed something of my suicidal thoughts. I was sitting next to the cash desk, the customers were looking at me and then I thought perhaps I had taken something. For the last five weeks I had had the feeling that I had done something wrong; my mother had been looking at me sometimes in a funny, piercing way.

It was about 9.30 in the evening (she had seen people whom she feared would take her away). I got undressed after all. I lay in bed rigidly and made no move so they wouldn't hear me; I was listening hard for the least noise; I believed the three would get together again and tie me up.

In the morning I ran away; as I went across the square the clock was suddenly upside down; it had stopped upside down. I thought it was working on the other side; just then I thought the world was going to end; on the last day everything stops; then I saw a lot of soldiers on the street; when I came close, one always moved away; ah, I thought, they are going to make a report; they know when you are a 'wanted' person; they kept looking at me; I really thought the world was turning round me.

In the afternoon the sun did not seem to be shining when my thoughts were bad

[1] Gerhard Schmidt, Z. Neur., vol. 171 (1941), p. 570.

but came back when they were good. Then I thought cars were going the wrong way; when a car passed me I did not hear it. I thought there must be rubber underneath; large lorries did not rattle along any more; as soon as a car approached, I seemed to send out something that brought it to a halt . . . I referred everything to myself as if it were made for me . . . people did not look at me, as if they wanted to say I was altogether too awful to look at.

At the police station I had the impression that I wasn't at the station but in the Other World; one official looked like death himself. I thought he was dead and had to write on his typewriter until he had expiated his sins. Every time the bell rang I believed they were fetching away someone whose lifetime had ended. (Later I realised the ringing came from the typewriter as it reached the end of the line.) I waited for them to fetch me also. A young policeman had a pistol in his hand; I was afraid he wanted to kill me. I refused to drink the tea they brought me as I thought it was poisoned. I was waiting and longing to die . . . it was as on a stage, and marionettes are not human. I thought they were mere empty skins . . . the typewriter seemed upside down; there were no letters on it, only signs which I thought came from the Other World.

When I went to bed I thought someone else was in it already because the eiderdown was so bumpy; the bed felt as if people were lying in it already; I thought everybody was bewitched; I mistook the curtain for Aunt Helena; I found the black furniture uncanny; the lampshade over the bed moved continuously, figures kept on swirling round; towards morning I ran out of the bedroom and shouted 'What am I? I am the devil!' . . . I wanted to take my nightdress off and run out into the street, but my mother just caught me . . .

The illuminated signs of the town were very scanty—for the moment I did not think of the blackout due to the war; it seemed to me extraordinary; the glowing cigarette-ends of people were uncanny . . . something must be the matter; everything was looking at me; I felt I was brightly illuminated and visible when others were not . . .

At the clinic I found everything unnatural; I thought I was going to be used for something special; I felt like a guinea-pig; I thought the doctor was a murderer, because he had such black hair and a hook nose. Another man outside pushing an apple-cart seemed like a puppet. He was walking so hurriedly, just like in the pictures. . . .

Later at home things were changed, partly they were smaller; it was not so homely as before, it had become cold and strange. My father had got me a book; I thought it had been written specially for me; I did not think I had lived through all the scenes it described but it was more that they seemed meant for me. I was annoyed that now they knew all this.

Today I can see clearly how things really are; but then I always thought something unusual was up, even on the most trivial occasion. It was a real illness.'

Ideas of reference can also be experienced during hashish intoxication, and in a remote way resemble schizophrenic ideas of reference:

'Feelings of uncertainty spread; things lose their self-evident nature. The intoxicated person feels defeated and finds himself in a situation of distrust and defence. Even the most banal question sounds like an examination or an inquisition, and harmless laughter sounds like derision. An accidental glance leads to the reaction—"stop gawping at me". One constantly sees menacing faces, one senses traps, hears allusions. New powers seem to grow under the intoxication, and ideas of reference spread to the inflated ego (Fraenkel and Joel). What then happens, happens because of oneself, not to one's detriment, but purely for one's benefit.'

(*bb*) *Delusional ideas.* These give new colour and meaning to memory or may appear in the form of a sudden *notion*—'I could be King Ludwig's son'—which is then confirmed by a vivid memory of how when attending a parade the Kaiser rode by on his horse and looked straight at the patient.

A patient wrote: 'It suddenly occurred to me one night, quite naturally, self-evidently but insistently, that Miss L. was probably the cause of all the terrible things through which I have had to go these last few years (telepathic influences, etc.). I can't of course stand by all that I have written here, but if you examine it fairly you will see there is very little reflection about it; rather everything thrust itself on me, suddenly, and totally unexpectedly, though quite naturally. I felt as if scales had fallen from my eyes and I saw why life had been precisely as it was through these last years . . .'

(*cc*) *Delusional awarenesses.* These constitute a frequent element particularly in florid and acute psychoses. Patients possess a knowledge of immense and universal happenings, sometimes without any trace of clear perceptual experience of them, and when there is sensory experience, pure awarenesses will often intermingle among the forms in which the actual content is given. When there is delusional experience of some emotional depth, content will usually appear for the most part in the form of awareness. For example:

A girl was reading the Bible. She read about the waking of Lazarus from the dead. She immediately felt herself to be Mary. Martha was her sister, Lazarus a sick cousin. She vividly experienced the events about which she read just as if they were her own experience. (The vividness was a feeling rather than a sensory vividness) (Klinke).

From the phenomenological point of view the delusional experience is always the same: besides sensory experience of illusory, hallucinatory or pseudo-hallucinatory contents, there is a kind of experience where sensory richness is not essentially changed, but the recognition of certain objects is linked with an experience totally different from normal. The mere thinking about things gives them a special reality—which does not have to become a sensory experience. The new and special significance may be associated as much with thoughts as with things perceived.

All primary experience of delusion is an experience of meaning, and simple, 'one-stage' delusional notions do not exist. For example, a patient suddenly has the notion that a fire has broken out in a far-away town (Swedenborg). This surely happens only through the meaning he draws from inner visions that crowd in on him with the character of reality?

A basic feature of the first experience of delusional meaning is 'the establishment of an unfounded reference' (Gruhle). Significance appears unaccountably, suddenly intruding into the psychic life. Later the identical experience of significance is repeated, though in other contexts. The trail is blazed and the preparedness for the significant experience then permeates almost all perceived contents. The now dominant delusion motivates the apperceptive schema for all future percepts (G. Schmidt).

### (c) *Incorrigibility of delusion*

Delusional experiences proper, false perceptions and all the other primary experiences we have so far described give rise to errors of judgment. They are the source for the great variety of delusional syndromes which we encounter in individual patients. After the creation of the primary delusion from his experiences, the patient often takes *a further step*, and *holds on* to his delusion as truth. He will maintain it as such in the face of all other experiences to the contrary and against all argument. He does this with a conviction far beyond normal, even perhaps stamping down on any occasional, initial doubt he may have himself.

*Psychological digression.* Normal convictions are formed in a context of social living and common knowledge. Immediate experience of reality survives only if it can fit into the frame of what is socially valid or can be critically tested. Experience of reality leads us to judgments of reality. Individual experience can always be corrected but the total context of experience is something stable and can hardly be corrected at all. The source for incorrigibility therefore is not to be found in any single phenomenon by itself but in the human situation as a whole, which nobody would surrender lightly. If socially accepted reality totters, people become adrift. What is left to them? A set of habits, survivals, chance events? Reality becomes reduced to an immediate and shifting present.

Incorrigibility however has another source as well. The fanaticism with which opinions are held in a discussion or over long periods of time does not always prove that their content is really believed in, but only that in the holder's judgment such opinions will have some desired effect, sometimes no more than his personal advantage, to which his instinctive drives unconsciously direct him. It is the behaviour which will show clearly enough what is held to be reality; since only the reality that is actually believed will compel to action. Fanatic opinions that are not believed in can be dropped at any time and in this sense they become corrigible. But genuine reality judgments which are the expression of a believed-in reality and according to which people in fact conduct themselves (e.g. belief in hell) are extremely difficult to correct. Should they be so, it will mean a revolution in the individual's whole conception of life.

Normal mistakes are also very largely incorrigible. It is astonishing how most people tend to maintain the realities they believe in during a discussion, although the mistakes they are making seem to the knowledgeable person little else but 'sheer delusion'. 'Delusions' on a national scale, as commonly discussed, are not really delusions but mass-beliefs that change with the times and are typical illusions. Only those that reach the highest ranks of absurdity deserve the term delusion—belief in witches, for example—and even that need not be a delusion in the psychopathological sense.

Speaking methodologically, the concept of incorrigibility does not belong to phenomenology but to the study of psychological performance and the psychology of meaningful connections. Phenomenologically, we have only to decide whether there is more than one kind of incorrigibility which may indicate different phenomena as the source.

We may sum up the position briefly as follows: *Errors in normal people* are the errors common to their social group. Conviction has a root in the fact that *all* believe. Correction of belief comes about not on the ground of any logical argument but through historical change. *Delusion-like errors* on the part of individuals always imply some segregation from what all believe (i.e. 'what one believes') and in this case the incorrigibility cannot be distinguished psychologically from the unwavering force of a true insight, asserting itself against a whole world. *Delusion proper* is incorrigible because of an *alteration in the personality*, the nature of which we are so far unable to describe, let alone formulate into a concept, though we are driven to make some such presupposition. The decisive criterion seems to be not the 'intensity' of the direct evidence, but the maintaining of what is evident to the patient in the face of subsequent reflection and external criticism. Delusion cannot be grasped as a change in one of the thought processes nor as an alteration in any one of our activities, nor as mere confusion, nor is it the same as the normal fanaticism of dogmatic people. One need try only to suppose an ideal case of a paranoic with a high level of critical insight—a born scientist, perhaps—who shows incorrigibility as a pure phenomenon in the midst of his general scepticism—well, he would no longer be a paranoic! Patients are in a state of clear consciousness and have continual possibilities for testing their ideas but correction of their delusion does not come. We cannot say the patient's whole world has changed, because to a very large extent he can conduct himself like a healthy person in thinking and behaving. But his world has changed to the extent that a changed knowledge of reality so rules and pervades it that any correction would mean a collapse of Being itself, in so far as it is for him his actual awareness of existence. Man cannot believe something that negates his existence. Such formulations, however, are only trying to make us understand what in its essence cannot be understood—i.e. the specific schizophrenic incorrigibility. We can only hold on to the fact that it is found where formal thinking is maintained, the capacity for thought undamaged and where there is not the slightest clouding of consciousness.

On the other hand we should look at *what* it is that is actually incorrigible. The patient's behaviour will show this more readily than any conversation with him. Reality for him does not always carry the same meaning as that of normal reality. With these patients persecution does not always appear quite like the experience of people who are in fact being persecuted; nor does their jealousy seem like that of some justifiably jealous person, although there is often some similarity of behaviour. Hence the attitude of the patient to the content of his delusion is peculiarly inconsequent at times. The content of the delusion strikes one as a symbol for something quite different; sometimes content changes constantly though the delusional meaning remains the same.

Belief in reality can range through all degrees, from a mere play with possibilities via a double reality—the empirical and the delusional—to unequivocal attitudes in which the delusional content reigns as the sole and absolute reality. During the play of possibilities, each individual content may perhaps be corrected but not the attitude as a whole and once the delusional reality has become absolute, incorrigibility is also absolute.

Once we are clear that the criteria for delusion proper lie in the *primary experience of delusion* and in *the change of the personality*, we can see that a delusion may be correct in content without ceasing to be a delusion, for instance —that there is a world-war. Such correctness is accidental and uncommon— mostly it appears in delusions of jealousy. A correct thought ordinarily arises from normal experience and is therefore valid for others. Delusion however arises from a primary experience not accessible to others and it cannot be substantiated. We can recognise it only by the way in which the patient subsequently tries to give it ground. A delusion of jealousy, for instance, may be recognised by its typical characteristics without our needing to know whether the person has genuine ground for his jealousy or not. The delusion does not cease to be a delusion although the spouse of the patient is in fact unfaithful—sometimes only as the result of the delusion.

### (d) *Elaboration of the delusion*

Thinking accompanies the first step which brings delusion about. This may be no more than the unsystematic, blurred thinking of the acute psychoses and states of chronic defect, yet even here patients look for some kind of connection. Or the thinking may be more systematic as in the case of better-preserved chronic conditions. Here the thought works over the delusion on the basis of the primary experiences, trying to link them harmoniously with real perceptions and the patient's actual knowledge. To do this sometimes calls for the full strength of an intelligent personality. In this way a *delusional system* is constructed which in its own context is comprehensible, sometimes extremely closely argued and unintelligible only in its ultimate origins, the primary experience.[1] These delusional systems are objective meaningful structures and methodologically we can assign them to the psychology of creativity. (Werkpsychologie).

### (e) *Delusion proper and delusion-like idea*

The term delusion should properly only be given to those delusions which go back to primary pathological experiences as their source, and which demand for their explanation a change in the personality. As such, they constitute a group of primary symptoms. The term delusion-like ideas is reserved by us for those so-called 'delusions' that emerge comprehensibly from other

---

[1] Examples of closely argued delusional systems may be found in Wollay, *Erklärungen der Tollheiten von Haslam* (Leipzig, 1889), pp. 14 ff. Schreber, *Denkwürdigkeiten eines Nervenkranken* (Leipzig, 1903).

psychic events and which can be traced back psychologically to certain affects, drives, desires and fears. We have no need here to invoke some personality change but on the contrary can fully understand the phenomenon on the basis of the permanent constitution of the personality (Anlage) or of some transient emotional state. Among these delusion-like ideas we put the transient deceptions due to false perception, etc.; the 'delusions' of mania and depression ('delusions' of sin, destitution, nihilistic 'delusion', etc.)[1] and over-valued ideas.

*Over-valued ideas* are what we term those convictions that are strongly toned by affect which is understandable in terms of the personality and its history. Because of this strong affect the personality identifies itself with ideas which are then wrongly taken to be true. Psychologically there is no difference between scientific adherence to truth, passionate political or ethical conviction and the retention of over-valued ideas. The contrast between these phenomena lies in the falsity of the over-valued idea. This latter occurs in psychopathic and even in healthy people; it may also appear as so-called 'delusion'—'delusions' of invention, jealousy, or of querulant behaviour etc. Such over-valued ideas must be clearly differentiated from delusion proper. They are isolated notions that develop comprehensibly out of a given personality and situation. Delusions proper are the vague crystallisations of blurred delusional experiences and diffuse, perplexing self-references which cannot be sufficiently understood in terms of the personality or the situation; they are much more the symptoms of a disease process that can be identified by the presence of other symptoms as well.

## (f) The problem of metaphysical delusions

Patients may display their delusions in some supra-natural mode and such experiences cannot be adjudged true or untrue, correct or false. Even when empirical reality is concerned it is difficult enough to be decisive, though some evaluation can usually be made. We can study the metaphysical experience in its schizophrenic manifestations as it is conditioned by the morbid process and yet realise that the metaphysical intuitions (the images themselves, the symbols) that have arisen in the course of these experiences have acquired cultural significance in the minds of normal people for quite different reasons.

For us reality is the reality of time and space. Past, present and future are real for normal people in the form of 'no longer', 'not yet' and 'now' but the constant flux of time makes everything seem unreal, the past is no longer, the future is not yet and the present disappears irresistibly. *Temporal reality* is not *reality itself*. This reality lies athwart time and all metaphysical awareness is experience and affirmation of this reality. Where it is truly felt, we call it faith. When it is externalised into something tangibly existing in this world (where it becomes mere reality again) we talk of superstition. We can tell how much people need this absolute hold on the reality of the world when we see the abysmal despair into which they fall should they lose it.

[1] Depressive delusions can only be attributed to affect comprehensibly if we presuppose in severe melancholia a temporary change in the psychic life as a whole.

Superstition we might say is the 'delusion' of normal people. Only faith, transcending in the world, can by virtue of its own unconditioned living and acting be sure of the Being which all our existence symbolises. Only faith can hover above both without fear of falling into bottomless confusion.

The shattering of the self is said to be mirrored in the schizophrenic experience of the end of the world. This is not sufficiently explicit. Experiencing the end of the world and all that this implies involves a deep religious experience—of a symbolic truth that has served human existence for thousands of years. We have to regard this experience as such and not merely as some perverted psychological or psychopathological phenomenon if we really want to understand it. Religious experience remains what it is, whether it occurs in saint or psychotic or whether the person in whom it occurs is both at once.

Delusion is the morbid manifestation of knowledge and error in regard to empirical reality, as it is of faith and superstition in regard to metaphysical reality.

## § 5. Feelings and Affective States

*Psychological Preface.* There is fairly general agreement as to what we mean by sensation, perception, image, thought, also perhaps what we mean by instinctual urge and act of will. But confusion still reigns regarding the word and concept 'feeling'. We may still ask what is meant by it in any individual case. Commonly the term 'feeling' is given to any psychic event that does not clearly belong to the phenomena of object-awareness, nor to instinctual excitation and volitional acts. All undeveloped, undefined psychic manifestations tend to get called 'feeling'. That is, everything intangible, analytically elusive, everything for which we can find no other name. Someone feels he does not care, or that something is not right. He feels that the room is too small or that everything is clear or he feels uneasy, etc. *This diverse set of phenomena* which we term 'feelings' has never been satisfactorily analysed from the psychological point of view. We do not know what constitutes the basic element or elements nor do we know how to classify, whereas with sensation the basic elements have been both well examined and classified. There are very few scientific investigations into feeling and we will mention them when necessary. On the other hand there is an extensive literature on the pathological phenomena of object-awareness as well as on the perversion of instinct.

It is difficult to know how we should set about it. However, psychologists[1] have laid some foundations for the analysis of feelings and we can get an orientation from the leading schools of thought, a methodological approach which will help us to evaluate more precisely what has been established so far. Extensive analysis of every different kind of feeling would only end in a vast array of trivialities.[2] First therefore we will review *the different ways* in which feelings have been *classified*:

[1] Geiger, 'Das Bewusstsein von Gefühlen', *Munch. phil. Ab.* (Th. Lipps zum 60 Geburtstag gewidmet). 'Über Stimmungseinfühlung', *Z. Asth.* (1911). Kulpe, 'Zur psychologie der Gefühle', *6 Psychol. Kongr. Genf.* (1909).

[2] For psychological discussion on feelings generally, at a superficial level, see Hoffding and Jodl; Nahlowsky, *Das Gefühlsleben*, 3rd edn. (Leipzig, 1907); Ribot: *Psychologie der Gefühle* (Paris, 1896) (in German, 1903).

1. *Phenomenologically*, according to the different modes in which they appear:

(*a*) Feelings that are an aspect of *conscious personality*, and define the self; these are broadly contrasted with feelings that *lend colour to object-awareness*, e.g. my own sadness in contrast to the sadness of a landscape (Geiger).

(*b*) Feelings that can to some extent be *grouped in opposites*; Wundt, for instance, distinguished pleasure and displeasure, tension and relaxation, excitement and calm. There are a number of such opposites: e.g. profound and shallow feelings (Lipps); feelings of shatterment, deep pain on the one hand and feelings of petulance or for the comic on the other.

(*c*) Feelings may be *without an object* and contentless (i.e. how one feels) or they may be *directed upon some object* and classified accordingly.

2. *According to their object* (Meinong, Witasek). Here the contrast is between phantasy feelings directed on to *suppositions* and reality *feelings directed upon actual objects*. Feelings of value may be directed on the subject himself or on to someone else; they may be positive or negative (pride-submissiveness, love-hate). Any classification by content, e.g. social feelings, patriotic feelings, family or religious feelings etc., leads not so much to a classification of feelings as to a classification of the innumerable contents, to which feelings of value may be attached. Language has uncounted resources at its disposal for this end but these are better suited for concrete description than for the purpose of a general phenomenological analysis.

3. *According to source*. The classification is made in accordance with different *levels* of psychic life, i.e. a distinction is made between localised feeling-sensations, vital feelings involving the whole body, psychic feelings (e.g. sadness, joy), and spiritual feelings (a state of grace) (Scheler, Kurt Schneider).

4. *According to the biological purpose*, the vital significance of the feelings, e.g. pleasurable feelings express the advancement of biological purposes, displeasurable feelings their frustration.

5. *Particular* feelings directed on specific objects or partial aspects of the whole are distinguished from *all-inclusive feelings*, where the separate elements are fused into some temporary whole, which is then called *the feeling-state*. Such feeling-states are characterised in various ways; for instance, there are irritable feeling-states, states of sensibility and of diminished or increased excitability. A 'feeling of being alive' arises on the basis of organic sensations as an expression of the vital state, of drives, needs, tendencies and of the organism as a whole.

6. The old and useful classification into feeling, affect and mood is based on the difference of *intensity* and *duration* of feeling. *Feelings* are individual, unique, and radical commotions of the psyche. *Affects* are momentary and complex emotional processes of great intensity with conspicuous bodily accompaniments and sequelae. *Moods* are states of feeling or frames of mind that come about with prolonged emotion which while it lasts colours the whole psychic life.

7. *Feelings* are distinguished from *sensations*. Feelings are states of the self (sad or cheerful); sensations are elements in the perception of the environment and of one's own body (colour, pitch, temperature, organic sensations). Sensations, however, show a whole scale of differences; they range from those that are purely object-bound to subjective bodily states. Vision and hearing are purely object-bound while organic sensations, vital sensations, sensations of stance and balance all predominantly refer to subjective bodily states. Between these two poles we find sensations referable to bodily states at the same time as they are object-bound, e.g. sensations of skin,

taste, smell. Hunger, thirst, fatigue, and sexual excitation are simultaneously sensations (elements in bodily perception) as well as feelings (in the form of pleasure and displeasure). Hence we can talk of *feeling-sensations* (Stumpf). Bodily sensations as feelings are at the same time aspects of instinctual drive, as with hunger, which impels to food, fatigue, which impels to rest, and sexual sensations, which impel to contact. Thus sensation, feeling, affect and drive show themselves an integrated whole.

In classifying abnormal feeling-states we need to make a preliminary distinction as follows: (1) those affective states which *emerge in understandable fashion* from some experience, even though they appear abnormally exaggerated and heavily coloured; (2) those affective states which defeat understanding and arise endogenously *as a psychological irreducible.* Explanation can only point to sources beyond consciousness (physical events, phases, periods, etc.). This helps us to distinguish *normal* homesickness, for instance, from *excessive but understandable* homesickness (sometimes leading to violent behaviour in young girls away from home), and both of these from depression *without external cause,* which is then subjectively interpreted as homesickness.

*Abnormal feeling-states of an all-embracing character* are represented by a rich terminology, e.g. grief, melancholy, cheerfulness, merriment, accidie, etc. Certain typical states can also be recognised: natural cheerfulness, bubbling hypomanic merriment, the gloomy mood of depression, the euphoria of General Paralysis with its contented complacency and the silly, awkward blandness of hebephrenia. Out of all the host of trivial feeling-states our aim is to mark down only those which are the more typical and noteworthy.

### (a) Changes in bodily feeling

In physical illness bodily feeling is bound up with all the innumerable sensations which general medicine recognises as symptoms: e.g. the fear of the cardiac patient, the suffocation of the asthmatic attack, the sleepiness of encephalitis, the general malaise of an initial infection.

Bodily feelings are basic to the feeling-state as a whole. In the psychoses and personality disorders there is often a change in feelings for which it is difficult to have empathy, particularly with schizophrenia. Self-description, however, gives us only a little information about the great variety of these vital and organic feelings.

*Kurt Schneider* sees a change in *vital feeling* as the core of cyclothymic *depression.* The misery of these vital depressions is located specifically in the limbs, forehead, chest or stomach:

A patient said: 'I always have an oppression in my stomach and neck; it feels as if it would never go away, it seems fixed; it makes me feel as if I would burst, there is so much pain in my chest.' Another patient described feelings of pressure in the chest and abdomen and said 'it is more a sadness'; another, speaking of her chest, said 'I have such a terrible misery there'. Besides this very physical sadness one will usually find other complaints of vital distress (Kurt Schneider).

## (b) Changes in feelings of capacity

We always have some feeling of our capacity; this gives us confidence in ourselves without any explicit awareness of the underlying feeling. In depression, patients get a *feeling of insufficiency*, one of their most common complaints. In part these feelings are an awareness of real insufficiency and in part they are unfounded, primary feelings. Awareness of being useless for the real world, of being incompetent and incapable of action, of being unable to make a decision, of wavering, of being clumsy, of not being able to think or understand any more, all these are the burden of many abnormal states, though real inefficiency need not exist; it can, however, be present in a moderate degree. Such complaints often appear with symptoms of an objective retardation, and are experienced as subjective retardation.

## (c) Apathy

This is the term given to absence of feeling. If this absence is complete, as can happen in acute psychoses, the patient is fully conscious and orientated, sees, hears, observes and remembers, but he lets everything pass him by with the same total indifference; happiness, pleasure, something positive in which he is involved, danger, sorrow, annihilation are all the same. He remains 'dead with wakeful eyes'. In this condition there is no incentive to act; apathy brings about aboulia. It seems as if that one aspect of psychic life we call object-awareness has become isolated; there is only the mere grasp of reason on the world as an object. We can compare it to a photographic plate. Reason can portray its environment but cannot appreciate it. This absence of feeling shows itself objectively in the patient not taking food, in a passive indifference to being hurt, burnt, etc. The patient would die if we did not keep him alive with feeding and nursing care. The apathy of these acute states must be distinguished from the dullness of certain abnormal personalities who are constantly at the mercy of innumerable feelings, only crude in quality.

## (d) The feeling of having lost feeling

This feeling of having no feeling is a remarkable phenomenon. It appears in certain personality disorders (psychopaths), in depressives and in the initial stages of all processes. It is not exactly apathy but a distressful *feeling of not having any feeling*. Patients complain that they no longer feel gladness or pain, they no longer love their relatives, they feel indifferent to everything. Food does not gratify: if food is bad they do not notice. They feel empty, devastated, dead. All 'joie de vivre' has left them. They complain they cannot participate in things, they have no interest. A schizophrenic patient said. 'There is nothing left; I am cold as a block of ice and as stiff; I am frozen hard' (Fr. Fischer). Patients suffer very much from this subjectively felt void. But the very fear which they imagine they do not feel can be recognised objectively in their bodily symptoms. Mild cases will complain about numbness of feeling, feelings that have got damped down, feelings of estrangement.

*(e) Changes in the feeling-tone of perception*

First there is a simple *increase* in the feeling-tone:

'Thoughts that otherwise I would have felt as merely unpleasant and brushed aside now brought a distressing, almost physical feeling of fear. The smallest pang of conscience grew into a near-physical fear, felt as a pressure in the head' '(Encephalitis lethargica,' Mayer-Gross and Steiner).

The following description of an early phase in an acute psychosis shows increased feeling-tone towards normal objects:

'The covered bath made a weird impression on me . . . the keys on the attendant's key-ring with their double hooks could, I felt, be used to pry out the eyes. I waited for the heavy key-ring to fall from the attendant's belt on to my head and when it kept clattering on the ground I couldn't bear it. The cells to which I was hastily consigned every evening and where I was left to my own devices were I felt deeply insulting in their emptiness and absence of every comfort and decoration . . . most painful of all were the feelings aroused by the wild, swearing talk of the patients. I really suffered from this far more than I would have done had I been well' (Forel).

There are also *alterations* in the characteristic *feeling-tone of perceived objects.* Similar changes may occur with mere sensations and appear as abnormal *feeling-sensations:*

'The feeling of touch has become most unpleasant. When I touch wood (they have given me poisoned pencils), wool or paper, I feel a burning sensation run through all my limbs. I get the same burning feeling in front of the mirror. It "throws out something" which rinses me with an acid feeling (that is why I avoid the mirror). The best things to touch are china, metal, small silver spoons, fine linen or my own body in certain places. . . .' 'In addition the obtrusive luminosity of a group of colours (flowers at a distance) strikes my senses as devilish and poisonous. They have a painful emanation, for instance, red, brown, green or black (printer's ink, deep shadows, black flies). Lilac, on the other hand, yellow and white are all pleasant to look at' (Gruhle).

'All my senses enjoy things more. Taste is different and much more intense than before' (Rümke).

*All the contents* of our object-awareness, forms, figures, nature, landscape and other people, have these characteristic feeling-tones for us. We can speak of a 'physiognomy of things' which expresses their psychic essence. We only have a very summary knowledge of the changes that may take place. In one instance the patient spoke of the outer world as having grown cold and strange. 'I can see the sun shining, but I do not feel as if it is'. In other cases a positive feeling for objects is present. A patient has a great feeling of tranquillity and his view of the environment is clear and full of feeling. Everything is pregnant with meaning, solemn and wonderful. He enjoys unthinkingly the impression of a world divine and far-removed (as in light fever, in 'periodic states', under opium, etc.). Nature is marvellous; the golden age is here; the landscape might be a picture by Thoma or H. von Marées. The sun is incomparably beautiful. (All this at the beginning of a psychosis.) Or we may find the patients feel the objects they perceive are ghastly, spookish, thrilling or horrific.

'Nature seemed infinitely more beautiful than before, warmer, grander and calmer. There was a more brilliant light in the air, the blue of the sky was deeper, the cloud-play more impressive, the contrast of light and shadow was much sharper. The landscape was all so clear, so brightly coloured and so full of depth. . .' (Rümke).

*Empathic feelings* towards other people must be classed as a special type among these feelings ascribed to objects. We may observe how patients either suffer from abnormally strong empathy or complain that people appear to them like automata or soul-less machines.

### (*f*) *Unattached feelings* (*free-floating feeling*)

The elementary break-through of experiences, which are not understandable in their genesis, is manifested in unattached feelings. If they are to become meaningful to the subject, these feelings must first search for an object or try to create one. The feelings simply arise in the first place and remain in force though they may never find an object. For instance, unattached anxiety is very common in depressive states, so is a contentless euphoria in manic states, so is obscure erotic excitement in early puberty, so are the feelings roused at the start of a pregnancy and in the early stages of a psychosis. Driven by an almost inescapable need to give some content to such feelings, patients will often supply some such content on their own. It is a sign of critical insight if feelings are actually described as lacking in content. Some of these contentless feelings are as follows:

1. *Anxiety* is both common and painful. Whereas fear is directed towards something, anxiety is free-floating and unattached. We can differentiate a vital anxiety as a specific feeling-sensation in the heart, the anxiety of angina pectoris, or as an anxiety of suffocation (e.g. the breathlessness in decompensated circulatory conditions). But anxiety may also be a primary psychic state, all-pervasive and dominating, analogous to vital anxiety and involving existence as a whole. There is every degree from contentless, powerful anxiety that leads to a clouding of consciousness and ruthless acts of violence against oneself or others, down to a slight, anxious tension where the anxiety is experienced as alien to the self and inexplicable. Anxiety is linked with physical sensations such as pressure, suffocation, tightness. It is often localised—precordial anxiety, for instance; sometimes too in the head. A patient felt the urge to poke into it physically as he might poke a painful tooth with a toothpick. But the existential anxiety, which is a fundamental of our human life as it manifests itself in marginal situations and which is a source of Existence itself, can no longer be grasped phenomenologically.

2. Anxiety is usually linked with a strong *feeling of restlessness* but this emotional state of inward excitement can occur on its own without anxiety. Retrospectively patients will call this feeling a 'nervous excitement' or 'fever'.

In a mild degree the state may occur in the form of a feeling that one has to do something or that one has not finished something; or it may be a feeling that one has to look for something or that one has to come into the clear about something. In florid psychoses this feeling of restlessness may be heightened to tension and a sense of oppression. Patients feel they cannot stand the massive weight of impressions any longer and want only distraction and peace.

A schizophrenic patient in an initial phase described his restlessness as new and different from the usual sort in which one cannot work, has to get up often or go for a walk. He said it was more tangible, so to speak; it pervaded his whole being and swallowed it up. He ran up and down in the room; he felt he could not escape. Going for a walk was quite out of the question in this state. 'It tortures me more than anything else in the world; I can't get out of its reach; I want to tear myself away but I can't; it only gets worse; an urge comes to smash everything to bits but I can't trust myself to start with something small; everything else would follow. I would start to lash around; if I only threw a glass on the floor, everything else would come on its own; the power of stopping myself is wholly undermined; I find it so hard to hold back I wish sometimes "if only it were all over".'

3. Abnormal *feelings of happiness*[1] are complicated by dimly experienced meanings which do not become objectively clear to the patient. They may range from purely sensuous feelings of pleasure to mystical ecstasies of a religious character. Feelings of sublimity[2] occur as phases in psychasthenics and as states of ecstatic intoxication in schizophrenic patients. Patients become filled with a remarkable enthusiasm; are touched deeply by everything; find everything moving and meaningful. During convalescence from illness, in mild feverish conditions, tuberculosis, etc., soft, world-embracing, sentimental states may occur. Schizophrenic experiences are described as follows:

'I woke up one morning with the most blissful feeling that I had risen from the dead or was newly born. I felt supernatural delight, an overflowing feeling of freedom from everything earthly . . . brilliant feelings of happiness made me ask "am I the sun? Who am I?" . . . "I must be a shining child of God" . . . "Uncle A. changed into God will fetch me . . . we shall fly straight into the sun, the home of all those risen from the dead . . . in my blissful state I sang and shouted; I refused to eat and no longer needed to eat; I was waiting for Paradise and to feast on its fruits' (Gruhle).

'Light clouds lifted me . . . it was as if every moment more and more the spirit was unwound from its bonds; a nameless delight and gratitude took hold of my heart . . . an entirely new and heavenly life began in me . . . I was enormously cheerful, I looked transfigured . . . I felt extraordinarily well and delighted with myself . . . my condition at that time was to be envied . . . I had a true foretaste of heaven in myself . . . my voice became clear and bright and I was always singing . . .' (Engelken).

Another patient called his rare feelings a 'lust of the soul'. He felt it to be divine and the content of eternal bliss. Such patients enjoy an entirely self-contained state of invincible delight, though bodily sensations appear to play a larger part than usual.

[1] H. C. Rümke, *Zur Phänomenologie u. Klinik des Glücksgefühle* (Berlin, 1924).
[2] Janet, *Psychasthenie*, vol. I, pp. 388 ff.

A schizophrenic patient in the early phases of his illness distinguished three types of happiness: (1) 'intuitive happiness'—in which he is productive; it is for him a full-blown and continual jubilation; symbolically he sees it as a sphere out of which other spheres emerge as a single solid mass; (2) 'bliss'—which is on a different level. It is like floating; awareness of the body is faint, he stands above it; (3) while 'intuitive happiness' comes often and 'bliss' is rare, he has once had an attack of happiness on the same level as the first type but this is better expressed symbolically as an ever-rising wave, which spirals upwards while imposing masses pile up one on the other. The feeling of happiness crescendoes . . . bliss, on the other hand, is a contrasting peace. It remains quite independent and contentless. Physical happiness is there alongside the psychic happiness but the physical remains more on the surface' . . . He felt as if the wave of happiness was at once dark on the outside, bright and empty within, a mere skin. It seemed something always straining higher and higher, existing for itself alone and with no relationship to anything. It faded out quickly in the end and left a state of psychic exhaustion. The feeling of happiness was contentless but bright; the other experiences of happiness were not so fine-spun, but much more articulate. The patient felt he could not stand this state again; he said it would be unbearable because it came from within and would destroy him bodily.

The following case illustrates how feelings of happiness link up with 'delusions of reference' and become a source for such phenomena: 'It seemed as if everyone could see how happy I was and as if seeing me made others happy. I seemed something divine; older people at the station kept looking into my compartment; each did his best to catch my eye; officers, officials, families with their children all ran in front of me hoping I would look at them. That is all very fine, I said . . . but I must know who and what I am . . . am I no longer myself, am I altered? Then I cried because I always had to be moving on, yet I felt infinitely happy. Even the animals were glad when they saw me; swans stretched their wings out in honour of me . . .' (Rümke).

### (g) The growth of private worlds from unattached feelings

These new and unfamiliar feelings press for some understanding on the part of the person who experiences them. Countless possibilities are contained in them which can be realised only when reflection, imagination and formative thought have created some kind of coherent world. There is therefore always a path which leads from these unimaginable experiences of happiness towards an attempt to render them precise. The experience of blissful feelings starts with a crystal clarity of sight though there is no real, clear content to communicate; the patients delightedly believe that they have grasped the profoundest of meanings; concepts such as timelessness, world, god and death become enormous revelations which when the state has subsided cannot be reproduced or described in any way—they were after all nothing but feelings.

Nerval gives a self-description which shows this *feeling of crystal-clear sight*, of profound penetration into the essence of things: 'It struck me I knew everything; everything was revealed to me, all the secrets of the world were mine during those spacious hours'. . . . A patient wrote: 'I seemed to see everything so clearly and distinctly as if I had a new and remarkable understanding' (Gruhle). Another patient said: 'It was as if I had some special sense like second-sight; as if I could perceive what I and others had never before been able to perceive'. (K. Schneider).

The patient of mine who described his three types of happiness while he was still critical and able to view his experiences without any delusion formation, later on developed other mystical and religious experiences from these. He sensed the attacks as 'metaphysical experiences' in so far as they contained 'a character of the infinite'. He also had certain objective experiences (vivid awarenesses, etc.) and said of them: 'I see something of infinite greatness, something that makes me shiver.' One day he said he had 'experienced God' and that this was the 'climax of his life'. He had 'obtained his meaning'. It had lasted a good hour. Emanations came from him and 'his soul expanded'. Excitement was incredibly strong. Finally there was peace and bliss with God and God poured into him. Comparing his former experiences of happiness with this he put the experiences of God alongside the happiness which seemed like an ever-rising wave, only now the crest had detached itself and become a sphere, expanding into the infinite. The experience had a 'cosmic character'. He said the symbolic significance was different from that of the earlier experiences of happiness. God was the obvious content but only as a form that could be felt. The patient said everything was quite incomparable, unimaginable, and had nothing in common with his ordinary percepts.... He made other formulations such as 'I come to God, not He to me. I am streaming forth ... it seems as if I might embrace the whole world but stay outside myself as if my spirit stepped forth to embrace God'.

*Feelings of absolution* are often linked with these feelings of happiness, this clarity of vision and this experience of God; the patient then quickly passes from this sphere of feeling down into concrete delusional ideas. Patients feel freed from sin; they feel holy, children of God and eventually Messiahs, prophets and madonnas.

These feeling-states are found not only in the early experiences of schizophrenia. They also occur in toxic states (due to opium, mescalin, etc.) and they make a classic appearance in the brief moments before an epileptic seizure; nor can they be wholly banned from the fields of normal experience, that is, no other specific symptom seems present. We cannot class all the elaborate descriptions of mystic ecstasies as psychiatric states.

Dostoevski gave repeated descriptions of his epileptic auras: 'And I felt that heaven came down to earth and engulfed me; I experienced God as a deep and lofty truth; I felt invaded by Him. "Yes, there is a God," I shouted; after that I do not know what happened. You can have no idea of the marvellous feelings that pervade an epileptic a second before his attack. I do not know whether they last seconds or hours but believe me I would not exchange them for all the lovely things that life can give.'

'Yes, one such moment is worth a lifetime ... in these few moments I understand the profound and wonderful saying: "there should be Time no longer"'.

'There are seconds when suddenly you feel the one eternal harmony that fills all existence. It is as if you suddenly feel the whole of nature within yourself and say: yes, this is the truth ... it is not only love, it is more than love; the clarity of feeling and the overwhelmingness of the joy are terrifying. In these five seconds I live a lifetime and would give my whole life for them ... development has no point since the goal is reached....'

The awakening of new worlds in the schizophrenic transformation of the individual goes along with an alienation of the natural world. Patients feel they have lost contact with things. They feel distant and lonely. 'What is there in the world? I don't seem to belong to it any more' (Fr. Fischer).

## § 6. URGE, DRIVE AND WILL

*Psychological preface.* Here, as before, we shall deal only with the phenomena of actual experience, and not with any mechanisms outside consciousness. Such mechanisms, e.g. motor mechanisms, carry into effect the instinctual impulses and volitions which we experience and help them to outward expression; they give these experiences simple effectiveness. Volitional impulses that come into being outside consciousness are either inwardly effective (as well-defined memory images) or externally effective (as motor performances). We will deal with the latter when we come to the chapter on objective phenomena. Here we are concerned only with the direct subjective experience as such.

In regard to the experience of instinctual drive and volition[1] psychology only gives us a few elementary concepts. From an over-all picture of the phenomenology of these experiences, we can visualise them as arranged in a *progressive series*, subject to interruption by the appearance of qualitatively new elements. Thus we can distinguish the different experiences of primary, contentless, non-directional *urge*; of natural *instinctual drive* unconsciously directed towards some target; and of the *volitional act* itself which has a consciously conceived goal and is accompanied with an awareness of the necessary means and consequences.

Urges, instinctual activity, purposeful ideas compete with each other as *motivations*; distinct from these motivations which provide the material as it were, we find *decision* which comes after weighing-up, wavering and conflict. This is the personal 'I will' or 'I will not'. This *volitional awareness* is an irreducible phenomenon, found alongside the experience of *instinctual activity* and the experience of being at *variance* or *in opposition*. We speak of will or volitional acts only when there is some experience of choice and decision. When such experience is absent, the instinctual drive goes into action uninhibited by any volitional act. We then speak of *instinctual behaviour*. If in the background there lies a possible volition, we experience a sense of being 'driven' or of being 'overpowered'. Without this, simple non-volitional, biological necessity asserts itself.

Besides these phenomena of urge, instinctual activity, conflict and volition, there is the awareness of drive and will as they operate through motor discharges or psychic effects. These effects are then experienced as *willed* or as *due to a special kind of impulse*, i.e. as coming from me, belonging to me, and different from other spontaneous phenomena such as muscle cramp. A special kind of *inner* volitional phenomenon is the voluntary or involuntary *giving of attention* which increases the clarity and significance of the content.

### (a) Impulsive acts

When instinctual activity takes place directly without conflict or the

---

[1] Lotze, *Med. Psychologie*, pp. 287–325. Th. Lipps, *Vom Fühlen, Wollen u. Denken*, 2nd edn. (Leipzig, 1907). Else Wentscher, *Der Wille* (Leipzig, 1910).

making of any decision, but still within the hidden control of personality, as it were, we use the term *instinctual act*. But if the manifestation is uninhibited, cannot be inhibited and is totally uncontrolled, we use the term *impulsive act*.[1] We speak of an abnormal impulsive act when, no matter how much empathy we exercise, the possibility of its suppression remains inconceivable. Such acts are common in the acute psychoses, in states of clouded consciousness and in states of retarded development. Instinctual acts but not pathological impulsive acts are some of the commonest acts of our everyday life.

A schizophrenic patient in the first stages of his illness reported impulsive behaviour in the following terms: 'We had had a party. On the way home I was seized by an idea out of the blue—swim across the river in your clothes. It was not so much a compulsion to be reckoned with but simply one, colossal, powerful impulse. I did not think for a minute but jumped straight in . . . only when I felt the water did I realise it was most extraordinary conduct and I climbed out again. The whole incident gave me a lot to think about. For the first time something inexplicable, something quite sporadic and alien, had happened to me' (Kronfeld).

With acute psychoses and certain transient conditions, we often find a number of unintelligible instinctual activities. Motor discharge is usually reached very quickly. A patient who seemed stuporous will jump out of bed, thrash about, bite, run against the wall; on the next day, he is accessible and knows what happened; he will say the impulse had been irresistible. Another patient suddenly hit the doctor in the chest in the middle of a quiet conversation; a little later he apologised; he said the impulse came suddenly and irresistibly with the feeling that the doctor was hostile. The simple *urge to move* (instinctual discharge through pleasure in aimless movement) and the *urge to do something* (discharge through a definite activity, handwork, etc.) are both common in acute conditions. The urge to move may appear on its own and be circumscribed, e.g. an urge to talk when otherwise perfectly still.

In encephalitis lethargica, particularly with young people in the acute stage and immediately thereafter, impulsive acts may be observed in the form of sudden aggressiveness and cruelty. Thiele[2] investigated these primitive urges in detail and described them as elementary, aimless and undirected tendencies to discharge which arise out of an unpleasant restlessness and tension. The urge takes shape only in its effects, according to situation and opportunity and turns into an action with a definite content. Such *urges*, like frustrated instincts, simply find an object; *instincts* always seek their object, whereas *volition* determines the wanted object.

### (b) Awareness of inhibition of will

Awareness of inhibition is a characteristic disturbance, which is experienced subjectively as an inhibition of instinctual activity (complaints about

[1] See Förster and Aschaffenburg, 'Impulsive Insanity', *Z. Nervenhk.* (1908), p. 350. Ziehen, *Mschr. Psychiatr.*, vol. 11, pp. 55, 393. Rauschke, *Charité-Ann.*, vol. 30, p. 251.
[2] R. Thiele, 'Zur Kenntnis der psychischen Residuärzustände nach Encephalitis epidemica', *Mschr. Psychiatr.* (1926), Beih. 36.

loss of interest, lack of desire, absence of motive, etc.), or as an inhibition of volitional drive (complaints of incompetence, inability to make a decision). Alongside this subjective inhibition we usually find objective inhibition, but not necessarily to a corresponding degree. The former can however be experienced intensively, without any objective inhibition at all.

### (c) Awareness of loss of will or access of power

The experience of total loss of will-power is a remarkable phenomenon. With acute, florid psychoses feelings of passivity and subjection are quite characteristic. Often we cannot decide whether we have here an experience of defective volition or an awareness of an actual, objective ineffectiveness of the will. The following is an illustration:

> The patient is in bed. She hears a thumping at the door. 'Something enters' and comes right up to her bed. She feels it and cannot move. It comes up her body right up to the neck like a hand. She is terrified and all the time is fully awake but she cannot cry out, raise herself up or sit up. She is utterly stricken.

It also happens to patients that without experiencing any content, and though they are *fully conscious, they cannot move* nor can they talk. People may think the patient is drunk and laugh at him. He may get annoyed but cannot answer back. Afterwards he remembers everything all right and shows quite clearly that all the time he was quite conscious. Such states have been in part described as *narcoleptic*. Friedmann[1] has described them thus: 'The eyes are upturned and fixed, the pupils are somewhat dilated and reacting; the power to think is arrested but consciousness is preserved. Posture is relaxed and immobile but more rarely there may be an automatic continuation of the immediately preceding activity. The patient usually awakes without any residual disturbance.' We also find reports of similar *paralysing attacks* among hysterical patients and particularly in the schizophrenic group. Complete consciousness is preserved. Suddenly—as if from a shock—the body fails to respond to the volitional impulse, either as a whole or only in a circumscribed area. The body is experienced as rigid and stiff, heavy, powerless, lifeless. The patient is usually overtaken by this condition when lying down, but sometimes when he sits or stands; it differs from a paralysis in its transitoriness.

Kloos[2] gives some patients' reports as follows: 'She tries hard to speak; it won't work; she can't get up from the chair, give any sign or communicate, as if she was gagged and bound; all the time she is frightened'—'She could not move mouth or limbs while praying; it was as if she were dying; she was not afraid; she thought she would wake up again; she went on praying in her mind; then it was all over. The next time, however, she felt real fear of death. On both occasions the whole body felt lifeless.'—'She felt she was tied; she could not lift her feet from the floor and had to stay just where she was (but only for a few seconds).'

[1] Friedmann, *Dtsch. Z. Nervenhk.*, vol. 30.
[2] Gerhard Kloos, 'Über kataplektische Zustände bei Schizophrenen', *Nervenarzt*, vol. 9 (1936), p. 57.

Here we are not dealing with motor paralysis nor with a psychogenic disturbance but with an *elementary event* during which the *volitional drive fails to get translated into physical movement.* We do not know where the disturbance lies. Phenomenologically, when we move, the last thing we experience is the actual effort together with the image of the goal to which our movement is directed. Pikler has analysed the situation.[1] If we exercise our will on some particular bodily part in order to move it, the conscious point of attack is not on the nerves and muscles but rather on the surface of that part of the body which will be most engaged during the movement (e.g. on the surface of the fingers, when grasping). The will has no dynamic impact itself but it impinges at the point where the movement is conceived. We are in the dark as to where this actual point of impact lies and where exactly we shall find the relationship between the psychological experience and the entirely heterogeneous and complex nerve/muscle process. It is only in pathological states that we see thus dramatically demonstrated the disappearance of something we have always accepted as a matter of course. There is *no paralysis* either to account for it. A failure of motor-impulse is being experienced; there is an absence of the normal, magical effect of the will on our physical movements.

This experience of utter powerlessness or ineffectiveness may also occur in respect of *controlling our own processes of thought and imagination,* which we normally take as a matter of course. Patients feel that something has taken possession of their head; they cannot concentrate on their work; thoughts disappear just when needed; inappropriate thoughts intervene. They feel sleepy and absent-minded. In addition to an inability to work, they have no wish to work. But they can be successful with mechanical activities and will often undertake these gladly; in this they differ from patients in states of inhibition and fatigue. Such phenomena are common in the initial stages of the process; intelligent patients will themselves say their condition is different from ordinary fatigue, with which they are quite familiar.

With some acute psychoses patients experience the very opposite of what we have so far described. They get an *immense feeling of power.* It is as if they could indeed do anything. Physically they feel giants in strength; a hundred people could not master them. Their power, they feel, has a remote extension. Linked with this sometimes are certain feelings of immense responsibility; an awareness that they are to perform world-shaking deeds:

Nerval described the following: 'I had an idea that I had become enormous, and through a flood of electrical power I would throw everything near me to the ground. There was something comical in the extreme care I took to hold my powers under control, to save the life of the soldiers who had captured me. . . .'
A schizophrenic patient wrote: 'All the people I speak to believe in me wholly and do what I tell them. No one tries to lie to me; most of them have ceased to believe

[1] Julius Pikler, 'Über die Angriffspunkte des Willens am Körper', *Z. Psychol.*, vol. 110 (1929), p. 288.

in their own words. I have an indescribable influence on my surroundings. I think my look beautifies other people and I try this magic out on my nurses; the whole world depends on me for all its weal and woe. I will improve and rescue it' (Gruhle).

Other patients will be surprised to find at the beginning of their psychosis that they have an *unusual power and clarity of thought*. Thoughts flow into their mind just as they want them with a facility they have hitherto never had and with a surprising copiousness. Now they feel capable of solving every possible problem as if it were child's play. Their mental powers have been multiplied a thousandfold.

## § 7. AWARENESS OF THE SELF

*Psychological preface*. Self-awareness is contrasted with object-awareness. As we have had to differentiate a number of modes of object-awareness, so we have to do the same for self-awareness, since the *modes in which the self becomes aware of itself* do not present any single or simple phenomenon. Self-awareness has *four formal characteristics*: (1) the feeling of activity—an awareness of being active; (2) an awareness of unity—I am aware at any given moment that I am a unity; (3) awareness of identity—I am aware I have been the same person all the time; (4) awareness of the self as distinct from an outer world and all that is not the self. Within these four formal characteristics, self-awareness displays a range of developmental levels from a plain, bare existence to a full life with a conscious wealth of sensitive experience. In the course of such development, the self grows aware of itself as a *personality*. Abnormalities of self-awareness show themselves typically as a lack of one or other of these formal characteristics. In the end we come to abnormalities in the awareness of personality, at which we will briefly glance.

### (a) *Activity of the self*

Self-awareness is present in every psychic event. In the form of 'I think' it accompanies all perceptions, ideas and thoughts, while feelings are passive, and instinctual drives are impelling states of the self. *All* psychic life involves the experience of a *unique and fundamental activity*. Every psychic manifestation, whether perception, bodily sensation, memory, idea, thought or feeling carries *this particular aspect of 'being mine'* of having an 'I'-quality, of 'personally belonging', of it being one's own doing. We have termed this '*personalisation*'. If these psychic manifestations occur with the awareness of their not being mine, of being alien, automatic, independent, arriving from elsewhere, we term them phenomena of *depersonalisation*.

1. *Alteration in awareness of existence*. A group of phenomena which represent defective awareness of one's own activity may be seen in what we call depersonalisation and derealisation, in the cessation of normal sensory experience of one's body, in the subjective inability to imagine and remember, in complaints of inhibited feeling and in the awareness of one's behaviour becoming automatic. This whole group of phenomena are obviously related

to each other. Here we shall quote only the descriptions of patients[1] who are aware of their existence as an *awareness of having lost the sense of self*:

Patients showing a mild degree of this phenomenon feel they are estranged from themselves; they feel they have changed, become mechanical; they will speak figuratively of a twilight state, they say they are no longer their natural selves. Amiel records the following in his diaries: 'I feel nameless, impersonal; my gaze is fixed like a corpse; my mind has become vague and general; like a nothing or the absolute; I am floating; I am as if I were not.' Patients also say: 'I am only an automaton, a machine; it is not I who senses, speaks, eats, suffers, sleeps; I exist no longer; I do not exist, I am dead; I feel I am absolutely nothing.'

A patient said: 'I am not alive, I cannot move; I have no mind, and no feelings; I have never existed, people only thought I did.' Another patient said: 'The worst thing is that I do not exist.' 'I am so non-existent I can neither wash nor drink.' It is not that she is nothing but she just does not exist; she only acts as if she did; she speaks of 'swirling'—doing something 'out of not-being'; nothing she did was out of a sense of 'I am' (Kurt Schneider).

The remarkable thing about this particular phenomenon is that the individual, though he exists, is no longer able to feel he exists. Descartes' 'cogito ergo sum' (I think therefore I am) may still be superficially cogitated but it is no longer a valid experience.

2. *Alteration in the awareness of one's own performance.* Loss of the sense of existence can also be conceived as a reduction in one's awareness of performing one's own actions, an awareness which normally accompanies every psychic event. In the natural course of our activities we do not notice how essential this experience of unified performance is. We take it for granted that when we think, it is we who think, a thought is our thought and the notions that strike us—and perhaps make us say not 'I think' but 'it occurs to me'— are still at the same time our thoughts, executed by us.

This general awareness of one's own performance can alter in a number of directions, which are quite incomprehensible, difficult to imagine and not open to empathy. With compulsive phenomena, where the patient cannot rid himself of haunting tunes, ideas or phrases, we can still find some measure of comprehension. The patient takes the distressing part of the experience as part of his own thoughts. But the thought-phenomena of schizophrenics is something quite different in that they talk about 'thoughts made by others' (passivity-thinking) and 'thought-withdrawal', using words coined by themselves, which psychopathology has had to take over. Patients think something and yet feel that someone else has thought it and in some way forced it on them. The thought arises and with it a direct awareness that it is not the patient but some external agent that thinks it. The patient does not know why he has this thought nor did he intend to have it. He does not feel master of his

[1] Janet, *Les obsessions et la psychasthenie.* 2nd edn. (Paris, 1908). Österreich, *Die Phänomenologie des Ich* (Leipzig, 1910).

own thoughts and in addition he feels in the power of some incomprehensible external force.

'Some artificial influence plays on me; the feeling suggests that somebody has attached himself to my mind and feeling, just as in a game of cards someone looking over one's shoulder may interfere in the game (a schizophrenic patient).

Just as the patients find their thoughts are '*made*' for them so they feel that these are being *withdrawn*. A thought vanishes and there arises the feeling that this has come about from outside action. A new thought then appears without context. That too is made from outside.

A patient tells us: 'When she wants to think about something—a business matter for instance—all her thoughts are suddenly withdrawn, just like a curtain. The more she tries the more painful it is—(a string seems pulling away from her head). Still she succeeds in holding on to them or regaining them.'

It is extremely difficult to imagine what the actual experience is with these 'made thoughts' (passivity thinking) and these 'thought withdrawals'. We just have to accept the account as outsiders, relying on the descriptions we are given of these otherwise easily recognisable phenomena, which are not to be confused with unusual thought-content, poorly grounded notions or compulsive phenomena.

There is still another abnormal mode in which thoughts are presented. No one speaks them to the patient nor are the thoughts 'made' nor does the patient oppose them in any way. Nevertheless the thoughts are not his own, not those which he usually thinks; they are suddenly implanted, coming like an inspiration from elsewhere:

'I have never read nor heard them; they come unasked; I don't dare to think I am the source but I am happy to know of them without thinking them. They come at any moment like a gift and I do not dare to impart them as if they were my own' (Gruhle).

Any mode of activity may acquire this sense of being 'artificially made'. Not only thinking is affected, but walking, speaking and behaving. These are all phenomena that exhibit *influences upon the will*. They are not the same as those of which people complain who suffer from personality disorders and depression and who declare it is as if they themselves were no longer acting but have become mere automata. What we are discussing here is something radically different, an *elementary* experience of *being actually influenced*. Patients feel themselves inhibited and retarded from outside; they cannot do what they want; when they want to lift something, their hand is held; some psychic power is at work. They feel as if they were pulled from behind, immobilised, made of stone. They suddenly find they cannot go on, as if they were paralysed and then suddenly it has all gone again. Their speech is suddenly arrested. They may have to make involuntary movements; they are surprised to find their hand is led to their forehead or that they have attacked someone else. They did not intend it. This is all felt as some alien, incomprehensible power at work. A patient of *Berᶎe* said: 'I never shouted, it was the vocal chords that shouted out of me.' 'The hands turn this way and that, I do not guide them nor can I stop them.' Here are phenomena which seem to lie outside our imagination. There is still some similarity with a volitional act, yet it seems to be an autistic, reflex movement which we have merely observed. Its performance is 'criticised' not executed by a self. The following passages from a self-description will make the matter clearer:

'The "shouting miracle" is an extraordinary occurrence; the respiratory muscles are put into motion, so that I am forced to shout out, unless I make an enormous effort at suppression, which is not always possible in view of the suddenness of the impulse, or rather I have to concentrate relentlessly on it . . . . At times the shouting is so repetitive that my state gets unbearable . . . since words are shouted my will is of course not altogether uninvolved . . . . It is only the inarticulate shouting which is really like a compulsion and automatic . . . my muscles are subject to certain influences which can be ascribed only to some external force. . . . The difficulties too, which get in my way when I want to play the piano, defy description—paralysis of my fingers, alteration of my gaze, misdirection of my fingers on the keys, quickening of tempo through premature movement of the finger muscles. . . .' We also find in this patient analogous experiences in the field of inner volition—'passivity thinking' (made thoughts) and 'thought-withdrawal', etc. (Schreber).

We also find that instinctual activities are experienced as 'made' in this sense, sexual drives in particular:

A schizophrenic patient describes suprasensual enjoyment with young girls with no physical contact . . . 'a pretty girl flirts in passing . . . attention is roused . . . one gets acquainted rather like a pair of lovers . . . after a little while she makes gestures towards her lap . . . she wants to arouse sexual stimulation from a distance telepathically without physical contact and bring about an ejaculation as with a real embrace'.

Another patient said: 'My character is not mine, it has been "made".'

## (b) The unity of the self

The experience of the basic unity of the self can undergo some notable changes. Sometimes, for instance, while talking we may notice that we are talking rather like an automaton, quite correctly may be, but we can observe ourselves and listen to ourselves. Should this dissociation last any length of time, disturbances will occur in the flow of thought, but for a short time we can ourselves experience without any disturbance that 'doubling' of personality which patients describe to us in much more elaborate terms.[1] This is not the old familiar situation in which we say 'two beings live within my breast' or where reason struggles with passion. Nor must we be misled by

[1] Janet, *Les obsessions et la psychasthenie.*, 2nd edn. (Paris, 1908), pp. 319–22. Österreich, *Die Phänomenologie des Ich* (Leipzig, 1910), pp. 422–509.

patients who interpret their compulsive ideas as a doubling of personality or announce that they conclude they have a double self for one reason or another (e.g. heautoscopic hallucination). Nor is the experience in question to be confused with the so-called 'double personality' which appears objectively in alternating states of consciousness. The real experience of *being in two*, of *being doubled* occurs when both chains of psychic events so develop together that we can talk of separate personalities, each with their own peculiar experiences and specific feeling-associations, and each perfectly alien and apart from the other. The old autobiographical sketch of Father Surin[1] gives a very vivid description, if we allow for the religious language in which it is cast:

'Matters have got so far that I believe God, because of my sins, allows something unique to happen in Church (the Father was practising exorcism). The devil leaves the body of the possessed person and rushes into mine, throws me on the ground and beats me violently for some hours. I cannot really describe what goes on; the spirit unites with my own and robs me of consciousness and the freedom of my own mind. It reigns in me as another self, as if I *have two minds*, one dispossessed of the use of its body and pushed into a corner, while the other intruder ranges round unchecked. Both spirits fight within the same body and *my mind is divided*, as it were. One part is subject to this devil, the other obeys its own motives or those which God gave it. I feel at the same time a deep peace and that I am in accord with God without knowing whence comes the raving and hate of Him which I feel inside me, a raging desire to tear myself away from Him that astonishes everyone; but I also feel a great and mellow joy which cries out as the devil does; I feel damned and afraid; as if my one mind is pierced with thorns of despair, my own despair, while my other mind indulges in derision and cursing against the author of my distress. My shouts come from both sides and I cannot decide whether pleasure or fury prevails. Violent trembling seizes me on approaching the Sacrament; it seems due both to distress at its presence and to adoration of it; I cannot stop it. One mind bids me make the sign of the cross on my mouth, the other mind stops me and makes me bite my fingers furiously. During such attacks I can pray with greater ease; my body rolls on the ground and priests curse me as if I were Satan; I feel joyfully that I have become Satan, not in revolt but because of my own miserable sins'. (The Father seems to have fallen ill in due course with a schizophrenic process.)

It is rare to get a description of these remarkable experiences of a double self, where the self is really one, yet experiences itself as two and lives discretely in both sets of feeling-associations, and knows them both. The fact of this double existence cannot be denied and every formulation of the experience always carries this contradictory quality.

## (c) *Identity of the self*

The third characteristic of self-awareness is the awareness of one's identity through the passage of time. We need only think of statements made by certain schizophrenic patients. They will speak of their previous life before the

[1] Ideler, *Versuch einer Theorie des religiösen Wahnsinns*, vol. 1, pp. 392 ff.

onset of their psychosis and say this was not their own self, but somebody else. A patient said:

> 'When telling my story I am aware that only part of my present self experienced all this. Up to 23rd December 1901, I cannot call myself my present self; the past self seems now like a little dwarf inside me. It is an unpleasant feeling; it upsets my feeling of existence if I describe my previous experiences in the first person. I can do it if I use an image and recall that the dwarf reigned up to that date, but since then his part has ended' (Schwab).

### (d) Awareness of self as distinct from the outside world

The fourth characteristic of self-awareness is the clear sense of the self confronting an outside world. According to rather obscure utterances of schizophrenics patients seem to identify themselves with the objects of the outer world; they suffer from what others do. If someone is spinning, they say 'why are you spinning me?' or, when a carpet is beaten, say 'why are you beating me?' (Kahlbaum). A schizophrenic patient said: 'I saw a vortex whirling before me—or rather I felt myself whirling outside in a narrow space' (Fr. Fischer). During mescalin intoxication one report reads: 'I felt the dog's bark painfully touching on my body; the dog was in the bark and I was in the pain' (Mayer-Gross and Stein). During hashish intoxication: 'Just now I was a piece of apple' (Fraenkel and Joel, s.102). In this same category we can place patients who for brief moments think they are vanishing; they are 'like a mathematical point' or they continue to live only in the objects around them. Baudelaire describes something of this sort in hashish intoxication:

> 'Sometimes one's personality disappears and objective reality, as with the pantheistic poets, springs up in its place, but in such abnormal fashion that the sight of external things makes you forget your own existence and soon you are flowing into them. You look at a tree bending in the wind. As a poet you see it as a perfectly natural symbol of yourself, but in a few seconds it has become really you. You ascribe to it your passion, longing and melancholy. Its sighing and waving become yours and soon you are the tree. So with the bird sailing about in the blue sky; it may first only symbolise the eternal longing to soar above human concerns but suddenly you have become the bird itself. Let us imagine you are sitting there smoking your pipe; you let your attention linger a little too long on the blue pipe-smoke . . . by some peculiar equation you feel yourself wreathing up, you will become the pipe (into which you feel yourself pressed like the tobacco) and credit yourself with the strange ability to smoke yourself.'
>
> A schizophrenic patient said: 'The sense of self had dwindled so that it was necessary to complement it with another person—rather like the wish for stronger selves to be near and protective . . . I felt as if I were only a little piece of a person' (Schwab).

We now add a few reports from patients about similar experiences, the basis of which must be some cancellation of the distinction we normally draw between the self and the outside world. It is a frequent remark of schizophrenics that *the whole world knows their thoughts*. Patients answer all questions by saying, 'Why do you ask me—you know it already':

Patients notice that other people know their thoughts as soon as they have them. Or, in a way similar to passivity-thinking and thought-withdrawal, they experience the feeling of being exposed to everybody. 'I believe I can no longer hide anything; I have experienced this over the last few years; all my thoughts have been guessed. I realise I can no longer keep my thoughts to myself.'

### (e) *Awareness of one's personality*

Once the merely formal awareness of self acquires content, we can speak of awareness of personality. This, in its totality of content, provides subject-matter for the psychology of understandable connections. So far as phenomenology is concerned, the basic characteristics are as follows:

1. The individual can have *two distinctive relationships* to *his own experience*. Many instinctual activities are sensed by the personality as a natural expression of itself and its momentary state. They are felt to be entirely understandable in terms of the personality and experienced as its own instinctual drives. This is so for quite abnormal, sado-masochistic drives, urges to suffer, etc. There are other instinctual drives, however, which the personality experiences as alien, unnatural, not understandable, not as its own. They are felt as something imposed. The phenomenological opposites of subjectively understandable and ununderstandable drives can be contrasted with drives that are objectively understandable and ununderstandable to the observer. The two sets need not, however, tally. Perverse sexual drives which may occur at the beginning of a process (for instance, in senility) can be subjectively experienced and recognised as the patient's own, whereas objectively they may be seen as something quite new, not understandable, and due entirely to the morbid process itself. On the other hand, instinctual drives which have become an irresistible habit may be subjectively experienced as something alien, whereas objectively they are regarded as quite understandable.

2. The feeling of *change in one's own personality* is a normal experience, particularly at the time of puberty. Then many different and stormy impulses arise in the psyche, and new experiences emerge from obscure depths. There is a strong awareness—sometimes painful, sometimes delightful, sometimes crippling, sometimes lending wings—that one has become another and a new person. The awareness of patients in the early stages of their illness comes very close to this. They are conscious of something new and puzzling; they feel they are different. They feel that their awareness of their own personality has become uncertain, that there is something alien against which they have to fight. At last there comes the awareness of being wholly overpowered. Some patients will say that they think differently, feel and sense differently from what they did before. Some profound transformation has taken place. Others say that after an acute psychosis the change which they feel is something subjectively pleasurable; they are more indifferent, less excited, not so easily

'moved to their depths'; at the same time, they talk more easily, they have less reticence and are more certain in their conduct. A patient wrote:

'I was in a state of great physical weakness for several years; because of this morbid physical state, I turned gradually into a passionless, calm and reflective person. This was the opposite of what one might have expected, in view of the influences at work (telepathic effects).'

A patient complained: 'She longs for herself but cannot find herself; she has to look for the person inside her'—'Two years ago I started to wither'—'I have lost myself—I am changed and without defence' (Gruhle).

3. *Lability in awareness of the personality* is experienced in all sorts of ways in the acute, florid psychoses. The following self-description illustrates this phenomenon clearly, and the patients themselves sometimes call it '*taking part in the play*'. The example shows well the awareness of lability at the same time as this is being experienced:

'I was in a state bordering on actual delusion, yet still clearly distinguishable from it. It was a state that recurred frequently in the course of my illness, when, half-driven by inspiration, half-knowing and wanting it, I created a part for myself which I played out like an actor, declaiming it; I lived myself into it and acted according to it, without considering myself entirely identical with the character.' Among the parts played were 'the personification of a wave', 'the prancing of a fiery young horse', 'a young sister of Queen Sulamith in the noble song', 'the daughter of Alfred Eschers', 'a young French woman' or 'agriculture'—in which the hospital courtyard was the estate (Forel).

In similar psychoses patients experience themselves as Messiahs, divine personages, witches, or as historical characters. In the paranoid psychoses (in which Bonhoeffer[1] has described the lability of this personality-awareness), we can see the patient elaborate the role—say that of some world-famous inventor—and maintain it tenaciously over a long period of time. During these fantastic transformations it may happen that the patients remain aware of their previous identity; they are still the same but are now Messiahs, etc.

### (*f*) Multiple personalities: dissociated personality

Such a doubling or multiplication of the self can take place that patients find themselves confronted by *entirely alien forces*, which behave as *if they had a personality*. They not only use devious means, with certain obvious purposes, but they have a definite character, friendly or hostile. At the most elementary level in the formation of these entities we find the so-called simultaneous hallucination of several senses. The personality which the patient visually hallucinates also talks.[2] Voices, visual hallucinations, delusions of influence, doubling of body-awareness, may all combine and shape themselves eventually

[1] Bonhoeffer, 'Klinische Beiträge zur Lehre von den Degenerationspsychosen', *Alt's Samml.*, vol. 7 (Halle, 1907).
[2] Specht, *Z. Psychopath.*, vol. 2.

into veritable *personifications*, a name aptly given to them by a patient (Staudenmaier):

*Staudenmaier*, Professor of Chemistry, described these personifications among his pathological experiences. He did not regard them (as the other schizophrenic patients did) as strange beings, but as '*emancipated parts of his unconscious*'. We will follow his account, which has certain affinities with that of Father Surin quoted above: 'Single hallucinations gradually emerged more definitely and returned more often. At last they formed into *personifications*; for instance, the more important visual images regularly combined with the corresponding auditory images, so that the emerging figures began to speak to me, gave me advice and criticised my actions. A characteristic defect of these personifications is that they really think they *are* what they represent or imitate and therefore they talk and act *in earnest*. For a long time I tried to elaborate them further.' Here are some examples:

A few years ago I was watching some military exercises. I chanced to see one of the Court personages at close quarters repeatedly and heard her speak. Later I had a vivid hallucination—as if I heard her speak again. At first I paid no attention to this frequently recurring voice and for a time it disappeared. At length I had the feeling more and more often and clearly that this personage was near me and the visual image, by constantly forcing itself on me along with the inner voice, became clearer too without at first becoming a true hallucination. As time went on personifications of other Court people appeared, particularly the personification of the Kaiser, then the dead Napoleon I. Gradually I was overcome by the feeling, a peculiarly exalted feeling, that I was dictator and ruler of a great nation; my chest swelled on its own, my whole posture became stiff and military—proof that the respective personification had gained considerable influence over me. For instance, I heard the inner voice speak in grandiose terms: I am the German Kaiser. After a time I grew tired; other images forced themselves on me and I relaxed. Out of all the royal personages who appeared to me, a concept of 'Majesty' gradually developed. My majesty greatly desired to be a foremost, or rather royal and ruling personage at least, and—as I became more enlightened about these personages—to see and imitate them. Majesty interests itself in military displays, cultivated living, good manners, rich food and drink, order and elegance in my home, distinguished attire, fine, erect military bearing, exercise, hunting and other sports and tries to influence my mode of life accordingly with advice, warnings, orders and threats. Majesty, however, is an enemy of children, of quaint little things, of jokes and making merry, seemingly because it knows the royal personages from their dignified appearance in public or from pictures of them. Majesty is also an enemy of comic papers and magazines with caricatures, and of water-drinking, etc. Physically I am myself somewhat too short for 'Majesty'. The personification 'child' plays a similar role to that of 'Majesty'; there is the childish voice, childish needs and pleasures; there is also the personification 'roundhead' who enjoys jokes and jolly things. All have distinctive voices and one can speak with them as if with different people, 'except that one has to remain within the special field they represent and keep everything else out. As soon as one starts with anything diametrically opposite, the whole idyll vanishes'. The clearly defined personifications were preceded in time by less well-defined and rather hazy ones. 'Sometimes devils seemed let loose. I saw devilish faces repeatedly for quite a long time all perfectly clear and sharp. Once when I was in bed I positively felt someone putting chains round my neck; then I smelt sulphur, and an eerie inner voice said, "You are now my prisoner—I shall not let you go—I am the devil himself". Threats were often launched at me. I have really experienced it all in myself. Those tales about evil spirits which modern people present as the horror fables of the middle ages and those reports of spiritualists about poltergeists have not been dreamt up out of nothing. The personifications work without relation to the conscious personality but each one of them tries to gain complete control over it. A lengthy battle goes on with them and also between them, since some seek to help the conscious personality. I often observe quite clearly how one or two personifications will help and support each other or how they will secretly conspire to fight against me, the old man—which is the nickname they always use—and annoy me (rather like the situation when telegraphists in a number of stations in a complicated network conspire together without letting the others know). But how they fight against each other and abuse each other.' 'Because of the far-reaching and sometimes pathological influences of certain centres and personifications I could observe how vigorously they fought and how powerfully they tried to force out the feelings and ideas they found unpleasant and assert their own wishes and ideas, so as to improve their position in the organism and make it more influential.' All personifications have something one-sided about them. They are not wholes, only parts which are able to exist as dissociated parts of the unconscious side by side with the conscious personality.

These descriptions show us the *attitude* which Staudenmaier took towards these phenomena. This becomes clearer, as follows: 'Inexperienced in these things, one certainly gets the impression that a mysterious invisible and alien personality is playing a game. This "inner voice" has been acknowledged from time immemorial, has been regarded as divine or devilish.' Staudenmaier, however, felt this to be false; he did feel *possessed* in the same way as the Saints in the Middle Ages, but not by alien powers, only by split-off parts of his own unconscious. 'I considered them as entities that had still got a certain independence of existence, although they were developed for certain partial purposes and were confined once and for all to a definite place in the organism. Because of their one-sided position and purpose, they have certain separate memories and separate interests which do not necessarily coincide with those of the conscious self. With nervous people particularly they often gain an extraordinary ascendancy over the affect and over the whole mode of life of the conscious self, since they are themselves capable of such diverse affects. If they are capable of learning, they can eventually develop, as with me, into very intelligent part-existences with whom one has then to reckon seriously.' Normal people get to know of the influence of their unconscious from the obscure feelings they experience; but Staudenmaier made contact with his dissociated personalities in articulate conversation and thus experienced his unconscious more vividly than is otherwise possible. He does not believe that these dissociated entities are in principle different from what is contained in the normal unconscious. 'There are a number of intermediary stages starting from the complete and autocratic psychic unity of normal people down to a pathological splitting-up and far-reaching emancipation of individual parts of the brain.' Staudenmaier 'took as evident that the human being represented a single psychic entity. We should not forget that we have been dealing here with a state that passed directly into the pathological. Still the *fact that such phenomena are possible remains of the utmost importance for any evaluation which we may make of the human psyche and its nature.*'

## § 8. Phenomena of Self-Reflection

*Psychological preface.* I am not only conscious in the sense of having certain inner experiences, but I am turned back on myself—reflected back—in consciousness of self. In the course of this reflection I not only come to know myself, but I also influence myself. There is not only something happening within me, but I instigate, arouse and shape a happening within me. I can, as it were, draw reality into me as well as evoke and guide it.

Human development in the individual and in history is not only a passive transformation as with all other biological happenings, but it is an inward effort of mind and spirit working on its own, driving itself forward in the universal dialectic of opposition and transformation.

For this reason, there is no longer any such thing as unmediated psychic life. Thinking and volition beget reflection and with the reflective process begins the indirect alteration of all direct experience. Once, however, direct experience ceases to be the sole determining factor, we not only find expansion, a general unfolding, and new dimensions of experience, but also interferences of an entirely new character. For instance, to take the simplest, basic immediacies, the instincts, not only can they be assisted by reflective purpose, but they can be thoroughly confused and obliterated by it.

Interference of this sort arises when the mechanisms that realise and co-ordinate reflection with immediacy do not take their natural course, which remains obscure but maintains all that is self-evident, beneficial and unproblematical in our lives, reflect how we may.

Human psychic life can no longer be an immediate experience such as that of animals or idiots. Should it become a purely elementary process, we should have to consider it disturbed; equally so if it were nothing but pure reflection.

The fact that the immediate phenomena we experience do not remain immediate but are constantly being transformed by reflection does not obliterate for most of us their immediate character, as indeed we have tried to describe it in all its great variety. But the fact of alteration remains a basic one and while we investigate phenomena we should keep our eye carefully on the possible changes wrought by reflection. In particular it may be the source for new psychopathological phenomena which we will illustrate by three examples: *Firstly*, purposeful reflection may lead to disingenuousness; in hysterical persons it may deceive us with what appear to be real experiences. *Secondly*, it may throw instinctual activity, including the bodily functions, into confusion and, *thirdly*, it may lead to compulsive phenomena, unique psychic experiences that are possible only on the basis of reflection and volition. In all these three instances purposeful reflection is indispensable for the production of the phenomena which clearly did not intend themselves.

The immense importance of reflection when it has contents to work on will be discussed when we come to the chapter on meaningful psychic connections. All the pathological manifestations which we review here as phenomena will find a natural place there. They are but moments in a person's life and their content needs to be understood in the context of that life. Here however we are concerned only with the phenomena of experience as such, and the various types and forms. We are not dealing with their content or their meaning.

## (a) Psychic life—mediated and unmediated by thought

Normal, everyday psychic life is always in some way rooted in reflection. In this it contrasts with psychotic, elementary experience. For instance, if we contrast delusion proper with an ordinary mistake, a vivid awareness with an 'as if' experience, melancholia with a neurotic depression after an unpleasant occurrence, hallucination with projected fantasy, the experience of a double self with the feeling of a 'divided self', an instinctual drive with a simple wish, or motor agitation with a meaningful motor discharge of emotion, we see a number of elementary, immediate and irreducible experiences on the one hand, and on the other something that has evolved and grown, something that is rooted in ideas and in living into these ideas with some intensity, something that is perhaps a little faint and secondary by comparison, though the momentary affect and visible passion may be striking. What is elementary and immediate cannot be influenced by psychological means, though the latter may influence anything that is mediated by thought. What is elementary is primarily without content and gains this only secondarily, but whatever has been evolved conceptually starts from content and operates in reverse. All that is understandable and has developed understandably stands contrasted with phenomena that are obscure in their causes, exist incomprehensibly and break into the psyche with an elementary force. Whatever is purely elementary in this way belongs to a morbid process.

Where the understandable development is a healthy one, there is nothing disingenuous or deceptive about it but it is the undistorted reality of psychic development following its proper course. Yet whatever is mediated through concepts may become a distorting factor. Deception, difficult to detect, can intrude subtly along hidden connections. The smooth, well-adapted existence of the animal ceases once immediacy is at an end. Animals live beyond truth and untruth, but I, the human being, experience life and cannot simply leave it at that. I believe I am myself but I develop intentions and grow disingenuous in imitation. People with pronounced hysterical endowment can reach extraordinary lengths in this respect so that their psychic life which is entirely derived and thought up, totally artificial and treacherous, can become for the time being an elementary experience, gripping and immediate. For instance, a young man suffering from schizophrenia lived with a woman hysteric who shared many of his hallucinations and anxieties. The patient said of her, 'If one gets caught up, one is nervous; once one has the actual experience, one is not at all nervous; in my case the whole thing is much quieter and clearer.'

## (b) Disturbance of instinct and bodily function

So far as our bodily functions are concerned, we live successfully because we rely all the time upon the unconscious guidance of our instincts. But these in their turn are developed by exercise, and refashioned and enriched by our consciously inspired activity. The details of this process are extremely complicated and we can never wholly disentangle them. Our biological inheritance and the acquisitions of our personal history fuse into one. But reflection, which is indispensable for the development and stability of both, may in itself create a disturbance.

Such functions as urination, walking, writing, sexual intercourse can no longer be carried out. The affected person feels he is losing contact as well as becoming ridiculous. He wants to be able to do these things but directing his attention to them only makes it worse. Fear of failure makes it worse still.

Anxious attention to health brings about hypochondriacal complaints. As the result of constant reflection on the body and its functions, subjective syndromes develop with partly objective effects. Finally, expectations and fears drive consciousness into a life which concerns itself chiefly with the body and which in the process of looking for itself, actually loses itself.

## (c) Compulsive phenomena[1]

1. *Psychic compulsions.* Experience of psychic compulsion is an ultimate phenomenon. I may feel under quite normal conditions that I am being driven, impelled or overpowered not only by outer forces and other people but by my own psychic life. We have to keep this normal phenomenon well in mind and realise that it is strangely possible for us to oppose ourselves, want to follow an instinctual drive, yet fight it, want and yet not want. Otherwise we shall not properly understand the phenomena described in psychopathology as compulsive ideas, compulsive drives, etc.

Normally the self lives freely in its perceptions, anxieties, memories and dreams. This is so whether it surrenders itself to them instinctively or whether it deliberately chooses what it will attend to, what it will make the object of its affections. Now should the self be no longer master of its choice, should it lose all influence over the selection of what shall fill its consciousness, and should *the immediate content of consciousness remain irremovable, unchosen, unwanted,* the self finds itself in conflict faced with a content which it wants to suppress but cannot. This content then acquires the character of a psychic compulsion. This is not the kind of compulsion we feel when we are suddenly distracted by something catching our attention, but it is a compulsion from within. Instead of the normal *consciousness of controlling* the sequence of events (Kurt Schneider) there arises a *consciousness of compulsion,* the person cannot free his consciousness if he would.

We do not speak of a psychic compulsion when in the course of ordinary instinctual experience our attention is drawn to one thing or another or some desire is awakened. Psychic compulsion is possible only where there is a *psychic life subject to a certain degree of volitional control.* Psychic events can become *compulsive events* only

[1] Compulsive ideas: see Friedmann, *Mschr. Psychiatr.*, vol. 21. Compulsive phenomena: see Lowenfeld, *Die psychischen Zwangserscheinungen* (Wiesbaden, 1904); also Bumke, *Alt's Samml.* (Halle, 1906) (he defines and restricts the old concept created by Westphal). Kurt Schneider, *Z. Neur.* (Ref.) (1919). Critical bibliography, also 'Die psychopathische Persönlichkeiten', 5th edn. (1942), pp. 65–75. H. Binder, *Zur Psychologie der Zwangsvorgänge* (Berlin, 1936). Straus, *Mschr. Psychiatr.*, vol. 98 (1938), p. 61 ff. Freiherr v. Gebsattel, 'Die Welt des Zwangskranken', *Mschr. Psychiatr.*, vol. 99 (1938), pp. 10 ff.

when they contain an experience of self-activity. There is, therefore, no psychic compulsion where there is no volitional control and no choice, as with idiots and very young children.

All psychic events that contain an element of deliberation can become characterised by compulsion, and we use the prefix 'compulsive' when we wish to emphasise any one of them. Where the self tries but is unable to withdraw its attention from some hallucination, sensation or anxiety, we may speak of compulsive hallucinations, compulsive sensations, compulsive anxiety, etc. *Compulsion is co-extensive with the range of the individual's volition.* Perception retains a compulsive character only as long as I cannot divert my sense-organs or close them against the stimulus.

Compulsion as so far described refers only to the *form in which psychic events appear.* As to content, this may be meaningful and integrated with the personality; for instance, the fear of confinement which a woman experiences not for the moment only but with her whole personality as a *justifiable* anxiety. However, in so far as she may try in vain to think of something else, she experiences this anxiety as a compulsion. Yet she may realise that her fear is in fact unjustified and refuse to identify herself with it, considering it *groundless and silly,* not *her* fear. The anxiety is compulsive in character, related in content to the self, a possible anxiety but essentially alien to the self. In other cases the content of ideas is entirely *nonsensical,* the alien quality comes forward in a drastic manner (the individual cannot take a walk without having injured someone behind him in the eye, unnoticed, with his umbrella). In the strict sense of the term, compulsive thoughts, impulses etc., should be confined to anxieties or impulses which can be experienced by the individual as an incessant preoccupation, though he is convinced of the *groundlessness* of the anxiety, the *senselessness* of the impulse and the *impossibility* of the notion. Thus compulsive events, strictly speaking, are all such events, the *existence* of which is strongly resisted by the individual in the first place and the *content* of which appears to him as groundless, meaningless or relatively incomprehensible.

We can gather these compulsive phenomena into two groups if we want to get some *comprehensive picture* of them. *Firstly*: compulsive phenomena in the wider sense, where the main characteristic is the feeling of subjective compulsion and the content is indifferent (formal compulsive thinking). An image, thought, memory or question may intrude into consciousness repeatedly. One is haunted by a tune, for example, but it need not be such an isolated content only; there may be an intrusive re-orientation of one's thinking; one has to count, for example, spell names, ponder insoluble and silly problems (rumination) etc. *Secondly*: compulsive phenomena in the narrower sense, where the further characteristic of 'something alien' is added and the contents acquire strong affective tone. This group may be subdivided:

(1) *Compulsive affects*—strange, unmotivated feelings, against which the affected person struggles without success. (2) *Compulsive beliefs*—the patient is compelled to consider something true although he is convinced it is not. (3) *Compulsive urges*—senseless urges out of keeping with the personality—e.g. to kill one's own child. Where these urges tend to recur repeatedly in groups we can speak of *compulsive states,* compulsive excesses, for instance, of which compulsive cleanliness would be an example.

2. *Compulsive belief.* The characteristic of compulsive ideas is that the individual believes what is often a meaningful content yet knows the content

is false. A *struggle* ensues between conviction and knowing the opposite to be true. We must distinguish this phenomenon from ordinary doubt and from firm conviction. To give an example:

Emma A. had been through many phases of an affective disorder. Each time she recovered completely. For some weeks she had again been ill, homesick and depressed and she was in hospital. Two men were teasing her, tickling under her armpits and touching her on the head. She objected to this: 'I am not going to flirt around in the hospital'. Then the thought occurred to her that the men might have assaulted her and she might be expecting a baby. This idea, which was quite baseless, came to dominate her more and more. Here are some of her comments: 'I put the idea away sometimes but it keeps on coming back.' Her thoughts revolve round the topic. 'All day long I turn over in my mind how it all happened; they wouldn't have had the nerve.' She is certain she is having a child but immediately afterwards she says: 'I am not quite certain, there is always a bit of doubt'. She tells the story to her sister and they laugh about it. She had to go to the doctor to be examined and resisted this because the doctor might laugh at her about it, 'such a stupid idea'. The doctor found nothing. This reassured her for a day but then she ceased to believe him, perhaps he only wanted to reassure her. 'I simply don't believe people any more.' She expected to miss her periods; when menstruation started she was reassured for the time but she was not convinced. 'I try to sort it all out for myself; I sit down and think . . . it can't be true, I haven't been a bad lass and then I think again . . . and yet I tell myself, one fine day it'll turn out to be true . . .' 'I go on like this all day . . . there is always a wrangle going on inside me. It may have been like this or like that, it's always to and fro.' She was extremely restless. She was always thinking she was big with child and that everyone noticed it—'I keep on thinking it will be terrible when it comes'. Sometimes the patient laughs about all this nonsense which she thinks. Asked about her illness, she denies she is ill but says, 'I know that it has always gone away before.'

We may say in conclusion that the patient's ideas all group round one central idea which keeps recurring in her consciousness involuntarily (compulsive thinking); the validity of these ideas forces itself on the patient in the face of her conviction to the contrary (compulsive belief).

These compulsive beliefs need to be distinguished from three other phenomena, that is from delusion, from over-valued ideas and from normal doubt. In the case of *delusion* a judgment is made which is held on to with full conviction, not only with a consciousness of validity but with a sense of absolute certainty. In compulsive belief, there is no question of absolute certainty. With *over-valued ideas* belief is strong, the topic itself is the only thing that matters and the psychic life is normal and unchanged so far as the individual himself is concerned, whereas in compulsive belief he considers his belief to be morbid. In the case of *ordinary doubt* a judicious weighing of the pros and cons leads to an indecision, experienced as a psychologically unified judgment on the situation. In the case of compulsive belief, however, conviction is felt simultaneously with a knowledge of the very opposite. As an illustration, we might take the *competing visual fields* in the stereoscope (Friedmann). There is a constant contest going on between a consciousness of validity and of non-validity. Both push this way and that, but neither can gain the upper hand. In normal doubt, there is not this experience of right and wrong, but as far as the subject himself is concerned, a single, unified act of judgment establishes the matter as undecided.

3. *Compulsive urges and behaviour*. When urges arise in us and the consequences of acting them out are of some importance, there may arise a conflict of motive. Decision is reached in two ways, either there is a feeling of self-assertion, conscious freedom or defeat, a consciousness of having to submit. This is a normal and universal phenomenon. In the latter case, however, there may be the added awareness of an alien urge which does not arise as one's own, foreign to one's nature, apparently meaningless, incomprehensible. In these circumstances if action follows, we speak of compulsive behaviour. If the urge is suppressed and does not issue in behaviour, we speak of *compulsive urge*. Often individuals who are experiencing such phenomena will comply with these urges, when they are harmless (e.g. move chairs, swear, etc.), but they will successfully resist criminal urges or those with distressful consequences, e.g. murder of a child, suicide (e.g. throwing oneself from a great height).

Compulsive urges can be partly understood as secondary compulsive behaviour emerging from other compulsive events, e.g. a man who has the compulsive belief that he has given some promise which he cannot fulfil may ask for a written certificate that he has not done so. This secondary behaviour includes many defensive acts taking place on the basis of other compulsive events, e.g. washing through fear of contamination. The behaviour develops into a ritual and is expected to serve as a defence against disaster, one magic against another; the performance grows all the more irksome because it never brings fulfilment. Performance becomes scrupulously exact, distractions must be excluded and there is an engagement of the whole mind. Every possibility of error arouses doubt as to the effectiveness of the ritual and increases the demand for further acts to make certain, and, if there is further doubt, there must be a full repetition from the start; in this way any definite result in the form of a successful completion of the whole behaviour becomes impossible. When the compulsive urges are surrendered to, there is, as in impulsive action, a vivid feeling of relief. If, however, they are resisted, severe anxiety arises or other symptoms such as motor discharges. To get rid of the anxiety, patients must once more carry out the meaningless ritual of harmless acts. Fear of suffering this anxiety is enough to arouse it, and within this vicious circle the phenomenon pursues its increasingly painful and self-aggravating course.

4. *Phobias*. Patients are beset by an irresistible and terrifying fear of perfectly natural situations and performances: for instance, fear of closed spaces or of crossing open places (agoraphobia). The phenomenon has been described as follows:

Patients suffer an enormous anxiety, real fear of death together with terror, when they want to cross an open space, find themselves in empty streets, or stand outside tall houses or in other similar circumstances. They feel oppression in the chest, palpitations, a sense of freezing, of being hot in the head, of perspiring, of being clamped to the ground, and a paralysing weakness in the extremities and a fear of falling.[1]

## SECTION TWO

## THE MOMENTARY WHOLE—THE STATE OF CONSCIOUSNESS

For the first time in our study of the phenomena of experience, we come to the idea of something complete, something as a whole, and we find it in a form par excellence, that is in the immediate experience of the total psychic state.

Phenomena do not originate in discrete fashion, and causes which give rise to single phenomena are rare. There is always a total state of consciousness which makes it possible for individual phenomena to arise. We have isolated phenomena by description and we have begun to arrange them in certain groups and in a certain order. This has to be done because it is only by making these clear distinctions that viewpoints on the whole are reached, which are productive, because well structured. But by themselves all these distinctions are incomplete.

When speaking of individual phenomenological data, we have temporarily pre-supposed that the total state of the psyche within which these data occur remains the same; we call this the normal state of awareness and clear consciousness. But in actuality the total state of psychic life is extremely variable and the phenomenological elements are by no means always the same but have individual permutations according to what all the other elements are and to what the total state may be. We see, therefore, that an analysis of an individual case cannot consist simply in breaking up the situation into its elements, but that there has to be constant referral to the psychic state as a whole. In psychic life, everything is connected with everything else and each element is coloured by the state and context within which it occurs. Traditionally this fundamental fact has been emphasised by distinguishing the *content* of consciousness (broadly speaking all the elements so far described have belonged to content) from the *activity of consciousness itself.* Each single element, every perception, image or feeling differs according to whether it occurs in a state of clear or clouded consciousness. The more the state of consciousness differs in its characteristics from the one we are used to, the more difficult it becomes to get adequate understanding of it as a whole as well as of the individual phenomena. Psychic life taking place in deep clouding of consciousness is generally inaccessible for phenomenological examination, or can be made accessible only with the greatest difficulty.

[1] Westphal, *Arch. Psychiatr.*, vol. 3 (1872), pp. 138, 219; vol. 7 (1877), p. 377.

It will therefore be of decisive significance in the assessment of all sub-jective phenomena to determine whether they are occurring in a state of clear consciousness or not. Hallucinations, pseudo-hallucinations, delusional ex-periences and delusions which occur in *clear consciousness* cannot be taken as part-symptoms of some transient alteration of consciousness; they have to be regarded as *symptoms of much more profound processes* within the psychic life. We can properly speak of hallucinations and delusions only when there is this clear state of consciousness.

There are many altered states of consciousness (like sleep and dream) which are quite normal and accessible to everyone; others depend on certain conditions. In trying to visualise the psychotic states we seek *comparison* with our own experiences (in dreams, while falling asleep, in states of fatigue) and some psychiatrists have collected experiences during self-induced toxic states (mescalin, hashish, etc.), so as to get first-hand experiences by means of 'model' psychoses of states that may be closely related to that of some mental patients.

*Psychological preface.* The term 'consciousness' denotes first of all the *actual inner awareness* of experience (as contrasted with the externality of events that are the subject of biological enquiry); secondly, it denotes a *subject–object dichotomy* (i.e. a subject intentionally directs itself to objects which it perceives, imagines or thinks), thirdly, it denotes the *knowledge of a conscious self* (self-awareness). Correspondingly *unconscious* means firstly something that is not an inner existence and does not occur as an experience; secondly, something that is not thought of as an object and has gone unregarded (it may have been perceived and therefore can be recalled later); thirdly, it is something which has not reached any knowledge of itself.

The whole of psychic life *at any given moment* is called consciousness; and con-tains the above three aspects. *Loss of consciousness* occurs when the inwardness of an experience vanishes and with it, therefore, goes consciousness, as happens in fainting, narcosis, deep and dreamless sleep, coma and epileptic seizures. But if some degree of inner experience is present we still speak of consciousness, even though our awareness of objects has become clouded and there is only a weak self-awareness, if it has not been obliterated. *Clear consciousness* demands that what I think is clearly before me and I know what I do and wish to do it; that what I experience is my experience, linked to a self and held together in a context of memory. Before psychic phenomena can be called conscious they must be remarked by the individual at some stage so that they can be lifted into clear consciousness.

We *imagine consciousness* as a *stage* on which individual psychic phenomena come and go or as a *medium* in which they move. As something psychic it naturally belongs to all psychic phenomena and has a number of modes. To keep our metaphor we may say for instance that the stage can shrink (narrowing of consciousness) or the medium can grow dense (clouding of consciousness), etc.

1. The field of clear consciousness within the total conscious state is termed the field of *attention*. This covers three closely connected but conceptually distinct phenomena: (1) attention as the experience of *turning oneself towards an object* may show itself as a predominantly active experience when accompanied by awareness of its own inner determinants. Or it may show itself as a predominantly passive experi-

ence when it consists rather in being drawn towards something or being fascinated by it. This creates the distinction between voluntary and involuntary attention. (2) The *degree of clarity and distinctness* of the conscious content is termed the degree of attention. This relates to the preferential selection of content. Liepmann spoke of this metaphorically as the energy of attention and Lipps conceived it as the application of psychic power to a psychic event. This clarity or distinctness of content is usually linked with the experience of turning towards something or being fascinated by it. But in pathological states there may not be this accompanying experience and these qualities therefore come and go and vacillate independently. (3) *The effects* of these two first phenomena on the *further course* of psychic life have also been included under attention. The clarity of the conscious content is chiefly responsible for rousing further associations, since such content is retained in memory with particular ease. Guiding notions, set tasks, target ideas or whatever we choose to call them, if grasped with attention in the first two senses of the word, undoubtedly have such an effect on the appearance of other ideas that appropriate and useful associations are automatically selected (determining tendencies).

It will be seen, therefore, that our momentary state of consciousness is not an even one throughout. Around the *focal point* of consciousness a *field of attention* spreads, dimming in clarity towards the periphery. There is only one point in clearest consciousness. From then on a whole series of less conscious phenomena extends in every direction. Usually these phenomena go unregarded but taken as a whole they create an *atmosphere* and contribute to the total state of consciousness, the whole mood, meaning and potentiality of the given situation. From the brightly lit centre of consciousness there is a general shadowing down to the obscure area where no clear demarcation remains between consciousness and the unconscious. Trained self-observation makes it possible to investigate the degree of consciousness ( = degree of attention, the level of awareness).[1]

2. The *state of consciousness as a whole*, our total psychic life at any given moment, may have different degrees of awareness from clearest consciousness through various stages of clouding to complete loss of consciousness. Consciousness may be pictured *as a wave* on its way to the unconscious. Clear consciousness is the crest, the crest becomes lower, the wave flatter, until it completely disappears. It is not however a simple matter of the one following the other. We are dealing with a changing manifold. We may find constriction of the field of awareness, diminished differentiation between subject and object and a failure to disentangle the encompassing feeling-states that are obscuring the thoughts, images and symbols.

*Alterations in consciousness* and *disturbances of the conscious state* are not uniform. They spring from a number of different causes, and may be brought about by concussion, physical illnesses that lead to psychoses, toxic states and abnormal psychic reactions. But they also can occur in healthy people, during sleep, in dreams and in hypnotic states. In the same way, altered consciousness has many modes. The one common factor is the negative one that all these alterations in consciousness represent some departure from the state of normal clarity, continuity and conscious linkage with the self. The normal state of

[1] Cp. Westphal, *Arch. Psychol.*, vol. 21. 'Über den Umfang des Bewusstseins': Wirth in Wundt's *Phil. Stud.*, vol. 20, p. 487.

consciousness, which is itself capable of very varied degrees of clarity and comprehensiveness and can be of the most heterogeneous content, remains as the focal point and round it in all directions we find that deviations, alterations, expansions and restrictions can take place.

*Techniques of enquiry.* There are always two ways of trying to understand patients and gain some insight into the psychic events taking place within them. We can try *conversation* and make every attempt to establish a psychic relationship between the patient and ourselves; we can endeavour to empathise with their inner experiences. Alternatively, we can ask them to *write down afterwards* what went on in their minds, and make use of these self-descriptions when they have recovered from their psychoses. The more the total psychic state has suffered alteration, the more we depend on these subsequent self-descriptions.

If the total state of mind is on the whole intact—though even so the most severe psychic disturbances may be present, such as delusion, hallucination, or change of personality, we say the patient is sensible. *Sensible* is the term we give to the state of consciousness in which intense affect is absent, the conscious contents have an average clarity and definition and the psychic life runs in orderly fashion determined by foreseen goals. An objective sign of this sensible state is orientation (the individual's present awareness of the orderly structure of his world as a whole); another sign is the ability to collect thoughts in response to questions and to remember things. This is the most suitable state of consciousness in which to reach a mutual understanding. As the total state alters, it becomes increasingly more difficult to get in touch with the patient. One condition for keeping some mental rapport with him is that we should be able to pin him down in some way, and get him to react to questions and set problems, so that we can judge from his reaction whether he has grasped them or not. Normal people can concentrate on any task which is set them, but with alteration in the total psychic state, this capacity steadily decreases. Patients may no longer respond to a question in any intelligible way, but repeated questioning may possibly elicit some reaction. One can then still pin them down on easy and neutral points, such as the place of birth, the name of a place, etc., but they may no longer respond to the more difficult questions and tasks, such as what do they think, etc. We may then be able to get them with visual situations and stimuli, but they will no longer react to verbal stimuli. To the extent to which we can pin patients down in one way or another, we can hope to embark with some degree of success on the path of direct understanding. If, however, they are deeply preoccupied with themselves, the sparse fragments of information divulged are rarely sufficient for us to arrive at any convincing view of their inner experiences.

## § 1. ATTENTION AND FLUCTUATIONS IN CONSCIOUSNESS

### (a) *Attention*

This determines the clarity of our experience. If we take the second of the above discussed concepts of attention—the clearness and precision of the psychic phenomena, the degree of consciousness, the level of awareness, we can see that, with each psychic phenomenon we discover in our patient, we need to know how much attention he gave and *at what level of awareness* the

phenomenon was experienced. Otherwise we shall not reach a full understanding. If he has nothing special to say, we may assume the experience took
place in a state of clear consciousness.

Sense-deceptions may occur along with the fullest attention or with complete inattention. For instance, some sense-deceptions can take place only at a
low level of attention and will disappear if full attention is directed upon them.
Patients complain that 'the voices cannot be caught' or that it is a 'hellish
dazzle' (Binswanger). Other sense-deceptions—particularly in subsiding
psychoses—are experienced only in a state of acute attention, and disappear if
the attention is directed elsewhere. 'Saying a prayer makes the voices go.'
Observing an object brings the visual pseudo-hallucination to an end. The
importance of the degree of attention in the case of sense-deceptions is beauti-
fully illustrated by patients suffering from alcoholic deliria, as investigated by
Bonhoeffer.[1] If the examiner keeps attention up to a moderate degree by
making the patient talk and reply, few sense-deceptions occur, but if attention lapses—a tendency of the patients when left to themselves—massive
illusions and scenic hallucinations reappear. However, when the examiner
forcibly directs attention to visual stimuli, numerous discrete illusions
appear in this field. With psychic 'passivity' phenomena, we sometimes find
a noteworthy low degree of consciousness. When the patient is occupied
he feels nothing of this, but if he sits around with nothing to do 'passivity'
phenomena appear—attacks of giddiness, compression in the head, attacks
of rage, whispers—which he can subdue only by a terrific effort of will—
sometimes shaking his fists. This is why such troubled patients seek company,
conversation, something to do or some other means of distraction (praying,
mumbling meaningless phrases), through which they hope to free themselves
from the 'influence' of the voices. Schreber experienced ideas as put into his
head when he sat around doing nothing, and called them his 'non-thinking
thoughts'. The following self-description illustrates the dependence of schizophrenic phenomena on attention, and on arbitrary encouragement or dis-
couragement:

'I felt as if I were continually among criminals or devils. As soon as my strained
attention wandered off from things around me, I saw and heard them, but I didn't
always have the power to deflect my attention from them to other tangible objects.
Every effort to do that was like rolling a millstone uphill. For instance, the attempt
to listen to a friend's conversation that lasted more than a few sentences resulted in
such restlessness (because these threatening figures towered over us) that I had to
take my quick departure. It was extremely hard to attend to an object for any length
of time. My thoughts would wander off at once to far-away places where demons
would at once attack me, as if provoked. At first this shift of thought, this giving way,
happened voluntarily and was sought by me, but now it happens on its own. It was a
sort of weakness; I felt driven to it irresistibly. In the evening when trying to sleep I
closed my eyes and would enter the vortex willy-nilly. In the daytime, however, I

[1] Bonhoeffer, *Die akuten Geisteskrankheiten der Gewohnheitstrinker* (Jena, 1901), pp. 19 ff.

managed to keep out of it. It was a feeling of being spun round until figures appeared·
I had to lie in bed awake and watchful until after many hours the enemy withdrew a
little. All I could do was to try not to encourage the thing by letting myself go.' At a
later phase the patient reports: 'Every time I wanted to I saw these figures and was
able to draw conclusions about my own state. To keep control I had to utter words
for inner protection; this was to make me more aware of the new self which seemed
trying to hide behind a veil. I would say "I am" (trying to feel the new self, not the
old); "I am the absolute" (I meant this in relation to physical matters, I did not want
to be God). "I am spirit, not flesh" . . . "I am the one in everything" . . . "I am what
lasts" (as compared with the fluctuations of physical and mental life . . .) or I would
use single words like "power" or "life".'

These protective words had always to be at hand. In the course of 10 years, they
became a feeling. The sensations which they aroused had so to speak accumulated so
that he did not have to think afresh every time but at times of particular instability
they had to be used then as now, in a somewhat altered form. The patient could see
the figures at any time he wanted and could study them, but he did not have to see
them. (However, after specific physical disturbances they came on their own and
once more became dangerous) (Schwab).

## (b) Fluctuations in consciousness

Mild degrees of fluctuation in consciousness may be observed in *the
periodic waxing or waning of attention* (Wundt). The crest of the wave of
psychic life never remains at the same height from moment to moment, but
changes all the time, however slightly. We may observe more noticeable
changes during fatigue, and more noticeable changes still and to a pathological
degree in those *periodic fluctuations of consciousness*[1] which sometimes dwindle
down to a complete absence of it. We have observed a patient in whom this
occurred within the course of one minute. In epileptic patients normal conscious attention, as measured by reaction to hardly perceptible stimuli,
fluctuates much more than in the case of healthy persons.[2]

Fluctuations of consciousness must be differentiated from *petit mal* attacks,
absences, etc., which lead to irregular interruptions of consciousness, accompanied by
slight motor phenomena. Nor should they be confused with the *interruptions of concentration and reactivity* frequently observed in schizophrenic patients (so-called
*blocking*). They suddenly cease to reply, stare in front, and do not seem to understand
anything. After a time (minutes or seconds) this ceases, only to recur again a little
later. Subsequently one can often find that the patients have been perfectly attentive
during the time they were inaccessible and remember the occasion. These interruptions occur for *no apparent reason* as an expression of the disease process or they may
be attributable to *affect-laden complexes*, which the examiner's questions have triggered off, or they may be understood as distraction by voices and other hallucinations.
In the last case, we may observe that the patients have grasped only poorly what the
examiner said.

[1] Stertz, *Arch. Psychiatr.*, vol. 48, p. 199. Janet, *Nevroses et idées fixes*, pp. 69–108. *Psychasthenie*, pp. 371–7.
[2] Wiersma, 'The psychology of epilepsy', *J. Ment. Sci.*, vol. 69 (1923), p. 482.

Fluctuations of consciousness down to the loss of it may be observed in personality disorders (psychopaths) and in many acute and chronic psychoses. The patients themselves complain that they lose their thoughts momentarily. 'The works have stopped.' Janet describes these as 'éclipses mentales'.

A proband describes such an experience under hashish:

'It feels as if I am always emerging from unconsciousness only to fall back into it after a time . . . meanwhile my consciousness has altered . . . instead of completely empty "absences", I now have something else like a second consciousness. This is experienced as a period of time on its own. Subjectively it is as if there are two separate sequences of experience each running its own course. The experimental situation seems unaltered; but there follows the experience of a long-drawn-out, undifferentiated existence in which I cannot keep myself separate from the experienced world. In spite of this, I experience this second state not as in a dream but in complete wakefulness. This alternating consciousness may explain my over-estimation of time, which is excessive. I feel as if hours must have elapsed since the beginning of the intoxication; the thinking process is extremely difficult and every sequence of ideas gets cut off when the next change in consciousness occurs.' [1]

### (c) Clouding of consciousness

Lowering, clouding or narrowing of consciousness occurs variously as the accompaniment and consequence of single experiences. On a long train journey we may doze and experience a low ebb of the wave-crest, an *emptiness of consciousness*, which we can interrupt at will. When there are *violent affects*, as in anxiety states and deep melancholia as well as in manic states, it becomes much more difficult to concentrate on anything external, contemplate anything, reach a judgment, or even think of anything. Answers to simple questions can only be given after a number of unsuccessful attempts and visible exertion on the part of the patient. For this reason, i.e. difficulty of concentration, the contents of delusion-like ideas go unscrutinised by the patient and there is no reality-judgment concerning possible sense-deceptions. Consciousness is completely filled by the affect, and judgment and attitude become very disturbed in an understandable way. This is even more the case in depressive states when primary inhibition of function is added. All the above states, however, deserve the name of abnormal consciousness, which may become a persisting emptiness of consciousness in the last-named instance.

### (d) Heightening of consciousness

We may wonder whether heightening of consciousness really is a fact; do we find abnormal alertness, abnormal clarity, and other abnormal phenomena of this order? Kurt Schneider considers heightened clarity of consciousness a necessary prelude for the development of certain compulsive states. 'This exceptional clarity of consciousness is well marked in cases of encephalitis with obsessional symptoms.' Of another sort are those numerous self-descriptions

[1] Beringer, *Nervenarzt*, vol. 5, p. 341.

of a mystic retreat into contemplation, which suggest a state of overwakeful-ness. Different again are the unusual brilliant states of narrowed consciousness occurring as an aura in epileptic attacks and described by Weber and Jung. One patient described it as if 'thinking became absolutely clear'. The authors point to Dostoievsky's own description of his aura 'as if there was a flare-up in the brain', so that 'the sense of life and self was increased ten-fold'.

Zutt[1] describes phenomena after the taking of Pervitin: overwakefulness, vivid interest, shortening of performance, shorter reaction-time and the con-quest of masses of material by apperception. At the same time he points out diminished powers of concentration, crowding of thoughts, diminution in the ability to order impressions or meditate deeply and a restless interest of an aimless character with an equally aimless drive to activity. This overwakeful-ness means a reduction in the precision and clarity of the external world, since the external world tends to retreat for tired and over-wakeful people. Zutt, therefore, constructs a polarity of consciousness between sleepiness and over-wakefulness, so that the peak of clarity lies in the middle. The above phen-omena once more show the ambiguity and enigmatic character of what we call a state of consciousness.

## § 2. SLEEP AND HYPNOSIS

### (a) Dreams

Hacker[2] has tried to clarify dream life phenomenologically for the first time by taking notes on his dreams for a whole year. He did this immediately on waking up, noting how his dream experiences appeared to him. The specific character of dream life showed itself in three ways: (1) *Elements* which are always present in waking life are now *in abeyance*. There is no true aware-ness of one's personality, so that acts take place which would be foreign to the individual in his waking state without this being noticed at all in the dream. There is no awareness of the past, no awareness of self-evident relationships between things, so that the dreamer may, for instance, talk to a doctor about his leg-muscles while the latter dissects him anatomically, or he may look at his own abdominal cavity without seeing anything queer about such a situation. There are, therefore, no volitional acts, with the consciousness of 'I really will . . .', if for no other reason but that the feeling of personality is absent and there is only a momentary self-awareness. The dream may become completely rudimentary and all that is left consists of a number of psychic fragments. Thus Hacker once found that at the moment of waking a few incomprehensible words remained in the dream, which he could understand only when he woke

---

[1] Zutt, 'Über die polare Struktur des Bewusstseins', *Nervenarzt.*, vol. 16 (1943), p. 145.

[2] Hacker, 'Systematische Traumbeobachtungen mit besonderer Berücksichtigung der Gedan-ken', *Arch. Psychol.* (D), vol. 21. Köhler, *Arch. Psychol* (D), vol. 23. Hoche, *Das traümende Ich* (Jena, 1927). E. Kraepelin, 'Die Sprachstörungen im Traum', *Psychol. Arb.*, vol. 5, p. 1.

up. There was not only no awareness of meaning but no awareness that they were words, and no sense of any object versus the self. It was so to speak sensory material left over which had not become fully objectified. (2) *Psychic connections vanish*. Psychic life so to speak goes into dissolution, gestalt-configurations, the linking tendencies of volition, all disintegrate. There is no representation in the present of past and future; the dream lives only in the moment, one scene follows another, and often the previous one is completely forgotten. Contradictory things are experienced without surprise consecutively or simultaneously. From such elements as are apprehended, no determining tendencies emerge, but the most heterogeneous things follow one another in a changing, haphazard flow of association. Among the general dissolution of connections the most surprising was the misapprehension of sensory objects. Hacker dreamt, for instance, that he was looking for some chemical substance for analysis; some one gave him his big toe, which seemed quite naturally a chemical substance. On waking up he could recall both the sense-experience of seeing the big toe, and the being aware that this was a chemical substance. This dissolution of connection between sensory material and awareness of appropriate meaning is a common phenomenon in dreams. (3) *Fresh elements appear*. These are the dream-images which we cannot call hallucinations, delusions or false memories. On the other hand these contents have a vividness which they would not have if they were mere images. New things arise in the form of remarkable identifications and condense and separate in an astonishing way.

Apparently Hacker never dreamt of coherent situations and events such as others have experienced in dreams with great vividness. He belonged to those who completely forget their dreams if immediately on waking they do not record the few remembered fragments which they can retain. Other people, however, can be haunted all day by dreams and remain vividly conscious of them. But in general the sensory richness, the actual experience of vividness is apt to be over-rated. This is shown by the following example in which the dreamer looks on and observes his experiences while dreaming:

A friend of mine, who had no psychological training and was not interested in psychology, sometimes thought to himself: 'it really seems that one sees things in a dream which one has never seen before. Perhaps one can learn in a dream of things which waking reality never shows. I want to look out for this in my dreams.' One day he recounted a recent dream: 'I must have slept a long time, when I realised I was dreaming without having to wake up because of this idea. I thought in my dream that I was dreaming and could wake up when I wanted to, but immediately I became conscious of the thought—No, I will go on dreaming—I want to see how this ends; I was clearly aware of the question—will I see something in my dream never seen so far in reality! I went on dreaming and seemed to take up a book to see the letters clearly; as soon as I brought the book near to my eyes the letters became blurred; I could not read anything; I took other objects to look at closely but I saw everything as one sees them ordinarily when one is in a room, with a general impression of detail. If I tried to see the details properly, they became blurred. After a while I really woke up and looked at the clock. It was 3.0 a.m. It surprised me to find that one could dream and yet be an observer at the same time.'

## (b) Falling asleep and waking

These allow for intermediary states to be experienced. Carl Schneider[1] describes the experience of falling asleep; everything grows fleeting, vague and loses its structure; thoughts, feelings, perceptions, images merge in confusion, glide away, slip about and get derailed, while at the same time we may have exotic experiences, sense deep meanings or the presence of the infinite. One's own activity merges into an accepting and a yielding until, in spite of the unity of consciousness, self-awareness completely dissolves away. During the phases of falling asleep, healthy people will often have what are, therefore, called hypnagogic hallucinations.

Certain *hallucinations at the time of waking* are very characteristically dependent on the state of consciousness. Patients have a feeling that they have been wakened by the hallucination, but once they are quite awake the hallucination has gone.

Miss M. clearly felt during the night that she was pulled suddenly by the hair at the back of the neck on the left, pulled with great force. At the same time, she saw a great flame flare up for a moment from the depths and then die down. She awoke immediately and once awake there was nothing more to be seen, but she knew this had not been a dream. It had been real and it had wakened her. It happened between sleeping and waking and it had disappeared altogether once she was completely awake. Similarly on two occasions at night when she was staying in the clinic something was done to her genital organs; certain movements were carried out quickly, as if she were having sexual intercourse. The moment she opened her eyes, she saw no one was there but she was certain it was not a dream and that it was being done by some evil force. On another occasion she saw the bedcovers lifting just when she woke up. Fehrlin reports: 'I suddenly woke up at midnight and felt myself embraced by a woman whose hair fell over my face. Quickly, she cried, you have to die . . . then it was all over.' With some patients this sort of thing repeats itself several times during the night and they are tired and unrefreshed the next day. The content of these phenomena proves to be manifold but they themselves always have this element of suddenness, something happens like lightning.

## (c) Hypnosis

Hypnosis is related to sleep and is identical in character. During hypnosis a particular kind of productivity arises; pictures are seen and memories are relived. There is no known principle on which we can grasp this state, as to what it really is. We can delineate it only by distinguishing it. It is not an understandable psychic change but a vital event of a peculiar kind which is linked with effective suggestion. It is a primary phenomenon of somato-psychic life, manifesting itself as an alteration of the conscious state.

---

[1] Carl Schneider, *Psychologie der Schizophrenen*, p. 12 u.a. 'Über das Einschlaferleben vgl.', Mayer-Gross in Bumke's *Handbuch*, vol. 1, pp. 433–8.

The changes in consciousness which occur during sleep, hypnosis and certain hysterical states are in some way inter-related but they can be fully grasped only if we know in what way precisely they differ.

## § 3. Psychotic Alterations in Consciousness

The alteration of consciousness in acute psychoses, in deliria and in twilight-states is certainly very different in each case. We need only to compare the reduced consciousness of organic processes with the dreamy perplexity of the acute psychoses, the confusions of deliria or the relatively well-ordered, coherent behaviour in some twilight states to get the impression that we are not dealing with one single type of disturbed consciousness. At the present time, however, we cannot formulate the differences comprehensibly. We will only describe the following types: *reduced consciousness (torpor)*, *clouded consciousness* and *altered consciousness*.

(a) By '*reduced consciousness or torpor*' we mean those states that lie between consciousness and unconsciousness; no *fresh psychic events* are being experienced, *only fewer*. Perceptions remain as dim as the memories. Very few associations appear and the act of thought can no longer be performed. All psychic events are slowed down and much more difficult. As a result patients take no part in things, are apathetic, apt to doze and show no spontaneity; when talked to, their attention is hard to rouse and cannot be sustained; they cannot concentrate and are easily tired but in pure cases appear *perfectly orientated*. There is a tendency to fall into a dreamless sleep or sink into a state of coma or sopor from which they cannot be roused.

(b) *Clouded consciousness.* *Florid events* are taking place and hallucinations, affects and partly coherent fantasy experiences are occurring to the extent that there is no longer any consistent, connected flow of psychic events. Psychic life *breaks up*, so to speak, and fragmented experiences take place disconnectedly. Only single, completely isolated acts remain and there is an entire splintering of consciousness. Contents become highly self-contradictory (there are, for instance, rapidly changing and opposing 'delusions') so that nothing can be remembered.

(c) *Altered consciousness.* The state is usually clearly demarcated from normal psychic life and *relatively coherent* so that patients possibly remain quite normal. Consciousness is restricted to certain areas only and nothing else is allowed to intrude that does not fit the inner set. Westphal gave the following description: 'There are states which may last a few minutes or hours in which consciousness is so deeply disturbed that the individual moves in a circle of ideas that appear quite detached from his normal ones. On the basis of these ideas and the feelings and wishes which are linked with them, he may carry out acts which are entirely foreign to the usual content of his thoughts and are unconnected with them. But the ability is not abolished to act coherently and to a certain extent logically.' The span of altered consciousness is different and split off in the memory from normal consciousness. Not only hysterical twilight states but also apparently elementary phenomena such as epilepsy belong to this group.

(*d*) The state of consciousness *during an aura* before an epileptic seizure[1] is an uncommonly brief alteration in consciousness before it merges into unconsciousness. During it the outer world disappears; the inner experiences become overpowering, consciousness narrows and in this restricted state it can yet have a moment of high illumination. Out of initial anxiety, and with full clarity of consciousness, ecstasy may rise to a pitch of unbearable terror during which unconsciousness and the fall of the seizure begin:

There are a number of *objective symptoms* for all kinds of clouding of consciousness in psychotic states, though they may not be present in every individual case. They are: (1) *Turning away from the real world*: Patients comprehend poorly, cannot fix their attention and act without regard to the situation. (2) *Disorientation*: This is closely linked with (1). (3) *Loss of coherence*: which makes the behaviour un-under-standable. (4) *Disturbance in registration and memory*: along with difficulties in reflection and subsequent *amnesia*.

## § 4. FORMS OF COMPLEX FANTASY EXPERIENCE

Alterations in the conscious state are frequently the soil for pathological experiences. At any time of day these states may appear briefly as a kind of sleep or, if of longer duration, as psychotic states which last several days or weeks. Hallucinatory experience is especially common (a differentiation between hallucination proper, pseudo-hallucination and mere awarenesses no longer becomes possible). While the patient is in this half-sleep, someone may approach his bed; he feels the actual approach, he feels the hand around his neck, feels suffocated. Or he lives among a series of vivid scenes, landscapes, crowds, mortuaries, graves. Very often the patients can feel this alteration of consciousness when it happens. They may feel it from the start, at the point where it overcomes them and also at the end, when they come round again: 'just now, as I dreamt it'. In mild cases they may be able to observe themselves in this altered state: they are peculiarly puzzled; they feel they cannot think, they have to remind themselves where they are and what they wanted to do. Hysterical people can more or less put themselves into a twilight state through an abnormal kind of day-dreaming.

These unreal contents of psychotic experience have their own context; they build up as it were a continuous world and fate for the patient. This context splits off from the world of real experience and becomes a transitory event, limited to a certain period of time (days, months or years). We will try to bring some order into these diverse and numerous experiences, and if we want to understand the peculiarities of an individual case, we shall first have to be clear about certain basic differences of a purely descriptive character:

[1] Weber and Jung, *Z. Neur.*, vol. 170, p. 211.

1. One set of experiences comes during *clouded consciousness*; the other—more rarely—may fill the psyche in states of *altered consciousness*, which do not exclude complete wakefulness. In the former, clouding is recognised in the general lowering of the mental activity, in the loosening of context and in the hazy memory which remains. Wakeful experiences on the other hand are of extreme clarity; they demonstrate a pervading connectedness of phenomena which brings the psychotic experience close to real experiences and they tend to be remembered vividly. Even incoherent experiences during wakefulness are well remembered.

2. One set of experiences occurs *in complete isolation* from the real environment. The psyche is in another world altogether and is without relationship to the real situation. The other set of experiences *intertwines* in a peculiar way *with real perceptions* and with the real environment, which is then misinterpreted and bears a different meaning as related to the particular psychotic experience.

3. In relation to the subjective attitude of patients towards their psychotic experiences, we find two contrasting extremes: Either the patient is nothing but *a spectator*. He is quite detached, passive, even indifferent. He sees everything clearly and faces the contents calmly as they emerge or pass before him as impressive visions, with complex elaborations in all the sensory fields. Alternatively, he is *actively engaged*. He stands in the mid-stream of the events; he is in the grip of powerful entities which, sometimes painfully, sometimes delightfully, toss his mind to and fro. He may be thrown from heights of bliss to depths of hell. He becomes a world-redeeming person and then the devil himself in most evil form. Whereas the first group of experiences have a pronouncedly scenic character, the latter are much more dramatic. To use Nietzsche's words, the former have more the character of dreams and dream-objects, while the latter are more like an intoxication.

4. As far as the *connectedness* of the particular content is concerned, this may vary from *completely isolated*, individual, false perceptions or awareness, etc.—hardly to be included among experiences in the sense in which we use the word—to a *continuous, progressive* occurrence, with definite circumscribed events, that denote phases and crises in the history of the psychosis. In rare, fully developed cases, we may see over long periods a sequence of phases in which the patient passes, rather like Dante, through hell, purgatory and paradise. Such connection as there is will either predominate in the concrete, rational content of the experience or in the confusion-like subjective state. Either we observe isolated experiences of fragmented situations occurring in a confused sequence or we see over a period one scene emerging organically out of another. Usually the patient seems completely submerged in the psychotic experience, in which he lives with all his senses to the full, but sometimes a particular sense, usually the visual one, seems more predominant.

5. *Contents* are either *sensorily vivid* and *complex* or in spite of the intensity of the experience they may be little more than *awarenesses* or pale images. As

to their significance, contents are either *ordinary* and simply relate to everyday experience (the patient, for instance, is concerned with his experiences at work and its possible irritations) or the contents may prove *fantastic*, such as never occur in reality. The patient stands at the crossroads of world events. He feels the world's axis at his side; tremendous cosmic movements are connected with his fate; mighty tasks await him; everything depends on him; he can do anything, even the impossible, thanks to his magnificent powers.

6. The experiences may be unified—the patients have only one reality, the psychotic one; or the experiences—particularly the fantastic ones—may occur while the patient lives in two worlds simultaneously, the real one which he can see and judge for himself and his psychotic one. He acquires a certain *double orientation* and can move among live realities more or less correctly, in spite of his cosmic experiences, but the psychotic reality is the real world for him. The actual external world has become an illusion which he can conveniently ignore to the extent that he knows: these are doctors, I am in the cells, they say I am religiously deluded. It happens that the patient in an acute psychosis is completely filled for a time with his psychotic experiences and forgets who he was, where he is, etc., but he is apt to be pulled out of this illusionary world by harsh events or certain profound impressions (admission to an institution, visits by relatives). An emphatic word may lead the patient back to reality for a moment. Then the double orientation reasserts itself; everything acquires double motivation, he himself is double or manifold. 'I have thought of an enormous number of things from many spheres altogether at once', said a patient. In typical cases the patient comes into collision with reality when he experiences supernatural processes which he expects to change something in the external world. Reality is to disappear and so on. Then occurs 'the experience of the catastrophe that fails' and this is followed by indifference which later on makes room for new contents to arise.

Differentiations such as these are very general and are mere viewpoints for analysis. We have no factually based order for the various forms of psychotic experience. Out of the immense variety that presents itself to us, we will limit ourselves to the description of a few selected types:[1]

1. *Daydreaming* can be found associated with other abnormalities. A man in prison imagines himself into the situation of fabulous wealth; he builds castles and lays the foundations of cities. He fantasies to such an extent that he cannot now differentiate clearly between reality and unreality. He draws large plans on waste paper and has vivid experiences of how he would behave in his new situation; how he acts and delights people. Fantasy such as this may start from an accidental notion but be carried on subsequently with an awareness that it is full reality. The individual buys a good deal he cannot pay for, for an imaginary mistress perhaps; he lives through the part of an inspector of schools and behaves so naturally during the school visit that he is not noticed

---

[1] Further material on these phantasy experiences can be found in W. Mayer-Gross, *Selbstschilderungen der Verwirrtheit* (die onciroide Erlebnisform) (Berlin, 1924).

until some all too obvious contradiction arises and puts an end to his fantasy. (Pseudologia phantastica.) With hysterical patients a certain alteration of consciousness may occur in the course of such daydreaming. The patients live through imaginary situations which they experience in the form of vivid hallucinations. The fantasies occurring during febrile illnesses, as described by Hoepffner,[1] are probably closely allied to such experiences.

2. *Delirious experiences.*[2] These are characterised particularly during alcoholic delirium by a strong sensory vividness, a low level of consciousness and therefore a lack of coherence. Content is quite natural and possible and corresponds to accustomed reality; it is almost always tinged with anxiety and consists in persecutions, maltreatments and often unpleasant and hurtful experiences.

3. *Illusory experiences* full of blissful tranquility that come to some people during hashish and opium intoxication have a peculiar character of their own:

*Baudelaire* reports the following description given by a woman: After taking hashish she found herself in an exquisitely panelled and furnished room (it had a golden ceiling with a geometrical grille). The moon was shining. She said: 'At first I was surprised; I saw enormous plains stretching in front of me and all around; there were clear rivers and green landscapes reflected in the quiet waters. (You may guess the effect of the panelling—reflected in the mirrors). As I raised my eyes, I saw a setting sun, like molten metal as it cools. This was the gold of the ceiling. The grille led me to think I was in some kind of cage or in a house open on all sides, separated from all these wonderful things only by the bars of my imposing prison. At first I laughed about the deception, but the longer I looked, the stranger the enchantment, the more living it grew, in all its clear and deceptive reality. Now the image of being locked in dominated my mind, without I must confess diminishing the pleasure I derived from the spectacle surrounding me. I considered myself imprisoned in this handsome cage for thousands of years among these enchanting landscapes and wonderful horizons. I dreamt as follows: The Beauty who sleeps in the forest is making expiation. I dreamt of her liberation. Brilliant tropical birds flew over my head and as my ears picked up the ringing of the horses' bells in the street, the impressions of the two senses fused into a single idea. I ascribed the wonderful tinkling sounds to the birds and I believed they were singing through their metallic beaks. They were chatting about me and glad I was a prisoner. Monkeys were playing and satyrs capered about delightfully and all of them seemed to be amused over the prisoner lying there condemned to immobility. However, all the gods of myth gave me a friendly smile as if they wanted to encourage me to bear the "spookery" patiently. All eyes were turned into one corner as if they wanted to touch each other with their gaze . . . I must confess the pleasure which I felt in looking at all these forms and brilliant colours and considering myself the centre of some fantastic dream; this took up all my thoughts. It lasted a long time. Did it go on till morning? I do not know. . . . I suddenly saw the morning sun in the room; I felt vivid surprise, and in spite of a struggle with my memory I could not tell whether I had been asleep or whether I had survived an ecstatic sleeplessness. A moment before it had been night; now it was

---

[1] Hoepffner, *Z. Neur.*, vol. 4 (1911), p. 678.
[2] Liepmann, *Arch. Psychiatr.* (D), vol. 27. Bonhoeffer, *Mschr. Psychiatr.*, vol. 1,

day . . . in that moment I had lived a long time, a very long time. My knowledge of time was in abeyance . . . so the whole night could be measured by me only in terms of the thoughts which filled it. Long as this seemed, I still felt it had all only lasted a few seconds; alternatively, it was so long it could not even find room in eternity.'

*Serko*'s self-description during mescalin intoxication is as follows: 'Seeing masses of colours, visual hallucinations with no connection in objective space; haptic hallucinations; disturbances of time-sense, a sentimental state of bliss, an enchanting fairy-tale atmosphere, due to the colours, the hallucinations, the disturbed time-sense, and with all this, a complete clarity of judgment and a correct reality-judgment.'

4. Surpassing all the forms of experience so far enumerated are the schizophrenic psychoses,[1] the acute experiences of which offer a continuity, richness and importance of content, which overshadow the rest. We have selected two cases of such experiences, which of course by no means exhaust the matter.

(*a*) The common schizophrenic experience at the beginning of the process is not a very connected one, but it is full of uncanny import, vague riddles and shifting contents, as follows:

Mrs. Kolb had been having delusions of reference for some time connected with her work as a seamstress. In September she felt different: 'I feel as if I am veiled, I believe I shall soon get to know something I don't know yet.'—She falsely believed that Mr. A. was going to marry her. She constantly thought something was being done in the shop for someone whom she was not supposed to know—perhaps it was a dowry for herself; she found more and more things . . . when she came home on Sunday she thought someone had been in the room and disarranged a few things. On Monday certain things at work did not tally; she had the impression that the cutter had been giving her wrong orders . . . everyone seemed conspicuous, but she did not know why . . . she was surprised about everything . . . the fact that her brother was fetching her made her pleasurably excited . . . she thought it odd that people greeted her in such a friendly way . . . she was surprised to see so many people passing in the street. At home she had an overpowering feeling of compulsion—'you have to stand still; you must stay put; do something special'. In spite of the warning by her sister-in-law that she ought to come and eat and not talk too much, she never budged. Finally, towards evening, she was taken to hospital. She felt this was a game. When she saw the barred windows she got frightened; she got an injection because of her excitement. Lots of girls were looking through a little window in her door when she was sitting in her room in the hospital; they were winking. Someone called from the ceiling 'you rascal'. In the garden she saw white figures in the dark; she stayed up all night because she felt she had sworn right at the beginning 'My God I am not going to bed'. On Tuesday, she was reading in the Bible. All afternoon she saw people in the garden going to a funeral; she thought it was a television show with her lover (some months before she had really seen a television show). Finally she herself played in it. Sister was giving some signal to the people in the yard. So the game ended. She suddenly saw a stove in the ceiling and a flat cross. She found the light of the lamp wonderful; in the middle were three stars; she felt in heaven; she

[1] Cp. my write-up of Dr. Mendel in *Z. Neur.*, vol. 14 (1913), pp. 210–39: a case with rich symptomatology.

was wondering how she could sing, something she had never done before. She had the idea of counting the points in the window. Then she was overcome by what seemed another power; she had to count up to 12,000; she kept hearing a knocking; there was always something happening. The letters in the Bible turned blue; her faith was being tested and they were making her into a Catholic. After sunset the sun changed to blood. The following night she remained standing at the window till she was frozen; she must remain standing because of her faith which they wanted to take from her. She saw a moving hand on the street; it was a devil. As she stood there she felt a power from above on her right; at this she always looked to the left; she had an idea that the power came from the right, there was also more warmth there and from above there was pressure on her chest. This was spiritual power not physical; she felt quite closed in; she could turn neither to right nor left nor look up. Many more peculiar and puzzling things happened, until after seven days it was all over.

(b) The following case offers a much richer experience. We see vividly the *new significance* of the perceptions and thoughts; the *bliss* experienced, the feelings of power, the *magic connections*, the unusual *tension* and excitement coupled with the inability to hold an idea, and the eventual transition into *confusion*.

The patient (Engelken) had had a love relation with William X. She had slowly slid down through degrees of depression and mania into her psychosis. After she was cured of the acute phase she described the further course of her illness as follows: 'I was crying terribly; I was quite beside myself; I called for people dear to me. It seemed to me I had everything collected round me. Then everything was forgotten; a sparkling cheerfulness appeared. The whole world was turning round in my head. I got mixed up . . . the dead and the living. Everything turned round me; I used to hear the voices of dead people distinctly, sometimes William's voice. I had indescribable happiness when I thought of bringing my mother a new live William; I had lost a brother of that name but the puzzle was too much for me; it was too great a muddle—I was terribly excited; I had an incredible longing for peace—my brother came towards me, frightened, looking like a skeleton, he seemed quite unaware of the things that were filling me—I cannot describe it better than by comparing it to intoxication with champagne . . . I saw other figures—a wonderful lady—I then felt like the Maid of Orleans, as if I had to fight for my lover, had to conquer him; I was terribly tired, but I still had inhuman force. They couldn't hold me down, not three of them. I thought at the time he was fighting in a different way, he was influencing people. I didn't want to be idle. The effective circle of my mental strength was shut, so I wanted to exercise my physical powers. Afterwards I was supposed to have cried, but I cannot remember this . . . I wanted to make the world happy through sacrifice . . . to dissolve every misunderstanding . . . 1832 was prophesied as important . . . I wanted to make it important. If only everyone was pervaded by the same sort of feeling as myself, the whole world would be a paradise. I thought I was a second Messiah; I thought I had to make the world happy and important through my love. I wanted to pray for sinners, to cure the patients, to awaken the dead. I wanted to dry their tears; when this was done and not before, I wanted to be happy with what I had. I called the dead as often as I could. I felt as if I was in the vaults among mummies whom I was to awaken with my voice. The picture of the Redeemer and his melted into one . . . so pure and mild he stood before me. Then he was the murderer of my father and like a distracted person for whom I should pray. I worked fearfully hard and my only recreation was to sing . . . every idea had first to be given order and sequence and then I was looking for a new one. My hair seemed to be the tie between us . . . I wanted to throw it at him so my inner voice would give me new thoughts for which I had to work. The smallest details had deep meaning for me. . . . The last French I did had been "Napoleon in Egypt". I seemed to experience everything I had learnt, heard or read. I thought Napoleon had returned from Egypt but not died of cancer of the stomach. I was the remarkable girl in whose eyes his name was written. My father returned with him too. He was a great admirer of him . . . and so it went on day and night until I was brought here [to the hospital]. I have made my escorts suffer terribly; they didn't want to leave me to myself and that I couldn't bear. I tore everything off to meet him unadorned. I tore my bows off, they were called butterflies, I did not want to beat my wings and declare myself a prisoner. Suddenly it was as if I were among strangers but you [to the doctor] seemed like a well-known good genius, I treated you as if you were my brother. Here I thought my fate is going to be decided . . . the people seem wonderful, the house looks like a fairy palace, but the joke went on too long . . . everything seemed cool and feelingless. I had to get to know more about this . . . I continually kept in contact with William X . . . he would give me a sign on the window or door telling me what to do and encouraging me to be patient . . . A lady from R whom I loved also spoke to me, I replied to her and I was firmly convinced she was here . . . I cannot tell everything that went on but it was a lively, active life . . . I would count it as the happiest time of my life . . . you saw what my condition was later on . . . It has remained a bit of a puzzle ever since . . . it took a good deal to tear myself away from this beautiful dream and come back to reason once more . . . The whole illness has left certain traces on my mind . . . I have to admit a certain loss of power; I might say my nerves were rather exhausted. I don't have any pleasure in mixing with people, no excitability nor any desire to do anything nor any power of reflexion. I remember my condition too vividly not to see how much is needed for me to make up.

# CHAPTER II

# THE OBJECTIVE PERFORMANCES OF PSYCHIC LIFE

## (PERFORMANCE-PSYCHOLOGY—LEISTUNGSPSYCHOLOGIE)

*(a) Subjective and objective psychology*

Chapter one dealt with psychic experiences and we were not concerned with those perceivable objective facts which, in an individual case, give us access to the other person's psyche. We have so far seen the psyche only 'from inside' but in this chapter we shall examine it, as it were, 'from the outside'. In the previous chapter we were engaged with *subjective* psychology and we now turn to what may be termed *objective* psychology.

The external objective phenomena of psychic life may be assessed in a number of different ways. They may be assessed as *performances* (Performance-psychology) or recorded as physical accompaniments or consequences of psychic events (Somato-psychology) or they may be understood as meaningful somatic or motor expressions of the psyche (Psychology of Expression), or as the observable facts of personal existence and conduct in the world (Psychology of the Personal World) or as perceived facts of human creativity (Psychology of Creative Work). Each of these psychological studies provides us with certain appropriate methods whereby we may gain access to different fields of psychically relevant facts.

In the present chapter our concern is with psychic *performances*. For the sake of methodological clarity, we shall keep 'performance' as our guiding principle in grasping the objective material of our investigation. Performance as such arises from the application of some general category; for instance, the *correctness* of a perception (e.g. spatial perception, estimation of time, an idea), or the correctness of memory, speech or thought, etc. Or it may be the *type* of perception that is assessed (e.g. whether predominantly of shape or of colour) or the type of apperception, etc. Or a *quantitative standard* may be set—the extent of memory, the amount of work done, the amount of fatigue.

*(b) The basic neurological schema of the reflex arc and the basic psychological schema of task and performance*

The traditional schema of neurology is the concept of an organism into which *stimuli* are fed. After *inner elaboration* (excitation) it reacts to these with movements and other objectively perceivable phenomena. This physiological excitation is of infinite complexity. The concept is of reflexes superimposed on reflexes in a system of interacting functions, ranging all the way from the patellar reflex to instinctive behaviour. The basic concept of the nervous system is that of the *reflex arc* underlying all psychic events and it contains the tripartite concept of centripetal (sensory) performance of the sense-organ, central event, and centrifugal (motor) performance to the end-organ. In the concept of the '*psychic reflex arc*' this schema is transferred into the psychic life. Thought processes are considered to belong to the central events. In the place of sensory stimulation there is a memory image, for example, and in the place of motor excitation, an image of movement. Here objective psychology has the closest contact with neurology because of the physiology of the sense-organs and of motor phenomena. Neurology teaches the complexity of the apparatus which underlies psychic life. Perception and memory depend on the intactness of this apparatus, and so does externalisation of the inner drives. The investigation of the higher levels of this apparatus takes us into the borderland between psychology and neurology, and its disorders are both neurologically and psychologically analysed in the agnosias, apraxias and aphasias. It is characteristic of such investigations into the psychic reflex arc that they always lead us to physically tangible and at the same time localisable functions as its groundwork.

In contrast to this schema of the reflex arc psychologists have long viewed living activity in quite a different light. There is a radical difference between the facts that appear when simple *stimuli* arouse somatic reactions and those which are deemed to be performances that fulfil certain '*tasks*'. In the latter case the object of investigation is no longer a physically tangible occurrence but a performance in an environment, a meaningful act, a reaction not to stimuli but to a situation. In such investigations we no longer introduce simple stimuli but set certain tasks, e.g. the recognition of briefly exposed objects, the memorising of syllables, adding up, etc.; we no longer register mere movements but evaluate performance according to duration, correctness and incorrectness. Task[1] and performance are the basic concepts, and the experiment of setting a task is the basic experiment of objective psychology.

The reflex apparatus and the apparatus of performance represent two different methodological viewpoints. Of neither can we say that they are life itself. On the contrary they are both artificially isolated, whether in the one case we think of the *mechanism* of an automatic event or in the other of a *performance as a whole*. In life they are both inseparable.

The *psychological point of view* of task and performance has therefore repercussions on the *neurological investigations*. It has been recognised that reflexes are artificial, isolated events of the experimental situation and that reactions in their normal context in real life cannot be explained in terms of reflexes. It is true there are reflexes, but only those people who are carried away by the concept of reflex activity will try to comprehend real life reactions

---

[1] Re the concept and significance of the set task see Watt, *Arch. Psychol.* (D), vol. 4, pp. 289 ff. Ach, *Über die Willenstätigkeit u. das Denken* (1905). Külpe, *Göttinger gelehrte Anzeigen* (1907), pp. 595 ff.

in these terms. As life adapts itself, as it acts purposefully for its own preservation and extension, as it unwittingly trains itself, learns, and takes on shape and form and as it keeps itself in constant movement, so must we conceive it, as if it were motivated by meaning, in terms of what has been called the teleological principle or the function of 'Gestalt' or 'integrative action' (Sherrington). The muscle movements are not a summation of reflexes but the meaningful behaviour of a live organism in an environment or a situation. 'Our psychophysical performances (as opposed to physiological functions) should not be represented as part of the schema of neurophysiological excitation but within a schema of relationships between an organic subject and its environment. Every act carried out is an adaptive performance of my body to my environment . . . for example, sensory stimuli on the vestibular organ act in such a way that orientation to a given situation is possible . . . so that coherence in behaviour is maintained' (v. Weizsäcker). The same author wrote as follows: 'When we analyse going up and down hills, the real performances occur in a continuous cycle of connectedness between organism and environment—environment and organism, but not in the way that we can put the two together as two parts of one whole, because the organism itself always determines what part of the environment will act on it and so with the environment, it determines what part of the organism will be excited. Every stimulus has already been selected and is thus not just given but fashioned. Every excitation is already an alteration of set and once more not just given but fashioned. We may term this cyclic interaction a Gestalt-circle' (Gestaltkreis).[1]

On the other hand the neurophysiological viewpoint of the reflex arc has repercussions on the psychology of performance. The basic concepts of neurology are *translated into psychopathological theory* and they offer a model and sometimes a very apt analogy. We will illustrate with some of the *basic concepts* of neurophysiology:

(1) *Fatigue*: reduction of function by constant exercise in time is something which may be observed in an analogous way from the highest levels of psychic life down to the lowest level of function of the nervous system. (2). *Practice*: is conceived to be a factor in the mnestic formation of the nervous system in general. Functions released by stimuli produce after-effects which facilitate the function and permit it to take place in response to other stimuli or in response to partial or weak stimuli. (3). *Excitation and suppression*: are the opposite poles in all nervous function. (4). *Inhibition*: is the name given to the weakening or suppressing effect on reflexes produced by the higher centres or other simultaneous stimuli. If we omit these other stimuli or exclude the higher centres, the reflex will immediately appear in full strength. *Facilitation* is the term used when no reaction appears following either of two stimuli but will do so only when both stimuli act together or within a short interval of each other. Each single stimulus is too weak but several similar weak stimuli summate in their effect. 5. *Shock*: is the term used when there is cessation of nervous function brought on by injury of all kinds (including very strong stimuli)

---

[1] *Nervenarzt.*, vol. 4, p. 529. v. Weizsäcker *Der Gestaltkreis* (Leipzig, 1940).

without destruction. After some time the ability to function returns spontaneously to the parts which have been affected by the shock.

All these neurophysiological concepts have found application in psychology, but so far with undoubted justification only the concepts of fatigue and practice, excitation and inhibition. The psychic factor is already important for reflexes; for instance, Pavlov's dogs. These were fed after a bell had been sounded and later on produced gastric juices in response to the bell alone (no food present). It is impossible to discern how far we are using mere analogies and how far the phenomena are identical. Are we to conceive the effect of upbringing as an inhibition or facilitation of reflexes; or are we to regard the increasing complexity of psychic performances such as memory or speech—in which complex performances clearly presuppose simple ones—as levels of integration in the morphology of the nervous system or as linked with the physiology of reflexes (their integrative action)? Are we to think of a depression as being brought about by the summation of all the little stimuli rising from a painful situation or are we to explain as shock[1] the violent emotional upheavals that are followed by complete flattening of all emotions.

This consideration of the nervous system helps us to draw a necessary distinction when we are enquiring into psychic life and trying to find causal explanations. The distinction lies between *phenomena* (which are experienced or visible as a performance) and *functions* (which are not themselves visible but manifest in the phenomena). Functions are not mere theoretical additions but actual facts of the performances and experiences. As such they are not in consciousness. The effect of a volitional act on the organs of movement, the effect of attention on the sequences of thought and of the act of thought itself on the play of language cannot be comprehended simply in terms of awareness. Complex functions take place when the simplest direct experiences and performances appear. The reverse is also true: simple functions, 'basic functions', are the condition for a far-reaching range of phenomena.

(c) *The antagonism between the two basic schemata*

The clearer our analysis is, the more our knowledge improves and the more we comprehend events as mechanically constructed by the elements of our analysis. We see reality, however, more distinctly, the more concretely we can perceive its complex unities, groupings and configurations. Both tendencies have their own specific point. Each fails should it try to be the sole foundation of our knowledge or aim at finding the complete answer. We analyse but in fact are never able to know the whole apart from its elements;

[1] A. Pick has done much work to make psychological phenomena comprehensible through analogy with the nervous system. He has collected a wealth of minute observations and has reported his views and methods in *Die neurologische Forschungsrichtung in der Psychopathologie* (Berlin, Karger, 1921). His numerous writings, highly detailed, are scattered all over and contain valuable things which are unfortunately embedded in a highly circumstantial presentation. It would be desirable to try to get at what is of real value by bringing some order into this work.

we get involved in endless complexities and the whole always remains more than the sum of its parts. We scrutinise things as wholes and, by the clearest representation of them, we see them more concretely, but in this manner we do not learn anything of their origin or function. Analysis therefore finally tends towards the grasping of original complex wholes from which the movement of the parts is derived while the perception of complex wholes tends finally towards analysis in order to comprehend them. The interaction of these two tendencies is founded in the nature of all living things which as we study it becomes capable of infinite exploration under these two aspects. This interaction calls for clear distinctions and clear relationships and does not allow for any confused mingling in which the one tendency substitutes for the other. Let us take a physiological example:

*Integration of the reflexes.* Reflexes exist in isolation only in the physiological schema, not in the nervous system in reality. Through mutual inhibition and facilitation the reflexes even in the lower levels of the spinal cord are integrated to a functional tissue within which they act in consonance, superimposed or antagonistically. They build themselves up into a hierarchy of functions which plays together as a whole. Sherrington demonstrated how complicated even peripheral reflexes, such as the patellar reflex, are in their relationships. Changes in posture of the leg or even that of the other leg exert an influence. Sherrington termed this manifold interaction of the reflexes 'integration'; the action may be inhibiting, facilitating or regulating and exists right up into the highest levels of the nervous system.[1] This integrative action of the nervous system makes reflex responses to stimuli appear extremely variable. Co-ordination of reflexes may be disturbed and illness may bring about a reduction in the hierarchy of functions.

With this kind of presentation there is a constant interweaving of the mechanism of mutual influence and modification of all the reflexes with the independent, original source of the whole complex pattern. For a moment it seems as if the whole might be comprehended from its parts yet, without the support of the entirely opposite viewpoint of a whole in its own right, such an explanation could only lead us into endless and astronomical complications. Such investigations make us feel that there is a primary independent source of all the complex unities and that this needs some method for its formulation. As a mechanism reflexes are parts of the totality of reflexes; from the point of view of a complex unity, they are members and the membership cannot be comprehended simply through the fact of being a part.

There are some noteworthy facts that dramatically demonstrate the existence of complex unities:

Good performance may be maintained in 'complicated' life situations and certain tests can demonstrate this experimentally, although isolated, artificial laboratory tests show serious defects of elementary functions of perception (for instance, in cerebral injury). A patient suffering from agnosia (psychic or 'soul' blindness) who cannot recognise shapes during a test may still be able to move quite correctly according to

[1] C. S. Sherrington, *The Integrative Action of the Nervous System* (Cambridge, 1906).

the situation, in his flat or in the street. There are people with encephalitis who cannot go forward but can go backward and even dance (E. Straus) or someone suffering from the rigidity of Parkinsonism may suddenly show a good performance during some ball-game, with a graceful pattern of movement (L. Binswanger). The defects are there in a hidden way and will show themselves up as failure in certain tests, but the ability of the whole is more than the sum of the individual performances.

Some exact experiment in biological research may often make us feel that we have grasped life in its original wholeness and that we have at last penetrated it through and through and yet in the end we find it is still only a widening of mechanistic insight, a widening which in comparison with the preceding simplicities may be truly magnificent but which is yet no penetration of life itself, only of its apparatus. Thus we have the 'co-ordinating factors' of Spemann or the genes of genetics. In the end we have comprehended only elements and the problem of the whole appears again in new form. The elements however may be complex unities themselves compared with other elements while at the same time they are also elements in a mechanistic style of thinking. This mutual interplay is a characteristic of all that we know in biology and psychology. We can keep things clear only if we know exactly what we are doing.

We should make ourselves conscious of the antagonism of these two tendencies and not forget them in our investigations. Only so can we protect ourselves from contradictory and futile polemics, which follow current fashion and play off one method against the other. There is a dislike for complex unities, for anything 'gestalt-like', since they defy reason, and we prefer to leave the arts and the poets to deal with matters unscientific. On the other hand there is also a dislike of elements and mechanisms and a desire to do away with these remote and artificial abstractions. One party despises interpretations derived from the whole, the other any interpretation of the whole from its parts. With many people today holistic and gestalt theories have the upper hand; there is a certain fear of still using such concepts as belonged to the old, mechanistic psychology of reflexes and association. It all seems so dull and retrograde. Yet in fact we still abide by these constructions and use them unwittingly. The old tendency to make them absolutes was false just as is the present tendency to make a fresh absolute. Neither way is wrong in itself, but we have to move in both paths deliberately, otherwise we shall not reach the real margins of our understanding nor the ultimate possibilities they imply.

### (d) Association-, Act- and Gestalt-psychology

The antagonism between mechanism and integrating unity, between automatic happening and creative shaping, between analysis into elements and discernment of things as a whole, has dominated biological and therefore neurophysiological thinking and turns up again within the sphere of psychological study. There is a vast psychological literature which discusses the various schemata of apprehension, by means of which we interpret psychic events in the form of psychic performances. The schools of thought which have developed one after the other (as the psychology of association, of intentional thought, or as gestalt-psychology) and which have all attacked each other, can in fact be brought together. We can make use of all of them, each one within its own limitations, as a means of describing phenomena and posing new questions for analysis. None of these psychologies can claim to explain everything or provide an all-embracing theory of psychic life as it really is. They fall down entirely as an explanation of the psyche, but show their value nonetheless if one employs them for a clear presentation of the relevant psychic facts. They cohere, they can be combined and do not have to contradict each other.

1. *Basic concepts.* The flow of psychic life is thought to be an *association of elements*, which group into complexes and as time proceeds call each other up into consciousness. These elements are called '*ideas*'. Our perception of the external world provides the content for these inner images. The psyche can turn to the external world through perceptions or it can surrender itself to an inner sequence of ideas. The ideas or images—the elements of this psychic flow—are built up into units by the *act* which intends an object in them. In these acts we apperceive certain constantly forming, structured units (Gestalten—configurations of perceived objects) and we experience intra-psychically similar structures among our own psychic events.

2. *The automatic mechanism of association.* We may investigate the flow of psychic life from two aspects. On the one hand we can understand how drives give rise to motive, how motives give rise to decision and deed; and we can understand how thought and thought-content arise from the purposeful consciousness of the person who is thinking. On the other hand we may try to give some objective explanation of how one element of consciousness 'follows' another automatically; how a mere sequence of psychic events rolls along mechanically. This automatic happening is the basis for the rest of psychic life, which it makes possible, and we can study it in isolation. Objective explanation of the existence and sequence of psychic elements can proceed either by referring to *concrete physical events*—the mechanism of perception, neurological localisation—or by the use of psychological concepts such as those which combine into a theory of *association mechanisms*.

We conceive the psyche as if it were broken down into innumerable elements, which move through consciousness one after the other as in a chain, and leave behind them certain extra-conscious dispositions, through which they may again become conscious. All psychic events appear either through external stimuli or through the actualisation or revitalisation of those dispositions that have been acquired through previous stimuli. The dispositions are thought to be linked among themselves. They never appear by themselves (independently arising images) but almost always through a stimulation of these linkages. The latter are of two kinds: primary, the same in all of us (association by similarity, or associations of a general character in virtue of some objective context), or they are acquired  and dependent on specific antecedent experiences, they are individually different (association by experience or according to the particular subjective context). Thus a psychic event may appear by associations of similarity, e.g. I see a red colour and I think of another colour, or by associations of experience, e.g. I perceive a smell and think of the house in Rome where I experienced a similar smell and feelings are aroused in me similar to those I felt then. The extra-conscious association-links which theoretically are considered to be causal remain by definition always unconscious; moreover, when a new image emerges we are by no means always conscious of the connecting link of objective similarity or of chance subjective experience. We have feelings and thoughts the origins of which we cannot discover even by thinking hard about them. Sometimes we are successful when some time has elapsed, as, in the example, we may explain the appearance of certain feelings by that earlier experience and the present olfactory sensation. Thus it is with most explanations of psychic phenomena in the case of patients. *We* find the associations. The patients are not aware and do not need to be (for instance, in the speech of aphasic patients and the flow of images during a flight of ideas, etc.).

This rather crude picture of *elements* and *association-links* will have to suffice. We try to explain what appears new in the flow of ideas by the principle of association but it is not only new things that are constantly appearing. Ideas that have been aroused tend to stay and after brief intervals will return by themselves. *Perseveration* is the term given to this tendency of psychic elements to linger on. From what has been said it will be clear that not only ideas but feelings, thoughts, aims and modes of reaction 'perseverate' as well.

3. *Constellations and determining tendencies.* This flow of ideas holds momentarily immense possibilities for the association-process. But only few of these possibilities come to pass. How does the *selection* of them take place? It is certainly not brought about simply by the latest idea but by the whole complex of antecedent experiences, through the influence of ideas which are far removed from the centre of consciousness, and of which we are only dimly aware, and even through ideas which are too weakly stimulated outside consciousness to reach it. The term 'constellation' is given to all these very complex conditions that determine the eventual direction of the associations. The various individual conditioning factors are said 'to constellate'. Besides this constellation of associations we find another quite different factor which is responsible for the selection of certain associations out of all the infinite number possible. Certain aims (master-ideas)—the awareness that the flow of ideas is to lead to a certain goal and satisfy the requirements of a particular task—bring about a preference for the *relevant* ideas if the individual has the necessary association-links. We can demonstrate this effect experimentally. The extra-conscious causal factors that are linked with this target-awareness are called the *determining tendencies* (Ach). We have to make a threefold distinction: (1) the awareness of the target, (2) the selection of suitable ideas—as can be shown objectively, (3) the determining tendencies which provide the theoretical explanation for this selection of ideas as demonstrated and which are thought to be linked with the target-awareness. Determining tendencies do not originate only from a rational awareness of the target. They arise from all kinds of ideas, from aesthetic images of some complex unity, from moments of mood etc.

4. *The chain of associations and the link by Act.* We are now acquainted with that objective explanation of the psychic flow of ideas which is based on the principles of modes of association (similarity or experience), the constellation of ideas and determining tendencies. Elements are linked by association and are called up in clusters or constellations under the influence of determining tendencies. To make any meaning-

ful use of these explanatory principles we need to know what are the elements that are being called up and between which links exist and are being created. When we begin to think of examples we immediately find that there are a number of extremely diverse elements: sensations as such, percepts and ideas, ideas as such, ideas and thoughts, ideas and feelings, feelings and entire thought-complexes etc. In psychic life everything can be associated with everything else. One might be inclined to the opinion, as many psychologists are, that all psychic life could be reduced in the last resort to a number of simple elements, sensations and simple feelings. All more complex functions are then built up from associative links. All associations at this level would be traced in the last resort to the links between the primary elements. This is a mistake due to the confusion of two quite different connections, the *associative link* and the *intentional link*. We must be clear about the difference because otherwise we cannot apply the concept of association correctly. With idiots and parrots we can establish an association between words and the perception of objects; on seeing the object, the word is said, without knowing that the two are linked by any meaningful association. Here the associative link causes one element to be aroused by the appearance of the other (i.e. perception and word). But if an individual grasps that a word means an object, we have here the experience of an intentional link. Word and object form a new unit now for him, whereas when mere associative links are in operation the context of the connection is present only to the observer, not to the individual who associates (in whose consciousness one element is following the other automatically). Speaking quite generally, we may say that innumerable psychic elements are grouped within one intentional act and are grasped as one comprehensive whole, and this, in contrast to the individual elements, gives rise to something new. One thought builds on another, on ideas and perceptions, and these all become unified for the subject eventually in his thought. This experience of unity seen from the point of view of association-psychology is again another element. Everything which is grasped *in one intentional act* and experienced as a whole is *an element*.

We are now approaching the answer to the question what an element means for association-psychology. We can design a visual schema to give us a proper view of the matter (*see accompanying diagram*, Fig. 1). The elements lie in horizontal layers, one on top of the other, in such a way that several elements of the lower layers can meet again at a higher level by means of the intentional Act; for instance, at the bottom there are elements of sensation, at the higher level, thoughts of relationship.

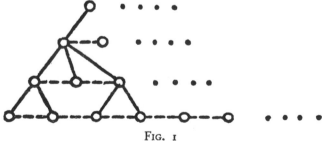

Fig. 1

○ Element
∧ Intentional link by Act
- - - - Association link

In the diagram, the intentional links have been drawn from above down; the association links are presented horizontally. Every intentional act in the higher layer is an element which associates, and at the highest levels most complicated intentional Acts are being associated together.

*Schema*

|  *Association link* | *Intentional link* |
|---|---|
| 1. Associations occur mechanically in sequence and stand side by side. | Intentional links build up one on another to higher wholes, which are again experienced as units.[1] |
| 2. Associations occur unconsciously; an association-link is not an object of experience for the individual associating. | Intentional links occur consciously; the link is an object for the individual who experiences it. |
| 3. The lower the level of intentional acts, the more frequent are the association-links, as observed, occurring in speech and conduct. | The higher the level of intentional acts, the more conspicuous to the observer are the meaningful connections of conscious psychic life. |

5. *Elements and configurations* (*Gestalten*). The unity of anything that has been comprehended by an intentional act and which has been carried out as a whole by means of its movement has been termed a configuration (*Gestalt*). We do not perceive sensations but all our perceptions, images and thought-contents appear to us as configurations. We do not carry out muscle contractions but a configuration of movements. The simple act of unitary object-perception would be impossible if the miraculous interweaving of all that has preceded it in our psychic life did not supply the influence which brings order into the scatter of individual facts. Sensations in the course of perception become members of a whole, muscle contractions become governed by ideo-motor schemata. We talk of word-pictures or movement-patterns in order to differentiate these configurations from sensations and contractions. The psychological study of perception and movement has examined these configurations in some detail, particularly with reference to disturbances in this field in the form of agnosias and apraxias. The function of configuration is, so to speak, the architectonic association of sensory and motor elements to make a meaningful unit of the perceived object and in the movement pattern; to make a meaningful unity also of sensory and motor patterns in general, wherever there is perception and motor activity, understanding of speech or the act of speech. According to this conception, configurations become the elements of every psychic event.

The *concept of elements* in psychic life never denotes 'ultimate' units but only units as they are seen to function according to some particular point of view. We shall, therefore, work with different units as elements according to the point of view we have for the moment adopted, so that what is an exceedingly complex construction from one point of view will become a single element for another.

(e) *The hierarchy of complex unities*

Beyond the reflexes, which only appear as isolated units under experimental conditions, lies the first complex unity—performance. Performance is the

---

[1] Beringer, *Spannweite des intentionalen Bogens.*

completion of a task which has meaning only as a whole. But every individual performance is once again a particular.

Beyond the *individual performance* lies the *total performance*. This complex unity influences the single performances of every individual. It may correct or modify them. Only the performance that is in harmony with the total performance will obtain full realisation. The total performance can be conceived from several points of view: as the *psychophysical ground* for the performance of basic functions; as the present state of the individual within *the flow of his psychic life*, or as that persisting capacity for performance, which we call *intelligence*.

However, this total performance is not the final thing. As a whole it is a tool for understandable personality. Although the personality itself lives in it, it always still remains a tool. If we talk of tasks to be performed, we may ask what tasks? for what end are they posed and by whom? The psychological study of performance presupposes the existence of meaningful tasks; but we have to turn to sources in human beings themselves when it comes to whether the tasks are grasped and assented to, whether the performance is seen as a means, and why these means are used. Hence the psychological study of performance never grasps the human being as a whole but only the *apparatus* which lies at his disposal. The psychophysical apparatus in all its developed thought-performances provides the basic structure for intelligible personality. One could construct the theoretical borderline case where the personality as a potentiality remains intact although there is every kind of disturbance in the performances of the psycho-physical apparatus and there is no further possibility of self-expression.

If we look at the contents objectively realised by human beings through the medium of task and performance, we see that mere performance is something extremely limited yet necessary. The machinery must function if the human nature which it serves is to reach realisation. The aspect of performance links the psyche most closely with the neurological apparatus. From this point right up to thinking proper there is a hierarchy of connected function, providing the tools with which man works.

## (f) *Experimental work in psychopathology*[1]

The psychological study of performance is also the main field for experimental psychopathology. At this point we can appropriately include some remarks on psychological experiment:

1. *The set task.* The basic structure of every experiment consists in the

---

[1] On experimental psychology see Kraepelin, 'Der psychologische Versuch in der Psychiatrie', *Psychol. Arb.*, vol. 1 (1896). Sommer, *Lehrbuch der psychopathologischen Untersuchungsmethoden* (1809).—For a survey, see Gregor, *Leitfaden der experimentelles psychopathologie* (Berlin, 1910). More recently Ernst Schneider, *Psychodiagnostisches Praktikum* (Leipzig, 1936). Papers in *Z. Neur.*, vol. 161, pp. 444, 511. Über Psychotechnik u. Eignungsprüfungen; Münsterberg, *Grundzüge der Psychotechnik*; F. Giese, *Handbuch der psychotechnischen Eignungsprüfungen* (Halle, 1925). W. Poppelreuter, 'Psycho. Begutachtung der Erwerbsbeschränkten in Abderhalden', *Handbuch der biol. Arbeitsmethoden*, Abt. 6.

setting of tasks and the observing of performance, reaction and the general mode of behaviour. Set tasks are of the following kind:

1. Recognising an object which is exposed for a very short time (use of the tachistoscope): *test of apperception*. 2. saying the first word that comes to mind in response to a stimulus-word;—*test of association*: 3. taking in and retaining certain test material—*test of attention, test of learning*: 4. looking at a picture and then giving a spontaneous description of it, followed by an examination on individual points, or reading a story instead: *test of powers of reproduction*: 5. adding up, making measurable movements. The performance is calculated and the many determining factors are investigated: *test of working capacity*.

*Example. Test of associations.* Association experiments[1] are often used because of the technical ease with which they can be arranged. Stimulus words are called out and the instruction given to react as quickly as possible with a single word, the first that occurs to one. Or the task is set to surrender oneself to ideas as they come and speak them out without thinking. The extremely simple procedure of the association test has shown itself to be fruitful, not so much through its exactness as in what it reveals objectively to the observer.

In association tests we observe: 1. *the length of time* of the individual reaction (measured with a stop-watch). 2. the correct or incorrect *reproduction* of the individual association when the test is over. 3. the number of associations falling into certain *categories* e.g. clang-associations, associated content etc. The classification of associations is made according to a number of schemata the value of which can only be assessed according to their particular purpose. 4. reactions with associations which are *qualitatively different*; e.g. egocentric reactions, whole sentence completions, definitions, verbal similarities, marked emotional colouring etc. The test reveals the *wealth* of associations at the disposal of an individual, though the conclusions gained by the test are not very reliable; the emotionally toned *complexes* that dominate the patient's life (shown by increased reaction-time, poor powers of reproduction, marked accompanying phenomena—a convincing but unreliable clue); *odd types of ideational processes*, e.g. flight of ideas, catatonic incoherence. These will occur spontaneously during the test as in conversation.

2. *The manifold nature of experimental observations.* Experiments abound in great variety. They range from simple aids to examination to complicated and costly techniques, from a simple recording of performance to the endless possibilities of accidental observations, from the sole observation of the experimenter to self-observation of the proband.

(*aa*) *Aids to examination.* There are some very simple experiments, such as having pictures described, or observing false perceptions that arise when there is pressure on the eyeball, having a story retold, having inkblots described (Rorschach) etc. Here we are not dealing so much with actual experiments as with technical aids to examination, which have proved to be valuable techniques for complementing the ordinary interview.[2] Rather more complex are

[1] Aschaffenburg, *Psychologische Arbeiten von Kraepelin*, vols. 1, 2, 4. Jung, *J. Psychiatr.* vols. 3, 4, 5. Isserlin, *Mschr. Psychiatr.*, vol. 22, pp. 419, 509. *Münch. med. Wschr.*, vol. 2 (1907).

[2] Such technical tests exist in great numbers, especially intelligence tests; for the examination of inaccessible patients see Liepmann, 'Kleine Hilfsmittel', etc., *Dtsch. med. Wschr.*, vol. 2 (1905).

the techniques for examining aphasias, apraxias, and agnosias. There are a series of carefully graded tasks in a number of situations, to bring out clearly and objectively the actual performance and the failures, which are kept circumscribed in relation to specific factors. (This has been subtly developed by Head.)

(*bb*) *Precise measurements*. The results are characterised by being in the precise form of figures and measurements. There are experiments with a series of tasks, learning experiments, experiments with the tachistoscope. In these there is always a quantitative assessment; experimental conditions are systematically varied and correlations between factors are established.

(*cc*) *Techniques for presenting the phenomena*. An attempt is made to write down everything the patient says during the experiment; behaviour is described, and performance recorded, the way the patient writes, how he moves. Here belong also the mechanical recordings of movement for 'objective' presentation, speech-recording and the use of film and gramophone.

(*dd*) *Self-observation under experimental conditions*. The purely objective tests ask for co-operation, accessibility and understanding of the task on the part of the patient or subject, but they need no particular psychological ability on his part nor any self-observation. Tests that require self-observation call for individuals who have this latter ability and who are able to carry out self-observations in an unbiased way. The results of such experiments belong as much to the study of objective performance as to phenomenology, e.g. in the explanation of failures in performance noted by phenomenological observation.[1] These experiments simply create suitable conditions under which through the patient's self-observation it is possible to become aware of certain psychic phenomena of a particular nature. Patients are asked what they experience when carrying out the tests. An effort is made to relate these phenomenological reports to the failures in performance, so that they may be interpreted psychologically; this applies especially to disturbances of perception and movement.

(*ee*) *Observations made during the experiment, but not as part of it*. Testing in psychopathology derives much of its value from the observations made during the actual tests. These are not like the experiments made in the natural sciences during which one simply registers and measures. The patient is placed in conditions under which he tends to disclose himself more quickly and more clearly than he will do in ordinary interview. The unexpected observations are especially stimulating for the examiner. Moreover, they are essential for the correct interpretation of the measurements obtained. It is only through observation that we can detect schizophrenic thought-blocking, whether affective pauses prolong the test, and whether the behaviour is due to laziness or stolidity. Purely mechanical test-results are useless here.

---

[1] The school of Külpe (Bühler, Messer, Selz) has developed this kind of test. Cf. *Arch. Psychol.* (D). For criticism see E. Müller, *Zur Analyse der Gedächtnistätigkeit* (Leipzig, 1911), pp. 61 ff. Wundt, 'Über Ausfrageexperimente', *Psy. Stud.*, vol. 3 (1907).

(*ff*) *The aim of experimental testing.* This is to measure *individual performance, basic function, intelligence, personality* or *constitution.* Whatever the test many functions must be intact for performance to be possible. We can only test certain psychic functions if the other functions are intact. This is why, for example, association experiments, reproduction experiments, tests of working capacity are equally applicable to the investigation of single functions as to the characterisation of the total personality, whether it be in its constitutional features (psychic tempo, sensory type, etc.) or as an individual form of personal expression.

(*gg*) Several tests attempt to *penetrate the unconscious*, and illuminate hidden aspects of the life-history, i.e. association-tests and the Rorschach.

3. *The value of experiments.* Experimental psychology is not equally valued by everyone. Some think it sterile and empty; others see it as the only scientific method we have. To a balanced observer it must appear irreplaceable as an experimental method in its own field, but we cannot concede it the right to consider itself as the only method. The main thing is to formulate our problems clearly and this needs an all-round psychological education. We should certainly try experiment where questions can be suitably answered in this way; otherwise we should look out for other methods, such as simple observation and the study of the patient's life-history and the use of cases, statistical methods, and methods of sociology.

Experiment creates objective facts which convince. Other methods do not do this as easily nor as quickly nor as obviously. Many psychic phenomena only become apparent when their relation to the patient is shown in this objective way. The distance created by the experimental situation may reveal quietly and impersonally what had been hidden during actual interview.

Furthermore the experiments of normal psychology as of sense-physiology have important results. They make us keenly aware how even the simplest phenomenological process contains extremely complex factors, not only in its somatic genesis but in the function and correlation of the phenomena brought out by the experiment but not yet explicable in somatic terms. Psychopathological experiments also confirm this. We always need to distinguish what the experiment really shows from the theoretical explanations we give of what is happening. Where no direct link with a physiological-somatic base appears possible, we would still like to find a psycho-physical apparatus functioning. This is achieved when the conceptual schemata of neurology become translated into psychology and concepts are formed such as those in the above-discussed schools of Association-, Act- and Gestalt-psychology.

## SECTION ONE

### INDIVIDUAL PERFORMANCES

Performances are classified according to the form in which they materialise. Everything that can be observed objectively, tested, investigated and called a performance of some kind will fall naturally into one of the groups which we are about to discuss. These are perception, apperception and orientation, memory, movement, speech and thought. Our concern is with particular failures of performance which can be directly observed. Description of these will always give us the performance-profile of an individual. First, however, we must make an inventory of the separate types of performance.

## § 1. Perception

Not all the stimuli that impinge on sensory nerve-endings reach consciousness. There are many centripetal nerves which elicit complex reflex responses without anything becoming conscious. The whole process remains automatic. As surgeons have found, the stomach and intestines are almost entirely devoid of sensation and yet within their numerous nerves reflex mechanisms of a most complicated kind occur. Maintenance of equilibrium, the performance of many movements (individual muscle contractions as well as complex synergies) happen without our awareness but we cannot draw any sharp dividing line between purely physical mechanisms and psychically conditioned events. Mere reflexes, as for instance breathing, can become conscious and conscious events can become automatic (for instance, the movements learned in riding a bicycle).

When we come to perception it is obvious that disturbances in the nervous system will affect perception in so far as the latter is based on the former. Thus, for example, we get anaesthesias, parasthesias, disturbances caused by morbid processes in the visual apparatus (hemianopsia, disturbance of visual perception through lesions in the choroidea etc.) and all the other anomalies described in neurology. These disturbances are subdivided physiologically according to their predominantly peripheral or central nature. The higher the level of nervous integration in which they are situated, the nearer we come to psychic events. It is true there seems no end to it, an infinite progression. Every new neurophysiological discovery, instead of setting foot within the psyche, simply enters a yet higher level of the neuro-mechanisms that underlie psychic life. However, when describing psychopathological disturbances in perception, we usually include the neurophysiological anomalies that affect the highest levels. *Sensory disturbances belong here, a few of the false perceptions* and above all *the agnosias.*

(*a*) We find *simple sense-deficiency*—congenital deafness, colour-blindness, anosmia—where sometimes no physical cause for the deficiency is known. We can find full descriptions in the textbooks of neurology, ophthalmology and otology of the manifold perceptual disturbances arising from local diseases of the sense-organs and of the nerve tracts up to the projection-area of the cerebral cortex.

(*b*) With the majority of *hallucinations* we do not know what causes or conditions their appearance. With some hallucinations, however, we do know some if not all the contributing causes (cp. pp. 377–89). Hallucinations follow diseases of sense-organs and certain localised conditions of the sensory cortex (peculiar elementary light and sound phenomena). We have also observed vertigo in diseases of the vestibular apparatus and hemianoptic hallucinations in particular with localised lesions in the occipital lobe. With other hallucinations we have noticed a certain dependence on external stimuli; in organs which are so disposed and can hallucinate almost spontaneously, it is possible to bring hallucination about by any kind of stimulus. With delirious and other patients visions can be elicited by pressure on the closed eye, as we all know. But all these effects are far too crude for us to penetrate to the extra-conscious mechanisms that underlie the hallucinations.

(c) *Agnosias*.[1] This is the term given to disturbances of recognition while sense-perception is intact. After a head-injury, the patient may be able to see the room and its furniture but cannot recognise the objects as furniture; she is perplexed, does not know what objects they are and of course does not know that they are *her* furniture.

She can therefore perceive but cannot make out the meaning of her perceptions. In agnosia, perceptions take place, with sensations present in the act itself, but what is then perceived is not perceived as a definite object, nor can it be recognised. Reproduction, which links up previous experiences and makes recognition possible in all perceptions, is absent here. Goldstein and Gelb have to some extent clarified what is actually present in consciousness in such cases. They have given us a description of a patient of theirs with a gunshot wound in the head:[2]

The patient has coloured and colourless blotches in a certain part of his visual field. He can see whether a certain blotch is higher or lower, to the right or left of another one, whether it is narrow or wide, large or small, short or long, nearer or further, but that is all, because the various blotches together create a confused impression and there is not, as with normal people, any impression of a specific, well-characterised whole. The patient could not recognise any shapes, neither straight nor crooked ones. When, however, he followed the shape with his hand, he could recognise it. Nor could he see movements properly. He reported: 'When I saw the train coming, I saw it about 5 metres away.' After that, usually, he saw nothing until it was suddenly standing in front of him. A moving train which 'he clearly recognised' he did not see moving; he concluded it was moving only from the noise; when he wanted to go for a walk with his sister-in-law, she went in front of him, and he followed her at a distance of 20 metres; he then thought his sister-in-law had stopped and was standing still and was 'very surprised that he did not overtake her'. The distance did not get any shorter . . . What he saw was only a 'now-here', 'now-there'; he never had the impression of movement as a normal person has it, that is, as something specifically different from individual, static position. In the tactile field, however, the patient had distinct perception of movement.

[1] Wilbrand, *Die Seelenblindheit* (1887). Lissauer, *Arch. Psychiatr.* (D), vol. 21, pp. 222 ff. Müller, *Arch. Psychiatr.* (D), vol. 24, pp. 856 ff. Liepmann, *Neur. Zbl.*, vol. 27 (1910), p. 609. Külpe, *Z. Pathopsychol.*, vol. 1, pp. 224 ff.

[2] Goldstein and Gelb, 'Zur psychologie des optischen Wahrnehmungs und Erkennungsvorgangs', *Z. Neur.*, vol. 41 (1918), p. 1. Fruitful translation of Gestaltpsychology into psychopathology is continued in *Z. Psychol.*, vols. 83, 84, 86 (1919–20), and in the continuous series of 'Psychological analyses of brain-pathology cases'.

Visual agnosia ('soul'- or psychic-blindness) occurs with the destruction of both occipital lobes. Actual facts do not support a relationship between these specific disorders of performance and any fine, localised cerebral lesions. Visual agnosias, auditory agnosias and tactile agnosias (stereoagnosias) are differentiated according to the sense-areas.

(d) Some of these perceptual anomalies which so far have only been treated phenomenologically can be recognised by objective tests and measurements, and can be explained as defective performances; for instance, some disturbances of the *time sense*. We have to distinguish between disturbances in the perception of time, which we can test, and disturbances in the experience of time (which so far we have only studied phenomenologically). So with *perception of space*, in a few cases it is possible to link this up with testable alterations in performance; for instance, a reduction of the visual field,[1] explicable in terms of a fatigue-phenomenon or a disturbance of attention and increased distractibility.

## § 2. APPERCEPTION AND ORIENTATION

Agnosias are disturbances of recognition, that is they are properly disturbances of apperception, but because they are confined to particular sense-areas, we have grouped them with disturbances of the perception mechanism. If we now discuss disturbances of apperception[2] in the narrower sense, we cannot make a very sharp distinction. What we mean now is a disturbance in all the senses at the same time, in so far as they are related to the psychic life as a whole. We can, therefore, differentiate disturbances of this sort from those agnosias which, similarly to disturbances in the sense-organs, occur as more peripheral anomalies in a normal person and attack only one of the mechanisms underlying psychic life. Whereas phenomenologically perception and apperception form a single whole, an objective analysis of the performance can differentiate the *mechanism of perception*, as the process whereby nervous mechanisms can lead to awareness of objective content, and *apperception*, as the process which brings about the absorption of such content into the body of our experience.

Apperception can be *slowed down*, or *remain in abeyance* in the face of difficult objects or lead to *false results*. These facts can be crudely observed in any interview, through reading a sample of short stories to the patient, or showing him a number of pictures.[3] The time required for apperception can, however, be measured in much finer detail, and so in cases of false apperception can the dependence on the constellation of the preceding inner associations. For this we can use experiments with the tachistoscope, an apparatus which exposes pictures, letters, words for very brief measurable periods. Investigations

[1] Klien, *Arch. Psychiatr.* (D), vol. 42, p. 359. Rehm, *Z. Neur.*, vol. 55, p. 154.
[2] Heilbronner, *Mschr. Psychiatr.*, vol. 17, pp. 441 ff. Kronfeld, *Arch. Psychol.* (D), vol. 22, p. 543. (Summaries), Gregor, *4 Vorlesung.*
[3] Heilbronner, *Mschr. Psychiatr.* (D), vol. 17, p. 105.

such as these lead to a tentative classification of disturbances of apperception into three groups, according to the source of the disturbance:

1. *Level of intelligence.* Apperception fails with the more difficult objects because of the persisting defective state. There is no body of knowledge with which the perception can be linked.

2. Apperception can be affected owing to disturbances in *registration* (e.g. in senility, in Korsakow-syndrome). Everything that comes into consciousness is immediately forgotten. Before anything more complex can be apperceived, however, what has been perceived must also have been retained. In this case this is already forgotten when the next part of what is to be apperceived appears.

3. Apperception depends upon the *state of consciousness* and on changes in the *mode of psychic activity.* In states of clouded consciousness there is an indistinct, often illusory, apperception, sometimes clear in detail but never clear as a whole. In manic states apperception is most changeable, following the flitting interest and the marked distractibility through chance constellations of ideas which may lead to falsifications. In depressive states apperception is inhibited and does not reach its goal though efforts are made, sometimes intensively. With the use of the tachistoscope and by exposing a series of letters, we can count the omissions and mistakes in apperception and measure reliability and distractibility objectively.

*Orientation* is a highly complex apperceptive performance. We can easily verify it in respect to the environment in the current real situation or else in respect to one's own person. We distinguish orientation in space and orientation in time, orientation in relation to the self and orientation in relation to others. Orientation in one direction may be intact when there is disturbance in others. For instance there is the characteristic symptom of delirium tremens, complete disorientation in place, time and environment but correct orientation in relation to one's own person. Disorientation, however, is not a particularly pathognomic symptom. It can come about in very different ways and its significance therefore may vary greatly. It is only the last, easily detectable, objective failure in performance in a chain of manifold acts of apperception. The following schema covers the different *modes of disorientation:*

1. *Amnestic.* Where there is a severe degree of disturbance in registration, there is a disturbance of apperception as a result of immediately forgetting what has just been experienced. Senile patients, for instance, think they are twenty years old. Women take their maiden name again, write the wrong year, think they are at school or at home when they are in the clinic, think the doctor, whom they never recognise, is a teacher, some official or the mayor etc. 2. *Delusion-like.* The patients are fully conscious but have delusions and therefore conclude, for example, that the date is three days out although they know everyone else finds the date different. They may conclude they are in prison, though everyone else considers the place is a hospital etc. *Double orientation* as it is called is connected with this. The patients are correctly and incorrectly orientated at the same time. They know, for instance, where they are, what time it is and that they are having a mental illness. At the same time this is only an appearance, the golden age has arrived and time no longer matters. 3. *Apathy.* The patients do not know where they are, what time it is, because they do not think of it,

but they are not wrongly orientated. 4. *Clouding of consciousness*. The patients only grasp details. Apperception of the real environment is replaced by the changing experiences of the disturbed consciousness, which cause a wealth of fantastic disorientations, analogous to dreams.

Disturbances in orientation occur in acute psychoses and many chronic states. They are easily recognisable and important for the assessment of the case. In each case it is necessary to make sure about all four dimensions of orientation. The finding that the patient is orientated or in which direction this is so will influence the whole of the further examination.

The disturbances of apperception have been differentiated and investigated according to their content—the failure to recognise people, for instance.[1] This phenomenon is an objective disorder of performance but it may be of very different kinds and origins.

Failure to recognise persons occurs where there is alteration of consciousness (deliria), where there is confabulation in amnestic syndromes, fooling about in manic states, altered perception (illusion), acute psychosis, or delusional perception in schizophrenia. The mode of experience is as heterogeneous as the cause.

## § 3. MEMORY[2]

*Psychological preface.* A threefold distinction is necessary.

(1) *Registration.* The ability to add new material to the store of memory. We then differentiate into learning ability (repeated presentation of material) and registration in the narrower sense (single presentation of material). (2) *Retention.* The big reservoir of lasting depositions, which can enter consciousness on appropriate occasions. (3) *Recall.* The ability to bring into consciousness particular remembered material at a particular moment under particular circumstances. Registration and powers of recall are actual functions; memory itself is a possession of lasting depositions. We can find pathological disturbances in any one of these three fields. They can all be described as 'disturbances of memory' but in fact they are each different in character. Normally, memory may be faulty with constant limitations and fluctuations as regards fidelity (reliability), duration, readiness and serviceability. Extensive psychological experiment has established certain laws which are of interest; there are laws of *memorising* (e.g. the dependence on attention, interest, whether one learns the whole or part, impairment by simultaneous evocation of other associations, generative inhibition). There are also laws of recall or *reproduction* (impairment by other simultaneous psychic processes, inhibition by associations which try to enter consciousness at the same time; effectual inhibition). We have to realise that there is

---

[1] Werner Scheid, 'Über Personenverkennung', *Z. Neur.*, vol. 157 (1936), p. 1.

[2] Ribot, *Das Gedächtnis und seine Störungen* (D), (1882). The following summarise the great experiments of Ebbinghaus and G. E. Müller: Offner, *Das Gedächtnis* (Berlin, 1909). G. E. Müller, 'Zur Analyse der Gedächtnistätigkeit und des Vorstellungsablaufs', *Erg-Bd.d.Z.Psychol.*, vol. 3 (1911 ff).

As regards psychopathology see Ranschburg, *Das kranke Gedächtnis* (Leipzig, 1911). K. Schneider, 'Die Störungen des Gedächtnisses', *Bumke's Handbuch der Geisteskrankheiten*, vol. 1 (1928), p. 508.

no such thing as memory in the form of a general ability to remember, but that memory consists in a number of *special memory factors*. We can sometimes find, for instance, an otherwise feebleminded person possessing an outstanding memory for time.

So far in this discussion of memory we have had in mind a mechanism, a machine which we can work well or badly. Memory, however, is also subject to *meaningful connection with affect*, significance, the desire to forget. Nietzsche once said: 'Memory declares that I did this; I could not have done this, says my pride; and memory loses the day.' It is one thing to deal with memory in respect of *things learned* (knowledge); it is quite another to deal with memories in respect of *personal* experience (recollection) and the latter may differ greatly in relation to the personality. Memories may be fresh, effective, significant, not at all remote, or may have become objective, a matter of history, a sort of knowledge, at one remove from the present personality. A number of these meaningful connections have been investigated experimentally: e.g. the relationship between the pleasantness or unpleasantness of an experience and retaining it correctly or forgetting it.[1] Pleasant experiences are retained better than unpleasant ones and the latter better than indifferent ones. It is an old saying that pain is soon forgotten. Memory is optimistic in that we tend to remember the pleasant parts most of all. Memories of severe pain after operation, during confinement or of violent affects soon fade. We only know finally that what we suffered at the time was very powerful, painful and unusual, but we do not keep any real memory of the experience itself. Are unpleasant experiences not so well memorised from the start or do we only recall them with greater difficulty? Or is it that we think of them less frequently and so forget them more quickly? We have to distinguish the forgetting of obligations, of unpleasant tasks, of embarrassing scenes, by simply not thinking of them, and that unintentional repression of unpleasant things, which may lead to an actual splitting off of the content (with impossibility of recall).

In discussing memory disturbances we must distinguish between those which result from abnormal states of awareness (Amnesias) and those which occur in normal states.

## (a) Amnesias

These are disturbances of memory which last over a *definite and limited time*, when nothing or only little (partial amnesia) can be remembered; the term also covers *experiences* not so well defined as to time. The following different situations should be noted: (1) there may be no disturbance of memory at all. There is a state of deeply disturbed consciousness in which *nothing could be apperceived* and therefore nothing could be registered. Nothing has come into the memory and nothing can therefore be recalled. (2) Apperception may have been possible for a while but registration was seriously disturbed so *nothing was retained*. (3) Transitory registration may have been possible during an abnormal state, but the memory depositions have been destroyed by an organic process. The clearest example of this is what happens with *retrograde amnesias*,

---

[1] Peters, 'Gefühl und Erinnerung', *Psychol. Arb.*, vol. 6 (1911), p. 197. Peters and Nemecek, *Fschr. Psychol.* vol. 2 (1914), p. 226.

after head injury, when everything experienced during the last hours or days before the injury is totally extinguished. (4) There may only be disturbance of the power to *recall* (*reproduce*). The memory contains the whole content but cannot evoke it. Under hypnosis, however, successful recall occurs. Such amnesias have been investigated by *Janet*.[1] His patients were unable to remember certain experiences (systematic amnesia), or some particular period of their lives (localised amnesia) or their life as a whole (generalised amnesia). If we observe such behaviour in our own patients we shall see that memory does play a conspicuous part. They do not behave as if they had really lost the memory depositions. They do not appear subjectively disturbed by the amnesia. Their attitude towards it is one of indifference and is full of contradictions. Finally the amnesia may lift, spontaneously, periodically or with the help of hypnosis.

Several of these four types of amnesia may appear in one case, but usually one or other predominates. Particularly characteristic is the way in which something belonging to the amnestic period tends to be *preserved*. An amnesia is very rarely complete and this or that particular can be *evoked*. We find two types of spontaneous memory:[2] (1) *Summary recollection:* the recollection of the essential points in a vague, undetailed way. (2) The recollection of a *mass of detail*, of small, unimportant points which stand unconnected, alongside each other. Sometimes the memory consists of these detailed small irrelevancies, but neither the relationships in time nor in context ever become clear. The above two types correspond to what can be evoked by stimulation or by the use of certain props to the memory: e.g. (1) by appropriate means, and most strikingly of all by hypnosis, we find we can evoke a whole systematic context, a whole complex, a whole set of experiences; (2) we can also sometimes evoke a large number of particulars, by arousing detailed images via the most diverse associative paths. The proper time order and the context can only be evoked with the utmost difficulty or not at all. Speaking categorically, we might say that the former method is appropriate for hysterical amnesias and amnesia after powerful affects, while the latter is more applicable for amnesias in epileptic and organic states, disturbances of consciousness etc.

The fact is worth noting that even *organically* caused amnesias can sometimes be lifted with the use of *hypnosis*. This has happened repeatedly in the case of epileptic amnesias[3], and also with a person who had had a retrograde amnesia due to hanging and who was revived.[4]

## (b) Disturbances of recall (reproduction), retention and registration

Besides the more circumscribed amnesias we commonly deal with

---

[1] Janet, *Der Geisteszustand der Hysterischen* (Vienna, 1894), pp. 65 ff.

[2] Heilbronner, *Mschr. Psychiatr.*, vol. 17, p. 450.

[3] Ricklin, 'Hebung epileptischer Amnesien durch Hypnose' (Diss., Zürich, 1903), *J. Psychiatr.*, vol. 1, p. 200. v. Muralt, *Z. Hypnotism usw.*, vol. 10 (1900), p. 86. H. Ruffin, *Dtsch. Z. Nervenhk.*, vol. 107 (1929), p. 271.

[4] Schilder, *Med. Klin.*, vol. 1923, p. 604.

disturbances of memory in the simple form of an exaggeration of everyday forgetting, of ordinary poverty of registration, etc. Here too we make the usual subdivision into the ability to recall (reproduction), the reservoir of memory-depositions (retention) and the ability to grasp (registration).

1. *Disturbances of recall (reproduction)*. Hebephrenics sometimes give a deceptive impression of poor memory when they talk past the point or suffer from thought-blocking; melancholics do the same when retarded and preoccupied with their own distress, and so do manics who show flight of ideas and lack of concentration.[1] In all such cases recall may perhaps be transiently diminished but the memory is there and after the disturbance has passed will appear unaltered. The patients have only been temporarily unreflective. We also find these disturbances in recall among psychasthenics. They know everything quite well, but the moment they want to use what they know nothing comes to them—e.g. during an examination. As to the hysterical inability to recall, we mentioned this among the amnesias. It is always related to a number of complexes and is not so much a question of momentary lapse of memory as the dissociation or splitting-off of some definite, circumscribed memory-complex.

2. *Disturbances of memory proper (retention)*. Our memory capacity is increased or fortified by our powers of registration, but at the same time it tends to disintegrate continually. As time goes on, the memories that have been laid down fade from us and we forget. In old age particularly and in organic processes, memory may undergo excessive disintegration. Beginning with more recent events, the patient finds himself robbed of the memory of his own past and his vocabulary suffers as well. Concrete terms disappear first, abstract terms and conjunctions etc. are preserved longer. Generalities and broad categories linger on, whereas everything that is directly observed and individual vanishes. Of personal memories, the most recently acquired disappear first, the more remote ones are engulfed more slowly. The memories of childhood and youth are retained the longest and sometimes are particularly vivid.

3. *Disturbances of Registration*. Patients no longer register though their previous memories are at their disposal. These disturbances have been investigated experimentally. In particular there is the test in which pairs of words are learned—be they nonsensical or meaningful—and the assessment of such performance has proved fruitful. A quantitative assessment of the memory disturbance becomes possible.

G. E. Störring[2] observed the case of an isolated, *total loss of registration* with no other disturbances than those consequent on this disastrous loss. The

---

[1] J. Schultz, 'Über psychologische Leistungsprüfungen an nervösen Kriegsteilnehmern', *Z. Neur.*, vol. 68, p. 326—of relevance to the failure of grasp and recall in depressions and neurasthenia.

[2] G. E. Störring, 'Über den ersten reinen Fall eines Menschen mit völligem isolierten Verlust der Merkfähigkeit', *Arch. Psychol.* (D), vol. 81 (1931), p. 257. For an earlier report on the same case see Grünthal and Störring, *Mschr. Psychiatr.*, vols. 74 and 77.

case has been excellently described and it is unique as well as uncommonly instructive:

A 24-year-old locksmith sustained gas-poisoning on May 31st, 1926. In 1930 he was examined. Memories dating from before May 31st were preserved. From then on nothing new had been added. Every impression vanished after two seconds. Any long question was forgotten by the time the questioner had reached the end of his sentence. Only brief questions could be answered. Yesterday for the patient was for ever May 30th, 1926; whatever seemed to contradict this, puzzled him for the moment but the contradiction was immediately forgotten. After his accident his fiancée married him. He did not know this had happened and therefore when asked 'are you married?' would say 'no, but I want to marry soon'. He said the last word of the sentence hesitatingly; he no longer knew why he was actually saying it. Looking through the window at the winter landscape, he could call the time of year 'winter', but if he covered his eyes he would say it was 'summer'—'it was so warm'. The next moment, looking at the fire he would say 'it is winter, because there is a fire'. During the usual examination of the skin with the use of painful stimuli, pinprick etc., each prick was immediately forgotten, though unpleasant sensation persisted. Thus he offered his hand unsuspectingly again and again but the unpleasant feeling summated until finally a sudden elementary fear and flight reaction ensued.

In so far as the whole experience of his former life was at his disposal, he apperceived correctly, recognised things correctly, judged correctly everything at the moment of apperception. He recognised people whom he had known before 1926. Those he met later, his doctors, for instance, struck him every time as strange, new people, in spite of his frequent meetings with them. He was not dull or 'dopey' but wide awake and attentive. He was fully there, observing, enjoying himself, spontaneous in movement and talk. His emotional life had remained the same; his personality, his reactions, values, likes and dislikes had not changed. Compared with the previous period there was a stronger intensity of feeling (his wife said he felt more deeply than before). Every situation was held isolated in his mind without incorporating past or future and every experience was sudden and therefore sharper. His feelings were less complicated than before, conditioned by the immediate past. He lived entirely in the present but not in time. Central feelings closely linked with his personality were more to the fore than peripheral, indifferent ones. His personality was strongly felt by those around him and he was found to be very likeable . . . He had been a tranquil man but his actions were now abrupt and hasty. He became outwardly restless before beginning; the feeling-drives had to reach an adequate intensity by summation before they suddenly triggered off. The patient was unaware of his memory disturbance and did not notice it. If he had noticed it, he would have forgotten it immediately but he did not even notice it, because every impression vanished by the time he wanted to reflect on it. Instead he became puzzled and restless in certain situations, not because he realised his forgetfulness but because he had a feeling that he intended to do something, while he no longer knew what he was to do or wanted to do, unless he was told again and again from second to second. The constant perplexity became set in his facial expression. Störring compared this situation with a wax tablet suddenly turned to stone; the old impressions were still readable but no more new impressions could be made.

The failure of memory-performance often affects registration and recall at the same time as it extinguishes the already existing depositions. The picture will get clearer if we describe the memory-performance as a whole and how particular behaviour is affected. W. Scheid[1], for example, gives us an excellent description of memory-defect in an alcoholic-Korsakow. Innumerable islands of memory appear, a random scatter of defects and an equally random scatter of successful efforts at registration. We may also note a complete loss of memory after some severely upsetting experience, though memory for small details may be retained. In every memory-performance the situation and the individual attitude are always important.

### (c) Falsifications of memory

So far we have described memory-lapses in respect of general knowledge and personal experience. We now come to a fundamentally different order of phenomena, which we have termed falsification of memory. This occurs universally and in healthy persons as well as the sick. Investigations into powers of reproduction or of giving evidence[2] have brought to light the surprising extent of these falsifications. These experiments, which, like most experiments, involve some kind of 'task', give a cross-section of the person's mental life and show many phenomena more clearly than the ordinary clinic examination can do, and can demonstrate it quantitatively.[3]

Falsification of memory plays a considerable part in mental illness.[4] We find boastful tales in paralytic patients, random spun-out fantasies in certain paranoid dements, who bring them forward as memories and tell them to others as such; we find falsifications of memory analogous to hallucinations (p. 64). With some conditions we feel we can well understand how patients after some serious disturbances in registration with simultaneous loss of old memories try to fill in the gaps with anything that springs to mind (confabulation). They still retain their intelligence, think and judge. They comprehend the situation but they cannot come to any proper conclusion as they lack the vital associations. They unwittingly invent what seems to fit the moment and although they may have been in bed a week, they will say they were in the market this morning or have been working in the kitchen etc.

W. Scheid observed real memories in the patient who was suffering from an alcoholic-Korsakow syndrome. (They arose in distorted fashion as in confabulation.) He experienced them, however, as if they were dream-memories, yet he doubted whether it was a dream or real after all: 'Did I dream that?'—Scheid describes the actual *experience of remembering*. Normally we remember the past as having happened at a certain time continuous with other

---

[1] W. Scheid, 'Zur Pathopsychologie des Korsakow-syndroms', Z. Neur., vol. 51 (1934), p. 346.
[2] Rodenwald, 'Über Soldatenaussagen', Beitr. Psychol. Aussage 2. Baerwald, Z. Ungew. Psychol., vol. 2. W. Stern, Beitr. Psychol. Aussage 1. Stöhr, Psychologie der Aussage (Berlin, 1911).
[3] Roemer, Klin. psych. u. nerv. Krankh., vol. 3. Eppelbaum, Allg. Z. Psychiatr., vol. 68, p. 763.
[4] Kraepelin, 'Über Erinerungsfälschungen', Arch. Psychiatr. (D), vol. 17 (1886), p. 830; vol. 18 (1887), pp. 199, 395.

events, and as preceding and following definite points in time. Some confabulations may possibly be experienced as memories of this sort, but generally they have much less degree of certainty; they are memories without any real background and lack temporal or causal connection with memory as a whole. It is true we can remember something without placing it in time and without a context, but then we are not sure whether it might not have been a dream, unless we can link it up with some other memories. So with the Korsakow patient. The lack of connections made him feel that his real memories had only been dreams.

## § 4. Motor Activity

From the point of view of the 'psychic reflex arc' all psychic events merge at last into motor phenomena, which assist the final inner elaboration of stimuli into the external world. From the point of view of *inner meaning*, subjective awareness of Will translates itself into movement. This volitional act is associated with an extra-conscious motor mechanism, on which the act depends for its effectiveness.

We can, therefore, examine the many, often grotesque, movements of mental patients from two points of view. Either we try to acquaint ourselves with the disturbances of the motor mechanism itself, which can sometimes show disturbances independently of any psychic anomaly and this is the approach adopted by neurology. Or we try to get to know the abnormal psychic life and the patient's *volitional awareness*, which these conspicuous movements exhibit. In so far as we know the meaningful connections, the movements become behaviour we can understand, for instance, the delight in activity shown by manic patients in their exuberance, or the increased urge to move shown by patients who are desperately anxious. Somewhere between the *neurological* phenomena, seen as disturbances of the motor-apparatus, and the *psychological* phenomena, seen as sequelae of psychic abnormality with the motor-apparatus intact, lie the *psychotic motor-phenomena*, which we register without being able to comprehend them satisfactorily one way or the other. Neurological phenomena are termed disturbances of *motility*; the psychotic phenomena are termed disturbances of *motor activity*. Psychological phenomena are not conceived to be primary motor phenomena but are to be seen as actions and modes of expression which have to be understood.

### (a) Neurological disturbances of motility

Motility and its regulation depend on three systems: the pyramidal system (if diseased, there is simple paralysis); the extrapyramidal system of the basal ganglia and brain stem (if diseased, there are changes in tonus, expressive movement, gesture and co-ordination —for instance, a disappearance of the automatic pendulum arm-movement when walking, choreic and athetotic movements); the spinal cord and cerebellar system (if diseased, there is ataxia, a disturbance in motor-co-ordination due to impairment of sensory factors). In psychopathology we must be familiar with these disturbances of motility so that we are not tempted to understand them psychologically. For instance, automatic movements such as forced laughter in bulbar paralysis are in no way expressions of psychic factors but the results of localised irritation in the brain.

### (b) Apraxias

Neurology climbs up from level to level in the nervous system as if it must come closer and closer to the centre of volitional awareness, the psyche itself. The apraxias are the disturbances at the highest level yet described.[1] Apraxia consists in the patient's inability to make the right movement in relation to his target-image, although his psychic life is intact and his motor-ability from cortex to periphery is undisturbed, that is, there is no ataxia or paralysis. He wants, for instance, to light a match; instead of doing this, he puts a matchbox behind his ear. The pattern of movement which would co-ordinate this gesture is not available to him. Liepmann localised this disturbance in the brain and has even observed it to occur unilaterally. The patient could carry out movements successfully with one arm but was apractic with the other.

The neurological disturbances in these apraxias have something in common with psychotic movements and normal activity. We can only recognise them as pure disturbances of the motor-mechanism when they occur in an otherwise *healthy individual* and when we can localise them anatomically in the brain. It is very likely that a whole series of extra-conscious functions are superimposed one on the other between these mechanisms of apraxia and the conscious volitional impulse. Our knowledge here has grown from below upwards but at present once we are beyond the boundary of the motor apraxias we find ourselves floundering about in an entirely unknown country.

### (c) Psychotic disturbances of motor activity

If for the moment we leave aside purely neurological motor-phenomena in mental patients, as well as other phenomena which seem to be expressive of psychic events and can be understood as normally motivated, we are still left with a large number of surprising phenomena which at present we can only register and describe and interpret hypothetically.[2] Wernicke distinguished *akinetic* and *hyperkinetic* disturbances of motor activity, and added the *parakinetic disturbances* as a contrast, meaning by this unsuccessful, inept activity.

1. *Description: Akinetic states.* (*a*) *Muscle tonus.* The jaws are firmly pressed together, the hands are clenched, the eyes tightly shut, the head kept rigidly just above the pillow. When one tries to move a limb, one meets with

---

[1] Liepmann, *Die Störungen des Handelns bei Gehirnkranken. Das Krankheitsbild der Apraxie. Drei Aufsätze aus dem Apraxiegebiet* (Sämtlich, Karger, Berlin).

[2] Kleist, *Untersuchungen zur Kenntnis der psychomotorischen Bewegungsstörungen bei Geisteskrankheiten* (Leipzig, 1908–9). Homburger, 'Motorik', in Bumke's *Handbuch der Geisteskrankheiten*, vol. 9, pp. 211–64.

resistance. Tensions such as these are basic for the term *catatonia*. However, at present catatonic symptoms denote rather more than these tensions alone, and include all the incomprehensible motor phenomena which we shall now proceed to describe. (*b*) *Flexibilitas cerea.* There is a slight, easily surmountable tension; the limbs can be put into various postures, like wax, and they will remain like this. This phenomenon is termed *catalepsy*. There is apparently a transition from this point to a meaningful phenomenon; patients will retain postures of an accidental nature or into which they have been put. They do not resist these movements, but permit them co-operatively. (*c*) *Limp immobility.* The patients lie immobile as in the previous descriptions; we can move all their limbs, sometimes with surprising ease. Afterwards they will flop down following the law of gravity. (*d*) *Bizarre, statuesque postures.* Kahlbaum compared some patients with Egyptian statues. They remain totally inexpressive, as if turned to stone; one will pose himself on the window sill, another stand rigid in a corner etc.

*Hyperkinetic states.* In states of motor-excitement, we speak of the pressure of movement. However, we usually know nothing about this 'pressure' and we would do better to resort to the more neutral expression 'motor-excitement'. Old writers would speak of 'furor' (Bewegungstollheit). Movements of this sort appear manifold, aimless and there seems to be no happy or anxious affect accompanying them or any other appropriate psychic change. If our immobile patients sometimes give the impression of Egyptian statues, these patients seem like soulless machines. When one investigates individual cases one gets the repeated impression that sometimes we are dealing with neuronal phenomena and sometimes with meaningful actions. At other times both seem to apply in that neuronal activity seems supplemented by expressive movements (Wernicke: complementary movements). But no general statement can be made of any validity. For the present we can only content ourselves with description of the movements we observe, and their different types.

Externally many of these movements *remind* us of *athetotic, choreic* or *involuntary movements* as we find them in patients with lesions of the cerebellum and cerebellar tracts. Patients make peculiar writhing movements of the body, roll around, stretch their backs, distort the fingers in bizarre fashion, fling their limbs about. Other movements give more the impression that they are *reactions to bodily sensations.* While the patients are writhing and contorting themselves, they put their hands suddenly on one side of their abdomen, press their hands on their genitals, pick their noses, open their mouth wide and grope in it, shut their eyes tight, lean over or hang on to something, as if they wanted to avoid falling over. Other movements again give more the impression of being *expressive.* All kinds of grimacing belong here, those grotesque gestures which have been long regarded as characteristics of madness, the faces of rapture and terror, or silly, childish facetiousness. Patients run their head against the wall, gesticulate, assume animal postures, or an ecclesiastical air; most of these movements are quickly interrupted and fresh ones take their place; or again certain movements are endlessly repeated over weeks and months. Dancing, hopping about, tripping around, affected little skips and jumps, gymnastics, innumerable rhythmic movements, can all be included here. A further group of movements might be subsumed under the category of *sterotypies linked in some way with sensory impressions*. The patients touch everything; turn things this way and that; outline contours with their fingers; imitate movements seen (echopraxia) or repeat everything they hear (echolalia) parrot-fashion. They say the names of all the objects they see. All these movements have in common that they are done uninterruptedly, in stereotyped repetition. Finally there is a group of movements which is characterised by complexity and *similarity to purposeful acts*. A patient jumps up and knocks someone's hat off. Another carries out a military drill. A third suddenly shouts out swear-words. We talk here of *impulsive acts*. They are extremely conspicuous when the patient has been immobile for days. He suddenly carries out such an act, only to relapse into complete immobility immediately afterwards.

We can occasionally make the observation for all the disorders of movement so far described that they are apparently *restricted to certain areas*. Patients may talk incessantly and senselessly but may otherwise be quite quiet in their movements or, inversely, there are other patients who are entirely mute when carrying out their peculiar movements. Increased muscle tonus is often localised to specific groups of muscles, for instance, eyelids and jaws are firmly shut while the arms can be moved quite easily.

One other observation is worth mentioning. In the akinetic states there is a great difference between *spontaneous* movements and those *made on request* (Wernicke: self-initiated and responsive movements). The otherwise immobile patient sees to his own toilet, will swallow his food, feed himself. When these spontaneous movements are present, the patient does not respond to any request at all. During testing, when one tries to get the patient to carry out some movement by request or perform a 'task', the patient may begin a movement and one has the impression that he has understood and has formed an appropriate target but the movement does not proceed. It is suddenly interrupted by another movement, or is simply suspended, or is replaced by widespread tension, or by some entirely contrary movement (negativism), or after prolonged hesitation, with much muscle tension and jerking, some small attempt is made at the requested movement and it is finally carried out perfectly correctly. We can observe all this if we simply ask the patient to raise his hand. During such tests, the patient seems to exert himself greatly, he flushes, perspiration breaks out; his eyes are turned on the examiner with a peculiar suddenness and with an inscrutable expression. In catatonic patients one can often see a last-minute reaction (Kleist). One has been at the bedside a long time. The moment one walks away, patients will say something; as soon as one turns back nothing further can be elicited. It is therefore an old practice with catatonic patients to keep one's ears open just as one walks away, so that one may at least catch the solitary piece of information that emerges. The patient who never speaks may write down the answer to some question, or an immobile patient may say he cannot move. But we get no more than an impression in these cases that we are dealing with mechanical motor-disturbances like motor apraxia, and manifestations of this sort are rare among all the many phenomena which still puzzle us and which for the time being we simply call 'motor' phenomena.

The original more circumscribed concept of 'catatonic' has been substantially enlarged to include all these incomprehensible phenomena of movement. The latter are very common in the large group of schizophrenic processes. The same phenomena are apparently found in low-grade idiots, as described by Plaskuda.[1] In the case of idiots, the commonest finding is a rhythmic movement to and fro of the trunk, torsion movements of the head, grimacing, clicking of the tongue, rattling movements of the lower jaw, whirling the arms, tapping, plucking, twiddling the legs, rhythmical jumping up and down, running in circles. Catalepsies with clouding of consciousness have been observed in physically sick children.[2]

2. *Interpretation.* We have already emphasised sufficiently that interpretation of all these phenomena is not yet possible. Wernicke's *neurological interpretations* as given in his teaching on the motility psychoses were applied by *Kleist* in the new teaching on apraxia, but despite excellent descriptive work he was not very successful. In some catatonic disturbances of motility it is possible, indeed probable, that neurological disturbances may constitute one factor. Here there would be nothing psychic but rather the disturbance of a mechanism with which volition is then confronted, but it could be linked with a disturbance in the pysche and in volition. There are anomalies of movement in genuine neurological diseases of the subcortical ganglia (corpus striatum) which are linked with certain psychic anomalies (lack of initiative) and comparison has been made with catatonia. But it is precisely the psychological differences that are conspicuous. Comparison can only be fruitful through a better description of what may be neurological, so that this can be used as a contrast for the clearer comprehension of catatonic psychic disturbance.[3] Disturbances of movement in post-encephalitics are externally very similar to catatonia and are very remarkable:

We find rigidity of muscles, lack of spontaneous movement. The clinical picture initially looks like a catatonic state: 'lying on the back with head bent forward; the head not touching the pillow. Lengthy retention of passively received postures whether uncomfortable or not; fixation of the final posture after action or the freezing of a movement in the middle of an action; when a spoon is taken to the mouth, the hand stops halfway, or the arms are kept rigid during walking. 'The inner state, however, is quite different from catatonia. Patients see their disturbance objectively;

[1] Plaskuda, *Z. Neur.*, vol. 19, p. 597.

[2] Schneider, *Z. Neur.*, vol. 22 (1914), p. 486, reviews the literature and discusses the onset of catatonic symptoms.

[3] Fränkel, 'Über die psychiatrische Bedeutung der Erkrankungen der subkortikalen Ganglien und ihrer Beziehungen zur Katatonie', *Z. Neur.*, vol. 70, p. 312. O. Foerster, 'Zur Analyse und Pathophysiologie der striären Bewegungstörungen', *Z. Neur.*, vol. 73, p. 1. The latter work instructs us on the purely neurological nature of these disturbances of motility due to lesions of the subcortical ganglia and how different they are from the genuine catatonic disturbances known to psychiatry.

though spontaneous movement is extremely difficult for them, they can carry out the same movements by request from someone else. Hence the patients try out psychological devices on themselves; they work themselves up, make themselves furious, or enthusiastic, to keep the movements up. Once their attention is distracted the tonus increases and movement becomes more difficult. The increase in muscle tonus is very disturbing when they want to fall asleep. When attention is directed towards the intended movement by someone else's will, relaxation and easing takes place. Reiterative phenomena are frequent; rhythmic distention of the cheeks, clicking of the fingers, rhythmical protruding and withdrawing of the tongue. The patients experience this inability to stop as a compulsion. The patients remain aware and thinking is orderly. They are orientated and not psychotic; there is no negativism, resistance or contrariness.

Severe cases of encephalitis are described in phrases very reminiscent of catatonia. 'Physically these people are almost completely blocked'—'Expression is immobile, they have staring looks'—'silent, speechless people, motionless as statues'. Many attacks of fury are reported, sudden apparently unmotivated shouting, crying without apparent cause, even spontaneous attempts to strangle someone near-by, especially in young encephalitics (Dorer).

Further descriptions deal with the interweaving of intended movements and those which are neuronally determined. Movements which patients will make after encephalitis epidemica seem to bring the limbs into positions which one sees in choreic or athetotic types of movement or in torsion spasms.[1]

*Psychological interpretation* has been offered by Kraepelin. The observations of restricted and interrupted movements, of last-minute responses, negativism, are particularly suggestive of possible understanding on the basis of the psychic mechanisms of idea and counter-idea, effort and counter-effort; with patients it seems as if every idea not only evokes a 'counter-idea', every effort a counter-effort, but the one actually encourages the other and lets it assert itself. The patient who wants to raise his hand, does not want to, for that very reason. Kraepelin called this state of affairs *'blocking'*. Many of the disturbances of movement described were then explained in terms of such 'blocking of volition'. He interpreted other movements as an expression of the *alteration in personality*. Every person exhibits his nature through his movements and the sick person shows his nature in his manneristic and bizarre movements, in a 'loss of grace'. Wernicke interpreted yet other movements as the sudden appearance of *'autochthonous'* target-images, psychologically unmotivated, and he supposed an *impulse to realise them*. Others he interpreted as automatic innervations, complemented by psychologically motivated movements (*Complementary movements*). Thus a jerk of the arm is complemented by some groping movement. Patients' self-descriptions sometimes give us insight into their own experience of these disorders of movement. We see that even the most surprising movements may have a psychologically understandable motivation, which of course does not exclude their having an organic basic as well:

[1] Rothfeld, *Z. Neur.*, vol. 114, p. 281.

A patient in an acute psychosis in which she was almost inaccessible kept tearing up her underwear and making countless incomprehensible movements. After the acute phase had disappeared, the patient wrote this about herself (Gruhle). 'I was in a dream-like state and had the idea that "if you are not ashamed to tear up your underclothes in the presence of a man, all people will get to Paradise. The man will make you his Heavenly Bride and you will be Queen of Heaven." That then was the *motive* for *tearing up my underwear*. Another idea I had was that as a divine being I must not wear any clothes, just as I must not eat anything.' Movements which might cause the onlooker some frightening moments meant for the patient harmless amusement (i.e. jumping around). 'As to my desire to fall, this had a variety of reasons. Sometimes I obeyed voices: "Fall down, Claudia" (her christian name). At other times the world would only be saved by my fall, because I would fall to my death by *falling* forward vertically on to my face. I never had the courage to do this and always landed on my knees or on my seat' . . . 'I forgot to explain my *tip-toeing*. I had lost weight and had a wonderful feeling of being light as a spirit, so that floating along on tiptoe gave me great pleasure.'

## § 5. SPEECH

*Psychological Preface.* From the viewpoint of the 'psychic reflex arc' language is only a particularly well-developed part of the total reflex arc. Understanding of language is a part of perception and apperception, speech a part of the motor phenomena. This viewpoint clarifies only a few aspects of language, not language itself.

Speaking should be differentiated from *uttering noises that are audible*. The latter may be involuntary expressions but as such are not speech. They are cries, interjections, whistles, etc., but not words, sentences. There is no intention to communicate. Speech only exists if meaning attaches itself to articulate words. Objective speech is a system of symbols, sanctioned by traditional usage, and used as a tool by anyone who grows up within the system.

We should also differentiate speaking from *expressive movements*. These are involuntary manifestations of the psychic self through gesture, voice and posture. Speaking, on the other hand, is a willed communication of an objective content, whether by gesture-language or voiced speech. If I speak, I have something to communicate to a listener which he will understand.

We also have to separate *speech* and *speaking*. Speech, as language, is an objective symbolic structure in which the individual who belongs to that language-group partakes to a greater or lesser extent. Speaking is *an accomplishment of the psychic reality of the individual*. Our concern here is with speaking as a psychological occurrence and not, as later, with language or speech as cultural products.

*Speaking* and *understanding* are closely linked. They take place in group intercourse. They occur as a communication of meaning and it is the meaning as such, not the language or the words, which is in the field of attention for both the speaker and the understanding recipient.

Man, when *isolated*, uses speech in order to make himself understand his own thoughts and wishes. Although speaking and thinking are not identical, every thought nevertheless develops in conjunction with speech. In the manual handling of objects and during the actual execution of meaningful work, our thinking is speechless, but in the objects themselves we find symbols and signs of an activity analogous to speech.

No thoughts can exist without roots in something concrete; abstract ideas are linked with symbols, the concrete meaning of which is not immediately present although it is with these that we think. The symbol is then a concrete minimum.

Abnormalities of *verbal production* whether spoken or written may be due to two quite different reasons. The verbal production may be abnormal because although *the speech apparatus is normal something abnormal is being expressed.* We see in the verbal products elementary disturbances of thinking, feeling and awareness which make use of normal language and turn its content and character into expressive phenomena. In spite of the intact speech we can recognise in the verbal product the striking manifestation of underlying psychic disturbance. In the second place, the verbal production may be *abnormal* because the *mechanism of the speech apparatus itself has changed.* Only when this is so should we speak of speech-disorders. These are not meaningful changes, because they are extra-conscious events. But we can psychologically understand and try to interpret all abnormal verbal products that are secondary to abnormal psychic life; their content and expressive character have some meaning for us. Apart from these neurologically and psychologically explicable products of speech we find, thirdly, certain inexplicable ones the analysis of which helps us to learn what are the *speech disorders proper.*

We differentiate disorders of *articulation* from *aphasias* and *speech-disorders in psychosis:*

## (a) Disorders of articulation

Speaking is a co-ordinated process of muscle movement. Disturbances in this field are termed disorders of articulation, in contrast to disturbances of the central speech-process that precedes the muscle movement. Disorders of articulation are *neurologically* conceived and are possible *without any psychic disturbance.* The actual word is malformed owing to the paralysis of individual muscles or some disturbance of innervation. It therefore comes out distorted (where disorders of articulation are not immediately observable, the patient can be tested by being asked to repeat difficult word-combinations—(e.g. Royal Irish Artillery, the swimming swan etc.) We find, for instance, syllables are bungled; speech is slurred; there is dysarthria; lalling in paralytics, scanning in multiple sclerotics. In addition there is *stuttering* which belongs to this group although it arises from quite different causes and may be psychologically conditioned. We use the term 'stuttering' for those clonic movements of the speech-muscles whereby consonants and vowels at the beginning of a word fall prey to constant repetition instead of becoming incorporated into the spoken word.[1] Corresponding to these disorders of articulation on the motor side are certain sensory disorders; for instance the failure of a deaf person to understand. Those who are *deaf and dumb* for congenital reasons or through early acquired deafness need to be differentiated from those who are *dumb but*

---

[1] Hoepfner, 'Vom gegenwärtigen Stande der Stotternforschung', *Z. Psychother.*, vol. 4 (1912), p. 55. Gutzmann, *Die dysarthrischen Sprachstörungen* (1911). E. Fröschels, *Z. Neur.*, vol. 33 (1916), p. 317. E. Fröschels, *Lehrbuch der Sprachheilkunde* (Leipzig and Vienna, 1931, 3rd edn.). (This not only deals with stammering but with aphasia.)

*can hear*; these are feebleminded persons who do not speak though they can hear and there is no speech disorder.

## (b) Aphasias

We find patients who no longer speak (cases of apoplexy, brain injury, cerebral tumour). In the old days they were often thought to be demented but one can see they would like to speak when one addresses them. They try to speak and torture themselves in trying to do so. Their whole demeanour shows their personality is still there. Other patients will speak but cannot understand. It was a great discovery to find that in these cases one was dealing with a speech disorder, a circumscribed disorder of the apparatus, not of the personality or the intelligence (though such disorders hardly ever appear without some change in the total state). Another great discovery was that in right-handed persons symptoms of this sort were due to destruction of the left lower frontal convolution or of the temporal area. These speech disorders are incredibly and most confusingly varied. Attempts have been made to reduce them to some order by endeavouring to erect a large-scale basic psychology of language (Wernicke). Speech was broken down into speaking and understanding, repeated speech and spontaneous speech, naming, reading, writing etc. Each of these elements were then ascribed a definite place on the left frontal cortex, so that these psychological structures became physically embedded in the brain-structures. From this emerged the 'classical teaching on aphasia'.

The aphasias are similar to agnosia and apraxia but related to speech. Patients hear but do not understand what is said (*sensory aphasia*). We may differentiate here between understanding the sound-pattern and understanding its meaning. Other patients can move all their speech muscles and can use them for purposes other than speech but cannot pronounce words (*motor aphasia*). Here too we should differentiate between inability to pronounce from inability to find the words (*amnestic aphasia*). In the first case the patient cannot repeat words, in the latter he can. Sensory aphasia depends predominantly on destruction in the temporal lobes; motor aphasia on destruction in the posterior part of the third frontal convolution. In both cases this is on the left side with right-handed persons.[1]

We need to differentiate the psychic processes which occur in *speaking* and *understanding*. On the side of understanding we need to distinguish: (1) merely hearing a noise, such as a cough, or some inarticulate sound; (2) hearing a *word-pattern* without understanding it, e.g. a foreign language which we do not understand. So also with written material, which we may be able to read but need not understand. Or a word-series, which we can learn by repeating but it remains meaningless to us; (3) understanding the meaning of words and sentences.

The following *schema devised by Liepmann* (slightly modified) gives us a tentative survey of the different aphasias:

He analyses the aphasias and differentiates components that are *psychic phenomena*

---

[1] The best exposition is that of Liepmann in Curschmann's *Lehrbuch der Neurologie*. Von Monakow surveys the literature in the *Ergebnisse der Physiologie*. A new, critical and excellent exposition of the subject is given by Thiele in Bumke's *Handbuch der Geisteskrankheiten* (1928, vol. 2).

(shown in the diagram as blank circles) and *psychic connections* (shown as dotted or interrupted lines), from the *non-psychic* components that are linked to *anatomical* cortical areas (shown in the diagram as solid circles) and the *anatomical fibre tracts* (shown by lines). Making use of this diagram we may conceive the connections (left ascending, sensory; right descending, motor) as interrupted, or the circles as either destroyed or cut off. In this way we can construct possible types of aphasia in great variety. Thus (*see Fig.* 2):

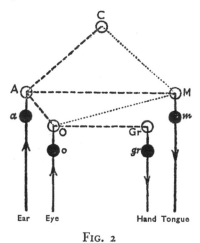

FIG. 2

1. *Anatomical components:*     a. acoustic projection area of the cortex.
                                     m. motor     „     „  „  „     „
                                     o. optic     „     „  „  „     „
                                     gr. graphic part of the motor projection area of the cortex (innervating the hand).
2. *Psychological components:*  A. acoustic component (word sound-pattern—Wortsinnverständnis).
                                     M. motor-speech components.
                                     O. optic components.
                                     Gr. graphic-motor components.
                                     C. meaning of words ('conceptual' components).

The test performance (sometimes called functioning) of aphasic patients becomes comprehensible only if the following paths are intact:

Spontaneous speech:        C—A—M—m—Tongue.

Spontaneous writing:      C—|     O—Gr—Hand.

Speech-comprehension:   Ear—A—C

Reading-comprehension: Eye—O

Repeating: Ear—A—M—Tongue.

Copying: Eye—O—Gr—Hand.

Writing to dictation: Ear—A—O—Gr—Hand.

(above: M with diagonal line to A and vertical line)

Reading aloud: Eye—O—A—M—Tongue.

From gr and m downwards destruction is responsible not for aphasic but articulatory disturbances (dysarthria, anarthria). Destruction from a to o upwards is responsible for deafness, tone-deafness, partial deafness and so with weak vision, blindness.

The following types can be elicited from the manifold and individually varying aphasias:

*Pure motor aphasia:* M is destroyed or isolated. Understanding of speech is preserved, so are reading and writing. But spontaneous speech is destroyed and the power to repeat and read aloud. This is a rare type and we more commonly get 'complete motor aphasia'. Through the involvement of M through O—M in all functions which require the pathway O—C, reading and writing are also disturbed, whereas copying (without M) is preserved. Such patients tend to be taciturn; at other times they are explosive; they try to speak but quickly break off.

*Pure sensory aphasia:* A is destroyed or isolated. Spontaneous speech is preserved, but comprehension of speech and powers of repetition etc. are destroyed. This form is rather rare; *complete sensory aphasia* is more common. Normally, spontaneous speech requires the pathway via A, hence the present disturbance of it, not in the form of word-dumbness as in the motor aphasias but as paraphasia. *Paraphasia* consists in a distortion of words so great that we can no longer recognise any meaning from the series of syllables heard. This is because the word-sound-pattern (A) cannot be aroused in the usual way while the simultaneous free-floating sound-patterns (Mehringer and Mayer) which occur associatively lead to a number of distortions, switchings, reversals, anticipations etc. These patients are paraphasically talkative with neologisms. If they lose control, they appear manic. They are surprised and dismayed to find that no one understands them.

*Transcortical aphasias:* With these we have the pathway: Ear—A—M—Tongue preserved; powers of repetition of what has been heard are therefore preserved. With *transcortical motor aphasia* the pathway C—M is blocked. The patients cannot find words, the concepts of which they possess, but yet they recognise and pronounce the word when the name is given to them. In mild degrees we term this condition *amnestic aphasia*. With *transcortical sensory aphasia* patients can repeat everything, but the meaning of the words escapes them.

Important *objections* have been raised against the total picture as presented by this classical theory of aphasia. The psychology used is exclusively that of association-psychology, which is hardly adequate and according to which discrete elements are only linked into units by virtue of association. The nature of speech, however, cannot be understood in terms of such a psychology, since the essence of speech is awareness of meaning. The unity of verbal meaning is shattered by a division into sensory, optic, acoustic, kinaesthetic and motor elements. Speech takes place at a fundamentally higher level of functioning in the form of impulse to movement and reception of sensations. This accounts for the fact that the clinical picture presented by aphasia cannot be classified into acoustic and motor speech-disturbances, as alexia, agraphia etc. There are a few cases it is true which with the help of the diagram may be very satisfactorily described. Most cases, however, would have to be forced within the framework. The theoretical schema is a deductive one and the individual clinical pictures are so constructed. The fruitfulness of the construction has shown itself up to a certain point—as happens in the natural sciences—but then we come to a halt. The discrepancy between clinical cases and what is presupposed grows noticeable. The construction here—in contrast to the theories of natural science—is of limited heuristic value and has utterly exhausted itself. Initially a small clearing has been made in the phenomenological confusion and there is some intelligible description of phenomena not properly understood in their nature. There can be no further elaboration or fruitful application and it is necessary to discard the theory as a whole and in principle to make room for a new and better comprehension growing out of other premisses.

The new approach has its origins in Wernicke himself, who formulated the term 'verbal concept' to express the basic function within which his sensory and motor elements were inseparably linked into unity. These unitary 'images of speech' were later seen as functions of a cortical speech area without any specific localisation of the motor, sensory and other elements.

Head[1] went furthest of all. He discarded the whole schema. Classification of speech disorders into disorders of speech, reading, writing, and understanding, hardly corresponds to the clinical facts. There are no basic psychic functions which are localised and correspond to these performances. Head himself started by improving the methods of examination, and in many decades of experience he enlarged and enriched these into an imposing and intelligible schema of investigation. His new interpretation of the findings avoids any dogmatic theory. He takes the disturbances of symbolic formulation or of any behaviour in which verbal or other symbols play a part in mediating intention into execution. Even though one cannot break language up into elementary functions (sensory, motor, etc.) we cannot really do without some typical syndromes which will present us with a meaningful picture. Head therefore develops four groups of aphasias: verbal, syntactic, nominal and semantic. He limited himself to this field, and remained closer to reality than the classic theory. Yet he pays for this by not giving us the impression of any simple or radical comprehension of the whole. He does not sketch psychological theories in the brain-space but presents clinical syndromes without theory. The question has to be left open whether these are just clinical pictures or whether behind them lies some really relevant function, waiting to be discovered. Head helps us to come closer to the reality of language and its disturbances than we have ever done before. He is not obsessed with untried psychological presuppositions or brain-mythology. We have yet to see what

[1] Head, *Aphasia and kindred disorders of speech* (Cambridge, 1926). Last, *Nervenarzt*, vol. 3 (1930), p. 222.

meaning his particular categories have, and how far they will help us towards firm, realistic and meaningful concepts. Head's success can only be judged by specialists with large numbers of cases at their disposal. The cases reported in the literature are insufficient. No one has yet succeeded in giving so seductive and lucid a picture as the old classical theory—deceptive though that lucidity seems to be.

It is of general psychopathological interest to find that in the examination of some aphasias we come across great fluctuations in performance within very brief spaces of time:[1]

Performance decreases as the patient grows tired with the examination. Sometimes a low ebb is reached and then after a brief interval this is overcome. The fluctuations may be related to the concentrated attention which the patients give to the tasks. As is the case with all impairment of function, speech in this case can only reach performance if there is a high level of attention. We should also expect aphasic patients to be considerably disturbed by affects, such as embarrassment, surprise etc. A situation which makes clear demands can interest and stimulate them and they can have remarkable success. Quite apart from this we cannot rule out the possibility of occasional spontaneous 'fluctuations in brain-function' (see above, p. 142).

## (c) Speech disorders in psychoses[2]

These disorders include certain verbal performances which at present cannot be explained in terms of neurological mechanisms; nor can they be simply understood as a form of expression or as the communication of abnormal psychic contents. We have to deal with a territory of interest to both sides. For the moment we only need to record the actual psychotic speech phenomena. They form a group of 'objective' symptoms on their own:

1. *Mutism and pressure of talk.* From the purely formal point of view, content apart, these phenomena correspond to immobility and excitement in the motor field. *Mutism* may be intelligible as a deliberate silence, or as an expression of psychic inhibition, or as the effect of some hysterical mechanism, but in many cases none of these interpretations seem to apply and we have to accept the phenomenon as incomprehensible for the time being.

Motor excitement in the speech apparatus, which we term *pressure of talk*, gives rise to most varied phenomena. Irrespective of their affective state, patients keep on talking about all sorts of senseless things without bothering really to communicate. They keep on all day long, uninterruptedly, and for several days or weeks the talk runs on; sometimes they speak quietly and the voice never rises above an indistinct murmur; sometimes they perform incredibly by shouting until they become hoarse, though this does not impede them. Some seem to address themselves, and talk themselves into it; others talk quite mechanically. There is frequently a tendency to rhythmical emphasis. In most cases we do not know what is the subjective experience during

[1] Stertz, *Mschr. Psychiatr.*, vol. 32, p. 363.

[2] Heilbronner, 'Sprachstörungen bei funktionellen Psychosen mit Ausschluss aphasischer Störungen', *Zbl. Nervenhk.*, vol. 1906, pp. 472 ff. Liebmann and Edel, *Die Sprache der Geisteskranken* (Halle ,1903)—a shorthand record of verbal productions.

these motor-speech discharges. *Self-descriptions*, however, do tell us of two different types of experience: (1) There is the experience of a real pressure of talk, like an instinctual drive; it is of varying degree; some patients can suppress it altogether; others have to give in and feel it an unpleasant and morbid experience. Other patients give way without any inhibition. (2) Others experience what seems to them spontaneous activity of the speech-apparatus; and look on the performance as a spectator. For instance, the case described on p. 124 will give us an example. Here is another described by Kandinsky:

> Dolinin suddenly felt his tongue starting to pronounce loudly and very fast a number of things that should not have been said; this was not only involuntarily but definitely against his will. At first the patient was startled and worried by this unusual event. It is hardly pleasant to feel some concrete, wound-up automatism inside oneself. When he began to realise what his tongue was saying, he became horrified; he found himself admitting to guilt as a political criminal, ascribing to himself plans he had never had. Yet he had no power to curb the utterances of his suddenly automatised tongue.

These are apparently clear-cut cases and there is a whole series of such phenomena ranging in clarity down to cases where the phenomena are the same but there is no such dichotomy between the self and the actual flow of talk.

2. *Where does this pressure of talk get its content from?*[1] (1) *The speech-apparatus itself* may function on its own with a stream of repetitive phrases senselessly reproduced, Bible-quotations, verses, numbers, months of the year, tunes, meaningless phrases in grammatical form, agrammatical constructions, clang-associations, word-compounds, inarticulate sounds. (2) There may be *perseveration*, which we now know to be a deficiency symptom, a 'getting entangled or stuck'. We can see this happen with aphasic patients in certain situations which we can predict. Pressure of talk which draws its material from perseverating content is bound to 'get stuck' in the end. In this case we speak of *verbigeration* (Kahlbaum). The patient is apparently talking and making a conversation but repeats separate words, fragments of words and phrases, meaningless phrases, in a monotonous tone; nothing significant is ever said nor does there seem any relation to the patient's experience. Kandinsky remarked that patients often feel vividly the compulsive character of this impulse to verbigerate, analogous to the states of shouting, mentioned above, and the automatic speaking of Dolinin.

One of his patients used the phrases 'involuntary speech', 'parleying with myself' or 'my self-parleys'. Even when he wanted to ask for something, he had to express himself in this particular form: 'selbstparlage, selbstparliere, excuse me . . . selbstparlage, selbstparliere, excuse me . . . selbstparlage . . . excuse me a Papiros . . . must not smoke oneself . . . I want to smoke myself . . . but by selbstparlage . . . selbstparlieren . . . I selbstparliere to you . . . give me a smoke . . .'

---

[1] Heilbronner, 'Sprachstörungen bei funktionellen Psychosen mit Ausschluss aphasischer Störungen', *Zbl. Nervenhk.*, vol. 1906, pp. 472 ff.

We must distinguish between these apparently *automatic* verbigerations and those which are affectively toned and in particular due to *anxiety*. In states of gross anxiety patients repeat the same matters over and over again in a puzzled way 'God, God, what a disaster . . . God, God, what a disaster . . .' and so on. (3) If unproductive patients look around for material for their pressure of talk they can obtain this from external *sense stimuli*, if they do not get it from automatisms of the speech-apparatus or from perseveration. Acoustic impressions are simply repeated (echolalia), a senseless name given to every object. (4) We should distinguish *flight of ideas* from all three previous sources, because of its sheer *productivity*. The pressure of talk that flows from this is marked by rich content and extremely varied associations, sometimes by its wit and apt turns of phrase. Flight of ideas and distractibility both need pressure of talk if they are to manifest themselves objectively; otherwise they will remain purely subjective feelings (an inner flight of ideas, an inner distractibility). Conversely, flight of ideas is by no means a condition for pressure of talk. The latter is often similtaneously present with an inhibition of talk, and in patients suffering from dementia, pressure of thought without any flight of ideas is particularly common. (5) The term 'confused speech' covers many different modes of speech. The form may seem coherent and yet no meaning may be communicated or understandable,[1] as the sentences, or interrupted fragments of them, are being uttered. Some of these constructions certainly have no meaning for the patients themselves; others are only unintelligible for the observer. The following extract from the letter of a catatonic patient suffering from this confusion of speech shows a relatively high degree of intelligibility:

For analogous and natural reasons I am disclosing to you the fact that I have passed various examinations, which rest upon fresh advances of the time and relate to all the natural rights to freedom. Self-help is always the best and cheapest. We know what national pride is, and I know the honour concerned, and what knowledge is, is my secret. Respect for my cause, which is related to the above. 'Eye and hand for the Fatherland' . . . My affairs must be taken roundly. With this I would inform you that I am already known here as the first public prosecutor . . . (Otto).

With confused speech we can compare *incoherent* productions, which no longer show any sentence-formation. Although the content can be understood, the following letter of a catatonic patient to his wife well illustrates this phenomenon:

In the house there, is he lying at home ill? yet . . . [untranslatable] 'anspruchlos, inderesenlos von dem was gekommen? doch was to geslagen an den? Ich. der Muller. Nachts unruig gewesen. Stimmen horen traurige. Ja Schwager da in F. Wir bilden eine kurze underdung von der Achmrika. Frau Kinder sesund. ja nun alen da. wie geth. gut mir auch sehr gut. das freuet mich.'

[1] Otto, *Ein seltener Fall von Verwirrtheit* (Diss., München, 1889). He gives a detailed description of an exceptional case of confused speech.

3. *Disturbance of conversational speech.* Description so far has been concerned with phenomena exhibited by the patient on his own. Another picture arises if we look at the *play of question and answer* in the conversational situation between examiner and patient. This is the occasion for the symptom '*talking past the point*' (Vorbeireden). With aphasic speech disturbances (particularly with the sensory aphasias) patients spontaneously utter garbled sounds with an awareness on their part that they mean something (Paraphasia). Here however the *paralogia* has intelligible content and is manifestly related to the question and answer, but although the intellectual competence may be there, answers are incorrect and there is no proper solution of the tasks set. The patient performs all the multiplications, for instance, except that he adds one digit more: $3 \times 3 = 10$, $6 \times 7 = 43$, and so on. How many legs has a cow—5, etc.'[1] There seems no single psychological interpretation for this phenomenon. It arises as a symptom of 'pseudodementia' in hysterical states, when illness fulfils the patient's wish (in prison, for example) or it appears as a form of negativism or an expression of the silly joking of hebephrenia.

4. *Psychological interpretation.* Attempts are made to explain psychotic speech psychologically, particularly the phenomenon of confused speech. *The principle of association* is invoked with recourse to sensory and ideational material, the one stemming from the apprehension of sensory stimuli, the other from the actualising of memory-dispositions.[2] The problem is whether all the verbal constructions can be explained in terms of association; or do 'freshly arising' structures occur? Elements link through similarity (e.g. clang-associations), through being experienced, through their related content etc., and perseveration adds itself to the initial elements. Syllables, words, bits of sentences, an intended 'meaning', etc., all function as 'elements' in this respect. Contamination is one of the concepts specially belonging to association-psychology and is used for the classification of abnormal speech-structures. This denotes the fusing of one word-element from two other such elements (e.g. sur-stonished, for surprised and astonished). In the same way, words and syllables suffer permutation, some are tacked on as affixes, others as suffixes.

§ 6. THOUGHT AND JUDGMENT

Thought is contained in all our performances from the act of perception to speech itself. Judgment is said to be disturbed only when perception, orientation, memory, movement and speech are otherwise in order or when we can distinguish between specific disturbances in these and what has occasioned the false judgment.

---

[1] Julius Hey, *Das Gansersche Symptom* (Berlin, 1904). Ganser, *Arch. Psychiatr.* (D), vols. 30–8. Raecke, *Allg. Z. Psychiatr.*, vol. 58. Henneberg, *Allg. Z. Psychiatr.*, vol. 61. Pick, *Mschr. Psychiatr.*, vol. 42, p. 197 (Vorbeidenken—Vorbeireden).

[2] Kraepelin, 'Über Sprachstörungen in Traume', *Psychol. Arb.*, vol. 5. Pfersdorff, *Zbl Neurol.*, vol. 1908, *Z. Neur.*, vol. 3 (1910), etc. Mehringer and Meyer, *Versprechen und Verlesen* (Stuttgart, 1895).

The performance of judgment is measured against objective truth. Where the judgments of an individual deviate from what is generally held as valid and he holds obstinately to their content although it interferes with adaptation, the question arises whether among other things there is a morbid cause affecting the judgments themselves. There is a difficulty here because the same characteristics might apply to the judgments of exceptional people who creatively open new ways of thought. If, therefore, a disorder is suspected merely because the judgment runs counter to current beliefs, this clearly will not suffice and we have to try and assess the situation in some other context before we can decide that a disorder of judgment is really there. Judgments that deviate from generally held opinions provide us with objective, if superficial phenomena, disregarding for the moment whether they may be false or true. The problem is what characteristics must judgments have for us to say that they are examples of disordered performance. We have to distinguish *disorders of intelligence* and *thought-disorders* from *delusion*. We shall deal with the first two in the next section and will discuss the latter here.

Delusion presents us with one of those great riddles which can be solved only if we define our facts clearly. If incorrigible wrong judgments are termed 'delusion', who will there be without delusion, since we are all capable of having convictions and it is a universal human characteristic to hold on to our own mistaken judgments? Nor can the prolific illusions of entire peoples and persons be given the title of 'delusion', since this would mean treating a basic human characteristic as if it were an illness. We should rather address ourselves to the problem of what it is that occasions the incorrigibility and causes us to recognise certain modes of wrong judgment as delusion.

As a psychopathological concept, delusion can be considered in four ways: as a psychological performance, in its actual phenomenology, with an understanding of how it comes about and with an understanding of it as a meaningful whole.

(a) As a *psychological performance*, it is delusion only where intelligence is undisturbed and there is no disturbance in the immediate state of consciousness either, so as to occasion the wrong judgment. The patient's thinking-apparatus and power of judgment are in order but there is a factor in his thinking which affords him unshakeable evidence when other people, even other patients, can see the mistake. Since thinking is in order in delusion and even used ingeniously to serve it, we can hardly speak of delusion as a thought-disturbance. To consider it from the point of view of psychological performance may be the first step, but it leaves us simply with the negative result that delusion is not really a disturbance of performance. It springs rather from some deeper source, which is manifested in the delusional judgment but has none of the characteristics of a judgment in itself.

The following is an example of the elaborating thought-performance which takes place in delusion: a schizophrenic patient (a factory-hand, who later became a policeman) experiences typical 'passivity' phenomena; there are movements of his limbs and he hears voices. He thinks of remote hypnosis and telepathy. He suspects and reports someone to the police. He arranges for a private detective to make enquiries and finally convinces himself that his suspicions are unfounded. He writes: 'Since no one can have been influencing me and I am sure I am not suffering from any false-perception, I have to ask who can it be? The way in which I am plagued and tortured and the hidden meaning in all these conversations and bodily movements suggest that there is some malicious supernatural being at work. He influences and plagues me continually and hopes to destroy me. Are my experiences of the same order as those of mental patients or are they unique? For humanity's sake I feel I should state my conviction that if they are of the same order, then the doctor must be wrong in thinking that the voices which patients hear are hallucinations. Whatever it is in my own case, whether it is the same experience as that of a mental patient or something exceptional, the conclusion is in either case that life goes on after death' (Wildermuth).

(b) *Phenomenologically*, we observe in delusion an experience that is radically alien to the healthy person, something basic and primary, which comes before thought, although it becomes clear to itself only in thought. This primary experience, moreover, is not limited to a single experience which breaks through into consciousness simply as one phenomenon among others, otherwise the patient could criticise and master it. The primary event has to be related to some radical change of personality since, otherwise, the insurmountable character of the delusion and its essentially distinctive incorrigibility would be quite incomprehensible.

(c) We may well *understand from the context* how a delusional belief liberates an individual from something unbearable, seems to deliver him from reality and lends a peculiar satisfaction which may well be the ground for why it is so tenaciously held. But should we also try to make the actual formation of the delusion, as well as its content, understandable, any diagnosis of delusion becomes impossible, for what we have grasped in this case is ordinary human error, not delusion proper. Philosophy is always trying to reach that state of mind where all mistakes can stand corrected, and to exercise that unprejudiced, large and perceptive affection for the world, that openness of reason, which can tolerate what is real and true and, when no decisive answer is possible, can endure doubt, and which always remains ready to communicate and prevent the rigidity of fixed opinion. But we are still far from that ideal state and are tied to the interests of our existence and to all that makes it bearable; here is the root of all our common mistakes to which, in their exaggerated form, we give the term 'delusion-like' mistake, although we are not really dealing here with delusion proper.

(d) *Delusion proper* shows itself *as a whole* primarily in the fact that it creates a new world for the deluded person. It expresses itself through its style but a living being is revealed as well. Delusion draws its content from the world which it shapes so pervasively for the patient, and, as it grows more elaborate, it becomes a cultural creation.

In whatever way we consider delusion we are presented with the *external* fact that delusion is a *defective performance* when measured up against objective truth—provided we have this measure. As a defective performance in this sense, we can consider it from the point of view of *content*: delusional ideas may be either of a *personal* relevance or of an impersonal, *objective* nature. In the former case they will concern the individual himself; they are the delusions of spite, persecution, inferiority, sin, poverty, etc; in the latter case, the delusional ideas are of more general interest; they may be revelations, delusions of invention, theses in defence of theories (e.g. the identity of Bacon and Shakespeare), so-called fixed ideas, objective enough in their content but completely monopolising the individual. Patients behave as if the whole meaning of their life rested on this one idea and superficially they in no way differ in this from great creative personalities who expend themselves on their own ends, but the difference lies in the extreme narrowness of idea and the atmosphere of slavish confinement. Both types of delusional content are linked together in that the objective content tends to become an extremely personal affair, e.g.: defence of justice becomes for the querulant the defence of his own particular rights. Any classification of delusional content would have to include all the interests that life can offer and all the contents of our minds. It seems as if everything in our human world can be remoulded into delusion-like forms, which (as distinct from delusion proper) may pass over into 'normality' at any point, so that as the mind pursues its course, these delusion-like creations pursue their own, a sort of parody of it, as it were. In psychopathology therefore we must be careful not to put all incorrigible mistakes under the heading of delusion proper. But when faced with actual delusional worlds, we need to think afresh about the meaning of truth, so that in any given case our assessment of reality can be justified.

Delusion is a word that is *commonly used for a number of quite different phenomena.* It is, however, a mistaken judgment, and a judgment by externals only, that allows the same term 'delusion' to be applied to such completely different phenomena as the so-called 'delusions' of *primitive peoples* and the 'delusions' of *demented persons* (paralytics) and of *paranoics.* Primitive peoples have a psychic life that is differentiated to only a slight degree. We characterise this in relation to their beliefs, and we say that they have not yet learnt to distinguish perception and fantasy as arising from different sources. A number of diverse logical processes all possess for them the same evidential quality; for instance, they will conclude by analogy, on the basis of purely external criteria. With the demented, paralytic patient, psychic life has disintegrated in ways characteristic for the organic, cerebral disorders and these cannot be compared with the undifferentiated state of primitive man. In paralytic changes every image obtains reality, every idea seems correct without regard to wish or purpose, often without effect and consequence. Every content appears real. This gives rise to unrestricted delusions of grandeur which shift constantly and can even change into their opposite. In the case of *paranoics,* we are again dealing with something quite different. The individual shows a high degree of differentiation, sharp powers of criticism and an ability to think, but none of this interferes with his belief in the content of his delusional ideas. He has had certain experiences and for him they carry as much, if not more, weight than anyone else's. He integrates these experiences with others and he builds up his delusional system quite seriously and with deep involvement and holds unshakeably to it. Contrary ideas do occur to him, but he brushes them aside disparagingly. He does not lack power to differentiate the discrete sources of knowledge but he insists on his own source, whether supernatural or material.

## SECTION TWO

## THE TOTAL PERFORMANCE

*Disturbance in each individual performance* affects the individual's total state. The effect may be quite catastrophic, although the disturbance need be limited to only one function as we have described. It may be a disturbance of registration, a severe aphasia, a motor disturbance etc. The individual's total state is changed but this can be fully grasped in terms of the demonstrable, separate disturbance. Inversely, each individual performance may change in quality and meaning through its dependence on *the sum-total of the performances*. If we consider this, each individual performance then becomes the symptom of a total event, which we cannot directly perceive. We no longer simply register a series of defective performances but the defects are formed into a group. This is done in various ways, depending on how we ourselves regard the total event. We may see this either as the *psycho-physiological basis* of the individual performance manifesting itself in the defects as a whole, or as the actual *mode of psychic being* which prevails at the time, or as the individual's permanent capacity for performance, which we call the *intelligence*. All these several totalities are phenomena that occur in states of clear consciousness and when there is no clouding or alteration of awareness.[1]

If individual performances are not the products of an isolated apparatus but already parts of a *total apparatus of performance*, this latter itself is not an independent closed unit either, but an instrument of the individual whose mind shapes the instrument it uses, while in its turn it remains dependent on the instruments given and their potentialities for its realisation. All mental performances have this in common that they can be measured against a norm of 'common awareness'.[2] This confines them to one area of human existence, which is clearly enough defined, but never exhibits the whole human person, the man as *such*.

### § 1. The Psychophysical Basis for Performance

We have no insight into the basic function of vital, psychic life. Our urge to premature comprehension has often driven us to conceive some such whole,

---

[1] K. F. Scheid, 'Die Psychologie des erworbenes Schwachsinns (1919–1932)', *Zbl. Neur.*, vol. 67, p. 1.

[2] Cp. my lectures: *Vernunft u. Existenz* (Groningen, 1935), pp. 31 ff.

but without success. We still ask questions, however, and it appears that we can dimly discern some all-embracing foundation for our biological existence. Areas of questioning are as follows: *defective performance* in *brain disorders*, the facts that emerge from the establishment of *a work-curve*, and *individual variations* within the countless types of performance. In all these cases research is constantly directed to what may lie at the root of these manifold appearances and what may be considered the vital, foundation occurrence.

## (a) *Basic psychophysical functions*

Investigations of defective performance following organic brain lesions have shown that—even if the lesion is localised in the brain—the disturbances of performance are often characterised by more than one, single defective performance. This tempts us to look for some comprehensive psychophysical basic function which manifests itself not only in one single type of performance but in indirect fashion in a whole number of defective performances. We would like to see what is common to them all, on what does this great variety of disturbances rest, what pervades them all. It is a comprehensive whole since we find it appearing in many phenomena and it is also something elementary, a basic function, one basic function among others.

Basic functions, however, cannot be directly demonstrated as can single defects of performance. *Our method* is to try and penetrate into the context of the disturbance by first using the *self-descriptions* of patients, brought out systematically by talking to them, and then by observing the paths of the still intact performances. If one knows where and how the patient experiences his difficulties, the disturbance lays itself open to us, even though objectively the performance is still intact. Objective observation and patients' self-descriptions together help us to get to know *the paths* and detours of their performance and we can compare it with the normal. In this way we can get to the central, essential point of the disturbance. We then compare the manifold performances of the patient, and hope that if there is something common to them all, we shall find it. *Research of this type*—followed by Gelb and Goldstein, Hochheimer, Benary, and so on—brings results. We will quote as an example a famous case of psychic blindness (soul-blindness) using the actual report of the authors:[1]

At 23 years of age the patient was wounded at the back of the head by splinters from a mine. He could no longer recognise shapes and movements in space (cp. p. 170 the descriptions of the same patient). Close examination showed that, even after performance had improved, the defects as a whole could not be wholly understood in terms of the visual agnosia.

One could talk freely with the patient and not notice anything conspicuous. He

[1] W. Hochheimer, 'Analyse eines "Seelenblinden" ' from *Psychol. Forsch.*, vol. 16 (1932), p. 1. On the same case Gelb and Goldstein, *Psychologische Analyse hirnpathologischer Fälle* (Leipzig, 1920), vol. 1. Benary, *Psychol. Forsch.*, vol. 2 (1922), p. 209. Goldstein, *Mschr. Psychiatr.* (1923), vol. 54.

had a letter read to him which he had written himself a short time ago to the doctor. He listened but did not recognise his own letter. The letter was then shown to him and he did not recognise his own handwriting, except when he read the signature. . . . 'Well, that is my signature!' . . . 'I would never have recognised it!' . . . Throughout long conversations with the patient, behaviour was quite inconspicuous, until some task came up, like the recognition of the letter, and the behaviour changed. The defect in performance was startling, and the man who usually talked cheerfully and unruffled became taciturn and tense.

In one investigation there were a number of listeners sitting around. After one hour the patient was asked: 'Do you see the others over there?' Reply: 'Now, yes!' The patient's attention is limited strictly to what it is directed to; no two elements exist for him simultaneously in his environment. To the question 'How did you get on in the winter?' he replies: 'I can't say that right now, I can only say what takes place now.' Past and future are not accessible to him and he cannot imagine them. He does not imagine at all and it is the same with everything that is not immediately present to him. 'I can name something but not imagine it.'

What is a frog? . . . 'Frog . . . a frog? . . . what is a frog . . . frog . . . quak, quak, it jumps!' . . . What is its colour? 'Frog . . . frog . . . a tree-frog . . . oh, colour . . . tree—green . . . the tree-frog is green. Well!' The patient is not able to invoke mental images himself in contrast to images emerging involuntarily. In place of inner representation he uses talking towards it to invoke his reply.

Tell us something! . . . 'I can't manage that, someone has to say what do you know of that and that . . .' When greeting: Any news? . . . 'What for instance?' or if you ask 'What happened last time?' . . . 'When, where . . . oh a lot of things, I don't know' . . . Can you remember anything we have done here? 'There was so much' . . . 'for instance?' This 'for instance?' was a favourite stereotype response of the patient. There was no point in directing him to indefinite matters; he could only be aware of something concrete; he could not answer general questions.

The conversation was about stealing: 'At any rate nobody stole from me' . . . The investigator recounted the theft of a watch from someone at the railway-station. When he says 'railway-station' the patient starts and interrupts. . . . 'Yes, railway-station, stolen at the station, that's right'. 'Something was stolen from me there . . . my big trunk.' Memory traces are not at his disposal, he always needs a stimulus-word. Unless a word fits like a latchkey, the past experience remains inaccessible. The patient does not know that he knows and he cannot dispose of what he has.

The patient depends on things cropping up within him spontaneously. He only manages with what occurs to him unwittingly; he cannot will things to appear and cannot spontaneously turn his attention to the contents of his own mind. Instead he has to be helped out by the spoken word and what accompanies it. The ego-impulse is supplanted by a word that rouses impulse and this replaces the acts of self-recall.

The patient's speech is therefore like an automatically released gramophone record. There is nothing there but mere words: memory images have given place to verbal memory.

Questions only rouse him to performance when he speaks them himself. The words then either start off an automatic progress to the target or bring the patient into some vivid concrete situation in which further things occur to him. Action becomes acting with the help of arbitrary words. However, not only words stimulate the patient, but also *perceptually concrete things*, e.g. a magnet put before him. He does not speak spontaneously; his speech consists only of replies to definite questions directly concerned with some object, or of responses to an object directly laid before him.

This patient knows of his disturbance. He is not just at its mercy and he *finds ways* of substitute performance. He recites Schiller's 'Glocke'; he is asked the meaning of it and whether he can imagine the content of the poem. He replies: 'But that's just it . . . I can't take part in my thinking . . . when I want to tell something, it just comes into my brain . . . it happens haphazardly . . . the words come just like that . . . but if one is asked the meaning . . . that is the difficulty.' The meaning? . . . 'No, it flows off; it's all right, one grasps it . . . then it is gone . . .' He tells us of his dependence on various 'props' . . . 'a word or a few words to help me hang on . . .'

We are struck by his intelligence in spite of this exceptional and primary disturbance; he is very clever in formulating and surprises us with the promptness and crispness of his phrases.

We record here only a fraction of the findings. The sum of them should lead us to the common factor. The basis of the disturbance is still obscure but the investigators had the compelling impression that it was something unitary. They *tried to formulate the basic disturbance*, using concepts which have unavoidably a more restricted meaning than they carry nowadays:

1. The patient *cannot 'visualise'*. Something is lacking which is equally necessary for recognition and for evoking previous perceptions in his imagination. It has as much to do with the structure of perception as with the recovery of memories. The patient with visual agnosia, it is true, appears to have the obvious disturbance in one sense-area only, but underlying this is some general factor. He was asked if he could imagine some music; he said 'No; with opera for instance, I am only in it again when the music has started.' If the patient is to live in it the situation must always be a concrete one.

2. The patient *cannot perform by apperceiving* a number of things *simultaneously*; he can only proceed by taking them in successively, in particular by talking himself into them. He fails when it is necessary to constellate a situation simultaneously as a structured whole, but he achieves fair, even good, results when all that is needed is to deal successively with the material. We may conclude from this that there is a basic function which appears when there are 'simultaneous configurations' (Simultangestalten); that is, the function of 'simultaneously beholding a totality of processes'.

The taking-in of a situation plays a predominant role in visual activity so any disturbance there becomes dramatically obvious. However, the unifying character of the structural organisation of sight is but one instance of *the unity of simultaneous structures in space*, or even in the spacelessness of our minds. Everywhere this unification is of the same character and it leads us to suppose it as the basic function which manifests itself in perception, imagination and thought. The concept of what is visual in this context should not be overstretched.

3. The patient can perform only *what he can represent to himself through his*

*own movements.* Hence the constant movement he makes when he is listening, comprehending, thinking and hence the talking which becomes his means of solving a task. There is a 're-organisation of the total performance'. He succeeds if the target can be reached by means of talking or moving about, but, when this is not possible, his failure is complete. What seems *objectively* the same performance is actually the performance of a radically different function, *the path* to the performance is different. In healthy people there are a number of paths to performance, with sick people these are limited. In this case, the only means at our patient's disposal was movement. His high level of intelligence is shown by his resourcefulness in finding substitute performances. At the same time one thinks one can descry a basic function which strikes our notice only when people are ill: *the close connectedness of all psychic life with motility,* with actual movement and with images of movement (Ribot, Kleist); we could compare here the central importance of movement in the cosmology of many philosophers (Aristotle, for example, or in more modern times the system of A. Trendelenburg).

4. The inability to visualise, the inability to hold simultaneous configurations, and the restriction to continuous movement are three formulations which all must converge on the same basic function. The general disturbance created, when this function is upset, is termed '*reduction to the concrete*'. Patients cannot inwardly comprehend what is possible, what is abstract or merely thought, nor can they use these generalisations in order to reach some performance-target. Hence they find a detour for the performance by making a connection with something concrete, actual objects, real situations, spoken words and formulae. They tend to avoid life-situations which they cannot meet adequately; they try to preserve an automatic conduct and in spite of profound defects they may get on reasonably well provided they are intelligent.

In the above-described cases (so-called agnosia) there has been a disturbance of a basic function; many other basic functions may of course be disturbed. The following are some examples of this:

1. In the *aphasic* patient the central disturbance is that of speech. In the above-described case of psychic blindness speech had proved to be the last effective aid towards performance.

2. There are possible defects at a vital level where the instinctual regulation of hunger, thirst, satisfaction and all the rest of the bodily rhythms is indispensably linked with the whole course of our consciousness. W. Scheid remarks in connection with his Korsakow case: 'such vital regulation obviously plays an important part in the time-orientation, by subdividing the day'.[1]

3. Disturbances in *conation* (see p. 485)[2] form another different group.

4. *Perseveration*[3] or 'getting stuck' is a phenomenon we observe in organic defect states, aphasias, dementias. This is perhaps a pointer to yet another basic function.

[1] Cp. Börger-Prinz and Kaila, *Z. Neur.*, vol. 24 (1930), p. 553.
[2] Cp. A. Hauptmann, 'Der Mangel an Antrieb', *Arch. Psychiatr.* (D), vol. 66 (1922).
[3] Heilbronner, *Mschr. Psychiatr.*, vol. 17, pp. 429 ff., vol. 18, pp. 293 ff. Brodmann, *J. Psychiatr.*, vol. 3, p. 25. Roenan, *Z. Neur.*, vol. 162, p. 51.

Constellations of ideas remain long after the normal span of appropriateness. This shows particularly in the set tasks, when there is inappropriate reaction. For instance, a word continues to stick and is given as answer repeatedly when quite out of context; or the word 'swan' may be a correct response to the picture shown but will then be said for all the others; or again, it can happen that after the first time a clock is never read again correctly but the patient gets lost in details though the actual ability to tell the time is unimpaired. Such *leit-motifs* will dominate all reactions for days on end. In many cases perseveration is a secondary phenomenon and when psychic life is defective it takes the place of the correct performance. Heilbronner found that perseveration increased as set tasks grew harder. In other cases we can understand the perseveration in terms of interest, emotional complexes etc. Yet in other cases it appears to be an *independent phenomenon*. Certain contents almost persecute the person and dominate him in such a way that it is difficult to dismiss the idea of spontaneous excitation (e.g. during fatigue).

5. The ruinous *disorder of thought* appearing in *Huntington's Chorea*[1] points to another basic function. With choreic patients, although the motor apparatus can function normally, it becomes impossible for them to hold on to what they intend, nor can they keep to their goal, conscious or unconscious. Just as their movements deviate, derail, and spontaneously occur so it is with their thought processes, which get side-tracked, derailed, interrupted by other thoughts and generally confused. 'It has simply vanished!'—'I think of something else, nothing at all to do with it'; 'I knew it was different, I have just messed it up' . . . 'I make so many slips of the tongue, I speak so much nonsense, don't I?—things that have nothing to do with it, is that not so?' . . . 'Now I've jumped again . . .' In brief, all performances requiring controlled motor-behaviour, e.g. body-movements, speech, thought, etc., are disturbed by involuntary impulses interfering with them. Impulses never reach their goal, they are always breaking off and renewing, but many break off for good. At the same time choreic patients in the beginning do not show any loss of intelligence level nor any inability to think—it is only at the end that dementia sets in. It is the steering that has failed; they do not find the things they look for, nor can they keep steadily to what they think and wish.

6. Zucker[2] applied the method of functional analysis to schizophrenics. He gave performance tests and linked these with the patients' self-descriptions. He investigated the modes of their imagination (by asking them to imagine things or stories; by comparing the two different experiences of having spontaneous hallucinations and of imagining somewhat similar contents; by observing the relationship between hallucinations and the deliberate reconstruction of them in the imagination, etc.). He found the imaginary creations were not very successful, became more difficult to produce, arrived more slowly, alternated between clarity and indistinctness and tended to break off and vanish. He thought one could detect here various degrees of disturbance of function, leading to the experience of thought-withdrawal, and from that to the breaking off of thoughts on the one hand and talking past the point and incoherence on the other.

[1] Hochheimer, 'Zur Psychologie des Choreatikers', *J. Psychiatr.*, vol. 47 (1936), p. 49. 'Kritsches zur medizinischen Psychologie dargestellt an Chorea', *Literatur. Fschr. Neur.*, vol. 8 (1936), p. 455.
[2] Konrad Zucker, 'Funktionsanalyse in der Schizophrenie', *Arch. Psychiatr.* (D), vol. 110 (1939), p. 465.

In all these investigations we find the presupposition of a threefold differentiation: 1. phenomena that can be experienced (Phenomenology); 2. certain well-defined performances (study of psychological performance); 3. basic functions. All these three categories are inter-related in such a way that the two first spring from the third, the basic function, which can be recognised as such only by means of the particular performances and experiences. Performance itself is clarified by the experience.

In the search for basic functions a tendency grows of simply not accepting mere concrete failures of performance as such; e.g. disturbance of registration is no longer just this but a disturbance in set or flexibility of set, which results in a disturbance of reproduction that looks like a defect in registration.[1] This method however becomes questionable once we begin to make explanations with the help of hypothetical basic functions. The analysis of performance then becomes a theoretical practice. We do not reach any clearer comprehension of grouped performances so that we apprehend the structure of our facts more clearly, but well-known facts are simply used to stimulate our interest in thinking out what may underlie them. The method loses all its fruitfulness if we merely stay satisfied with *a most general concept of basic function*, as, for instance, *gestalt-formation*. Disturbance of gestalt is always there, a concept general to all performance, as general as the concept of intelligence and valid thinking. Description of the gestalt-changes in the psychic structure is always a good method, but deductions from gestalt-formation as a basic function are meaningless, because far too general. The broad formulation of a disturbance in *the mental attitude that objectifies and predicates seems to be absolutely correct but unfruitful in its application. The investigator then only goes on saying the same thing once more.*

The search for basic functions must be distinguished from (1) the examination of *particular, concrete defects in performance and their consequences*, e.g. disturbances in registration. We should not stretch the general rule too far, that all disturbances of performance are disturbances of the whole. Precisely by contrast to this the search for specific disturbances and consequences remains alive. (2) Speculative analysis of *some vitally important basic event, glimpsed in its metaphysical setting* and seen as the source of understandable psychic experience and behaviour (v. Gebsattel, Straus, cp. pp. 453 ff). In the case of the basic functions under discussion, we observe the path followed by the performance and, combining analysis of performance with phenomenology, we investigate methodically until the basic function itself becomes self-evident in the separate phenomena.

We cannot doubt the importance of this approach for research. It is the only method which offers insight into the way performances are related to each other. It involves the use of phenomenology for the analysis of performance, an analysis of performance itself according to the path it takes, the proper fathoming of the re-organisation and the comprehension of defects in the context of intact performance or of what may be left of the total functioning. This stands out all the more strikingly in virtue of the defects themselves. The investigators concerned have extravagant

[1] Grünthal *Mschr. Psychiatr.*, vol. 35 (1923).

hopes and tend to look down on all that has gone before. It is a mistake, they think, to presuppose isolated performances and handle them like building-bricks. Defects are only crude findings; a host of failures may be noted but tell us nothing. Measurement of defects may be the beginning of some rough orientation but, if nothing more is done, there will be no understanding of the altered psychic structure of the individual. To ascertain the actual performance that has become difficult or impossible for the patient is only the first step. It is much more interesting to find out what the patient experiences as difficult. Only the analysis of experience by self-description will reveal the essential nature of defective performance. Progress in psychology is blocked by the use of such generalised terms as intelligence, attention, memory. Disturbances of intelligence (dementia), attention and memory as terms do not disclose the unique basic disturbance nor the basic mode of behaviour.

Now there is a good deal of exaggeration in all this. Investigation on these lines has not brought the findings one might reasonably expect, on which a *theory* could be constructed that would make 'crude' descriptions and attempts at classification superfluous. These interesting studies show a peculiar lack. In spite of much subtlety and skill investigation has on the whole got lost in the sand. Much has been seen in passing, but no really conclusive result has been achieved. A genuine beginning has been made, a method established and the techniques of enquiry once gained can never be lost. But so far the investigatory work has got a certain pointlessness and there is a lack of any clear, concentrated effort to end this. In research of this type decisiveness is in abeyance and vacillation is taken as satisfactory in the guise of caution, but it may just as well reflect the many possible interpretations of the individual results.

Furthermore, for the time being the whole approach is limited to defective performance in cases of organic brain lesions. Here it has been of great significance in helping us to see that circumscribed brain lesions rarely lead to equally circumscribed psychic failures; at most a number of performances are more or less affected. We cannot yet see clearly to what extent we may find basic psychological functions, over and above the organic functions disclosed by the cerebral disorders so far defined.

### (b) *Work-performance*

Performance turns into 'work' when it is carried out as a steady effort for a practical purpose, absorbs the person as a whole, depends on his getting tired and refreshed, and is generally subject to quantitative measurement. The *psychophysical organism* with all its powers engages in a great complexity of work-performance and thereby manifests certain of its *basic qualities*.

Work-performance may be objectively observed, quantitatively assessed and the effect of varying conditions noted. In this way we are beginning to uncover the factors responsible for the essentially mechanical element in work-performance.[1]

[1] The experimental basis was laid by the work of Kraepelin and his school. Kraepelin, 'Die Arbeitskurve', in Wundt's *Philosophische Studien*, vol. 19 (1902), p. 459. A critical exposition as to the importance of the findings for assessment of work-performance in life-situations. Max

The kind of work asked for in experimental investigation is nearly always the addition of single digits. We seem to know very little about the differences due to differences in occupation, e.g. work that is predominantly mental in contrast to work that is predominantly physical.

In our analysis of work-performance we should differentiate clearly between *subjective* phenomena, such as feelings of weariness and pleasure in the work, from *objective* phenomena, such as fatigue and suitability for the work. Objective work-performance is well illustrated by the *work-curve*, in which the abscissa show the time and the ordinates the quantity of the work unit. From this we can observe certain components such as the *fatigue-curve*, which at first goes down and then, after intervals of recreation, mounts again quickly; we can also read another important curve, the *practice-curve*, which at first rises quickly, later more slowly and then, after intervals, falls off.[1] In addition there is the *incentive-curve*, which shows a rise at the beginning which can be interpreted as the initial effort of will; we also find peaks at the end as well as at the beginning of the performance. Then there is the habituation-curve which shows reaction to distracting stimuli. At first it rises steeply but then flattens out and remains fairly level.[2] Fatigue and practice seem the most important components.

*Fatigue*[3] is contrasted with recuperation, and these are aspects of the psychophysical apparatus of fatiguability and recuperability. In the latter case the period for recovery is of very varying duration. It will depend on whether we are dealing with simple fatigue, explained by the effect of certain toxins, or with exhaustion, explained by the using up of substance. We also distinguish between muscle-fatigue and nerve-fatigue. It is an open question whether there is such a thing as general fatigue or only partial fatigue for certain work-performances. Kraepelin believes there is only general fatigue.

*Practice*[4] is the increase in ease, speed and evenness of performance by repetition. This is achieved partly through a *mechanisation* of psychic performances which at first are more deliberate but gradually become more reflex-like and mechanical. This means that we must assume there are changes in the physiological mechanism that effect practice. Capacity to become practised in this way and to make use of such practice varies with different people. Kraepelin therefore differentiated between what he called practice-ability and trainability. Whereas fatigue is a fleeting and transitory phenomenon, training-practice always leaves lasting residual effects.

The dispositions which have been enumerated as fatiguability, recuperability, practice-ability, trainability, distractibility, habituation and responsive-

Weber, 'Zur psychophysik der industriellen Arbeit', *Arch. Sozialw. u. Sozialpol.*, vols. 27–9. Kraepelin reports on further trials in 'Arbeitspsychologische Untersuchungen', *Z. Neur.*, vol. 70 (1921), p. 230.

[1] O. Graf, 'Die Arbeitspause in Theorie u. Praxis', *Psychol. Arb.*, vol. 9 (1928), p. 460.

[2] Kraepelin, 'Die Arbeitskurve', in Wundt's *Philosophische Studien*, vol. 19 (1902).

[3] M. Offner, *Die geistige Ermüdung* (Berlin, 1928), 2nd edn.

[4] B. Kern, *Wirkungsformen der Übung* (Münster, 1930).

ness to stimuli, are all to be conceived as *basic qualities of the psychophysical mechanism* (Kraepelin says of the personality).

Under *morbid* conditions all these qualities may suffer change. Kraepelin has examined their dependency on food-intake, sleep, intoxication (alcohol, coffee). With cerebral lesions we find an enormous slowing-down of the work-performance along with great fatiguability.[1] One finds other cases in which there is very little ability for performance, or practice-ability, and little fatigu-ability because there is virtually no effort; in this case the insufficiency is psychologically conditioned. With the neuroses (particularly after accidents) analyses of the work-curve have been made by Specht and Plaut.[2] It is possible to differentiate between the quick fatiguability of neurotic patients, the lack of determination in hysterics and the intentional poverty of performance shown by determined simulators. Usually with neurotics we have to confine our-selves to *subjective analyses*. The two main components are, on the one hand, adverse sensations and unpleasant feelings during effort, which tend to in-crease with the difficulty of the task, and on the other the feeling of 'not wanting', of weakness and of not being able to go further. Weakness of will depends on the unwitting acceptance that compensation will be lost if there is return to work. The excitement of the compensation proceedings tends to increase complaints and in particular the weakness of will (Compensation neuroses). It is not so uncommon to find that the examination shows decreased performance as the only objective symptom these patients have.

Concrete examination of work-performance together with certain currently held beliefs has led to a certain emphasis being put on the 'basic qualities of personality'. In this connection it must be pointed out that in fact only mechanical, automatic, learnable 'performances' are in question here, tasks that everyone can do and which can be quantitatively assessed, in short just those tasks that are commonly found rather a burden. The work-curve cannot be applied to qualitative performances, nor to productive activity, nor in particular to art, science and the general conduct of life. We shall value its contribution, however, as an objective demonstration of the way in which our nervous apparatus functions, that apparatus on which our life as a whole rests.

### (c) Individual variations in performance

When Kraepelin in his analyses of the work-curve spoke of 'basic qualities of the personality' as shown in the various degrees of fatiguability, recuper-ability, trainability etc., he laid the foundations for a system which was capable of considerable elaboration. *All performances* which can be demonstrated ex-perimentally reveal *individual differences*. These can in part be measured, and

[1] Busch, *Z. Neur.*, vol. 41, p. 283. 'Work with head injuries', Langelüddeke; *Z. Neur.*, vol. 58, p. 216. Ergograph tests, Bappert, 'Zur Frage der körperlichen Leistungsfähigkeit bei Hirnverletz-ten', *Z. Neur.*, vol. 73, p. 239.

[2] Specht, *Arch. Psychol.* (D), vol. 3 (1904), p. 245. Plaut, *Münch. med. Wschr.* (1906), p. 1274, *Neur. Zbl.* (1906), p. 481.

in part we can arrange them in typical polarities or opposites, or they may show a multipolarity.

For instance, 'types of imagery' have been differentiated: there may be individual preference for the visual, acoustic or kinaesthetic sense in imagery and memory; an individual may be an eidetic and an eidetic of a particular type. Similarly we find different types of memory, speech, thinking, perceiving and moving; different speeds, different rhythms, etc.

We are dealing with very heterogeneous matters. The one thing in common is that they all emerge from objective performance tests. Differences are looked for with the intention of finding certain basic psychological qualities due to what have been called constitutional variations in human beings. This does not give us the individual whom we understand, the aspect of personality which we call character, but the biological individual who is revealed in his performance.

One much discussed problem is that of right- and left-handedness. Right and left is a fundamental orientation in space for our bodies. It is a morphological feature of the body itself. There seems a very specific problem involved in whether a person prefers right or left in his movements. In any case left-handedness is regarded as a constitutional characteristic which is not appreciated as a physical sign but only becomes objective during performance. Attempts have been made to understand this in terms of personality development and structure, while others consider it only a chance finding.

*The facts*[1] appear to be as follows: Left-handed people are almost always in the minority. Incidence is stated to be 4 per cent in Russia, 13 per cent in Alsace-Lorraine, in Stuttgart 10 per cent of boys, 6.6 per cent of girls. 25 per cent of the stone-age tools discovered are said to have been made by left-handed people; the inhabitants of Celebes are said to be left-handed as a majority. Argument rages as to whether left- or right-handedness is an advantage or of no importance. Leonardo da Vinci and Menzel were both left-handed. Left-handedness shows strong hereditary trends and appears correlated to speech disorders. 61 per cent of boys and 81 per cent of girls with severe speech disorders were found to be left-handed (Schiller). 'The dominance of one cerebral hemisphere is necessary for the development of the higher centres, especially the speech centre', so that the effort to train both hands to equal skill is not a desirable one.

## § 2. THE ACTUAL FLOW OF PSYCHIC LIFE

The total present state can be considered from a number of standpoints: as an alteration or clouding of consciousness (pp. 137 ff.), as fatigue and exhaustion (pp. 465 ff., 206) or as the particular world in which the respective

[1] Maria Schiller, 'Probleme um die Linkshändigkeit', *Z. Neur.*, vol. 140 (1932), p. 496. H. Bürger, *Nervenarzt*, vol. 2, p. 464, on the whole problem of 'right and left'; a research report.

life goes on (pp. 280 ff). Each mode is linked as a whole with the others but our knowledge can only grow by making distinctions. Alterations in the present state (of consciousness and of the biological whole) and in the person's relevant world (of intelligible, meaningful wholes) must be kept distinct from alterations in the psychic flow itself, which is to be discussed in what follows, and which manifests itself particularly in the way in which thinking is connected or disconnected. We are forced, however, to analyse it as a defect in, or reversal of, certain normal performances taken as a whole. The changes involved have some very old designations: e.g. flight of ideas, retardation, disorganised thought. In diagnosis a distinction is made between the manic-depressive changes (flight of ideas, retardation) and the schizophrenic ones (disorganisation of thought). Yet the flight of ideas can grow into disorganisation and schizophrenic states can show a classic flight of ideas.

## (a) Flight of ideas and retardation

Below we give an illustration of what is meant by flight of ideas[1] and retardation. The examples are highly heterogeneous:

A patient produced the following in 'conversation' with his doctor in which *objectively* a flight of ideas was present: She was asked whether she had changed at all in the last year. She said 'Yes, I was dumb and numb then but not deaf, I know Mrs. Ida Teff, she is dead, probably an appendicitis; I don't know whether she lost her sight, sightless Hesse, His Highness of Hesse, sister Louisa, His Highness of Baden, buried and dead on September the twenty-eighth 1907, when I get back, red-gold-red . . .' With such patients the trend of thought is haphazardly interrupted. They start doing this and that and keep losing their target, but they are always busy about something and have a great number of notions. They cannot stick to the point and constantly lose themselves in side issues. They will then lose the thread and cannot recover it. They never finish what they begin, they jump from one thing to another, are breathless and led on by superficial connections. In contrast, the patient with *retardation* behaves in the opposite way in almost every respect. He shows no initiative, never begins anything, finds it hard to utter even one word, ponders over a question but nothing occurs to him.

What the patient *subjectively* experiences can sometimes be elicited by self-description: Patients, particularly in schizophrenia, will describe one mode of flight of ideas as a *crowding of thought*: Mrs. S. complained 'I can't hold on . . . it all dances round and round inside . . . I can't group anything together . . . I have no will . . . oh dear, what a lot of nonsense it all is . . .' A patient of Forel said . . . 'A whole uninterrupted string of ideas ran through my head . . . like clockwork . . . idea chased idea with the oddest associations . . . yet some kind of connection seemed there from link to link of the whole chain . . . what ideas have not tumbled about in my head . . . and what funny associations cropped up.' 'I kept on coming back

[1] Heilbronner, *Mschr. Psychiatr.*, vol. 13, pp. 272 ff.; vol. 17, pp. 436 ff. Liepmann, *Über Ideenflucht* (Halle, 1904). Aschaffenburg, *Psychol. Arb.*, vol. 4 (1904). Külpe, *Psychologie u. Medizin*, pp. 22 ff. L. Binswanger, *Über Ideenflucht* (Zürich, 1933). By flight of ideas, we mean here the disturbance in the actual flow of the total psychic life, not the mere verbal production of someone who actually need not be caught up in a 'flight of ideas'.

to certain ideas and images . . . droit de France . . . tannin . . . Barbara . . . Rohan
. . . they were like milestones in the headlong chase of thoughts . . . I said them
quickly, like a password as it were . . . the particular one which they had reached
at certain points in my daily life, on entering the hall, at the opening of the side-
room door, at mealtimes, when someone approached me and so on . . . I did it so
as not to lose the trend and get a certain hold on the mad thought-sequences which
were overwhelming me.'—A schizophrenic reported: 'my thoughts increased in
speed, I could no longer grasp individual ideas, I thought I would snap at any
moment; I only felt the movement of my thoughts, I could not see their content
any longer . . . in the end I was not even aware of the thoughts . . . I was empty . . .'

A 30-year-old patient with a post-encephalitic state described the inner change
in his thoughts with comparable phenomena. 'I cannot sit still for five minutes
without thinking of something; thoughts go faster than I can speak; I know the
answers before I say them . . . it is as if a film was reeling off in my mind . . . it
all goes like lightning and I seem to get hold of every detail . . . when I don't
answer at once and you think I have not understood, everything is repeating itself
. . . I can't answer at once . . . all day it is like this, when I think, it occurs again
and again and again' (Dorer).

The following self-descriptions show milder degrees of *retardation*: 'my mood
was constantly changing . . . my good days were characterised by interest, carrying
out what I wanted to do, personal stimulation, proper judgment of things and people
and of myself, and with a certain tension; I looked for company and took pleasure
in everything. The change of mood was not so sudden but progressed a little every
day. On the other bad days, I *lost interest, felt stupid*, indecisive about things and what
should be my attitude. I tried hard to hide these defects, and sometimes I could
manage to evidence something of what I was like on my good days. My handwriting and manner of walking changed. Latterly there was also a *complete indifference*, and a failure to take in anything. Theatres, concerts, made no impression on
me; I couldn't talk about them any more; I lost the trend in conversation and I
could not link one idea to what had gone before; I was insensitive to jokes and
points made in conversation; I didn't catch them.' (In the following year this patient
showed paranoid deterioration.) Other patients complain, 'I have lost my memory
and cannot follow a conversation . . .' 'I feel paralysed . . . I have no mind any
more . . . I am completely stupid . . . I can't recall what I have read or heard . . .
my will has gone . . . I haven't a trace of energy or drive . . . I can't make up my
mind to do anything . . . it takes all I have just to move, etc.'

1. *Interpretation of flight of ideas and retardation.* We might say these
phenomena are all characterised by the opposites of *accelerated or decreased
tempo*. But this does not take us to the central point of the disturbance. The
acceleration of an otherwise normal process would be a sign of health while
slowing up in what is an otherwise undisturbed psychic process appears in
epileptic personalities for example without any similarity to the phenomena of
retardation which have been described. Perhaps the opposites of *excitement* and
*inhibition* come closer to the point, but even though these can describe one
aspect of the total process they are still indefinite. If we really want to get at
the structure here it is best to make use of the contrast between *mechanical,*

*associative, passive flow of ideas* and *active, purposeful thought-processes* (governing ideas, determining tendencies). Associative processes bring in material, active processes order the thought. We see at once: on one side there is inhibition or excitation, a wealth or poverty of *associative* events, and on the other a retreat of active goal-formation along with its *determining tendencies.* When determining tendencies are diminished (because no goal-awareness exists, and therefore exercises no influence and in addition changes too fast) the flow of ideas is only guided by the constellations of the associative elements. Consciousness is fed by external sensory stimuli as well as images evoked by accidental constellations following all kinds of different associative principles. This gives us the objective picture of flight of ideas. The word 'idea' in 'flight of ideas' does not only refer to 'images' but to everything that can be called an 'element' in the general chaos of association. In the same way the goal-forming ideas are not just ideas but all those factors which bring about a selection and structuring of psychic content; the logical (perceived) necessities of the situation (speech, conversation, communication, task). Making use of this schema we can derive any number of subjective and objective types of retardation[1] and flights of ideas.

2. *Types of disturbed psychic flow.* (*aa*) *Classical flight of ideas.* Associative processes are excited; there is a massive flow of content into consciousness. In itself this might only imply increased mental productivity, but there is a crippling of determining tendency and gradually this disappears altogether; there is no longer any constant selection among the associations and they all get mixed up through chance conditioning, association of ideas, verbal associations, clang-associations etc.

So far there is no satisfactory or complete explanation of flight of ideas. It is not the result of some acceleration in the flow of our ideas; nor is it the result of pressure of speech. We cannot make it intelligible as a mere quick exchange of associations (e.g. clang-associations) nor as the predominance of inferior modes of association (loss of conceptual modes). The source of the phenomenon seems to lie in unknown extra-conscious processes; the performance has to be viewed as a whole, taking both sides of the thought-process into account, that is, the processes of association and the determining tendencies.

(*bb*) *Classical retardation.* This is the exact opposite to flight of ideas so far as associative processes are concerned. Autonomy over psychic content is limited. The content is not destroyed however as in dementia. No associations appear; nothing enters consciousness. There is a tendency towards a complete blank. Should a few sparse associations appear, the determining

---

[1] I have given the rendering of the traditional theory, although it has been sharply criticised and dismissed (by Hönigswald, L. Binswanger). Even in flight of ideas, every idea, every element, contains an act of thought. These are not just automatic happenings; there is still an 'I' 'thinking'. Correct as this may be, it is no objection to closer analysis. The older theory is a valuable description, not a theory as to what is happening, which in any case still remains obscure. The experience itself lies in this opposition of thought and the material on which it works, and we do wrong to dismiss the whole thing.

tendency, as with flight of ideas, is extremely weak. Patients cannot concentrate. At times a reaction may be staged after long-drawn-out effort, but often the patients are completely mute, and linger for a long time in deep stupor.

(*cc*) *Conjunction of flight of ideas with retardation.* It seems that these two phenomena can appear together. Flight of ideas may be rich or poor in content, speech may be profuse (pressure of speech) or extremely scanty (mute).

Where patients are aware of this disturbance in their psychic process flight of ideas is described by them as a pressure of thoughts, and the retardation as a subjective inhibition. Seen as a whole it appears as thought retarded with flight of ideas.[1] The patients complain that they cannot cope with the mass of thoughts, the painful chase of images which storm through their mind; or they may complain that they can no longer think, not another thought comes. Should the patients also be aware of a loss in determining tendency, they will still try hard to bring some order into their thoughts and experience the complete ineffectiveness of their attempts to form controlling ideas. They experience a simultaneous excitement, pressure of thought, brought about by increased associations, and retardation through their incapacity to keep hold of a single, coherent thought in the middle of this hectic chase.

(*dd*) *Distractibility.*[2] Where determining tendencies have failed or are insufficient, flight of ideas comes about, provided the thought-process consists mainly of an increased production of associations. Where, however, the process is haphazardly conditioned by *external impressions* we use the term *distractibility*. The patient will immediately notice and name and include in his talk, for instance, a number of objects, something one holds in one's hands, a watch, a key, a pencil, or something one does—one knocks, plays with the watch, jingles keys. But the next minute, he is off on something else, a spot on the wall, the doctor's tie, anything noticeable in his environment. It is obvious that flight of ideas and distractibility will commonly occur in conjunction, but they do not always do so. A patient may be entirely unproductive in association, but every external stimulus may catch his attention, and reversely with other patients whose whole process of ideas seems to consist solely of associations linked in a typical flight of associations that cannot be interrupted by any external stimuli.

Distraction does not occur with every stimulus. One can often notice a certain selection of areas of *interest*, or of a certain *coherence*. This partially understandable kind of disturbance passes over by transitions into the opposite extreme, distractibility by *any stimulus whatsoever*. Every object is named indiscriminately, every word repeated, every movement imitated. In cases of pure distractibility, should some understandable element appear, it seems to us an 'echo-symptom', a purely automatic event. In the former case, the stimulus picked up by the distracted attention is still being elaborated by the patient in a way that seems abnormal, but in the latter case all that appears left is an unchanging, automatic reaction. It would be better

---

[1] Schröder, *Z. Neur.*, vol. 2.
[2] Heilbronner, *Mschr. Psychiatr.*, vol. 13, pp. 277 ff., vol. 17, pp. 431 ff.

then not to talk of distractibility but to keep this term for those cases where we get the impression that the patient is conscious of some change in the direction of his attention, he observes and is then again distracted, in a way for which we can have empathy.

## (b) Confusion

Schizophrenic patients complain of fatigue, a loss of concentration, of a falling-off in their intellectual performance, poor memory. The meaning of these manifold complaints grows better 'defined when the observer can find objective disorganisation and actual disturbances of the thinking process. Beringer[1] selected a number of cases whose thought was not so disorganised as to make self-description impossible. He noted that the subjective reports (unlike many of the complaints of manic-depressive patients in regard to their retardation) were well correlated with the objective findings:

The patients complained: thoughts are so fleeting, as if cut off, connections are lost, thoughts are so rushed. It becomes worse when patients are left to themselves and better when they have something to do or are engaged in conversation. A patient said: 'I forget my thoughts so quickly; if I want to write something down, it has gone . . . the thoughts fall over each other . . . they are no longer clear . . . they go off like lightning . . . and another comes though I had not thought of it a moment before . . . I feel absolutely muddled . . . I can't control my thoughts . . . they are confused . . . they glance by, though I know they were there . . . there are always side thoughts beside the main thought . . . they confuse me and so one never gets anywhere . . . it gets worse . . . it's all criss-cross . . . everything mixed up and meaningless . . . even I have to laugh but I can't . . . I feel robbed of thought . . . everything I see and think seems to have lost its colour, it seems shallow, dull . . .' 'The university has shrunk to my cupboard . . .'

Much of this painful criss-cross experience is the lot of the patient who is passive; where he is active, he experiences the difficulties of his thought-processes and their extreme poverty.

When we try *tests of performance*, the patient may co-operate and try to do them, but we find a reduced power of registration, a marked deterioration in comprehending the logical structure of a story, the failure to recognise the nonsensical as such and greater difficulty in completing gaps in sentences, etc. The patient who gave the above clear description could not write a simple request to someone he knew: he had to write 14 pages, started afresh several times, but never achieved his end.

Carl Schneider[2] gives a very subtle description of such disordered schizophrenic thinking; there is 'Verschmelzung'—smelting or fusing, the bringing together of heterogeneous elements, 'Faseln'—mixing, muddling up actual definite but heterogeneous elements, 'Entgleiten'—snapping off, the unintentional breaking of the chain of thought, 'Entgleisen'—derailment, the interpolation of thought-contents in place of the true chain of thought, etc.

---

[1] Beringer, 'Beitrag zur Analyse schizophrener Denkstörungen', *Z. Neur.*, vol. 93 (1924).
[2] Carl Schneider, *Psychologie der Schizophrenie* (Leipzig, 1930).

In an effort to try and visualise this type of thinking—or rather this kind of psychic flow as a whole—comparisons have been made with the kind of thinking that occurs during fatigue or while falling asleep (Carl Schneider), or with archaic thinking of primtiive people (Storch). But there can be no more than comparison. During fatigue or falling asleep, the primary change is the change in consciousness; in archaic thinking we see a stage in the historical development of the human mind (as a product of culture not as biological inheritance). In schizophrenic thinking however a primary disturbance of a peculiar type is taking place in the psychic flow and this is our one empirical fact.

## § 3. INTELLIGENCE

Intelligence is the term given to the individual's totality of abilities, those instruments of performance and purpose available to him for adaptation to life.

### (a) *Analysis of intelligence*

We have to differentiate the preconditions for intelligence, the inventory of actual knowledge and intelligence proper. As *preconditions of intelligence* we may assume registration and memory, degree of fatiguability, mechanisms of motor phenomena, mechanisms of the speech apparatus etc. There often is a confusion between these preconditions and intelligence proper. The individual who has no memory, cannot speak, or tires very quickly, naturally cannot display his intelligence. But the cause then lies in the disturbance of some circumscribed function, as a result of which there is a disturbance in the manifestation of the intelligence, not in the intelligence itself. If we want to analyse anomalies of intelligence and differentiate them, it becomes very important to chisel out from the whole concept of intelligence those limited and basic psychophysiological functions which we have earlier on discussed. Liepmann speaks with pride of the advances made by 'separating out aphasia and apraxia from the undifferentiated morass of dementia'. In the past, aphasia had often been mistaken for dementia.

In the next place, we must not confuse *all that we have in our mind, our knowledge*, with intelligence. It is true that where there is great knowledge, we can conclude the existence of certain abilities which must be there to acquire what is not solely a reproduction of memory. But even then, we still find a far-reaching independence between mere learning ability and intelligence proper (the capacity for judgment). It is possible to learn a whole host of complicated matters, so that learning ability is again often confused with intelligence. In psychopathology, comparison between the actual store of knowledge and what is still left of ability sometimes provides us with a criterion for assessing acquired defect as opposed to congenital mental deficiency. In the latter case, the amount of knowledge and the ability are more appropriately related to each other. Very slight knowledge is usually a sign of mental deficiency, and vice versa. We can therefore in extreme cases indirectly base our judgment of mental deficiency on a test of knowledge. Such a test is of more value to us, however, in determining those contents which provide the individual's working material. Actions, attitudes, behaviour are intelligible only if we know the extent of this material, the picture of the world which the mind has built; only so can we converse. The smaller the mental estate, the more we can observe that words mean one thing for the speaker and another for us. The words he uses go in their objective meaning beyond what he wants to say. They may deceptively suggest that he has more knowledge than is the fact. The size of one's mental estate depends not only on learning ability and interest but on the milieu from which we derive and in which we live. If we know the average level of knowledge within the different social classes, this is of considerable help when we come to assess the individual. Usually one overestimates the average extent of knowledge.[1] Rodenwaldt found in a majority of soldiers a complete lack of social orientation, ignorance of their political rights, even of the law of the land. They did not even know the country a few miles away from their village. There was scarcely a trace of any knowledge of history. More than half of them did not know who Bismarck was. Usually in any test of knowledge one must take the *schooling* into account, as well as the *general life experience*. This latter (in the form of knowledge acquired from spontaneous interest or in the course of work) gives us a much better criterion for intelligence. Recent investigations, however, rather surprisingly show that the majority of people have only a most superficial acquaintance with their own occupations.

Finally we come to *the intelligence itself*. It is a difficult matter to comprehend. It is almost impossible to calculate the many different criteria we use to assess someone as intelligent. Obviously there are a great many different abilities which can perhaps be isolated out precisely, and it seems probable that there is not just a series of greater or lesser degrees of intelligence but a ramifying tree of many different abilities. We may doubt whether there is a general intelligence, a general capacity to perform, a 'central factor of intelligence' which must disclose itself in every respect. But there is always a strong inclination to assume that such a factor exists. It is this which the older psychology called the power of judgment.

However that may be, the phenomena of intelligence are immensely varied. We find lively people with a *quick grasp* but who mislead through their very flexibility, yet are taken for exceptionally intelligent people. On test they appear as only average and superficial. Then we find a level of *practical intelligence* where there is quick and correct choice of many possibilities and an apt adaptation to new demands. Then there is an *abstract intelligence* which in

[1] Rodenwaldt, 'Aufnahmen des geistigen Inventars Gesunder als Massstab für Defektprüfungen bei Kranken', *Mschr. Psychiatr.*, vol. 17 (1905). J. Lange, 'Über Intelligenzprüfungen an Normalen', *Psychol. Arb.*, vol. 7 (1922).

moments of decision becomes almost feebleminded but can achieve great mental feats when working quietly on its own. 'Doctors, judges, politicians may know theoretically many beautiful principles of pathology, law and statesmanship and can teach them, but in the application of them they may show themselves utterly futile. There may be a natural lack of judgment; they can see generalities in abstract but cannot decide whether the concrete case fits; or they have never been sufficiently trained by example and actual work to make judgments of this sort' (Kant).

Clinically we have not got much beyond a few very general aspects of intelligence. We lay much emphasis on the *capacity to judge*, on *the ability to think*, on *a flair for the essential*, on the ability to grasp viewpoints and ideas. In a difficult test the person who says he does not know something or cannot do it seems more intelligent than someone who goes off into irrelevant detail or tries to talk himself out of it. As well as the capacity for judgment there is *spontaneity* and *initiative*, which also count. In response to requests someone may well show intelligence in being able to judge, but when left to himself, he may sit around, an apathetic and very dull individual.

### (b) Types of dementia

The concept of intelligence, viewed as the whole of a man's mental endowment, means that an analysis will only elicit particular features which in themselves never quite meet the intended concept. We therefore have a much better idea of the characteristics of particular types of intelligence than of intelligence as such. We shall now try to describe some types of disturbed intelligence, as follows:

1. *Fluctuation in output.* Intelligence means for us in general a lasting disposition, and dementia a lasting defect. If we cannot get an intelligent performance from people in acute psychoses, confusional states, stupor, flight of ideas, retardation, we do not say there is any disturbance of their intelligence. This can only be stated if intelligent performances cannot be elicited in settled, orderly, accessible states, that is in the absence of acute disturbance. When this is present we do not even hazard a judgment on the patient's intelligence, what it was before and what it will be in the future. However, it is not always easy to make this distinction between the transitory and lasting disturbance in every case. Disturbances such as diminution in mental output in intellectuals, artists, scientists, or the transient, more lasting or permanent disturbances that occur in psychasthenic persons, are by no means easily classified. Passing phases when patients feel their inadequacy strongly are quite common. Memory they feel has gone; they cannot think any more. These feelings of inadequacy are justified in fact; the patients are really unable to concentrate, they read mechanically without getting the meaning, they have to think all the time how to set about things, and constantly watch themselves instead of what they are doing. Thus they really lose sight of their work as a whole; they have no spontaneous ideas and without these work comes to a halt. Such

people have suffered a loss in productivity which may be transient or lasting. Inversely may come phases of exceptional productivity, of the richest creativeness. In all such cases we are dealing not with changes in the intelligence as a whole but with changes in productivity. Phases such as these are usually to be found in depressive and hypomanic states.

2. *Congenital subnormality.* There is a steadily descending range of capacity, running from the limited productivity of a concrete, reproductive intelligence, to the lowest grade of mental subnormality. Slight degrees of this are termed feeblemindedness, moderate degrees imbecility and severe degrees idiocy. Here we are dealing with a psychic life that suffers impoverishment in all directions, with a low degree of differentiation. We can conceive it as a variation of human constitution in the direction of below average. As we get lower down, psychic life approximates more to that of animals; although the necessary instincts are well developed, experience does not move beyond the individual sensory experience and nothing fresh can be learned. No concepts are formed and planned, conscious behaviour is impossible. As they have no general viewpoints, such individuals are quite unable to form ideas, or advance ideals. Their life is spent within the narrow horizons of accidental, daily impressions. Yet at the lowest as at the highest level of human differentiation, we can see mental endowment is not unitary but consists of many unevenly developed abilities. We often see imbeciles who show special aptitudes, or even mental abilities such as arithmetical skill or a one-sided appreciation and memory for music.[1] At present we cannot distinguish psychologically the congenital mental defect due to organic lesions,[2] from those forms of congenital mental defect appearing as an abnormal constitutional variation.

3. *'Relative mental defect'.* In theory we can separate the congenital fashioning of the intelligence from that of personality but in actuality we cannot always do so. There are odd individuals with an apparently high performance-ability, coupled with an astonishing incapacity; Bleuler called this situation 'relative mental defect' (Verhaltnisblödsinn)[3] because the individual's endowment is in no recognisable relationship to the level of aspiration and there is consequent inevitable failure. There is a disturbed relationship between the intelligence and the aspirations. The disproportionate drive poses tasks for the intelligence and brings the person into situations with which he cannot cope. Such people are often equipped with an excellent mechanical and verbal memory, and appear to superficial observation as versatile thinkers, but on closer view they are 'masters of confusion'. They are incapable of 'finding useful directives from experience whereby to manage their affairs'; they suffer from an incorrigible self-overestimation, and a total absence of self-criticism. In conversation a fine flow of uprushing associations is let loose in a kind of 'drawing-room

[1] Witzel, 'Ein Fall von phänomenalem Rechentalent bei einer Imbezillen', *Arch. Psychol.*, vol. 38.

[2] Sollier, *Der Idiot und der Imbezille* (Deutsch, 1891).

[3] Bleuler, *Allg. Z. Psychiatr.*, vol. 71 (1914), p. 537. L. Buchner, *Allg. Z. Psychiatr.*, vol. 71.

idiocy' (Salonblödsinn), in an urge to be somebody and impress others. There is an impression of a flight of ideas but this is not so really. It is an understandable self-expansion coupled with an immense number of ideas, but they are controlled only by language facility and powers of mechanical memory. Ideas are not developed, only a chaotic knowledge displayed. Shallow, verbal witticisms take the place of responsible evaluations and attitudes; 'speak, rather than think' is the guiding motto. There is an intoxication with one's own wit, instead of any directed thinking, but the wit is only a reproduction of what has been read. Such people can deceive through their 'belief, reminiscent of pseudologia phantastica, that all they say is their own'. The chosen content is usually the most high-sounding problem.

4. *Organic Dementia.* We have to differentiate acquired, organic dementia in all its many forms from congenital feeblemindedness and schizophrenic defect. The organic process usually destroys in a far-reaching manner the *preconditions of intelligence,* such as memory, powers of registration, sometimes the apparatus of speech, so that, for instance in senile dementia, we get clinical pictures where a person forgets his whole life, cannot speak properly any longer and can only make himself understood with difficulty. But from his behaviour and general conduct we can still see evidences of an educated man; he has retained his sense for the essential and under certain circumstances some power of judgment.

In other cases of arteriosclerosis, paralysis and gross degrees of epileptic dementia, the process in the brain leads to progressive deterioration of the whole intelligence. Finally the patient loses all power of judgment, any inclination to go for essentials, less indeed than a congenital mental defective. At the same time patients, as they talk, will bandy about fragments of previously acquired experience, so that a different picture arises from congenital mental deficiency, and one gets the picture immediately of an organic disorder. Apperceptive power is seriously reduced. They are guided by accidental impressions and have no effective counter-ideas; they lack all initiative and find themselves at last in the severest states of mental devastation where they can only vegetate physically.

All organic dementias of severe degree show characteristically a lack of insight. Only when the organic process is essentially restricted to the preconditions of intelligence (memory, etc.) does any sharp awareness of illness exist (e.g. in arteriosclerosis). In senile and arteriosclerotic dementia there is at the beginning, in contrast to paralytic dementia, an acute feeling by the patient of his own regression.[1]

5. *Schizophrenic 'dementia' (deterioration).* If with the organic dementias we find it difficult to separate personality from the intelligence, the schizophrenic deterioration or dulling of the kind from which the majority of chronic mental

---

[1] Eliasberg and Feuchtwanger give a psychological analysis of a progressive dementia after brain-injury. *Z. Neur.,* vol. 75 (1922), p. 516. Patient's total attitude and the disintegration and impoverishment of the situation is shown.

hospital patients suffer presents us with an even greater problem. Perhaps the intelligence remains quite intact in these cases and the changes are due to alterations in personality alone. It would be of fundamental importance for our understanding of these illnesses if it were possible to separate this latter type of case—which forms the majority—from those cases where a true disturbance of the intelligence could be demonstrated. In fact we do not find a disturbance of memory and the other preconditions of intelligence, there is no loss of knowledge, but there is a deterioration in thinking and behaviour which has been described as silly, hebephrenic. We also find a lack of grasp on the essentials, at least for what can be said to be essential in the social, objective and empiricially real world. We have characterised schizophrenics by their lack of contact with reality and have contrasted them with paralytics, who in spite of severe destruction manage to maintain contact with their reality, in spite of disorientation too and reduction in awareness (Minkowski). The complete heterogeneity of the organic and schizophrenic 'dementias' is confirmed, the one in all its ruin, still a natural ruin, the other a crazy distortion. With the schizophrenias there is also in many cases a loss of spontaneity, a twilight living, which can be interrupted only by strong stimulation, to which very surprisingly they may respond. Instead of giving a general description we will quote a mild case of this deterioration, to bring out the peculiarities of this kind of loss of judgment. The remarks of the patient should not be read as intentional witticisms(!):

The patient, Nieber, is well orientated, in his senses, lively, chatty and jovial, always on the alert for smart and apt remarks; he is not acutely disturbed. On admission he implores immediate discharge; if one discharged him today he could call at the clinic occasionally. However, he goes off to the ward without difficulty and never brings the question up again; instead of this he speaks of his intention in the near future of making a dissertation at Tübingen for a doctorate in engineering . . . 'I shall give in it the blueprint of my life; I shall get the doctorate for sure unless I intentionally make some mistakes'. He wants to be employed by the clinic as a photographer; he asks for several private rooms for himself; he wants to be transferred to the first-class accommodation; but he never follows his requests up. He has a number of constantly changing activities which are soon relinquished and forgotten. He writes poetry, applications, letters to authorities, to doctors, to other hospitals, to titled people; he writes a 'dissertation'—'The toilet-paper'—extempore essay by H. J. Nieber. Here are some extracts from this voluminous manuscript: 'Essays have already been printed and printed about the immortality of the may-fly, about the risks of the shot-gun, about the disputability of Darwin's theory of descent. Why should an essay on toilet-paper not find a recognition and reward? I think the price of 30 M. is not too high for a volume full of writing. The social and political side of this subject will get particular attention . . . I therefore enclose a table which will offer a welcome aid to local politicians and the National Economy when it comes to discussion . . .' The patient draws with infinite care a cheque show-ing all the usual ornamentation and sends it to his previous hospital in payment for the food he had had . . . 'It seems to me the sum of 1000 M. is adequate for board and lodging including doctors' fees.' In conversation he always surprised one by his peculiar phrases: 'Psychiatry is nothing else but the investigation of the rights and benefits of the law in relation to persons . . .' 'I hold the view that mental illnesses do not exist' . . . 'Psychiatry has to offer an existence to people who are born for a working life . . .' One may feel like interpreting such talk as leg-pulling of those in the environment, but in fact this is not so. The patients' whole life is like this and is carried on in the institutions for decades without any efforts in earnest on their part.

6. *Cultural subnormality*. We distinguish between congenital mental sub-normality and dementia that is acquired as the result of a morbid process, including in this latter category the organic and schizophrenic dementias. This is a division according to aetiology, which coincides with differences in the psychological characteristics. Of quite different origin, however, is the mental 'subnormality' which clinically appears due not to congenital causes or any morbid process arising from illness, but very largely due to the *abnormal cultural environment in which* the patient lives. It is a socially conditioned defect: 'bad upbringing, inadequate schooling, lack of stimulation, narrowing of interest to breadwinning, and maintenance of the vegetative self, malnutrition, irregular living—all these circumstances are liable to bring about gross defects in knowledge and judgment and an extremely egocentric and morally poor attitude' (Bonhoeffer). We may find many different kinds of defect due in this way to the milieu, in tramps, for instance, in prostitutes, in wealthy people who from childhood upwards have never done or experienced anything much, in people who have had to live in sanatoria for various chronic illnesses and in long-stay mental hospital patients of all types.

7. *Emotional stupidity and pseudo-dementia*. Defects in intelligence are confused sometimes with acute states and with the changes that take place in depression, hypomania and confusional conditions. They can also be easily mistaken for some failure in emotional reaction, emotional stupidity (Jung). This can occur in examinations, for instance, but also during a medical investigation or any other upsetting situation in people who are so disposed. Lastly, we may take for a disturbance of intelligence what is really a pseudo-dementia, a state of prison-psychosis; this can last sometimes for a long period with consciousness unclouded. It is due to hysterical disposition reacting to the impact of a prison-complex, and there is always recovery.

(c) *Examination of intelligence.*[1]

How do we assess the intelligence of anyone? It must be based always on his *actual performance* and on his behaviour in the test-situation when given set tasks to do. Considering the narrow grooves in which most people pass

[1] Jaspers, *Z. Neur.*, ref. teil. 1 (1910), p. 401. Stern, *Die psychologische Methoden der Intelligenzprüfung u. ihre Anwendung bei Schulkindern* (Leipzig, 1916), 2nd edn. Über die Untersuchung von Kindern nach der Methode Binet-Simon. Cf. Berichte von Bobertag, *Z. angew. Psychol.*, vol. 3, pp. 230–59; vol. 5, pp. 105–203; vol. 6, pp. 495–518 (1909–17). G. Kloos is good, see his *Anleitung zur Intelligenzprüfung* (Jena, 1941).

their lives, a single lifetime is not enough to draw out the capacity of the intelligence to the full. The most important source for our assessment remains the *personal life history* and the *actual performance*. But we cannot remain satisfied with that. We like to feel we have made a reliable judgment, even if exploration has to be brief. We explore as much as we can, though the *incidental observations* of clinical practice sometimes give greater insight than the most carefully planned investigation. The observations arise from the *ordinary doctor's interview*. We put certain questions as doctors and long experience has shown their value (asking for differences, between a mistake and a lie, knowing and believing, etc., arithmetical problems not previously learnt, cp. pp. 140-155), questions as to how the patient sees his own situation, how he judges things from his occupational life and his own personal circumstances, etc.). Finally, *complex methods* have been worked out. For instance, the patient should fill in some text meaningfully, putting in words and syllables which have been purposefully left out (Ebbinghaus—completion test), or one asks the patient to describe pictures from memory (Stern—memory test). Patients are asked to repeat stories that have been told them etc. The results are assessed quantitatively, if possible (or numerically).

Up to now such investigations have yielded us the following: assessment of ability in any one field depends on the tests also being in that field. We cannot draw definite conclusions from the completion test, or memory test for instance, as to performance in other fields. We can indeed form some sort of picture of a person's intelligence if we use all the available sources (personal history, conversation, tests), but we cannot assess it in relation to all possible contingencies. It would be utopian to suppose that we can offer any opinion as to what work, at any rate a young child, is best fitted for through the use of an intelligence test, unless the concern is with some relatively simple task or with a plain property of the psychophysical apparatus. Quite often some surprising success or failure in the subsequent course of life will alter the judgment then made. In some extreme cases it may be possible to limit the future possibilities for those of very poor ability; it is also practicable to select experimentally from a large number of people those best fitted for a certain job, if one will allow for a proportion of mistakes. The method is certainly a sure one for detecting colour-blind people; but when it comes to selecting people for professions in the same way, one runs into the danger that experimentally the most intelligent individuals may well prove to be unfit.[1]

In all quantitative assessments of intelligence the individual's maximum performance at any one time should be distinguished from how his correct, competent and worthwhile responses are related to those that are incorrect, incompetent and of no value. It can happen that someone may be regarded as not very intelligent from the latter point of view yet perform extremely well from the former, and vice versa.

[1] Cf. my *Idee der Universität* (Berlin, 1946), Achtes Kapitel.

# CHAPTER III

# SOMATIC ACCOMPANIMENTS AND EFFECTS AS SYMPTOMS OF PSYCHIC ACTIVITY

## (SOMATOPSYCHOLOGY—SOMATOPSYCHOLOGIE)

There are a large number of physical, objective phenomena which appear without any operation of the individual's will. There seems to be no conscious intent. Nor can we take them for meaningful, objective 'performances' nor for any intelligible psychic expression. They follow certain psychic events or occur simultaneously with them. They are physical findings that have or may have some relation to psychic events but they do not portray them nor reveal them in any sense which we can understand. To start with they are nothing else but non-psychic, objective, somatic facts.

*Body–psyche relationship.* In every human being we see the unity of body and psyche appearing as a living whole. We have the fact of the individual as a unity in the shape of a body which either is a psyche, or has a psyche or produces the appearance of a psyche. On the other hand, this undoubted body–psyche unity does not itself appear as a recognisable object. All that we see, think and comprehend is something already separated out from this unity, something particular, and we are faced with the problem of what in fact is its relation to the unity as a whole. It follows that if we regard all psychological and somatic analysis with suspicion, any talk of body–psyche unity not only becomes sterile but positively cripples our thought. The unity of body and psyche is only true as idea. As such, it keeps our analysis from assuming an absolute value and helps us to maintain the findings as relative knowledge. At the same time it fosters the question of what is the relationship of everything to everything else in somatic and psychic life. The unity itself remains dim and incomprehensible or beyond reach as an object of knowledge, but we should think of it as the only idea that can guide our knowledge of life, which is only a knowledge of particulars, and has only the limited certainty of the particular.

(a) *Separation of body and psyche.* The separateness of body and psyche may appear a perfectly clear and obvious notion, which needs no further explanation. But it always leaves us with the question *what* is body and *what* is psyche?

For example, *psyche* means direct inner experience (the material for phenomenology); it means whatever it is that produces meaningful function or appears as human expressiveness; it means the unity of the 'I', the self, the underlying psychic substance, etc.

*Body,* for example, means the morphological shape of life; visible, purposeful movement; the chemical, physical, biological processes; foci in the brain, etc.

If everything is termed psyche, this does not make the psychic whole any more empirically comprehensible than the body would be, if we term it the vague something that embraces every spatial event. We only get an empirical object, if we chisel out clearly from the whole a version that is neither entirely of the body nor entirely of the psyche.

If in some way we manage to separate what belongs to the body and what to the psyche, we are still left with the problem of their *relationship*. This only becomes a fruitful question if it takes the form of something we can objectively test. If it is put as a general problem or a problem of principle, it reduces us to absurdities. Both of these questions must be discussed further:

(*b*) *Enquiry into the relationship of body and psyche.* The relationship of the physical and the psychic is rooted in a number of facts which we can formulate broadly while still using the concepts of body and psyche in a fairly undefined way:

*Physical* things affect the psyche (e.g. poisons, sickness, brain-injury, etc.).

*Psychic things* affect the body; either in the realisation of deliberate intentions (motor activity) or in unintended physical effects—heartbeat, blood-pressure, metabolism, etc.

*Psychic things* appear to be understandable in the physical phenomena (e.g. the psyche expresses itself in the body's posture and movement).

*That* there is a relationship seems to be a common, empirical fact, witnessed by all. This confirmation then leads us on to certain versions of what at any time may be thought to be body and what to be psyche. *How* any relationship is possible and what exactly happens within it eludes our observation. For instance, when I move my hand in writing, I know what I intend and my body obeys me. We can partly demonstrate how this happens in terms of the neurological and physiological events, but the ultimate act of all, the translation of psychic intention into a physical event is at present as inaccessible and incomprehensible as magic, though the magic is one of fact not of illusion. The same things have to be said of all psychic and bodily connections.

(*c*) *The relationship of body and psyche in general.* If we want to grasp the relationship of body and psyche in the form of some general principle, we shall find ourselves caught up in metaphysics in such a way that we shall get landed in absurdities. We have to be dualists, accepting a parallelism of psycho-physical events or some form of interaction; otherwise we have to be monistically materialist (the psyche becoming an incidental epiphenomenon, a property of the body) or else we have to take the path of the spiritualists (the physical being only a manifestation of some psychic substance, which alone is real). Any of these ideas will land us in impossible consequences. The empirical investigator can usually fall back on the category of interaction, in so far as psyche and body are treated separately; the psyche acts on the body and vice versa, without any need to state thereby anything as an absolute or final principle.

There have been metaphysical difficulties ever since Descartes parted body and psyche, as absolutes. He introduced the difference for the first time of inner and outer, between psychic states that are experienced and the physical processes in space. He saw these as two incommensurable realities, each one observable by itself, describable and open to enquiry; res cogitans and res extensa. Descartes' clarifying separation retains its value in the radical difference we make between the description of psychic experiences (phenomenology) and the observation of somatic events. But error began to creep in when the term 'psyche' was confined solely to the conscious inner experience and the term 'body' to the mechanically explicable, material event in space. It crept in too when these aspects of an extremely superficial division were treated as if they were true substances. Reality in its abundance is essentially neither a psychic inner experience nor a physical process in space, but it is something occurring in the medium of both, as meaningful performance or as an expression which we understand, as behaviour, as the human world, or as mental creation. Once the dualistic division had grown into an absolute, there was no longer any room for such abundance. Descartes' division has indeed its application, and any analysis that follows his methods will yield us facts, though the sphere of application is limited and disappears altogether when we reach the encompassing nature of life itself.

Descartes wanted to surpass the old, and in its own way magnificent, conception of life as it had been held from *Aristotle* to *Thomas Aquinas*. This involved the concept of a hierarchy contained within the unity of psychophysical being and ranging from the vital levels of the psyche through the levels of emotion to the level of thought. Within the one, immaterial human soul lies the 'substantial form' of the human body. The body is, so to speak, ennobled and the psyche embodied at one and the same time. There is no assertion in principle of any basic difference in the nature of what is physical and what is psychic.

Today the study of the psychology of Thomas Aquinas is still rewarding. It gives us a prototype on a grand scale and his classifications are still worth reflecting upon. We will take one particular point: Aquinas differentiated sensual knowing and sensual striving (which are both directly dependent on the physical) from reasoning and spiritual striving (which are indirectly dependent on the physical). He divided the sensual field into: (1) The external senses, touch, taste, smell, hearing and sight. (2) The inner sense-capacities, among which we find the *general sense*, which brings the individual sensations into consciousness and covers everything that belongs to the senses—movement and rest, unity and multiplicity, size and shape. It is the mid-point where all the senses are gathered up into a unity. Then there is the *power of imagination* which steers our impressions and reproduces them in image and fantasy. There is also *sensual judgment* (instinctive drives, instinctive evaluations, which transcend perception and carry their own judgment with them; they participate, as it were, in reason) and there is *sensual memory* (which stores all those sensual experiences that carry a time-signal). (3) Sensual striving (the 'appetitus concupiscibilis, irascibilis') and the passions.

The basic concept of the body–psyche whole can be greatly modified but it has never lost its fundamental feature—that of a *oneness* that is recognisable and absolute, whereas Descartes' newer philosophy took *two* substances as absolute. The older view pictured the whole in a way that preserved the abundance of reality without abandoning the unity of body and psyche and it continued to see the physical in everything psychic and the psychic in everything physical. For this reason, it has, right up to the present day, *often been revived in opposition to the views of Descartes*. A recent example of this is Bleuler's use of the term 'psychoid', which was to denote something common to somatic and psychic life alike: the function of memory, integration, the purposeful character of living structures and forces. The defect here, as with all such schematic ideas, is that a comprehensive viewpoint of this sort may indeed provide us with an ideal construct but this cannot be investigated nor can we use it in order to obtain new knowledge. *The one absolute* of the substantial Being of body–psyche unity *opposes the other*, that of the two absolute modes of Being, body and psyche. Both theoretical standpoints, that of Aquinas and that of Descartes, have to be discarded. Truth demands that we do away with *all* absolutes in favour of definite, though always partial, knowledge which has to proceed step by step and never finds itself wholly in possession. The completeness of the whole can never be encompassed by the time-bound nature of human knowledge. Knowledge is only true within that part of space accessible to us. If we want to know the transcendental whole, which has both physical and psychic effects and is primarily both, we find it has vanished from us into the clarity of particular facts which are comprehensible but which are never the whole itself.

(*d*) *The coincidental manifestation of body and psyche as a fact for investigation.* Everyone *experiences* within himself this coincidental existence of body and psyche. This experience, in the form of bodily sensation, provides us with the material for phenomenology and somato-psychology. We see the part played by physical sensation in the perception of our own bodily events and also in our feelings, drives and sufferings. This experience, however, is no means for obtaining a generally valid knowledge of body–psyche unity, but, in so far as it is an experience, it becomes material for our knowledge of body–psyche relationships.

Again, psyche and body are one for us in *expression*. When we see a happy, human face, we do not divide body and psyche, nor do we have two different things in some relation to each other, but we are presented with a whole, which we only separate secondarily into physical phenomena and something inward and psychic. The fact of seeing someone's expression is a primary phenomenon of the way we grasp our world. It is a fact of infinite richness, enigmatic in principle, but always there, present and real. If we want to talk of the coincidence of body and psyche as a fact for investigation, it is only in this fashion that we shall encounter it. After we have separated body and psyche, we never find again what was once present as a real phenomenon, both medium and material of some specific (understandable) actuality, present to us before we start to reflect.

However we differentiate the physical and psychic life, we may indeed find empirical relationships which follow the separation, but we never think of an actual coincidence of body and psyche or any identity between the two, let alone see it.

If we wish to inscribe psychic structures into the somatic structures and maintain their identity, we become involved in purely theoretical notions that lack objective reference and on closer inspection seem absurd: for instance, we may think that memory images are planted in the ganglion cells and psychic associations in the fibres; or that psychic configurations are of the nature of physical configurations in the brain and are rooted there; or that the basis of freedom lies in what are statistically erratic, atomic events. The assumption that what is physical and what is psychic coincide somewhere in the brain is pure fantasy, and must always remain an untestable hypothesis, which stems from Descartes' idea of the pineal body as the seat of the soul (which is there like a rider on his horse). It is a vague, general truth that the psyche is tied to the body, but how and where this connection takes place fragments into a multitude of possibilities awaiting exploration. The negative position is certainly valid, that there is no one exclusive place for psychic reality; there is only the most diverse set of relationships and connections between what is psychic and what are indispensable somatic determinants. There are it is true certain very circumscribed areas in the nervous system the destruction of which will cause immediate or early death. There are others the alteration of which will bring about unconsciousness or sleep and yet others the disturbance of which alters or abolishes individual functions (e.g. speech). There are also relationships of another kind which pertain to the functioning of the neurohormonal endocrine system; for instance, hormones have an effect on the psychic moods and drives or psychic events may evoke the inner secretion of certain hormones with effect on body and psyche. There are other relationships too, of a different sort, between psychic type and body-build. Still, *no seat for the psyche is to be found*, neither in a crude localised sense, nor hormonally, nor atomically nor in ultramicroscopic events. Leibnitz's insight is still valid today, as regards our mechanical knowledge of the body: If we could enter the machine of the brain, as we might a factory, and could observe objectively the very smallest, and ultimate events, we would not find anything else but physical parts in active contact with each other, never anything like a perception or anything that might serve to explain one. To sum up, coincidence (and that restricted to what is an understandable manifestation) exists only at the point where in primary fashion we see and experience the psyche in the body and the body in the psyche. If we have separated body and psyche and are investigating their relationship, no such coincidence is to be found.

(e) *Areas for research into the body–psyche relationship.* The result of the above presentation is that only those fields of investigation present a body–psyche problem where either the unity of the two is affirmed as a primary object or where the method of separating them presupposes a definite form in which they are to be conceived.

Beyond this there are many areas for research where neither separation nor unity are a problem nor do they enter the subject-matter. They are areas where human actualities are investigated that exist in their own right without having to be related to this problem at all. Thus in psychopathology we deal with a host of subjects in which this question of body–psyche unity or division is altogether irrelevant for our enquiry, as for instance, behaviour, performance, creativity, meaningful connections, personal histories, and the majority of social and historical questions.

Relationships between the body and the psyche are investigated:

(1) *In the study of expression* (Ausdruckspsychologie)—where physical characteristics and movements are seen by us as meaningful (pp. 253 ff.).

(2) *As a causal relationship*—where we look for some answer to the question—which modes of bodily existence affect the psyche and how? (pp. 463 ff.).

(3) *In the enquiry into body-build and constitution.* How far are these a basis for psychic characteristics? (pp. 633 ff.).

(4) *In the somatic consequences of psychic events.* We shall be dealing with this in the present chapter (Somato-psychology). These are the most superficial of body-psyche relationships, and compared with such matters as psychic expression, they carry minimal meaning, but we shall see how even here under abnormal conditions a certain meaning may be inferred from particular understandable connections.

In somato-psychology we classify our findings into three groups:

(1) *General basic psychosomatic facts.* Body sensations, continuous somatic accompaniments, sleep, hypnosis. As such they exist or can be produced in every human being. We will describe them and some of the disturbances that arise in this field.

(2) *Physical illnesses dependent on the psyche.* Some illnesses arise through the psyche, others are purely somatic disorders not wholly independent in their course from psychic events.

(3) Noteworthy *somatic findings in the psychoses*. These cannot be explained in terms of any known organic illnesses, though they look very like them. We can only record them for the time being. Possibly we are dealing with symptoms of organic illness as yet unknown responsible for the psychosis in question; possibly the relationships here are of quite a different order.

## § 1. THE BASIC PSYCHO-SOMATIC FACTS

### (a) Body-sensations

Bodily events are seen objectively by the outside observer in the form of visible signs. The somatic facts are established by methods of clinical and physiological examination. Everyone, however, with the help of his own body-sensations, can become his own observer. His body becomes an object to him. With the help of body-sensations he can observe his changing bodily state. There is something more here than the mere sensation of an external something; there is the feeling-sensation of one's own existence. The fact that body-sensations make perceptible something which I can then observe as something that confronts me gives rise to certain questions: first, whether there is an authentic coincidence between body-sensations and actual body-processes and, if so, how far does it extend; secondly, how far does the perception of one's own body reach (since the majority of organic processes are imperceptible and take place outside consciousness); thirdly, have the somatic complaints, descriptions, perceptions of patients any validity for our knowledge of the body?

An authentic coincidence rarely occurs. Apart from sensations due to primary organic processes, there are sensations brought about by organic changes which constantly accompany psychic life or arise psychogenically in a specific way; for instance, sensations of warmth and cold with vasomotor effects on the skin, leaden feelings during muscular relaxation, stomach-ache during psychogenically accelerated peristalsis. Lastly there are a host of body-sensations with no demonstrable physical cause brought about by attention, expectation, worry, etc.

Normally the range of body-sensations is not very wide, but the extent to which they are perceived can be enormously enlarged. Intensive direction of concern inwards—as described by J. H. Schultz during 'autogenic' training —leads to 'the discovery of organic experiences' which are not dependent on suggestion nor are they an illusory elaboration of normal sensation, but testable extensions of real bodily perception.

Patients tell us of innumerable *subjective sensations*. The somatopsyche is basically being referred to here. The 'organ-sensations', 'bodily sensations', 'pains', 'unpleaasnt sensations', 'vital feelings' of which they speak can all be divided into three groups:

1. *Hallucinations and pseudo-hallucinations*. These have been discussed on pp. 64 ff.

2. *Bodily processes* in the organs or in the nervous system; these are already *subjectively felt* and noted by the patients, although they *cannot yet* be *objectively* confirmed by the examiner. In spite of possible deception and the uncritical attitude of the average person, there is some point in the examiner investigating these subjective symptoms closely, taking into account the patient's ability to be objective. He may get certain hints of organic events or uncover the psychic source of the sensations which from the organic point of view are illusory.

3. Most people do not view their body-sensations with detachment. Rather they are apt to falsify their account through fear and other psychic reactions. These falsifications are in themselves a new reality. Psychic changes are connected with sensations which apparently have no physical basis, unless it be in the postulated somatic substratum of psychic life. These sensations are wholly dependent on psychic events. Hysterical and other similar sensations provide an example.[1] *Pains* are of special interest. Severe pains need not be felt. With wounded men arm-amputations can be carried out on rare occasions in the absence of narcotics, where there is a state of battle heroism, and the patient tells the story of his courage. Martyrs have painlessly endured torture and death. Severe pains may arise without any organic base; we can understand them as symbols, as unconscious means, as anxiety. Attentiveness and worry can increase pain, objective observation can diminish it, distraction can make it vanish.[2]

In general we may say that reports (especially of neurotic patients) on bodily sensations are of the nature of clinical findings, but hard to evaluate as a source for any knowledge of psycho-physical events. If we were to trust them as genuine sense-perceptions, as if they were real observations, it would mean treating the fantasies of neurotic people in the same way as observations of fact.[3]

*(b) Constant somatic accompaniments*

In all normal psychic processes, particularly where there are affects, we

[1] Samberger, 'Über das Juckgefühl', Z. *Neur.*, vol. 24, p. 313. Oppenheim, 'Über Dauerschwindel', *Neur. Zbl.* (1911), p. 290.

[2] F. Mohr, 'Schmerz u. Schmerzbehandlung', Z. *Psychother.*, vol. 10 (1918), p. 220.

[3] V. v. Weizsäcker, 'Körpergeschehen u. Neurose.', *Internat. Z. Psychoanalyse*, vol. 19 (1933), p. 16. He tries to 'link methodically anatomical-physiological knowledge with psychoanalytical findings'. He tries to explore the psycho-physical connections through the fantasies of a psychopath with a disturbance in micturition. He tests the 'supposition that the patient through his experiences has told us more about the process than we could ever perceive'. The patient in his analysis 'gives us only a picture, but in important points a very apt picture of organic events'. We should accept 'that the patient's ideas, pictures and formulations have illustrative value for something which he does not directly experience, namely the activities of his nervous system'. V. v. Weizsäcker believes that his method 'establishes the psychoanalytic method and the major part of its theory' and that 'we can now dare to approach psychoanalytic findings from another point of view'. I cannot accept this particular supposition of his and on reading his report and interpretation of this case of disturbance of micturition, I needs must remain unconvinced.

can observe physical accompaniments or can confirm them with the help of experimental apparatus, even down to the slightest of psychic stirrings:

In shame or fright we find blushing and blanching. Disgust leads to vomiting, emotional upset brings tears; fear makes the heart beat, knees tremble, the face pale; cold sweat break out, the throat go dry, hair stand on end, pupils dilate, eyeballs protrude. In states of anxious tension, there is diarrhoea or the increased need to micturate.[1] Many other affects also increase the amount of urine. Psychic upsets inhibit secretion of the respiratory mucosae, salivary glands and lachrymal glands (in melancholia also).

Scientific apparatus[2] enables us to make exact observations of changes in respiration, heartbeat, blood pressure, blood-volume (by displacing the blood through various localised vaso-constrictions or dilatations), of fluctuations in a galvanic current taken from the skin, of pupillary changes. The dependence of gastric secretion on psychic influences is shown by its inhibition where there is listlessness, or during sleep, and the increase of secretion when food or something pleasant is imagined visually or heard.[3] When we are investigating patients these physical accompaniments, if we watch the changes of intensity and course, will help us very greatly as a clue to the underlying psychic events. Thus there is an interest in learning whether during stupor consciousness is not entirely empty or whether something may not still be going on in the patient's mind.

Gregor[4] gives a thorough evaluation of psychogalvanic reflex phenomena as a means of assessing psychic events in mental patients. If electrodes are placed at two points on the skin, on the hands for example, and a circuit established, the body yields a weak, galvanic current; the fluctuations of this current can be recorded as a time-sequence and plotted as a curve. The fluctuations are partly physically, partly physiologically and partly psychically determined. Through refinements of technique and critical observation it is possible to separate the latter fairly convincingly from the rest. The curve is studied either as a *resting-curve* or in the way it *fluctuates* when external stimuli are applied. Characteristic resting-curves emerge with either

[1] Bergmann and Katsch, *Dtsch. med. Wschr.* (1913). They watched sudden blanching in the abdominal wall and immobility of the intestines in animals, using a celluloid window. This occurred in states of unpleasant stimulation. The mere sight of food being offered started peristalsis.

[2] Wundt's *Physiological Psychology* gives the older work. Lehmann, *Die körperlichen Äusserungen psychischer Zustände* (Leipzig, 1899). More recently E. Weber, *Der Einfluss psychischer Vorgänge auf den Körper* (Berlin, 1910). Veraguth, 'Das psychogalvanische Reflexphänomenon', *Mschr. Psychiatr.*, vol. 21, p. 397; vol. 23, p. 204. Leschke summarises in 'Die körperlichen Begleiterscheinungen seelischer Vorgänge', *Arch. Psychol.* (D), vol. 21 (1911), p. 435; vol. 31 (1914), pp. 27 ff.

[3] Following Pavlov's discovery of this dependence, there have been many investigations, e.g. Schrottenbach, *Z. Neur.*, vol. 69 (Bibliography), p. 254.

[4] Gregor and Gorn, 'Zur psychopathologischen u. klinischen Bedeutung des psychogalvanischen Phänomens', *Z. Neur.*, vol. 16 (1913), p. 1. Cp. also Gregor and Zaloziecki, *Klin. psych. u. nerv. Krankh.*, vol. 3, p. 22. Gregor, *Arch. Psychol.* (D), vol. 27 (1913), p. 241. 'Die Beeinflussung des psychogalvanischen Phänomens durch Suggestion in der Hypnose stellte' F. Georgi, *Arch. Psychiatr.* (D), vol. 62 (1921), p. 271.

diminished or increased psychogalvanic reactions to stimuli. There is also a differential response according to the type of stimuli (bell, pain caused by pinching the skin, doing sums, calling over emotive words—affective tone due to 'complexes').

Gregor confirmed the following findings:

1. The different types of resting-curve may be interpreted as expressions of inner psychic events, though so far this is not very clear. Gregor terms the steeply rising curve the 'affect-curve'. 2. Diminution or abolition of psychogalvanic reaction is found in chronic affective dullness (many catatonic end-states, paralyses, epilepsies and the arterio-sclerotic dementias), in temporary states of affect-loss, i.e. diminished affective responses during treatable melancholia, also in catatonic stupor and finally during certain phenomena of inhibition and exhaustion of a psychasthenic kind. 3. An increase in psychogalvanic reaction is found during arithmetical tests, which denotes greater effort in states of inhibition. 4. There are varied reactions to different stimuli; inhibited psychasthenic persons react most strongly to arithmetical tasks, dements (e.g. many paralytics, epileptics) will react most strongly to physical pain.—Notable among the special findings is the fact that reactions of normal strength are shown in congenital mental subnormality, even of low grade, which is not the case in acquired forms of emotional dulling. There is also the fact that with hebephrenia and paralytic excitement of a hypomanic character, all reactions are in abeyance, whereas in true hypomania they are always clearly and vigorously present.

*Pupillary movements* also accompany affective psychic events; and indeed in the absence of any outer stimuli, the pupil nearly always shows what we call *pupillary unrest* (Pupillenunruhe). This accompanies psychic activity, fluctuations in consciousness, attentiveness and mental effort. It corresponds to the psychogalvanic resting-curve. The pupils always dilate in response to psychic impressions, during any mental effort, during affect, and particularly in response to painful stimuli. When there is extreme fear, the pupils are maximally dilated and will not react to light. During sleep the pupils are small. With severe dementias and particularly with dementia praecox (Bumke's phenomenon),[1] pupillary unrest and reactive dilatation of pupils both disappear.

Other accompaniments of psychic events show themselves in the *blood-pressure*,[2] the *pulse-rate* and respiration,[3] in *plethysmographic* investigations[4] (where fluctuations in blood-volume of individual body-parts, the arms for instance, are recorded). During fear the blood-pressure rises enormously, and we also find a rise in mania and melancholia, especially in the latter. Pulse rate increases during mental effort, and feelings of displeasure; it shows temporarily during states of attentiveness to stimuli, in fright and tension as well as in states of pleasure. We note an *increase in excitability* in vaso-labile 'neuropaths', Basedow's disease, exhaustion, and convalescence. Typical of catatonia are: the tense vascular system (appearing plethysmographically as volume-rigidity) the rigid iris-muscles (fixed pupils), increased tonus

---

[1] Bumke, *Die Pupillenstörungen bei Geistes-und Nervenkrankheiten* (Jena, 1911), 2nd edn.

[2] Knauer, *Z. Neur.*, vol. 10, p. 319. Enebushe, 'Von der vasomotorischen Unruhe der Geisteskranken', *Z. Neur.*, vol. 34, p. 449.

[3] Wiersma, *Z. Neur.*, vol. 19, p. 1.

[4] de Jong, *Z. Neur.*, vol. 69, p. 61 (detailed literature on plethysmographic curves). H. Bickel, *Die wechselseitigen Beziehungen zw. psychischem Geschehen u. Blutkreislauf mit besondered Berücksichtigung der Psychosen* (Leipzig, 1916) (record of blood-pressure and volume).

of the voluntary muscles. (All these symptoms should be regarded as due to auto-nomic innervation and not as psychic events—de Jong.)

Weinberg[1] took recordings with the plethysmograph, the electrocardiograph, and noted electrogalvanic phenomena, respiration and pupil reaction. All reacted simultaneously and persistently in response to *every* psychic event—e.g. the mere ringing of a bell—so that 'the raising of the conscious level' through the stimulus brings about phenomena which depend on increased 'sympathetic stimulation'.

Berger[2] discovered a minute electric current emanating from the brain. The recording of this—electroencephalogram—showed various waves, indi-vidually distinct and characteristic for the particular person. These waves are an index of physiological events that are also closely related to psychic events. There is a big difference in the waves during the waking state and in sleep. Consciousness, attentiveness, indeed any activity is reflected in an alteration in the wave forms.

Physical accompaniments of psychic events appear in great numbers and we have only enumerated a few. They do not tell us much, except that they illustrate the universal link of psyche and soma. The concept that all these phenomena are consequences of psychic events is too one-sided. The relation-ship, as soon as it occurs, is a mutual one, acting back on the psyche itself. We can only comprehend the details of this happening by a better understanding of physiological relationships. These are always circular: the psychic event causes a series of somatic phenomena which in their turn modify the psychic event. We can scarcely see this in the swiftly moving accompaniments that we have discussed. Investigations of inner secretion gave clearer results in the case of events that lasted a longer time, from half an hour to a lengthy time-interval. Psychic excitation or inhibition, for instance, travels to the smooth muscles of the vessels relatively quickly, the effects on the endocrine glands are much slower. The circle is obvious—psyche, autonomic nervous system, endocrine glands, hormone production, effects of the hormones on somatic events and of both on the nervous system and psyche. Doubtless there are any number of such circles. During experimental recordings we can only objectively define one link at a time. The understanding of the whole enlarges with a better understanding of these physiological circles; how they summate and interact. To begin with we only know isolated samples. But often they may give us a clue as regards the complex psycho-physiological interaction; there can then follow almost exclusively animal experiments which help us to more precise physiological theories. We find that *psychic life*, as much in its smallest stirrings as in its moments of violent emotion, is *in its very last ramification intimately linked with somatic events.*

Somatic accompaniments *change* in intensity and in the mode of their

[1] Weinberg, *Z. Neur.*, vol. 85, p. 543; vol. 86 (1923), p. 375; vol. 93 (1924), p. 421.
[2] H. Berger, *Arch. Psychiatr.* (D), vol. 87 (1929), p. 527. *Allg. Z. Psychiatr.*, vol. 108 (1938), p. 554. R. Jung, 'Das Elektencephalogramm u. seine klinische Anwendung', *Nervenarzt*, vol. 12, p. 569; vol. 14 (1941), p. 57, 104.

appearance within the one individual, and as between individuals. It is customary to say: vegetative reactivity is not a constant. Blushing, lachrymal and salivary secretion, dermographic phenomena, heart-reflexes, etc. vary enormously in degree. Also toxins like adrenalin, pilocarpin, atropine vary greatly in the strength and fashion of their effects. We may speak of a *constitutional disposition* of the autonomic nervous system and find that its reactivity has very little to do with the psychic development of a person, or conversely we may believe we have found a correlation between basic types of body-build and temperament.

Detailed investigation gives us a multiplicity of findings; e.g. with some people psychic excitement is accompanied by congestion of the nasal conchi. There is a mutual interaction between the nasal conchi and the genitalia. One may be lucky and succeed in intervening therapeutically—by physical or psychological means—in this circuit of autonomic-psychic effects when it is disturbed, but the methods are somewhat unpredictable.

### (c) Sleep

*Physiological preface.*[1] Sleep is not a universal phenomenon (it is something quite different from the change that takes place in all biological processes as day alternates with night). But waking and sleeping are not specifically human attributes, as a waking consciousness is found in all warm-blooded vertebrates. Consciousness depends on the functioning of a vital, animal state of a very primitive kind. Even in the decerebrate dog, the sleep-waking rhythm persists. It is very probable that the function linked with consciousness and sleep is localised in the brain stem (perhaps in the grey matter of the third ventricle).

Sleep is necessary for life. It is a respite for the brain. Prolonged suppression of sleep (which is scarcely possible) causes death. We spend one-third of our life sleeping. Sleep is not paralysis but rest. It is also essentially different from narcosis; the latter does not refresh. Narcotic drugs have a refreshing effect not because they cause loss of consciousness but because of the natural sleep which they induce. On the other hand hypnotic sleep is a genuine sleep, differing from natural sleep only in the rapport sustained with the hypnotist, but it is not a difference in principle as rapport may also be made with someone dreaming in normal sleep, if one talks with them. Sleep is a function of the nerve centres which are the source for all somatic changes that occur during sleep: the slowing of respiration, of circulation, reduction in metabolism and body temperature, diminution of certain glandular secretions, reduced reaction to stimuli, immobility. During sleep, however, in contrast to narcosis, unconsciousness, etc., the psyche remains in touch with meaningful stimuli. The soldier who sleeps through the rattle of gunfire can be wakened by a distant telephone or a mother by the least noise from her baby; most extraordinary of all, but undoubtedly a fact, is punctual awakening at a certain predetermined time (our inner clock).

A distinction is made between *duration* and *depth* of sleep. People who need very little sleep, usually sleep deeply. Deep sleep refreshes more quickly than a light

[1] U. Ebbecke, *Handbuch der Physiologie* (Bethe and Bergmann), vol. 17 (1926). Pötzl, *Der Schlaf* (München, 1929); H. Winterstein, *Schlaf u. Traum* (Berlin, 1932).

sleep. The average duration of sleep in the first year of life is 18 hours; from the 7th to the 14th year it is still 10 hours; then up to the 50th year 8 hours; over 60 years it falls to 3–4 hours. The *depth of sleep* has been measured by a *curve*, which is arrived at by measuring the intensity of the stimulus needed to waken the individual. Normally the greatest depth occurs one to two hours after falling asleep; it then rises slowly and a light sleep is maintained until morning. The curve that shows the greatest depth towards morning is an abnormal one. A connection has been found between the sleep curve of the morning-worker (normal) and the night-worker.

Sleep is brought about by *physiological* and *psychological causes*:

Objective fatigue and subjective tiredness are preparatory. Severe fatigue in any one organ manifests itself in all the others. Fatigue toxins spread throughout the body; the longer the waking state, the greater and more compelling the tiredness becomes, until it is impossible to keep awake any longer.

If, as is usual, tiredness is not so great, the main condition for sleep is a situation that reduces stimuli to the minimum: darkness, quiet, a peaceful mind, a relaxed position, absence of muscle tension. The complete exclusion of stimuli induces sleep. A patient of Strümpell who had suffered extensive loss of sensation in various organs, would fall asleep at once as soon as one closed his remaining right eye, and stopped up the one hearing ear, his left one. Under normal conditions a complete exclusion of stimuli is impossible. The more excitability is reduced by fatigue toxins, the easier it is to sleep but first of all there has to be the additional auto-suggestion made by consciousness: 'I want to fall asleep; I shall fall asleep'. The preparatory physiological and suggestive psychic factors act together.

Among the physiological determinants of sleep, the following are probable from experience:

*The importance of an inhibition of reflexes:* Pavlov observed that dogs in a state of great attentiveness were overcome by insurmountable fatigue. He thought that inhibition is a localised sleep; sleep an extended inhibition. Concentration of one's attention on one object only is possibly the cause of hypnotic sleep, and can be related to this finding. Sleep has a relationship to the *brain-stem*. Animal experiments (e.g. cats fall asleep during electrical stimulation of certain brain-stem areas), as well as experience with encephalitis lethargica, point in this direction. It looks as if certain blocking points were localised in the brain-stem which inhibit excitation without blocking it out entirely. These are activated when we want to fall asleep and have brought about the appropriate situation, or else they enforce sleep upon us, when we are very tired.

*Sleep-disturbances*[1] are very various; they may affect falling asleep, waking, the mode of sleep, and may appear as insomnia.

*Falling asleep* is usually a rapid matter, taking only a few seconds. But with people who suffer from nervous symptoms it is very often a long-drawn-out affair. We can then observe several phases and a number of specific phenomena.[2] A state of somnolence develops with a steady increase in tiredness,

---

[1] See Gaupp, Goldscheider and Faust, Wiesbaden (*Kongr. inn. Med.*, 1913) for the nature and treatment of insomnia.

[2] Trömmer, 'Die Vorgänge beim Einschlafen', *J. Psychiatr.*, vol. 17, p. 343.

then suddenly, almost traumatically, there is a transition into a state of dissociation. These sudden eclipses into sleep may recur repeatedly, with a slight re-awakening into somnolence, and along with this a consciousness that wavers between sleep and waking. During that time pseudo-hallucinations are common and sometimes actual sense-phenomena (hypnagogic hallucinations). Visions appear and disappear in a flash, broken phrases and words are heard or whole scenes experienced which can no' longer be distinguished from dreaming proper and merge into it.

Auto-suggestion is one of the factors in falling asleep and this may fail. The intense struggle to sleep is coupled with doubt as to whether sleep will come, and this prevents it: 'to will yourself to sleep is to stay awake'. Willing must turn into suggestion, it must agree to wait, it must become passive in its activity. It must not try to enforce sleep but must learn to abandon itself to it. Normal *waking* is also rapid. The person is at once clear and collected. Disturbances in waking show themselves by a prolonging of this process., so that a state of sleepiness (drunk with sleep) intervenes between sleeping and waking.[1] This state can be so abnormal that the person can perform actions automatically without knowing anything about it.

The *quality of the sleep* is sometimes abnormally deep, so that patients sometimes feel as if they had been dead. It may however be abnormally light and the patients never feel refreshed, but have vivid, restless and anxious dreams, and feel as if only half of their being had been asleep, the other half had stayed awake and watched.

*Duration of sleep* may be very lengthy, for instance, in some depressive states. The patients are always wanting to sleep and sometimes sleep twelve hours uninterruptedly. On the other hand we find sleep abnormally curtailed. The patients go to sleep but are awake again soon after and then lie awake all night long. Or they only manage to get off to sleep towards morning.

There are many kinds of *insomnia*, and also many causes for it. We do not know whether there is a type of insomnia due to some localised lesion in the brain-stem. The place from which excessive sleep originates may also bring about insomnia when the pathological stimulus is of a different order.

Sleep sometimes shows unusual motor phenomena ranging from shaking, chewing, grinding the teeth, to talking in one's sleep, and alterations in awareness similar to hypnosis, with somnambulism and surprising behaviour with subsequent amnesia.

*(d) Somatic effects in hypnosis*

Experience with hypnosis teaches us how widely the psyche affects the body. The observation of the physical effects of hypnotic suggestion caused so much surprise that at first it was all felt to be deception. However, the finding of far-reaching physical effects due to suggestion have been established beyond doubt. Reddening and blistering with subsequent scarring of the skin have

[1] Pelz, 'Über eine eigenartige Störung des Erwachens', *Z. Neur.*, vol. 2, p. 688.

been brought about by suggesting that a hot coin is laid on the skin. Similarly, fever has been produced and postponement of menstruation. There have been specific alterations in gastric secretion through certain types of food being suggested, changes in metabolism due to the suggestion of emotional situations, pancreatic secretion after imaginary eating under hypnosis, the cure of warts.[1] Some of these are exceptional phenomena which only succeed in rare cases and remain somewhat controversial, such as the blister formation and the subsequent scarring. Others however are effects that are easily and frequently obtained.

Identical with these hypnotic effects are the physical effects that have been described by J. H. Schultz. He induced certain conditions through auto-suggestion and called the whole practice 'autogenic training'. It is surprising to hear that one is able in certain individual cases to increase or decrease the pulse rate enormously from 76 to 44 and up to 144.[2] The extreme possibilities of this procedure have not been exploited in western countries but we find it in India. It may be that the famous 'stigmatisations' (e.g. St. Francis of Assissi), analogous to the blisters raised under hypnotic suggestion, may be understood as produced by auto-suggestion of this kind.

Hypnosis achieves its effect through realistic, concrete images which exert their power by dominating feeling and mood. The patient carries out the normal reaction to the suggested situation, e.g. metabolism is increased because it is suggested that it is cold in the snow. The autonomic nervous system takes its cue from the experience—which is an imagined one—in spite of the quite different actual situation with its real stimuli. It is not possible to raise temperature, increase gastric juices or metabolism by direct suggestion; we can only do it through some suggested situation, which if real would have these effects.

Hypnotic effects can partly be comprehended as conditioned reflexes in the Pavlovian sense (Hansen). The image of food, when realistically present, provokes the gastric secretion. When the food is repeatedly shown to the dog but never given to him to eat, the conditioned reflex of gastric secretion fails to appear. In the same way, somatic effects of hypnotic suggestion will not appear if they are repeatedly tried out during the day but with no subsequent realisation. If genuine reinforcement of the conditioned response is permanently absent, the reflex disappears. The unconditioned reflex remains the reason why events may be influenced by the psyche. These physiological interpretations, however, by no means exhaust the totality of psycho-somatic relations.

We cannot assess how far psychic influences can affect the body. Up to

[1] Kohnstamm and Pinner, *Verh. dtsch. derm. Ges.*, vol. 10 (1908). Heller and Schultz, *Münch. med. Wschr.*, vol. II (1909), p. 2612. Schindler, *Nervensystem u. Spontanblutungen* (Berlin, 1927) (stigmatization). Pollak, 'Zur Klinik der Stigmatization', *Z. Neur.*, vol. 162 (1938), p. 606. Fieber, Mohr, *Münch. med. Wschr.*, vol. 2 (1914), p. 2030. Kohnstamm, *Z. Neur.*, vol. 23, p. 379. Eicheberg, *Dtsch. Z. Nervenhk.*, vols. 68–9 (1921), p. 352. Re menstruation: Kohnstamm, *Ther. Gegenw.* (1907). Re warts: Bloch, *Klin. Wschr.*, vol. 2 (1927), p. 2271. Metabolism: Grafe, *Münch. med. Wschr.* (1921). Gastric secretion: Heyer, *Arch. Verdgskrkh.*, vol. 27, 29 (1920/1). Pancreas: Hansen, *Dtsch. Arch. klin. Med.*, vol. 157 (1927).

[2] J. Schultz, *Das autogene Training* (Leipzig, 1932), p. 75.

now research finds this field an expanding one. There is, in a complex way which remains difficult to evaluate, a psychic factor present in many physiological processes. Surprising effects can be achieved by the psyche and severe disturbances of physical processes may be traced to this source.

*v. Weizäcker* (Aertzliche Fragen: S 31. Leipzig, 1934) writes: 'We would do better to press research to try and make something of the puzzles that lie before us, instead of gazing at the miracles of stigmatisation, hysteria and hypnosis as exceptions of the rule. As exceptions they release us from suspecting anything analogous in pathological symptoms.' v. Weizäcker wished to make all illness understandable. But is it true that all somatic illnesses—even the severe, organic ones—are penetrated by the psyche? Could this be shown convincingly, not only would new fields of human knowledge open up, but a radically new sort of knowledge of physical events would be constituted. I doubt however, that this is possible yet suspect that there are rather close boundaries here, in spite of everything. The question, however, retains some justification.

## § 2. Somatic Disturbances Dependent on the Psyche

The whole body may be conceived as an organ of the psyche. When the body is seriously sick, psychic excitement may do damage through associated organic stress. But this is a rare and borderline case. Psychic effects usually work through mental content and determining tendencies. These are pathogenic only when the psyche is sick. It can then happen that if the psyche is disordered this will show itself in physical effects. The physical disorders connected with the psyche are extremely varied and not well understood. We will first clarify the facts and then discuss the interpretation of them.

### (a) *Main categories of psychically determined somatic disturbances*

1. *Faints and fits.* Both can occur as an immediate result of psychic excitement. But both are also known to be conditioned by purely organic causes. In particular we differentiate organic, epileptic seizures from psychogenic hysterical seizures:

*Gruhle*[1] describes *psychogenic* seizures. For instance, 'A well-built man is walking quietly up and down the long corridor; he suddenly groans, grabs into the air and sinks down (he does not fall headlong). At first he lies on the floor, breathing heavily; his hand has torn open his jacket and shirt. Suddenly the convulsion starts, now with one arm, now with both, he threshes fairly vigorously about him. His body arches up and down, the legs bend and buckle or stretch out, now one, now the other or both together. We might characterise the movements as kicking. The face is contorted, the eyes firmly closed, but sometimes rolling wildly. If given a pinprick, kicking increases for the first few times, then ceases; pupillary reaction is difficult to test, as the patient throws his head about or shuts his eyes tight. If one manages to control this, pupils are usually found to be widely dilated (as in anxiety or pain), and they react poorly. Sometimes the patient wets himself, usually if he has been a bed-

[1] Gruhle, *Psychiatrie für Ärzte.* (Berlin, 1922), p. 93, 2nd edn.

wetter. The statement is often made that there is something theatrical about these attacks, but this is frequently not the case. After five to ten minutes, the movements diminish and gradually cease. The exhausted man, covered in sweat, passes into a long sleep and wakes up with only a patchy memory for events.'

Gruhle describes the contrasting picture of the *epileptic* seizure as follows: 'The epileptic seizure starts suddenly; the patient may indeed notice the signal (the "aura") for such a seizure (sensation of a gust of air, seeing red, seeing things small or large, seeing sparks, frightening enlargement of objects, rushing sounds, ringing, smells) but he is unable to speak. He may stagger forward a few steps as if pushed hard, then the seizure overtakes him. As he falls his face contorts, the mouth is screwed, foam forms on the lips, often blood-stained saliva comes from the mouth (from biting the tongue), the eyes are fixed, staring, turned one side or the other, a few violent twitches run lightning-fashion over the face, the head is turned to the side or jerks violently a few times in this direction, there is a grinding of the teeth, various muscle groups, sometimes all the muscles, are maximally contracted for a few seconds, a peculiar gurgle or groan comes from the mouth, breathing is very difficult. Then the spasm loosens. Repeated clonic jerks run through the musculature and the convulsion proper follows. A few 'wiping away' movements are interspersed. Perspiration covers the body, the face is blue or white as chalk; urine is voided; the pupils are fixed, the corneal reflex has gone; the patient does not react to stimuli but sometimes there is a certain unrest of the body after very strong and painful stimuli. The whole thing rarely lasts longer than five minutes. Often the seizure merges directly into deep sleep. On waking the patient is exhausted and weary. He complains of headache and is depressed; he does not remember the attack at all (there is total amnesia).'

The attack is the main symptom of the epilepsies. Seizures, however, occur not only in epilepsy but also in schizophrenia and almost all organic brain disorders. Seizures are essentially organic.[1] They are, therefore, quite different in kind from psychogenic attacks, which are very varied in appearance and have been artificially cultivated in all clinics up and down the country, particularly in the time of Charcot, Briquet and others in Paris, and have been the subject of elaborate description (attitudes passionelles).

2. *Organic dysfunctions.* Psychic events may now and then influence almost all physiological functioning of the organs. Under certain circumstances of a psychic nature, a particular experience or some long-lasting emotional state, there will follow: stomach and intestinal disturbances, cardiac disturbances, vasomotor disturbances, disturbances in secretion, disturbances of vision, hearing[2], voice[3], menstruation (cessation or premature commencement). In neurotic persons one often finds dysfunction which cannot be related to any

[1] Psychopaths show a rare reaction which has been described under the name 'affective epileptic seizure'. Bratz, 'Die affektepileptischen Anfälle der Neuropathen u. Psychopathen', *Mschr. Psychiatr.*, vol. 29 (1911), pp. 45, 162. Stahlmann, *Allg. Z. Psychiatr.*, vol. 68, p. 799.

[2] W. Kümmel, 'Entstehung, Erkennung, Behandlung u. Beurteilung seelisch verursachter Hörstörungen bei Soldaten', *Beitr. Anat. usw. Ohr usw.* (von Passov and Schaefer), vol 2 (1918), H. 1–3.

[3] K. Beck, 'Über Erfahrungen mit Stimmstörungen bei Kriegsteilnehmern', *Beitr. Anat. usw. Ohres usw.* (1918).

definite psychic event but which must have some connection with psychic abnormality, judging from the frequency with which the two go together.[1]

Many neurological phenomena belong to this group, where they appear without any organic base: paralyses and sensory disturbances (their configuration follows the imagination of the patient, not the anatomical structure), tics, contractures, tremor, vertigo etc. We should refer to the neurological texts for all the innumerable variations of these bodily phenomena, particularly in hysteria.[2]

One of the most striking effects of psychic commotion is the sudden greying of the hair, as reported by Montaigne; there is also the sudden appearance of an alopecia areata.[3] Psychogenic fever was for a long time doubted, but it must now be considered an established if rare phenomenon.[4]

In spite of the close psychic connection patients *regard* these somatic disturbances as something entirely alien, as if they were purely a physical illness. Hysterical phenomena can be observed appearing by themselves or accompanied by every kind of organic or functional disorder of the nervous system.

Most of these somatic disturbances are called *Organ-neuroses*. This does not mean that some organ can become neurotic of itself. It is the psyche that is neurotic; it, so to speak, chooses this or that organ and manifests its disturbance through it; it may be the organ itself is a *locus minoris resistentiae* and therefore more vulnerable or it may be that in the context of psychic meaning some particular organ appears 'symbolically' the more important. For a long time organ-neuroses were diagnosed far too freely. It was forgotten that the ground for such a diagnosis rested less on the positive findings but on the negative one of an absence of somatic findings. It was therefore correct to talk of the 'gradual reduction of the organ-neuroses' through the development of more exact methods of medical examination. The concept needed to be limited but not dropped entirely.[5]

This restriction of the organ-neuroses was accompanied by a development in the opposite direction: a growing recognition of the significance of psychic factors in disorders that were primarily somatic and organic.

---

[1] Wilmanns, *Die leichten Fälls des manisch-depressiven Irreseins u. ihre Beziehungen zu Störungen der Verdauungsorgane* (Leipzig, 1906). Dreyfus, *Nervöse Dyspepsie* (Jena, 1909). Homburger, 'Körperliche Störungen bei funktionellen Psychosen', *Dtsch. med. Wschr.*, vol. 1 (1909).

[2] Cf. Briquet, Charcot, Gille de la Tourette, Richer, Möbius, Babinski and the summary given by Binswanger, *Die Hysterie* (Vienna, 1904), and by Lewandowsky, *Die Hysterie* (Berlin, 1914).

[3] Poehlmann, *Münch. med. Wschr.*, vol. 2 (1915).

[4] Cp. Glaser, 'Zur Kenntnis des zerebralen Fiebers', *Z. Neur.*, vol. 17, p. 494. Summary by Lewandowsky, *Hysterie*, pp. 63 ff. 'Die Dissertation von Weinert,' *Über Temperatursteigerungen bei gesunden Menschen* (Heidelberg, 1912). This contains references from a related group of problems.

[5] von Bergmann, *Dtsch. med. Wschr.*, vol. 53 (1927), pp. 2057 ff. 'An old clinician has said that nine out of ten gastric patients have nervous dyspepsia; nowadays not even the inverse ratio is accepted.' 'The concept of neurosis or neurotic seems to me a comfortable way out in a vast number of cases where the full nature of the illness has not been properly understood.' 'In the majority of cases, the diagnosis of neurosis is in practice a wrong diagnosis.'

3. *Dependence of primary somatic disorders on the psyche.* Even organic disorders are not entirely independent of the psyche in their course. There is a
general acceptance of the fact that physical disorders may be influenced by
psychic factors. It is very difficult to separate what is determined physically
and what is determined psychically. The psyche looks for certain prepared
channels in the body to produce its pathological effects. If, for instance, pains
in the joints have existed due to a past arthritis these pains can be psychically
continued after recovery or they can be reinvoked. In nearly all physical illnesses the psychic state during the period of convalescence is by no means unimportant. Therefore what can be influenced by the psyche is not necessarily
a psychic condition nor need it be wholly psychogenic.

Another problem is whether organic illness accompanied by anatomical
changes can *have a psychogenic source.* It seems this can be so:

Glycosuria is common in states of anxiety and depression.[1] *Diabetes* can start
after some psychic commotion, and may be worsened through it.

Acute onset of *Basedow's diseases* has been observed following severe fright.
Kohnstamm[2] reports a case showing how big a part psychic complexes play in this
disorder. The onset may occur only a few hours after the fright but this is very rare.
Usually a long period of sorrow, worry or anxiety precedes the onset; the strong
psychic influences during its course have been universally accepted.[3]

*Colitis membranacea* (Mucous colitis) also may come on after psychic commotion
and can be cured by psychic means.

The general view is that *asthma,* though facilitated by a somatic disposition,
depends on psychic factors for its manifestation, course and cure. Medical research
has shown that somatic disposition and events are decisive but the attacks and onset
of the disorder can be precipitated psychically, and psychic factors may also be
responsible for cessation of attacks. The relationship here does not mean that the
psyche itself is disordered. Asthma like other physical accompaniments may be due
to normal psychic excitation. However, as only a relatively few people suffer from
asthma, we can best conceive it as a morbid somatic disposition and not a type of
psychogenic reaction as are the majority of somatic accompaniments.[4]

The view has been put forward that from a purely reactive, nervous stomach-
disturbance there can be a development through chronic functional anomalies into
*ulcus duodenale* (duodenal ulcer), so that a man who gets an ulcer as the result of
constant business strain might not have got it if he had lived a more restful life.

Alkan[5] gives some examples of how somatic effects that are at first functional may lead to organic, anatomic disorder:

Lasting contraction of the smooth muscles in the attacked area create pressure
and anaemia and thereby cause necrobiotic lesions, particularly so when the secretions at this point (the gastric juices) are psychogenically reinforced (as would be the
case with ulcus ventriculi and colitis ulcerosa).—Spasm in tubular organs leads

[1] Mita, *Mschr. Psychiatr.,* vol. 32, p. 159.     [2] Konnstamm, *Z. Neur.,* vol. 32, p. 357.
[3] Rahm, *Der Nervenarzt,* vol. 3 (1930), p. 9.     [4] Hansen, *Der Nervenarzt,* vol. 3, p. 513.
[5] Leopold Alkan, *Anatomische Organerkrankungen aus seelischer Ursache* (Stuttgart, Hippok-
rates-Verlag, 1930).

to muscular hypertrophy of the upper parts with dilatation (oesophageal dilatation, hypertrophy of left ventricle in hypertension). Lasting spasm or paroxysm in tubular organs leads to chemical changes in the accumulating secretions (single cholesterol stone in the gall-bladder, obstructive oesophagitis). When infection is added, which would not harm where the flow is free, inflammation will occur after obstruction. Psychogenic alteration in the secretion of the endocrine glands may lead to anatomical changes in the glands (psychogenic diabetes, and Basedow's disease).

The psychogenesis of organic disease is established only over a small field. We lack factual confirmation over a wide area. Latterly V. v. Weizsäcker[1] has posed some fundamental questions and tries enlarging them by case histories. He finds it hard to be convinced because firstly, positive and negative cases can be found side by side. For instance, if one finds positive evidence of psychogenicity in one case, the next case fails to show it and nothing psychic can be found of any importance. Secondly, we are ignorant of the significance of inner organs for psychic life, whether, for instance, the liver has anything at all to do with indignation and envy. Thirdly, the relationship between the physical and the psychic factors seems an extremely irregular one. He thinks, however, that in cases of angina tonsillaris, diabetes insipidus etc., it is possible to recognise how the illness plays some decisive role in the crucial moments of life. He does not intend to offer any insight which could be conceptualised and generally formulated; his subject-matter is purely biographical.

The influence the psyche exerts on organic illness may be very extensive. The subjective state can be improved by suggestion and hypnosis, and suggestion on its own is of utmost importance in all kinds of therapy. Objectively some surprising results have been achieved. The nexus of organic and psychic factors can strike one as grotesque. For instance Marx[2] reports a case from the Cushing clinic:

A 14-year-old boy is admitted with severe diabetes insipidus; he drinks up to 11 litres (22 pints) a day. It is found that the boy had started masturbation and felt that excessive drinking cleansed him and dissolved his conflict. Through psychoanalytic treatment he recovers to such an extent that he now only drinks about 1·5 litres. One morning he is found dead in his bed; post-mortem findings were a large tumour of the brain-stem. In this case the thirst, as a symptom of organic disturbance of the nervous system, became related to the instinctual life of the patient and to his thinking, in so far as he struggled to gain the mastery of his masturbation. The relationships were so tightly interwoven that because of it a therapeutic influence could be exerted both on the thirst and the polyuria.

4. *Functional disturbance of complex instinctive behaviour.* There are many physical functions which can be disturbed without the patient experiencing anything at the time of the disturbance other than what any patient may feel

[1] V. v. Weizsäcker, *Studien zur Pathogenese* (Leipzig, 1935).
[2] H. Marx, 'Innere Sekretion', *Handbuch der inneren Medizin*, von Bergman et al., vol. 6, 1, p. 422.

when confronted with a bodily discomfort. There are others, however, where complex functions are involved, and volition as well. Here the functional disturbance is in obvious relation to the psychic disturbance appearing at the same time. Functions cannot be carried out as the patient experiences anxiety, inhibition, sudden passivity feelings or confusion. The same thing happens whether he is walking, writing, urinating, or having sexual intercourse, etc. Writer's cramp, disturbance of micturition, sexual impotence or vaginismus are the result.

Traces of such disturbances are universal. One blushes, just when one does not want to, walks or talks awkwardly, when one thinks people are watching. Even reflexes can be influenced. Attracting attention may increase both coughing and sneezing reflexes, particularly the latter, but they can also be suppressed for the same reason. (Darwin's bet with his friends that snuff would no longer make them sneeze; they tried hard, tears came into their eyes, but Darwin won his bet.)

### (b) The origin of somatic disturbances

There is a very tangled relationship between the psyche and massive attacks, organ disturbance, and complex behavioral functions, even if sometimes it appears relatively simple in the individual case. In spite of what individually seems so plausible, the total relationship of body and psyche still remains obscure and extremely complex. Extra-conscious mechanisms are obviously numerous. Organs and physical predispositions have to meet the psyche half-way. It looks as if the psyche chooses the organs in which to manifest itself by dysfunction, or as if it chooses the functions into which its own disturbance can enter, like an interloper, as it were.

The several *physiological links* can to some extent be guessed: nowadays we view the autonomic nervous system together with the endocrine system as the media between the central nervous system, so closely linked with psychic events, and the body. This neuro-hormonal system regulates the activity of the organs outside our consciousness. Through the brain it must be accessible to the psyche and under certain circumstances far-reaching effects are possible. Those people whose autonomic nervous system is particularly excitable and responsive to the slightest psychic influence have been called by Bergmann 'vegetativ Stigmatisierte' (people with autonomic stigmatisation).

Many explanations have been offered in individual cases. Thus anaemia of the brain caused by contraction of the small cerebral arteries has been advanced to explain fainting for psychic reasons (through terror, sight of blood, overcrowded rooms, etc.).

The ways in which somatic disturbances arise lend themselves to the following descriptive schema:

1. A large number of organic dysfunctions occur purely *automatically*, such as palpitations, tremor and others. Examples are disturbances in the

digestive system after emotional upsets, abnormal subjective sensations, alteration in appetite, diarrhoea or constipation. We can only note them and record the phenomena as with the physical phenomena that accompany psychic events.

2. Somatic disturbances have a *tendency to become fixed* if they recur, and sometimes even if they only happen once. When psychic commotion has ceased, they linger on and the individual senses these disturbances as physical illness which recur on the most diverse occasions (habituation reactions); or a reaction which is roused for the first time by some powerful emotional event (localised pain, cramp) may recur later on when something of a similar kind is experienced, lesser in degree but reminiscent of the initial event (analogous to Pavlov's conditioned reflex).

Disturbance of function can develop and fixate in areas that by chance happen to be active during an affect. An upsetting message comes over the telephone, the hand holding the receiver feels as if paralysed, 'writer's cramp' sets in and so on. An actual tiredness caused by playing the piano and felt in the hands and arms becomes connected with affects of jealousy and competition and then appears as an independent complex of sensations which will arise on any occasion, e.g. when simply listening to music, should this also give rise to feelings of envy at another's ability.

3. In the foregoing cases there is no connection between the content of the psychic experience and the particular somatic effects. It is only that they appear together simultaneously. For an explanation one has to resort to increased or abnormal irritability due to the morbid state. There are, however, a large number of somatic phenomena, the *specific quality of which can be understood in terms of the experience, the situation or the personal conflict*. For example, unpleasant sensations and dysfunctions arise, which we term hypochondriacal, through specific attention being directed to a particular function, through careful observation of some slight disturbance perhaps, through definite worries and fearful anticipations. In the beginning such disturbances are only fears, in the course of time they become real. Such somatic disturbances, where the content can be understood in terms of the preceding psychic content, may also appear quite suddenly, e.g. paralysis of the arms after a fall, deafness after a slap, etc. These diverse phenomena have several things in common: (1) an *understandable* connection between cause and effect; (2) an effect on bodily functions that *otherwise are independent of our will and imagination*, e.g. sensation, menstruation, digestion; (3) the formation of a *vicious circle*. It seems that in healthy people the cycle of 'body-psyche-process of living' involves reflex increase in feeling through the somatic accompaniments of feeling, and a fuller realisation of meaning as feelings mount. With patients, everything (e.g. automatic and chance instinctual disturbances) can become the prey of psychic determinants which so modify it that the slightest disturbance may then turn into a serious illness. This mechanism is probably present in us all to

a slight degree and it is termed the *hysterical mechanism*. In some people it is more developed and dominates their whole life, in others it appears only when they are ill (e.g. in organic disorder) or under duress.

The term '*hysterical*' is used in a number of ways. *Psychogenic* is the broader concept. *Hysterical* is used for the fundamental characteristic of phenomena into which meaning has slipped, there is meaning but it is hidden, and there is some distortion, displacement, self-deception or deception of others involved. These dysfunctions are motivated by events that contain a dishonesty somewhere. The body then becomes an organ of double speech, and like speech is used to hide or disclose. This is done subconsciously, however, not consciously and only instinctual purpose is at work.

We can subsume these three groups under three commonplace categories: *automatic physical effects*, *fixed reactions* and *hysterical symptoms*. All three are closely related to each other. Purely automatic physical sequelae as well as hysterical symptoms can get fixated, and where somatic dysfunction becomes fixed through psychic stress, the hysterical component can hardly be distinguished from the purely automatic ones.

In the individual case we usually find ourselves dealing with all three factors which we can only separate out in theory or in the borderline case. The following is a case of Wittkower's:[1] 'An eighteen-year-old girl witnessed a railway disaster in which a worker was cut to pieces by a passing train. She felt nausea among all the excitement and did not eat for days; she vomited every morning during the first lesson at school. Since that time she has a railway phobia, anxiety and crying attacks. She also has compulsive phantasies about dismemberment in which she sees herself or a relative as the victim.'

The third group—*somatic phenomena which are understandable in a psychic context*—need fuller discussion. This does not apply so much to those that we have just discussed: (1) physical effects of anxious scrutiny, worry, fearful anticipation; (2) simultaneous linking of somatic events and psychic commotion on the first occasion and on repetition (analogous to Pavlov's conditioned reflex): e.g. a psychic trauma causes diarrhoea, vomiting, asthma, which can recur afterwards on the slightest stimulus; (3) detachment of what were originally psychically determined somatic phenomena, and their subsequent independent existence and development. The physiological aspect of this is still obscure but the psychological aspect is quite simple and clear.

The dependence of *vital processes* on *psychic mood* needs no further discussion either. The whole psychic condition, whether elated or hopeless, cheerful or depressed, tending to activity or withdrawal, plays on the somatic state uninterruptedly. We have long experienced the fact that illness, even that of organic origin, depends very greatly on psychic attitude, though it is hard to prove this in detail. The will to live, hope and courage are of the greatest importance. We can have the same experience in everyday life. Subjective

---

[1] Wittkower, *Nervenarzt*, vol. 3, p. 206.

tiredness is lost if the work is enjoyed. Fresh experiences and hopes can bring about an enormous increase in strength and effectiveness. The tired hunter springs to life when at last he sights his game.

In all these understandable phenomena we have tried to see the *specific somatic content as psychically meaningful*; we have tried to see the somatic event as an essential in the psychic and social context of the individual. In this the respective relationship between body and psyche has remained unconscious yet in principle open to consciousness; if the patient gains understanding of the connection, this reverts back with healing effect on the somatic phenomena, always provided there is a change in the psychic attitude along with the mere intellectual understanding. And here we have reached the field of interpretation which is most seductive but dangerous to enter. There is no doubt that fundamental knowledge may be gained here, but nowhere else do genuine evidence and gross deception go so closely together. A wealth of possible experience seems to offer itself but with it come confusing ambivalences and mistaken acceptances of the first interpretation that comes to hand.

Here are a few examples from the extensive literature which deals with these questions:

1. Hysterical phenomena in the narrower sense—paralyses, sensory disturbances, etc.—are connected with images, intentions and goals which have disappeared from consciousness. How they do this is difficult to understand but they are not completely inaccessible to consciousness. Simulations can lapse into hysteria, and then we should cease to talk of simulation.

2. This psychic rearrangement has been made comprehensible as an escape of psychic energy, e.g. the discharge of repressed sexual wishes, by means of a conversion into somatic phenomena which symbolically indicate the source. Alternatively the phenomena may serve as a displacement or substitute for direct but forbidden gratification (Freud).

3. The psychic unconscious events are further differentiated. The patient may punish himself by a symptom for some instinctual wish or act which is against his conscience; he may surrender his will, grow weak and unresistive and more readily accessible for any kind of illness to which he is exposed.

4. Organs have a language which expresses what the conscious will does not say: kidney haemorrhage, fluor albus, eczema of the vulva, are thought to be expressions of resentment against cohabitation and when the corresponding situation improves will vanish.

These are not objective relationships of body and psyche but have only been deduced. They are plausible and the time of onset and cessation of the trouble seems to indicate a possible connection and in many cases a certain one. Yet all this is still very far away from phenomena genuinely expressing an objective unity of body and psyche.

It has been asked why after emotional disturbances or long-lasting conflicts there seems to be some kind of *organ choice*: sometimes the heart and the circulation, sometimes the intestinal tract, sometimes the organs of respiration.

The accepted answer is that there is some organ inferiority, either constitutional or due to illness, that is the organ is in some way prepared, a locus minoris resistentiae, which meets the distress half-way. A gall-bladder disorder will channel the likelihood for breakdown.

Heyer[1] goes beyond this and gives quite a different answer:

Somatic states which may be psychically conditioned are:—in the intestinal tract, nausea, swallowing of air; in the circulation, anxious tension; in the respiratory system, asthma, phrenocardia. All these states are of symbolic significance; they are not only experienced physically but are felt to be meaningful.

Organs are *hidden speech* which the psyche understands and through which it talks. *Vomiting* is an expression of resentment (Napoleon is said to have vomited when told he would be taken off to St. Helena). *Air-swallowing* means to swallow down something, e.g. something humiliating, which one cannot contest. *Anxiety* means one is afraid for one's own life, for its very basis, for its full realisation. *Asthma* means one cannot stand the air, that is the atmosphere which has arisen through situations, conflicts and particular people in particular places. *Phrenocardia* (heart-neurosis) in which the diaphragm contracts and pain and palpitation follow, means a fixation of inspiration, a kind of tension not followed by release. (In the sexual act, tension and excitement are not followed by release and satisfaction.) In all these the person expresses some actual unbearable aspect of his life symbolically through his organs without knowing that he does so.

To try and reach clear understanding, Heyer distinguished what he called *life-spheres*: the *vegetative sphere* (digestive system); the *sphere of animal life* (life of the blood; blood, heart and circulation)—the *respiratory sphere* (breathing). Each sphere has a specific nature which is connected symbolically with psychic actualities. 1. 'The intestinal life is plant-like, peaceful and dark, deeply unconscious, the basis of existence.' Through this intestinal life movements travel in waves, much as the waves of the seasons pass through nature. 2. 'The life of the blood is that of hot passions, affects, of temperament and of instinct; it is the sphere of the sexual drives.' The dominating movement here is not of waves but of contraction and expansion. We can compare the life of the roaming and hunting animal. 3. Respiration also has a polarised nature; there are sequences of tension and relaxation, very close to a moment of ego-life. 'The light, easy quality of the breath, its relation to air and ether gives us a feeling of height, freedom, limitlessness, which we receive hardly at all from the vegetative and animal spheres of our being.' The bird is a symbol for air and breath.

The different life-spheres (organ-systems of digestion, circulation and respiration) are thus linked with certain 'basic', 'archaic' or 'universal' feelings which always preserve their separate character. Thus conversely 'these specific psychic movements express themselves through the corresponding organ-system'. We will confine ourselves to the main example given: In the circulation, the carrier of the animal life of drive and passion, the basic dysfunction is anxiety, arising through the infirmity of the elements of life (as in coronary sclerosis, anaemia, etc.) and through suppression of the blood, that is of urge and passion. Anxious tension is the person's loss of unity with the animal in his blood, he feels anxiety lest the animal in him has grown too weak, or anxiety lest it may be too powerful and devour him. Therefore

[1] Gustav R. Heyer, *Der Organismus der Seele* (München, 1932).

these are 'circulation-neuroses' which occur 'not only in people who do not follow the will of the blood (or of their sexuality) and repress it, but in those equally who dissipate their mental self in nature'. These neuroses of circulation therefore are fostered in 'conflicts with the untried world of earth and urge' no less than in a neglect of 'the illuminating human mind'.

This quotation shows how theories of this sort weave a complex web of concepts: (1) vital, physiological relationships, such as that between the heart and anxiety, sexuality and anxiety; (2) possible symbolic interpretations in which organs are experienced as a symbol for what is psychic; (3) a mystical symbolism, in which expression is given to a metaphysical interpretation of life. The interweaving of these heterogeneous elements is not without its charm, but from the scientific point of view it is insufferable. A vast inextricable confusion is created from obvious empirical facts, which are extremely difficult to isolate and grasp clearly. Patterns of possible experiences, of understandable connections with somatic phenomena, are mixed up with speculative meta-physical and cosmic interpretations. What emerges as true is only the general, indefinite reminder that the occurrence of a body–psyche relationship and all the facts that demonstrate it cannot be even approximately exhausted by our customary simple schemata and most certainly cannot be sufficiently compre-hended in this way. There is no scientific value in this psychotherapeutically nourished, fantastic configuration, justified though it may be as a negative kind of appeal against being too satisfied with the simplicities of physiological causation.

v. Weizsäcker's far-reaching studies on the subject of psychic pathogenesis in severe organic illness are wide open to this kind of interpretation, without his being necessarily in full agreement with it. Sometimes he seems to adopt it but he is careful to refrain from any too precise interpretation, being in favour of a biological approach, in which somatic events play a part in the dramatic unrolling of the psychic and social situation, but his study offers no universal fixed form of understandable connection, which could be used to provide a scientific theory of causation. His case-histories can be read with some wonder; it seems that anything is possible, but in the end we know as little as when we started.

## § 3. SOMATIC FINDINGS IN PSYCHOSIS

The final group of somatic symptoms to be observed in patients cannot up to now be related to anything psychic whatsoever. They are rather physical signs of morbid physical processes which are perhaps at the same time the source of the psychic illness, or at any rate are in some relation to it. These are not symptoms of definite physical disease (cerebral processes) but we will class them as somatic signs, physical symptoms of psychosis, without being able to recognise them as signs of any known disorder. Thus first and foremost in the group of the schizophrenias we have to record certain increased reflexes, changes in the pupils, oedema, cyanosed hands and feet, strong, peculiar smelling perspiration, the 'greasy face', pigmentations and trophic disturbances. All that can be directly observed has long been methodically complemented by special findings: for instance, body-weight, amenorrhea. In the last ten years physiological investigation has been pursued with all the refinements of modern medicine. Some of the findings are random findings accumulated into a limitless host; others provide a clear picture of the somatic phenomena produced by the physiological processes in psychosis. Here are a few examples:

## (a) Body-weight

Fluctuations in *body-weight* can reach an extraordinary degree with schizophrenic patients; it is a somatic symptom of varying significance. There may be a fall into complete emaciation and deep marasmus in the acute psychoses and a great gain in weight during convalescence from the acute phase, so that changes in body-weight may be an important indication of which way the illness is going. The increase in weight takes place during the return to health as well as at the start of the lasting state of dementia which can follow after an acute phase. (Increase in weight without any psychic improvement is therefore an ominous symptom.) In the latter case there is sometimes a notable over-eating, and a bloated, fat habitus. Loss of weight is seen in severe psychic shock, in worry and in long-lasting depressive states, and in nervous disturbances of all kinds (loss of 20 lb. or more). In the particular case it is not easy to decide how far the change in body-weight is an accompaniment of a morbid physical process that is also responsible for the psychic disturbances, and how far this change is a direct consequence of psychic events themselves. It seems that both types of relationship are there. I used to observe a patient with a traumatic neurosis who always lost several kilo. during his stays in hospital, in spite of eating the excellent food, perhaps because the situation always caused him extreme distress.

Reichardt[1] investigated the relationship between body-weight and cerebral or psychotic illnesses. He found body-weight and mental state showed a far-reaching independence, so that no definite correlations could be established. For instance, he observed severe fluctuations in some acute psychoses, but in general he found the weight-curve stationary in states of mental deficiency and end-states; frequent endogenous increases and decreases of weight in brain diseases, for instance, in paralyses, and a particular, excessive weight-loss in catatonic syndromes. As distinct from those that last over long periods, brief fluctuations in weight have been found to be due to fluctuations in water retention.

[1] Reichardt, *Untersuchungen über das Gehirn* (Jena, 1912), Part 2, 'Hirn u. Körper'. O. Rehm, 'Über Körpergewicht u. Menstruation bei. akuten u. chronischen Psychosen', *Arch. Psychiatr.* (D), (1919), vol. 61, p. 385.

*(b) Cessation of menses*

This occurs frequently in psychosis. Haymann[1] found it took place as follows:

| | | |
|---|---|---|
| in paranoia . . . . . . . . | 0% | of cases |
| in hysteria, psychopathic and degenerative states . | 11% | ,, |
| in manic-depressive insanity . . . . . | 34% | ,, |
| in dementia praecox . . . . . . | 60% | ,, |
| in paranoid types . . . . . . . | 36% | ,, |
| in hebephrenic types . . . . . . | 50% | ,, |
| in catatonic types . . . . . . . | 93% | ,, |
| in paralysis, tumours and other organic brain disorders | 66–75% | ,, |

Menstruation disappears in the majority of cases only after the psychic symptoms have appeared. In a large number of cases cessation of menstruation coincides with the onset of a loss in weight. When weight increases, the menses reappear. (This is so whether there is recovery or a final defect state.)

*(c) Endocrine disturbances*

In scattered cases the Cushing-syndrome is found with schizophrenia. As the latter progresses, the former tends to vanish. A hypophyseal tumour had been excluded. This finding only shows that schizophrenic processes tend to invade the field of hormonal activity.[2]

*(d) Systematic physiological investigations to find clinical pictures with typical somatic pathology*

Numerous metabolic investigations have been made, examinations of the blood, analyses of the urine, etc., but they all so far show equivocal findings. In some circumstances they may give valuable hints but for the most part they tend to be interminable and barren of results. In some cases of schizophrenia, for example, particularly with catatonia, and also in paralytic stupor, the metabolism was found to be slowed down. Other findings have been elicited with the help of modern metabolic studies of the pathology in such conditions as paralysis, schizophrenia, epilepsy, circular psychosis.

The unusually painstaking and thorough work of *Gjessing*[3] opened a new chapter. He did not set out to collect a large amount of data in order to make statistical comparison (such a method can only give indications, but is not any use as a research method itself). Instead he made a series of investigations of a few patients daily over a long period of time, so that he could observe changes

---

[1] Haymann, 'Menstruationsstörungen bei Psychosen', *Z. Neur.* (1913), vol. 15, p. 511.

[2] S. Voss, 'Das Cushingsche Syndrome als Initialerscheinung bei Schizophrenie', *Z. Neur.*, vol. 165.

[3] R. Gjessing, 'Beiträge zur Kenntnis der Pathophysiologie des. katatonen Stupors usw.', *Arch. Psychiatr.* (D), (1932), vol. 96, p. 319, 393; (1936), vol. 104, p. 355; (1939), vol. 109, p. 525.

in their physical state and compare these with changes in their psychosis. He did not try to investigate a single physiological phenomenon but a composite whole, which included examination of the blood, urine, faeces, metabolism etc. Lastly he selected his individual cases carefully; there had to be an absolutely definite diagnosis and they had to be typical cases and show an individual suitability for investigation. He gives exact reports on individual cases. Among them are a few, very conspicuous, classic cases:

Catatonic stupor starts suddenly; the emergence from it is critical. In the pre-stupor state there is slight motor restlessness. During the waking period he found diminished B.M.R. and a diminished pulse rate, lowered blood-pressure, reduced blood-sugar, leucopenia, and lymphocytosis; retention of nitrogen. (This picture occurring during the waking period Gjessing called the 'retentionsyndrome'.) As stupor began he found: marked, autonomic fluctuations (change in size of pupils, pulse rate, colour of face, perspiration, muscle-tone). During the stuporose period he found: raised basic metabolic rate, raised pulse rate, blood-pressure, blood-sugar; slight hyperleukocytosis, increased nitrogen secretion. (Gjessing called this picture 'the compensation syndrome'.) Symptoms returned periodically alternating with the stupor that lasted 2–3 weeks.

Gjessing found similar phenomena in states of catatonic excitement. Many cases of stupor and excitement however follow an altogether irregular course. The author always found that there was retention of nitrogen, autonomic changes, nitrogen excretion—with the nitrogen retention occurring during the waking period.

The idea is to obtain a physiological-chemical syndrome which will show some inner consistency and correlate with definite forms of catatonic stupor and excitement. Gjessing refrains from causal explanation (whether the psyche or the soma is the determining factor). He only suggests that we are dealing with the results of periodic stimulation of the brain-stem. In abnormal states the waking nitrogen retention is reversed; during stupor or excitement, there is as it were a recovery from nitrogen retention.

After this there were further investigations and new problems were demonstrated. This was all very different from the kind of disease entities usual in general medicine but without any corresponding morbid findings of a causal nature.

Jahn and Greving[1] found concentration of the blood, increased formation of red blood-cells (increase of erythrocytes and of early forms: the marrow of the long bones in section showed red instead of yellow) with a reduced destruction of red blood-cells—a unique finding. They attributed this finding along with the other somatic findings to a flooding of the blood with some poison—a poisonous substance stemming from the albumen metabolism which had the same effect as histamine in animal experiments. The cases concerned were the cases of fatal catatonia which had already been described at some length.

[1] Jahn and Greving, 'Untersuchungen über die körperlichen Störungen bei. katatonen Stuporen u. der tödlichen Katatonie', Arch. Psychiatr. (D), (1936), vol. 105, p. 105.

The classical picture of *fatal catatonia* was described as follows:[1] Unlimited motor restlessness appears to increase without inhibition to the point of self-destruction, while the physical strength develops tremendously. There is severe acrocyanosis. The moist skin of the extremities is cold and shows many places where pressure or knocks have caused confluent petichiae which soon turn into yellow spots. The initially raised blood-pressure falls; the excitement settles down. The patients lie weakly in bed with an expression of inner tension and sometimes with clouded consciousness. Although the skin is cold, the body temperature may be raised to 40° C. Section does not give any clear picture of the cause of death and no changes which would point us to any important cause of the illness.

K. Scheid[2] describes another picture, in schizophrenia: He found marked increase of sedimentation rate at certain periods coupled with high temperature, and the symptom of increased rate of formation and destruction of red-blood corpuscles. Both new formation and destruction generally kept in balance; when haemolysis was stormy, there was a marked anaemia. There were no signs of any serious physical disorder underlying the febrile episode.

We are always dealing with particular pictures or some narrowly circumscribed type, never with a recognition of the somato-pathology of schizophrenia as a whole. Comprehensive laws are therefore not to be found, and we are left with the rarity of the classical case and the many current contradictions. For instance, Jahn and Greving find a lack of blood-destruction in fatal catatonia while K. F. Scheid[3] found an increased blood-destruction in catatonic episodes; a lowering of the haemoglobin content and the appearance of breakdown products of haemoglobin.

It is natural to think of a physical disorder which conducts itself basically like all other physical disorders. *In support of this* are the severe somatic symptoms and, on the psychological side, the similarity between schizophrenic experiences and experiences with mescalin (and other poisons). This points to some agent, which will be discovered eventually as the cause. *Against* such a hypothesis however are the lack of pathological anatomical findings which would indicate the cause and, in addition, the unusual deviations in the somatic findings, such as the type of circulatory disorder which is present. The fresh findings are impressive. Their significance is not yet clear. A decisive factor is whether the same disorder can in principle occur in animals or whether the whole illness is specifically human. In any case it is a phenomenon of human nature, a process in that substratum of human life where psyche and soma are as yet inseparable.

[1] Stauder, *Arch. Psychiatr.* (D), vol. 102, p. 614.
[2] K. Scheid, *Febrile Episoden bei. schizophrenen Psychosen* (Leipzig, 1937). Cf. 'Die Somato-pathologie der Schizophrenie', *Z. Neur.* (1938), vol. 163, p. 585.
[3] K. F. Scheid, *Nervenarzt.*, vol. 10, p. 228.

## CHAPTER IV

# MEANINGFUL OBJECTIVE PHENOMENA

*Introduction.* Meaningful objective phenomena are what we term the sensory phenomena which we understand as expressions of the psyche. They consist of the human physiognomy (shape and countenance), involuntary gestures, speech and writing, artistic productions and conscious purposeful behaviour. These phenomena are, however, highly heterogeneous and are scarcely comparable. Thought, art and purposeful actions have an objective meaning which is not a psychological one as such and any understanding we may have of it does not necessarily imply an understanding of the psyche. We can for example understand the meaning of a sentence in a rational way without necessarily understanding the man who utters it; we need not even think of him. There is an objective world of the mind in which we move without thinking of the psyche at all and from this springs the spirit of enquiry into psychological matters. Hence we divide our meaningful phenomena into several different spheres:

1. The human psyche is expressed through the body and its movements. This *expression* is involuntary. It becomes objective to the observer but not to the individual who is thereby understood (Section I).

2. The individual lives in *his own personal world*—by means of his attitudes, behaviour, actions and the shape he gives to his environment and social relations. What he is appears in his actions and in his activity and these provide him with a known content (Section II).

3. The individual *objectifies this content* for himself in speech, productive work and ideas which form a world of the mind. He takes a firm hold on what he has materially understood, produced, created and intends to create (Section III).

These three spheres signify contents which concern us not only from the psychological point of view; in fact to begin with there is no psychological interest at all. If we are to study them psychologically this requires first of all an inward appropriation of these contents and an unerring capacity to perceive them with understanding. Apart from this there are no limits to such a study. The highest mental creation can still be questioned as to its psychic origins; what involuntary elements are being expressed, what is its effect on the psychic life and what significance has it as a footing for the psyche, etc.? The realm of the understandable is of course not exhausted by this psychic aspect of the understandable and we should remember that from other points of view the mind is regarded as a world of meaning divorced from the psyche and the human individual considered a free and rational creature. However, as psychopathologists we are only interested in the understanding of objective meaning in so far as this is a precondition for our psychological understanding of such a meaning as it exists in the psyche of an actual individual. In the psychology of expression indeed the direct perception of another person through what he sees and says depends entirely on the cultural breadth of the psychopathologist's personality. It is not surprising that many content themselves with ordinary trivialities while others feel very much the limitation of their understanding and access to other minds. Confronted with the individual they grasp a good deal yet they do not penetrate completely and a certain reserve descends.

In all three spheres of meaningful objective phenomena we can observe certain particular elements that belong essentially to a whole which is not visible to us in the same way as a single objective fact. As regards the phenomena of expression, this whole is the unconscious *Formniveau* (Klages—level of development); as regards the existence of the individual in his own world, it is the *configuration* or '*gestalt*' of this world (Weltgestalt) and as regards the objectification of ideas through knowledge and productivity, it is the *total consciousness of a single mind*.

Each sphere has its own particular principle, but for the most part all three go together. All three, for instance, have something of the expressive character that is the dominant principle of the first sphere. When a thought-content, purpose or practical intention exists objectively in the world, we find that from the psychological point of view there is no such thing as mere reason or pure purpose. All psychic manifestations are pervaded by an expressive atmosphere: thoughts are spoken in a certain way, there is the tone of voice and the style of speech; goals are obtained in a certain way, there is a particular kind of body-movement or a particular individual mode of behaviour matched to the concrete situation. Further it is just this person who has this thought, has just this or that purpose, reflecting perhaps an expression of personality or some particular pattern of mood. 'Performance' which in itself is not expressive takes on in the individual an expressive aspect: motility is harnessed to expressive movement, speech acquires expressive personal tone and form, the working-performance becomes a personal gesture through its rhythm and style.

Let us remind ourselves of the basic classifications of individual phenomena: subjective phenomena—experiences—which are studied by *phenomenology*; objective phenomena, either meaningless or meaningful; if the former they are studied by *somato-psychology*; if the latter, we either assess and measure them as performances (*performance-psychology*) or we understand them, either as human expression (the *psychology of expression*) or as life in a particular world (the *psychology of the personal world*) or as mental productions (the *psychology of creativity*).

We have a psychological need to give things *objectivity and meaning*, and in addition our intentions are always based on something unintentional and impulsive. This primary impulsiveness can be differentiated into:

1. An *urge to expression* in the narrow sense of involuntary, undirected 'giving vent' to psychic stirrings. The degree of expressive facility differs in the individual and in the race.

2. An urge *to present the self* which brings an element of half-intention, since the individual validates himself in the presentation either for some real or imaginary onlooker or for himself alone. This self-presentation is a basic human characteristic and an indispensable and positive factor in everyone's life. But there can be self-deception; form, setting and gesture are then no longer a direct outcome of living but take on a life of their own. As a string of shifting immediacies or in the shape of some rigid mask they come to sub- stitute for life itself.

3. *A need for communication*—human beings desire to relate themselves to others in mutual understanding. At first there is only the need to understand objective contents, ideas directed to objects, practical purposes and practical theories. Later the person needs to communicate himself. Language is found by the individual ready-made, a remarkable, enigmatic instrument of com- munication for him to use.

4. *An urge to activity*, to direct behaviour and grasp the situation and every- thing that is waiting to be done. But whichever direction this primary impulsiveness takes it will always be associated with meaning and thus dis- tinguished from the purely vital drives.

For all meaningful phenomena the rule holds that most is to be learnt from *cases that are unusual, well differentiated and complex*. These illuminate the rest and experience is enriched not so much by the number of cases we have seen as by the depth to which we have penetrated in any one case. Individual cases, therefore, have a principle of importance which is essentially different from what they have in the somatic sphere where it is always 'a case of . . .' In the psychological study of expression, the single case can be of exceptional importance simply as an example on its own.

## SECTION ONE

## EXPRESSION OF THE PSYCHE THROUGH BODY AND MOVEMENT

### (PSYCHOLOGY OF EXPRESSION—AUSDRUCKSPSYCHOLOGIE)

*(a) Somatic accompaniments and psychic expression*

When we speak of somatic accompaniments of psychic events we simply register a relationship (for example, between fear and dilatation of pupils). We register it and make it part of our knowledge. But if we speak about the expression of psychic events, we imply that we understand the somatic phenomena in terms of what the psyche wishes to express, e.g. laughter is an immediate understanding of something funny. Expressive phenomena are always *objective*, in so far as they can be perceived by the senses, and manifest themselves as matters of fact, which can be photographed or recorded. On the other hand, they are always *subjective* since actual perception of them does not make them expressive; this comes only when there has been understanding of their meaning and importance. Insight into expressive phenomena requires therefore rather different evidence beyond the simple registration of purely objective physical facts. It has been said that all our understanding of expression rests on conclusions drawn by analogy from one's own psychic life and applied to that of others. Conclusions by analogy are a myth. The fact is rather that we understand quite directly, without any need for reflection; we understand in a lightning flash, at the very moment of perception. We understand an expression we have never seen in ourselves (it could be that it is a future man who studies himself in a mirror). Then there is the fact that children who cannot yet speak will understand gesture. Lastly, even animals understand expression to a limited extent. The psychological process of empathy has been invoked to explain the understanding of expression. Whether this explanation is true or false, it remains a psychological problem, not a methodological one. The phenomenon of understanding expression is always a direct one, our consciousness recognises in it something final and immediately objective. We do not see ourselves in the other person but the other person or his meaning as existing in their own right, the other's experience, which in that form we have never had. All the same we are *not to take* understanding of expression as *something simply right and valid just because of its immediacy*. Even in the case of mere sense-perception this is not so; each particular is governed by our knowledge as a whole; and there are deceptions in the sensory sphere. It is the same with the understanding of expression, except that deceptions are more numerous and control more difficult—conclusions by analogy come secondarily; each individual expression is capable of many possible meanings and only understandable in relation to some whole. We also show a wide range of difference in the vividness and breadth of our understanding of expression. Understanding is linked with one's own possibilities of experience, one's own history, and one's own measure of learning, its width, depth and general complexity. For this reason we find that where there is a certain mental poverty, there tends to be a denial that the understanding of expression can have any validity. There is a commonplace use of it and a certain violence done to it within the confines of the individual's prejudices. We must not forget that any knowledge we may have of the psychic life of others has come to us through the understanding of expression. Performances, as such, somatic accompaniments as such, even our understanding of mental content as something merely objective, all teach us to recognise the psyche but only from outside.

A *basic mistake in method* is to *confuse our concepts*; for instance, calling all somatic accompaniments and sequelae the phenomena of expression. It is true they are this but only in so far as they can be 'understood' as psychic expression, as in a gesture. Increased intestinal peristalsis prompted by affective changes is not an expressive movement but simply a synergic accompaniment. The frontier of understandable expression is not well demarcated. Dilated pupils as phenomena of fear are not 'understood' by us, but if we know of this fact and notice it several times, this knowledge seems a direct perception of fear in the pupils; this is only so, however, if the fear is simultaneously grasped as a genuine expression. A dilated pupil as such has no inner link with fear in our minds. It can have other causes, atropine, for example, which come to mind just as quickly. Similarly if someone constantly needs to go to the lavatory. In the appropriate situation and with other genuine expressive phenomena present we know that some strong affect is at work; otherwise we would be inclined to think in terms of some purely physical disturbance.

### (b) Understanding the expression

We perceive in form and movement a direct manifestation of psychic events or psychic mood. If we reflect on this type of seeing we are bound to doubt its importance for the comprehension of empirical reality. We are making use of a symbolism that is universal; we are seeing quite directly everyone's person and movements of adaptation, not as mere mathematical quantities nor as sensory qualities, but as something living, carriers of mood and significance. For clarity's sake it is as well to review *the different ways in which we see shape and form*:

To begin with we need to extract some clear forms for observation out of all the confusion of the phenomena, and to look for favourable conditions in which to descry what we may call the basic phenomena, basic configurations, simple forms, etc. Next, there is need for analysis. We need to see what these configurations are, how they change, develop and summate into a whole. Here the path of investigation diverges.

Either we resort to *mathematics*, that is think or build constructs in terms of quantities and derive our basic forms in this way. If successful, we become as it were a second creator of forms and shapes, which we contrive, handle and survey. Knowledge thus gained is thought of in mechanistic terms, limits are set and endlessness controlled by the use of mathematical formulae.

Or we try to stay close to *the real shapes and forms*, which will not submit to mathematical handling because their nature is infinite. We study morphology (Goethe), observe the growth of forms and their endless transformations, try and help ourselves with diagrams, and delineate types. But we use all these simply as pointers on the way, so that we can find some language for nature's 'blueprints', the primary configurations, whether of animals or plants, without making any attempt to deduce them (a mistake Haeckel made in his general morphology). The basic forms are not spatial and therefore subject to mathematical definition as such, but they are shapes that live. Their inner structure which can be mathematically explained is only one of their aspects. Morphology is not deductive but tries to lead us towards a pure apperception through a process of dynamic and structured seeing.

What we see in this way is the totality of basic characteristics belonging to the spatial phenomena of our environment. Clear vision is always accompanied by a 'feeling'—an overtone, betokening *the meaning, the sense of the forms, their psyche.* Something inward, as it were, reveals itself directly present in the external form, whether this is the aesthetic–ethical effect of mere colour or at the other extreme the emotional appeal of animal forms or the human shape.

We would like to put this 'soul of things', their psychic quality, into words, understand it, and make it a fruitful concept at which we have arrived methodically. The path of investigation diverges once more.

Either we mistranslate this quality into a rational meaning, something we can know, and we say that things, forms and movements signify something. The '*signatura rerum*' then represents a physiognomy of the universe of which we can make use to control everything through an immense system of meanings in which things are simply the signs. This leads us to a superstitious pseudo-science, the rationalism of which offers a striking analogy to the mechanistic explanations of the world, which it successfully applies, but it differs from these in the fundamental deceptions on which it rests and its lack of general validity (e.g. astrology, medical pharmacology derived from the 'signatura rerum', etc.).

Alternatively, we can stay close to the '*soul of things*', their psychic quality. No interpretations are made but we open our senses to living experience, to the perception of the inward element in things. Goethe's 'pure reflective gaze' accompanies a contemplation of form which *does not know but sees,* and this vision of the inward life of things (Klages uses the term 'Bilder') forms the substance of our union with the world. This union may be of unlimited depth; it comes as a gift with every step we take and cannot be methodically developed; it remains bound up with everything that reveals itself to a receptive attitude and an unfeigned preparedness to accept. This mode of perceiving with its empirical clarity comes to us late in time. Hitherto it has been embedded in superstition and delusion and it has been continually exposed to self-defeating efforts at defence through rational argument and systematic theory, which has attempted to bring it within the boundaries of reason.

The understanding of expression has its place within this universal world of psychic perception, this 'vision of the soul of things'. The psychic quality, the inward element, can be seen in the outward form and movement of the *human body,* made visible to us as expression. But this psychic quality is something radically different from the psyche of the nature-myths. Psychic expression as we understand it in men is something *empirically real.* It is accessible to us, present as something that *responds;* we treat it as an *empirically real force.* The decisive question then arises; which phenomena are an expression of real pyschic life, which are merely conditioned by chance somatic events? And which are only an expression in the sense that a branch has a form, the cloud has a shape, and water has a flow? Sensitivity for form and movement is a precondition for our perceiving *expression at all,* but something more is needed if this is to develop into any knowledge of an *empirical psychic reality.*

It is easy to give a theoretical answer. *Empirical confirmation* is first achieved by making a demonstrable relation between the expression as understood and the rest of human reality accessible to us in speech, etc. Secondly, we can test one phenomenon of expression against another, and thirdly we can constantly relate every particular to some whole. The understanding of expression is the same as general understanding, in that the particulars may be meagre and deceptive and can only be rightly understood in terms of the whole which they have gone to form. This is the natural round of understanding and the psychology of expression follows the same rule.

Understanding of expression becomes most questionable when applied to individuals as a science of character. Anyone may come across this if he has had anything to do with graphology or with the study of physiognomy and gesture. Such studies when concretely applied are nearly always impressive, seem to succeed by inspiration and, though fashions fluctuate, are warmly acclaimed. In individual cases the interpretation is usually compelling unless the environment is especially critical. This seems due among other things to the fact that meaningful opposites are always linked and something is always right provided one can find the right dialectic in which to express it. There is also nearly always something striking in the person's mood or nature, which only needs to be emphasised and expanded verbally. Lastly one may be lucky and hit on something very personal, and the matters that are not correct are quickly forgotten. Our first acquaintance with characterology, graphology or the study of physiognomy may seem something of a revelation and especially seductive because such methods are often linked with some kind of natural philosophy. If we can avoid the seduction without losing sight of the genuine impulses which are part of it, we have made a step towards science and a liberal philosophy. The first basic experience of disillusion comes when, with graphology for instance, we find the most superficial of efforts is met with the most enthusiastic acceptance. We have to experience such embarrassing situations before we can be properly critical as psychologists.

## (c) *Techniques of investigation*

We can investigate the phenomena of expression in two different ways:

1. We can explore the *extra-conscious mechanisms* which condition the expression. In the case of speech we know of *disturbances* in the extra-conscious apparatus, appearing in the form of motor and sensory aphasia. Corresponding disturbances, known as amimia and paramimia, occur with gesture. For instance, when the patient wants to say 'yes' by nodding his head, he opens his mouth, but he cannot find the right movement. Finally, there may be spontaneous excited gestures which are not any expression of psychic states but only disturbances in the extra-conscious apparatus. Thus in certain cerebral diseases (in pseudo-bulbar palsy, for instance) we can recognise a forced laughter and crying following any kind of stimulus. In such cases, the neurologist is investigating disturbances in the extra-conscious apparatus of expressive movement. It is of course possible to do this with normal functioning if we record the movements exactly as if they were somatic accompaniments and analyse their somatic function. Duchenne[1] tried to do this with different kinds of facial expression, comparing them with the effects of electric stimulation

[1] Duchenne, *Mécanisms de la Physiognomie humaine* (1862).

of individual muscle groups. He wanted to find out which groups were concerned in each case. Similarly with the help of Kraepelin's writing-balance, it was possible to show that in the simple movement of making a full-stop, every individual has a specific and constant pressure-curve. Sommer demonstrated the movement of the face muscles during mimicry.[1]

2. The above gives us some knowledge of the extra-conscious mechanisms; we also add to our technical equipment for the recording of expressive movement (use of camera, film, tracing, etc.). But we have not added anything to our knowledge of the psyche. The second and more properly psychological investigation of expressive phenomena sets out to do just this. It hopes to *extend 'understanding'* beyond *this point.* In everyday life we all have the common experience of understanding expression and the investigation aims at making such understanding conscious; it seeks to increase and deepen it and delineate it properly. Something like this is clearly possible if we take an unprejudiced look at graphology. Much that is new can be learnt from handwriting—even though it is only one of the many modes of expression.

Some *technical preconditions* are needed for the deliberate study of expression and for any planned attempt to extend our understanding: *material has to be secured* from the stream of phenomena and collected in some way so that comparisons may be made at any time. Movements are very difficult to get hold of—they can only be filmed and this limits matters very much. In moments of psychic import the apparatus is not at hand or would be too disturbing. We have to fall back on description and on repeated observation of new cases as far as one can get repetition in this way. Sometimes we may make use of drawing. *Handwriting* has an advantage in that if the writer is relatively fluent it offers complicated movements that can be compared at any time. The bodily shape, the physiognomy, may be dealt with best by photography but even here we run into considerable difficulties.

We can see that only some of the phenomena of expression can be recorded by means other than description. Yet *clear and methodical description* is the first condition for any truly scientific grasp which will make the immediate understanding of expression conscious, control and expand it. In graphology scientific development became possible through the technically skilful, objective, complex and quite unpsychological analysis of the form of the handwriting (see Preyer's work); in the same way the scientific study of physiognomy was developed through accurate description of body-shape.

*(d) Summary*

Phenomena of expression may be divided as follows: (1) Material for the *study of physiognomy*: This is a study of facial and bodily form (body-build) in so far as both may be understood as the expression of a psychic life, manifesting itself in them. (2) Material for the *study of involuntary gesture*: This is a study of the actual changing facial and bodily movements, which are unquestionably an immediate expression of psychic events and rapidly come and go. (3) Material for the *study of graphology*: In handwriting the investigating

[1] Cf. Trotsenburg, 'Über Untersuchung von Handlungen', *Arch. Psychiatr.* (D), vol. 62, p. 728. Record of hand-pressure as a time-sequence in various individuals and under various conditions.

psychologist has before him a movement of gesture that has so to speak been 'frozen' and can therefore be examined all the more easily.

## § 1. THE STUDY OF PHYSIOGNOMY

This is the most problematic field of expression, and doubts have been felt whether it can even be considered as such. It should only deal with the persistent features of the physiognomy which have come about through expressive movements and appear as a *frozen gesture* (e.g. 'folds of thought' on the forehead). Only such phenomena allow for understanding. They can to some extent be portrayed as expressive gestures, and have no particular principle of their own.

If the psychiatrist thinks of the characteristic appearance of many of his patients, which often suggests his diagnosis at first sight, very little of this will strike him as the expression of anything psychic. *None* of the phenomena which reveal the *somatic process* in the *habitus* belong *to the field of psychic expression*:

e.g. the plump, swollen forms of myxoedema; signs of paralysis in the face, the limbs and the speech in G.P.I.; the tremor, sweating, high colour and puffiness of delirium tremens; the miserable, physical habitus of psychoses where there is severe physical illness; the emaciation, wrinkled skin, the dimness of the corneal margin and other signs of age.

If on seeing a hunchback we unwittingly ascribe to him a bitter and sardonic mentality, something else has entered the situation. He may have acquired his deformity in childhood through a lesion in his spinal column, and there is no psychic element, in any case. But sometimes such a deformity or some other physical suffering may entail *psychic consequences* such as the development of resentment and as it happens we wrongly suppose the hunchback to mean this. Or perhaps resentment is really there in face and bearing and the hunchback itself only increases the strength of our impression, but this is not what is meant by an expressive physiognomy. Generally we must imagine that from an early age the physical frame plays a part in shaping a person's self-awareness and general behaviour. All through one's life, what one feels about oneself and one's appearance is continually being supplemented by such items as whether one is small or tall, strong or weak or sickly, whether one is in any sense beautiful or ugly, even though originally this had nothing to do with one's psyche. The individual models himself according to his body and with its help and in its company there is psychic growth, so that body-form and psychic life become reciprocal even if at first they were apart. We also find that in different people body-form and character match in varying degree: in one case our whole impression is one of unity; in another, the nature is lean though the body is fat, and in another the phlegmatic temperament matches rather oddly with the bony frame. In every case primary somatic factors take effect in the body-form and the psyche comports itself in relation to these, but essentially they do *not* coincide with the psyche in the sense that they are an *expression* of it.

Leaving aside every gesture, every 'frozen' gesture, every physical trace of illness, everything we may have linked with the psyche as a primary somatic cause for an understandable psychic change, we find our total impression of the somatic phenomenon of an individual still leaves something to account for; that is, the persisting physical form of the individual, what we have called his *physiognomy*, the *unique individual quality* which has grown up with him and is only capable of a slow and limited variation as life runs on. Once puberty is past, it tends to settle finally, though sometimes this occurs rather later. In so far as the bodily habitus is not linked with the specific disturbance of any organ (with endocrine effects) such as in myxoedema, acromegaly, etc., but really exhibits the true fashion of the individual's life, we may call it his physiognomy. When we look at different kinds of physiognomy we can immediately picture an appropriate psychic life, indistinct perhaps but undoubtedly belonging and creating a certain psychic atmosphere. If we follow these impressions up and try to reduce this 'feeling' to some kind of knowledge, we find there are two ways of doing this, each different from the other in theory and method. We have to keep the two distinct if we want any clear discussion on these matters.

1. In regarding the physiognomy of an individual the nature of the psyche is perceived directly in the bodily form. Descriptions of body-build together with the relevant character-type have a striking evidential quality and they convince us immediately, like a work of art, when there is apt and revealing presentation by the expert. We certainly get the impression that things are in fact just as he says. But we may wonder whether this is a method of research or for any expansion of our impression. If there is something valid, the following would hold: A 'being' which cannot be divided into body and psyche develops from the basic constitution (Anlage) of man and every living thing. However valid such a division may otherwise be, it is not so here because the 'being' appears in what is physical; the same 'being' which is body and psyche and embraces both. Instead of the two standpoints of bodily, external reality, on the one hand, the subject of biological science, and on the other psychic, incorporeal existence as 'experience' with its inner relationships, we have the idea of a 'being' which could encompass them both but which always remains individual yet somehow typical, constituting the innermost character of man. There would appear to be some unitary characteristic present in all that could be read off from behaviour and bearing and—to take an extreme example—even from the shape of the ears. People with this orientation see in the latter something indistinct, incomplete but essentially characteristic. They tend to express all this in the form of epigrammatic and arbitrary judgments and speak of an ethical bump, a metaphysical ridge or a lecherous lobe, etc. We would do well to keep an eye on logical possibilities of this sort and be clear about them. If we discard the whole study as a fanciful sort of game and clarify our own minds about it, we can see to it that such ideas are not admitted as exact formulations. Yet genuine efforts of this

kind deserve interest and need not undermine our scientific facts. Those who claim to read the essential features of anyone in the way just defined might as well claim to see the essence of the universe in the symbols of nature—they are what we used to call 'natural philosophers'. The whole thing is really metaphysics. The kind of being which expresses itself simultaneously in human character and the shape of the ear must lie at so deep a level that it is inaccessible to empirical research. Suppose we try to apply such methods: someone has his character read from the shape of his ear; let us then check the assessment with all the biographical data we can find. We shall undoubtedly come across major successful performances of an unexpected kind as I found in my own investigations. These spring from the individual's unchecked direct intuitions. The absurdity becomes apparent of bottling up such human powers into a science of bumps, ridges, proportions, etc., so that we may read mechanically from the shape of someone's ear what a whole lifetime can hardly reveal, the essential nature of a man. We cannot objectify the intuitions that come to us of the nature behind the forms because what is involved is not the measurable aspect of a form but its undefined nature. The situation is not one of registrable individual forms and their measurement but of the mutual relationships of form and measurement. These relationships are not specific ones which can be measured but tail off into an indefinite potentiality which cannot be reduced to any rational dimension.

2. Completely different from the above is the method of *objective* research. It abandons intuitive understanding and tries to relate certain well-defined body-shapes and character traits. This is done simply by counting the *frequency* of simultaneous occurrences. The aim is not to find any essential connection, nor is any found; nothing comes to light as a psychic phenomenon but there is only *statistical correlation*. Even if only a few empirical cases of body-build fail to be associated with the expected psychic type or are associated with another or opposite type, this will exclude any important, necessary relationship between body-build and character or at any rate makes it questionable. Statistical correlations such as these only throw up the question, they do not give us any information about the nature of the relationship.

It seems in fact to be extremely difficult to find an exact correlation statistically because bodily form as well as character do not lend themselves *unequivocally to simple measurement and enumeration*. We can only see them in the form of types. But these types are not of a generic nature, and we cannot classify under them unreservedly. They do not appear in reality in pure form except very rarely and usually they are 'mixed'. We use them as a kind of 'yardstick', not as actual categories to which a case either belongs or not. Even in 'mixed' cases we cannot measure them as we can the protein content in urine and say so much of this type, so much of the other. Counting is too exact and there is nothing quantifiable. Different observers not in contact with each other are likely to come to different conclusions on the same material. However that may be, we are not dealing here with the question of physiognomy but with the kind of enquiry which asks what the relation of diabetes or Basedow's disease or tuberculosis is to dementia praecox. The only difference is that in these latter instances the relationships can be exactly numbered, and found to be either absent or present and if present to what degree. This cannot be done with the relationship between body-build and character; it cannot be exactly reckoned. Perhaps something as yet unrecognised lies behind all this, something which gives some colour to these unproductive investigations, but even if this underlying factor could be found by the first line of approach we should not be able to make it accessible to quantitative and exact research.

These two ways of investigation which we have just described are completely heterogeneous from the point of view of method. The first way lays itself open to a wide sweep of possible interpretations through the use of bodily forms as symbols, but after a while it narrows down dangerously into preconceived categories, unequivocal assertions and banalities. The second method makes an objective study of countable factors but in the process loses the form; there is a desire to be exact and exactness is shown, but one is reduced to simple elements, endless correlations and the heaping up of findings which only end in saying nothing. The symbolic nature of the study of physiognomy calls for some exact research to confirm it, but the process of doing this annihilates itself. Simple, objective factors might well be material for the study of physiognomy, but they happen to lack any obvious symbolic significance.

In this chapter we shall confine ourselves to the first line of approach which is the only truly appropriate study of physiognomy, and we will reflect on this remarkable way of viewing bodies, heads and hands. The *judgments made in this respect* may be conceived as *threefold*:

1. *Single forms.* Single features are generally conceived as character-symptoms and we take them as 'signs' in our conclusions as to a person's nature. This is as far as the study of physiognomy usually can go; where it aspires to be a science it only becomes absurd. All statements of the sort that such a study must make are quickly contradicted by actual experience. It is also somewhat grotesque to suppose that human characteristics should manifest themselves in such crude, measurable form; in character we are dealing with structures that are highly differentiated and do not lend themselves readily to conceptual formulation.[1]

2. Instead of using 'signs' as symptoms of human properties, we let ourselves experience the inward effect of significant form. We steep ourselves in *the morphological whole*. Nothing is deduced from this but we catch sight directly of something psychic which displays itself as a natural unity of head, hand and bodily form, and is seen as such by our inward eye. This can hardly stand as a scientific formulation or communication; it is more like an artistic translation, a portrait. It concerns itself with those slight, intangible deviations which can alter the whole cast of countenance, those features which cannot be

[1] *Phrenology* has a place here. The work rests on a theory of localisation of character-properties in certain cranial areas visible on the skull, from which one can see whether these characteristics are well or poorly developed. This theory, created by *Gall*, had much influence during the nineteenth century; it was unsuccessfully resurrected by *Möbius*, who made some experimental comparisons and claimed he could recognise a 'mathematical organ' in a prominence of the lateral forehead. (P. J. Möbius, *Über die Anlage zur Mathematik* (Leipzig, 1900)). See also Gustav Scheve, *Phrenologische Bilder* (Leipzig, 1874), 3rd edn. *Chiromancy* also has a place here, which deduces character traits from the hand (apart from fortune-telling). See v. Schränk-Notzing, *Handlesekunst u. Wissenschaft.* G. Kühnel, *Z. Neur.* (1932), vol. 141. F. Griese, *Die Psychologie der Arbeiterhand* (Vienna and Leipzig, 1927).

'caught' by any amount of calculation and thought, but only by the artist's eye, features that can be caricatured in the wide play of their peculiarities and eccentricities but do not alter the character essentially. It is obvious that the study of physiognomy is not a teachable science, anyhow at present; yet, thanks to the artist, we have any number of portraits, characterisations, non-conceptualised meanings, in the sphere of physiognomy.[1] So far we have an irreconcilable division between seeing a form and measuring a proportion or a quantity. In the case of crude connections measurement is more certain than our own assessment. In the case of fine morphological relationships, which matter in physiognomy, the eye is a much more sensitive and exact instrument.

3. Finally there is a *meaning* in bodily form *which goes beyond the psychological meaning*. This is grasped by the artist, who distorts the body-shapes according to his own inner vision, and chooses extended, thick, slanting or angular forms, without any caricature of some exaggerated psychic feature. The human form is drawn into the universal symbolism of all the forms and shapes of the world. Man is then seen as of metaphysical rather than of psychological importance. Physiognomy is of no relevance here. But the scientific problem still remains, where and how is the dividing line to be drawn between the specific symbolism of the human psyche, as revealed in the physiognomy, and the universal, metaphysical symbolism of the cosmos. It is this which casts doubt on the study of human physiognomy once it has taken the first step towards being a science with a set of communicable concepts.

An empirically valid study of physiognomy could grow only in the field described under point (2)—the symbolism of morphological wholes. Here we could try to produce a *methodical theory* and some training in the observation of the human physiognomy, or again, we could produce a *theory* of what certain physiognomic features may mean *in terms of psychic content*:

*As to method*, the innate ability to see meaningful form can be cultivated by the specific exercise of it, training the eye through description, by schematic illustration, by the use of carefully selected and contrasted photographs, by analysis of the work of great artists, and by instructing the student to observe living behaviour, and if possible measure it, for although numerical findings teach us little, they give good opportunity for intelligent seeing. The constant reward of this methodical approach is the factual experience of the observer, who finds he cannot have enough of this scrutiny of the human countenance. Even though his general scientific knowledge is not greatly enlarged, there is a steady broadening of his vision so far as human nature is concerned. He acquires a visual knowledge, if not a conceptual one.[2]

*In terms of content*, the significance of certain physiognomic features may be stated, some classification of basic types may be made, certain schemata of

---

[1] For the human face in Art, see Bulle, *Der schöne Mensch im Altertum* (München, F. Hirt, 1912), pp. 427–54 (bibliography, and in particular that concerning ancient physiognomists). Waetzoldt, *Die Kunst des Porträts* (Leipzig, 1908).

[2] Cp. the excellent analysis of L. F. Clauss, *Rasse und Seele*.

opposites and different dimensions may be drawn up, and every individual be classified accordingly. This systematic treatment of types of physiognomy has always been thought questionable:

Looking at the matter *historically* we find there is an extensive literature on this matter of the human physiognomy. There are ancient Indian writings, in which, for example, three types were distinguished (taking into account bone-structure, body-circumference, size of genitalia, hair and voice). These were expressed as animal types, the Hare, the Ox and the Horse. In ancient times such problems were also discussed in Europe.[1] A comparison of human and animal types always has something impressive about it which goes beyond the mere joke, but it is difficult to say anything serious about it. *In the eighteenth century* educated people were much preoccupied with the question of physiognomy,[2] and it became fashionable. Lichtenberg analysed the subject critically but did not refrain from dabbling in it himself.[3] Hegel endeavoured to grasp and settle it once and for all.[4] It was always tempting to advance the solid, comprehensible elements, i.e. human physiognomy understood as 'frozen' gesture, and to remain satisfied with this.

However, in the cultural world of *the romantics*, C. G. Carus[5] once more developed a learned and systematic theory of human physiognomy, which can be recommended for its careful comparative method to anyone interested in this subject. Carus wished 'to see and understand the whole world as a symbol of God, and man as a symbol of God's idea of the soul'. His symbolic system, therefore, draws into its context the whole cosmos as well as the fields of morphology and physiology. For him the symbolism is visible but not comparable; it is something direct that cannot be mediated. Carus studies 'the outcome of the creative acts of idea, the organisation and in particular the external appearance of the individual as a whole'. From this we needs must arrive at a clearer understanding of his inner psychic being and character. The moment of vision is conclusive, 'it is the capacity to discover the kernel in the husk, the nature of the psychic idea in the symbol of the form'. Carus wanted to turn this unconscious vision into a science and a practical art; he wanted to know what were the *basic principles* which could be applied to countless individuals, and what *practical skill* was needed to apply the principles in the individual case. In this general discussion, there is something most suggestive, which somehow confirms our own vague and imprecise experience, but when he tries to conceptualise this into a science, he meets the same fate as others in the field. When he comes to particulars, he ceases to be convincing. He tries measurement (organoscopy), describes body-surface according to its individual modelling (physiognomy), observes changes in form during the course of life (pathognomy). He draws into his net every scientific finding and anything that appears possible material from the physiognomic point of view. Thus he accumulates a wealth of data and tries always to keep the whole in view while he attends to the smallest detail. To him is due the creation of the first and up to now the only basic 'scientific' system for the study of physiognomy.

[1] See the literature quoted by Bulle.

[2] Lavater, *Physiognomische Fragmente* (Leipzig, 1775). Goethe, *Cottasche Jubiläumsausgabe*, 33, pp. 20 ff. Klages, *Graphologische Monatschefte* (1901), vol. 5, pp. 91–9.

[3] Lichtenberg, *Über Physiognomik wider die Physiognomen* (Göttingen, 1778).

[4] Hegel, *Phänomenologie des Geistes* (Ausgabe Lassons, pp. 203 ff.)

[5] C. G. Carus, *Symbolik der menschlichen Gestalt* (Leipzig, 1853).

*At present* there seems no attempt to study physiognomy which would allow comparison with these older attempts in the degree of their thoroughness, wealth of material and general depth of human understanding. Yet it is the fashion to talk about the physiognomy of things. Nowadays we look and interpret where we used to explain and comprehend or else scrutinise and question. In this way, many remarkable notions creep in which, though they teach us nothing specific, do not leave us totally unmoved.[1]

If we have grasped what has been said above about the methods and history of the study of physiognomy, we may still be doubtful whether scientific research can replace intuition with any definite findings, but we are not on that account prepared to ignore this whole field and let the subject drop. Even if exact knowledge is not possible, such studies are an education of our sensibility for form. Our responsiveness to form and shape is increased and cultivated through the presentation of forms as concrete, observable wholes, which we can fully accept without according them the status of empirical facts of general application. They create for us rather an 'atmosphere' without which we would be the poorer when we come to study our psychiatric realities. The artistic approach offers us something incomparable, but the psychiatrist on his side can always try to represent the forms he sees as 'types'. This has been done and we are impressed, though not by the theory, only by the 'art', which enriches our mode of observation but does not tell us what to think.

1. One such attempt was the once-famous *'theory of degeneration'*. It was supposed that in the morphological deviations of bodily form one could detect the degenerate nature of an individual (signs of degeneration, stigmata degenerationis). His character, his tendency to neurotic and mental illness, and in particular his criminal predispositions, were also revealed.

These morphological abnormalities were, for example: Bodily proportions that deviated markedly from average, e.g. too long legs in relation to the trunk; peculiar head-formation, like turret-skull; deviant bone-formation, e.g. too small chin, extreme smallness of the mastoid bone; dental malformation; high palate; malformations such as harelip; excessive or absent body-hair; special hairy moles; shape of the nose and ears (to which much attention was paid); attached ear-lobes, big and protruding ears, prominence of the Darwinian ear-fold, mobility of the ears.

This theory of degeneration tried to look into the deep substratum of life from which psychic and somatic phenomena simultaneously spring. The psychic degeneration—as shown in personality disorders (psychopathies), psychoses and mental defect—was also supposed to declare itself in the appropriate bodily deviations. This theory held something intuitively plausible for contemporary thought. But once it tried to make a scientific

[1] Rudolf Kassner, *Die Grundlage der Physiognomik* (Leipzig, 1922), an essay which deals with human physiognomy and certain experiences in an unmethodical way and reflects on the philosophical interpretations of the impressions.

theory out of this intuitive grasp of the human shape, it was applicable only within extremely narrow limits.

If we are going to talk of abnormal familial deviations (without thinking of progressive degeneration) we have to conceive of certain constitutions, which occur familially, and give these families a distinctive character which is recognisable sometimes through quite slight indications.[1] In such cases the signs of degeneration are connected with anomalies of the nervous system or other organ-systems. They are the result of faulty development and group themselves together in typical syndromes of morphological and functional signs (e.g. trembling, deafness). The most significant example is status dysraphicus.

It has often been emphasised that we frequently find stigmata such as these in healthy people and many severe psychic abnormalities are found without them yet this theory has had historical importance and however critically it is reviewed it still has a certain validity. We may reject it scientifically but we cannot be talked out of it completely. We cannot draw any practical consequences from it but we are unable to be wholly indifferent to the forms described. Degeneration is a concept which, if one wants to get hold of it firmly in relation to the empirical facts, melts away in one's grip. It seems to want to say something about the ultimate springs of life but fails to do so. It can however do one thing. It can keep interest and enquiry alive and supply us with a term for something which we see intuitively but for which no adequate theory is as yet forthcoming. In addition it means from the start that we abandon the study of physiognomy proper and treat the signs of degeneration as symptoms, thus exchanging the scrutiny of the human physiognomy for a naturalistic pseudo-science. Symbolism vanishes but the particular relationship of symptom to degenerative disease with which one is left cannot be taken as a medical fact and must definitely be disputed.[2]

2. Kretschmer[3] tried to relate body-build to psychic properties. His theory is a comparable one in its methods but very different in content. He distinguishes the dysplastic types, which occur in relatively few people and then three main body-builds: leptosome (asthenic), athletic and pyknic. The following are the main cues given by his descriptions:

(a) *Leptosome:* little increase in girth with undiminished growth in length, slender, lanky people; narrow shoulders, narrow flat chests; sharp costal angle, receding face owing to insufficient development of the chin, similarly a receding forehead, resulting in an angular profile, with the tip of the nose as the vertex; nose excessively long.

Associated with the above is a schizothymic character: corresponding to the thin, angular, sharp-nosed body we find an angular, cold, edgy nature.

[1] F. Curtius, 'Über Degenerationszeichen', *Eugen. usw.*, vol. 3 (1953), p. 25.

[2] Lombroso, *Due Ursachen u. Bekämpfung des Verbrechens* (D) (Berlin, 1912). Baer, 'Über jugendliche Mörder', *Arch. Kriminalanthrop.*, vol. 11 (1913), p. 160.

[3] Kretschmer, *Körperbau u. Charakter* (Berlin, 1921), 1940 edn., pp. 13, 14. Kretschmer and Enke, *Die Persönlichkeit der Athletiker* (Leipzig, 1936).

(b) *Pyknic:* squat figure, soft, broad countenance on a short, thick neck, tendency to put on fat; deep, round chest, fat belly, slenderly built motor-apparatus (shoulder-girdle and extremities), skull large, round, broad and deep but not high; well-modelled contours, harmonious proportions.

Associated with the above is the cyclothymic or syntonic character; a well-rounded, natural, open nature. Corresponding to the body-build, we find a balanced, warm-hearted, accommodating character; they are people who are active in their environment, frank and sociable, either on the serious side or rather cheerful.

(c) *Athletic:* broad, wide shoulders; a tall figure; strong bone-development; strong muscles; thick skin; heavy bony structure; large hands and feet; high fore-head; massive, high-vaulted head; strong, protruding chin; facial circumference—elongated egg-shape; broad cheek bones and prominent supra-orbital ridges. The facial skull protrudes in comparison with the cranium.

Associated with the above is a quiet, reflective nature to the extent of being cumbersome and clumsy. There is a poverty of responsiveness, and due to this the person appears very stable and his reactions massive. There is a dislike of move-ment, they are sparing of speech, and there is an absence of lightness and flexibility; this leads to what has been called the 'viscous' temperament. 'A spirit of heaviness lies over everything.'

Kretschmer's theory of the connection between body-build and character is only one section of a much more comprehensive conception of man as a whole, which will be discussed later on in this book (p. 641). Here we need say only one thing: These types are intuitively perceived forms, which enrich and clarify our seeing in the same way as Art does, but not as a concept would. We feel that we can see in the body-build—as we saw the psychic deviation in the morphological degeneration—a certain type of character which has been most vividly described by Kretschmer. But this enrichment of our vision does not have any empirical significance and does not allow us to draw any con-clusions. A single, well-defined case can empirically contradict any general validity it may seem to have, yet if we take the theory on its own terms it is not one which we would repudiate completely.

Kretschmer's book begins as follows: 'People think of the devil as thin, with a pointed beard. Fat devils have an admixture of good-natured stupidity. A con-spirator is hunchbacked and coughs behind his hand. The old witch has a thin and bird-like face. Where there is wine and merriment, who is there but the fat knight, Falstaff, with his red nose and gleaming pate! The woman of the people with her sound commonsense, stands hand on hip, sturdy and round as a ball. Saints look emaciated; they are long-limbed, pale and gothic. In short: virtue and the devil should have a sharp nose; humour a broad one.' He then takes as his motto for all this, Caesar's remarks to Cassius:

> 'Let me have men about me that are fat;
> Sleekheaded men and such as sleep o' nights;
> Yond' Cassius has a lean and hungry look;
> He thinks too much; such men are dangerous . . .
> Would he were fatter! . . .'

Conrad comments on the unsurpassed description which then follows of lepto-some and pyknic body-build and schizothyme and cyclothyme personalities. He says quite rightly—underlining what is unscientific, particularly from the point of view of the natural sciences—'Any attempt to improve on the picture would only dis-tort and spoil it, like touching up the painting of one of the Old Masters.' Max Schmidt expresses his enthusiasm also by saying, 'Kretschmer has given an almost inspired description of the two types. If one thinks of all the different schizophrenic and manic-depressive patients whom one has encountered in the past, and lets them pass through one's mind, they will fall quite effortlessly into these two types.' In Denmark—so the Danish author writes—we find two historic cases, Christian VII and Grundvig: 'These two personalities might well stand as a symbol for the two char-acteristic types of psychosis. Christian VII, the small, slender, asthenic leptosome, degenerate in colour and schizophrenic; Grundtvig, the large, broad, corpulent and pyknic cyclothyme.'

Indeed the descriptions affect us like *a work of art* and the impact is one of direct conviction. The achievement lies in the compelling force that makes the reader see with Kretschmer's eyes. But it is precisely this which poses the question: *exactly what does this truthfulness mean?*

Can we say with Conrad: 'We may be sure no fruity, comfortable or cheerful soul inhabits that lean, lanky and narrow-chested body, nor is there a dry, prim, sentimental soul in that fat, stubby-limbed and capacious frame.'? I do not think so. Such certainty belongs to intuition, to the study of physiog-nomy and to this extent no further investigation is needed. But empirically it is far from certain and there are constant contradictions by the individual case.

There have therefore been those who were not satisfied with direct, intuitive insights of this sort. Instead *they have counted* how often character-type and body-build coincide in this way. Mere *correlation* appears in the place of an *essential con-nection.* But this means we embark on a radically different course. Correlations can exist between phenomena which have no observable or essential relationship to each other. When we find correlations, the next question is 'why?' The unity of the human physiognomy cannot provide a cause, because its nature is not causal; it is a plasticity that we somehow understand. In the second place, if it were the cause, no exceptions must be found in the coincidence of the effects. The method of seek-ing correlations gives rise to a type of knowledge quite distinct from that gleaned from the study of human physiognomy.

The *paradox* remains: We know practically nothing, yet it is in the nature of the drive for knowledge to try and find some satisfactory shapes and forms even where there is no exact knowledge, on which judgment may be based; there is the urge at least to see. Anyone so engaged has to travel far before he can predict or schematise his findings. Lichtenberg said long ago: 'I have always found that those who expected most from the study of physiognomy, which is a practical art, were those with a limited knowledge of the world. People of wide knowledge are the best students of physiognomy and expect most of the rules to be broken.' 'The study of physiognomy, next to prophecy, is the most deceiving of all human arts that have ever been concocted by our extravagant minds.'

## § 2. Involuntary Gesture (Mimik)

The study of physiognomy concerns itself with *established bodily form* as a distinguishing characteristic of the psyche. The study of involuntary gesture deals with *bodily movement* as a manifestation of psychic life. In the study of physiognomy there is no principle which makes the connection between body and psyche understandable, and which could serve us methodically as a reliable criterion. In the study of involuntary gesture, however, such principles do exist. It is here and not in the study of physiognomy that we stand on the firm ground of insights that can be discussed.

### (a) Types of bodily movement

We have to make some distinctions in order to visualise clearly what is meant by involuntary gesture. We must first exclude those phenomena which we discussed earlier on, the *accompaniments and sequelae* of psychic processes, such as blushing, blanching, shaking at the knees, tremor, paralytic rigidity of the face in acute fear, etc. These are movements which we do not directly 'understand' but only link with psychic events through experience, without any inner glimpse of the psyche.

In the second place, we must distinguish *voluntary movements* from involuntary gesture. Voluntary movements have an intended goal, while the expressive movements of involuntary gesture are unintentional. Voluntary movements include gesticulations, signs and indications (e.g. shaking of the head, nodding, waving) which by convention say something (though the convention differs in different cultures). The movements are related to speech as an incomplete means of communication. Involuntary gesture proper, however, has got no intention and does not consciously want to communicate: it is a universal human form of utterance, understood in part even by animals, so it seems.

*Movements of involuntary gesture*: for instance, a cheerful expression of face, or a tense or sorrowful one, etc. These are involuntary and unintentional. All voluntary movements, however, have an aspect of involuntary gesture, none is quite like the other even if the same end is in view; they vary in the individual and according to the emotional state. The way someone looks at me, gives me his hand, the way he walks, the timbre of his voice, it is all involuntary expression; it contains a self-revealing, unintentional content alongside the one that is purposely intended.

Among involuntary gestures, we may further distinguish the following:

1. There are infinite nuances, a wealth of self-revealing movements, which *constantly accompany psychic events* and make them visible in the person's expression. They are transparently clear to others, and can be understood as the ceaseless play

of a secret, sensitive resonance in the features, look and voice. To some extent these phenomena are common to man and animals.

2. *Laughing and crying*[1] are in a class apart. They are reactions to a human crisis; small, somatic catastrophes in which the body, being so to speak at a loss, becomes disorganised. But the disorganisation is still symbolic—symbolism is present in all gesture—yet here the situation is not transparently clear to others because both responses are marginal. Laughing and crying are exclusively human, they are not shared by any animal, but for the human race they are universal.

3. There are certain movements which are *marginal as between movements of expression and somatic accompaniments*. In spite of their reflex character, they seem to have an element of expressiveness: yawning, stretching the limbs when tired. Animals share these movements too.

4. All movement can merge into *rhythmic* repetition. Klages[2] has dealt with the subject of the nature and universal significance of rhythm.

## (b) Understanding involuntary gesture—general principles

It lies outside our experience to say whether or not the morphological processes that freeze into the forms of human physiognomy have sprung from psychic impulses. On the other hand, however, it is our continual experience that bodily movements are linked with the psyche, with its mood, purposes and essential nature. The understanding of the movements of gesture has therefore a good basis which can be tested and communicated. This relationship between the psyche and that movement which is its 'expression' has been *reduced to certain principles*. These can render our immediate interpretations conscious, control them, relate them and finally expand them. The principles of expression have been recognised and formulated by eminent investigators.[3] They hold for all kinds of movement, voluntary and involuntary, self-revealing gestures of face, gait and posture and handwriting as the record of such movement. There are two main principles:

1. Every inner activity is accompanied by a movement which is an understandable symbol for it. Bitter feelings, for instance, reveal themselves involuntarily by movements connected with having a bitter taste in the mouth. Keen thinking goes with a firm, fixed gaze directed to the near-distance as if some object stood there. With involuntary gesture the person is not aware himself of the symbolisation, and the observer, directly perceiving the bitterness or the keen attention, does not know either in the first instance how he came to perceive it. Here we see a direct manifestation of the psyche. These symbolic processes have been investigated in great detail; Piderit has studied gesture, Klages uses a wider context and in the case of handwriting goes into the matter more minutely.

[1] Plessner, *Lachen u. Weinen* (Arnheim, 1941).

[2] L. Klages, *Vom Wesen des Rhythmus*. Pallat and Hilker, *Künstlerische Körperschulung* (Breslau, 1923, reprinted, Kampen and Sylt, 1933).

[3] Piderit, *Grundzüge der Mimik u. Physiognomik* (Braunschweig, 1868). *Mimik u. Physiognomik* (Detnold, 1867), 3rd edn., 1919. Klages, *Ausdrucksbewegung u. Gestaltungskraft* (Leipzig, 1936). Darwin, *Der Ausdruck der Gemütsbewegungen bei. Menschen u. Tieren* (1872). Hendel's

2. Movements are influenced by the personality which selects unwittingly their mode and form according to what 'suits' it, what it feels is fine, fitting, stylish, sound or desirable in some way. There is a drive for this *self-presentation* which uses '*key-symbols of the personality*' in shaping all involuntary gestures. Natural direct expressiveness then gets moulded by a more conscious expression, of which the person is himself aware. Klages was the first to grasp this—particularly in the case of handwriting—and noted the way in which complex personal and social ideals take on expressive shape.

3. Frequently repeated movements of gesture leave certain traces in the body, particularly in the face. The study of physiognomy, so far as it understands the traces of gesture, establishes certain forms of '*frozen*' *gesture* and so may be seen as part of the study of gesture, the only area in the whole study of physiognomy that has some empirical basis for further exploration.[1]

## (c) Psychopathological observations

1. We have only occasional, unsystematic descriptions of patients' involuntary gestures and the fixed forms of expression that arise from them. Here are a few, haphazard examples:[2]

*The passion for movement of manic patients*, who make aimless movements for the sheer sake of moving, out of 'delight' in it as such, and the drive to give vent to exuberant excitement; *pressure of movement in anxious patients* who are always seeking peace and respite, always trying to get rid of something, and run to and fro in desperation, push against walls and gesticulate monotonously.

The indestructibly exuberant features of manic patients, exactly like those of natural delight; the unnatural, silly, exaggerated jollity of *hebephrenics*, the painful dejectedness of cyclothymes appearing as a slight indication at the corners of the mouth and eyes; the profoundly downcast, passively resigned expression of the severe depression which turns into chronic *melancholia*; the cold, apparently empty expression of mute melancholics (even when the patients can talk about their distress it is not quite convincing); the distracted features and excited despair in the alarming anxiety of agitated melancholia.

The dream-like, absentminded expression of certain patients with *clouded consciousness*, who seem to be revelling in a number of imaginary experiences; the empty expression of many *hysterical twilight states*, which can change so easily into expressions of fright or worry or an ungenuine astonishment.

The empty, expressionless face of many *demented* patients, who sit around like human vegetables with a fixed expression (sometimes perpetually smiling, sometimes defiant, sometimes dull, sometimes tormented); *paranoid* patients who stalk about, dignified and grave, full of stoic calm and contempt; the sharp, piercing look of the paranoid woman; her suspicious, mistrustful, testing and dogged countenance; the sudden glance shot by some stuporous catatonics.

*Bibliothek*—phylogenetic viewpoint; he confuses expression proper with somatic accompaniments. Bühler, *Ausdruckstheorie* (Jena, 1933). Lersch, *Gesicht u. Seele* (München, 1932). Fischer, *Ausdruck der Persönlichkeit* (Leipzig, 1934). Strehle, *Analyse des Gebarens* (Berlin, 1935).

[1] F. Lange, *Die Sprache des menschlichen Antlitzes, eine wissenschaftliche Physiognomik* (München, 1937).

[2] Oppenheim, *Allg. Z. Psychiatr.*, vol. 40, p. 840. Th. Kirchhoff, *Der Gesichtsausdruck beim Gesunden u. beim Geisteskranken* (Berlin, J. Springer, 1922).

The shifting, soft, melting expression, the swimming eyes of *hysterics*, their flirtatious, half-conscious, highly exaggerated looks.

The inconstant features and restless eyes of *neurasthenics*. The torn, tormented look of some *early hebephrenics* behind which surprisingly little psychic content is to be found.

The loutish look of the ineducable, the brutal, animal expression of true moral insanity; 'the sad eyes of the trapped animal' which Heyer noted in the childish, retarded inmates of his institution.

Homburger described many of the 'motor forms of expression'.[1] Heyer described the state of certain personality disorders (psychopaths)—'hard, tight individuals, every movement well controlled, nothing soft, supple, biddable or easy about them; the whole bearing boardlike'.

Besides observations on bearing and movement as significant psychic expression, attention has also been paid to the way in which expression in its turn affects the psyche. Stance and posture are accompanied by an inner posture and atmosphere. Hence the possible significance for the psychic state[2] of physical exercise and physical culture. We have a particular case of this in the body posture during sleep.[3] 'Everyone has his sleep ritual or likes to ensure certain conditions without which he cannot sleep' (Freud).

2. *Laughing and crying* are of special interest. This phenomenon can occur as a physical compulsion in cases of bulbar paralysis. There is no psychic motivation. Schizophrenics are often seen to laugh; melancholics are tearless; depressives may sob loudly but get no relief.

3. *Yawning*[4] is a complex movement which occurs involuntarily and seems akin to stretching. It occurs spontaneously on waking, during fatigue and boredom. It seems a purely physical event but under certain conditions can be an expressive movement. Landauer[5] takes stretching as purely physiological but has no evidence for this. We can think of a series of such reflexes including sneezing which never become expressive movements in this way.

4. For a long time attention has been directed to the *rhythmical movements* and *stereotypies* of mental patients. Comparisons have been drawn between the *rhythmical* movements of idiots and demented patients and the circling movements of wild animals in captivity. But so far no real analysis has been made.[6] Kläsi[7] has defined *stereotypies* as 'manifestations which are repeated over a long period always in the same form. They are separated off from the person's total activity; that is, they are automatic and neither express a mood nor are they at all appropriate to any objective purpose.' They are diverse in *origin* and meaning. They may be remnants of once meaningful movements or may spring

---

[1] Bumke's *Handbuch der Geisteskrankheiten* (1932). Also *Z. Neur.*, vol. 78 (1922), p. 562; and vol. 85 (1923), p. 274.

[2] J. Faust, *Aktive Entspannungsbehandlung*, 2nd edn. (Stuttgart, 1938).

[3] H. Thorner, *Nervenarzt*, vol. 4 (1931), p. 197.

[4] E. Levy, *Z. Neur.*, vol. 72, p. 161.

[5] Landauer, *Z. Neur.*, vol. 58, p. 296.

[6] Cp. Fauser, *Allg. Z. Psychiatr.*, vol. 62 (1905).

[7] Kläsi, *Über die Bedeutung u. Entstehung der Stereotypien* (Berlin, Karger, 1922).

from a delusional world; they may be rituals, movements of defence against bodily hallucinations, and so on.

Since Klages the concept of rhythm has taken on a definite and narrower meaning in contrast to 'beat'. Rhythm is living, infinitely variable expression; beat is mechanical, arbitrary repetition. Langelüddeke[1] has investigated schizophrenics, manic-depressives and patients suffering from Parkinsonism and has taken Klages' point of view.

## § 3. HANDWRITING

Handwriting is particularly suitable for the investigation of movements of expression because it is a fixed form and can thus be more thoroughly examined. Simulation usually plays little part. In the majority of people there is a great deal of play-acting in their other expressive movements, from movements of embarrassment (scratching the head, twiddling buttons) which like certain laughter is intended to cover up something, right up to gestures confirmed by constant exercise and habit. These have no special meaning but surround the person with a wall of conventional expression behind which the real self hides. In handwriting, however, we see much less of this. The disadvantage is that valuable results can only be obtained when the handwriting is well established and to some extent formed. It would take us too far afield if we were to discuss the details of graphological understanding in respect of character, temperament and mood, and the regular changes that take place under different affects, during personality development, in abnormal mental states and under different experimental conditions.[2]

As with all understandable phenomena that can only be understood as a whole, every individual feature of the writing has such complex relationships and possibilities that only a most thorough and detailed examination will give us anything like a clear picture. The essay of Klages[3] shows us how even the pressure used in writing can lead us on to the psychology of the whole personality, provided we regard the effort as a movement of expression. The older method of interpreting certain special 'signs' in the handwriting has been completely discarded.

The writing of *mental patients*[4] has been investigated chiefly from the

---

[1] A. Langelüddeke, 'Rhythmus u. Takt', *Z. Neur.*, vol. 113 (1928), p. 1.

[2] Klages, *Die Probleme der Graphologie* (Leipzig, 1910); *Handschrift u. Charakter*, 2nd edn. (Leipzig, 1920); *Graphologischen Monatshefte* (München, 1897–1908); and *Graphologische Praxis* (München, 1901–8). Preyer, *Zur Psychologie des Schreibens* (Hamburg, 1895, 1912). G. Meyer, *Die wissenschaftlichen Grundlagen der Graphologie* (Jena, 1901). R. Saudeck, *Wissenschaftliche Graphologie* (München, 1926); *Experimentelle Graphologie* (Berlin, 1929).

[3] Klages, *Zur Theorie des Schreibdrucks*, Graphol. M. 6 and 7.

[4] Köster, *Die Schrift bei Geisteskranken* (Leipzig, 1903). Erlenmeyer, *Die Schrift* (1897). Goldscheider, *Arch. Psychiatr.* (D), vol. 24. Kraepelin's *Psychologische Arbeiten*. Lomer, 'Manisch-depressives Irresein', *Z. Neur.*, vol. 20, p. 447. *Arch. Psychiatr.* (D), vol. 53, p. 1. *Allg. Z. Psy.*, vol. 71, p. 195. Schönfeld and Menzel, *Tuberkulose, Charakter u. Handschrift* (Brünn, Prague, Leipzig, 1934). Jakoby, *Handschrift u. Sexualität* (Berlin, 1932). Unger, 'Geisteskrankheit u. Handschrift', *Z. Neur.*, vol. 152 (1935), p. 569.

point of view of neurological disturbances. It has also been investigated from
the point of view of content, but hardly at all as a form of psychic expression.
*Paralytic handwriting* has been described a long time ago: we get omissions,
reduplication of letters, mistakes of meaning, tremor and ataxic phenomena in
moving the pen. Certain *dementing processes* show themselves strikingly in the
handwriting: repetition of the same word or letter in an otherwise orderly
script, fantastic flourishes and ornamentation of a manneristic and stereotyped
kind. In many *organic dements* the writing finally disintegrates into a completely
unformed scribble. Disturbances such as *agraphia* are analogous to aphasia:
otherwise healthy patients can no longer read words or write them or can do
neither. They write meaningless letters and syllables, in the same way as
patients with sensory aphasia speak paraphasically. In *manic* and in *depressive*
states the writing shows typical changes in size, pressure and form (G. Meyer,
Lomer).

## SECTION TWO

## THE INDIVIDUAL'S PERSONAL WORLD

### (PSYCHOLOGY OF THE PERSONAL WORLD—WELTPSYCHOLOGIE)

We contrast the phenomena of expression with those other meaningful
objective psychic phenomena in all of which there is a meaning conceived,
intended or carried out by the individual himself. The meaning has to be understood before the psyche is understood. In this sense we understand the objective meaning, the rational content, the intended purpose and the aesthetic
vision in the sense-data of speech, written words and behaviour. Just as the
precondition for seeing anything at all is a sensitive capacity for the perception
of movement and form plus a certain trustworthiness of impression, so there
is a precondition for understanding the meaning of these objective mental
products whenever they occur. The precondition is a broad understanding of
the world of the mind and a wide experience. To acquire broad understanding
is only the first step; *having taken it,* we can proceed to comprehend meaning
directly as essentially the expression of an individual psyche. The same problems are encountered here as we met when considering the psychology of
expression.

We divide these objectified meanings into *action in the world* and *pure
mental creation.* To obtain clear concepts we must now describe action and
creation in a methodical manner, just as we described handwriting, movement
and bodily form. The more fundamental the content, the more we have to
leave the everyday world of common sense and look for appropriate scientific
concepts and an appropriate methodology (e.g. linguistics, aesthetics, the
humanities, etc.). But up to now psychopathology has confined itself only to
the simplest objective manifestations of this sort.

All these objectified meanings have an aspect which we can understand as an involuntary expression of the psyche, something which we could call their particular tone, melodic line, style or atmosphere. To this extent *everything may be said to be mere expression* and therefore—as language itself indicates—have a 'physiognomy' in the widest sense. Goethe interested himself in Lavater's study of physiognomy. He enlarged the meaning to include the entire range of human phenomena:

The study of physiognomy 'deduces the inner from the outer' but what is the 'outer' in Man? Surely not just his naked form, his unintended gestures which denote the forces within him and their interplay? A host of things modifies and shrouds him: his social status, his habits, his possessions and his clothes! It would seem extremely difficult, if not impossible, to penetrate all these different layers into his innermost self, even find some fixed point among all these unknown quantities. But we need not despair . . . he is not only affected by all that envelops him; he too takes effect on all this and so on himself and, as he is modified, so he modifies all that is around him. Clothes and furniture help us to deduce a man's character. Nature forms man, man naturally transforms himself. Set in the vast universe, he builds his own small world within it, makes his own fences and walls, and furnishes everything after his own image. His social status and circumstances may well determine his surroundings but the way in which he lets himself be determined is of the greatest significance. He may furnish his world indifferently, as others of his kind, because this is how he finds it. Indifference may grow into neglect. But he may also show eagerness and energy, he may go on to higher levels or (which is not so common) take a step back. It will not be held against me, I hope, that I try in this way to enlarge the field of physiognomic study.

This organic, comprehensive view of human beings and of the way in which they behave in their own world supplies the background for every individual analysis. For this we must first differentiate our concepts as follows: taking the *individual findings* one by one, we can distinguish *behaviour*, in the form of attitude and gesture, how a man presents himself to himself and others; *the way he has shaped his environment*—his choice of clothing, dwelling and his physical environment; *the whole way he lives*—how he acts, the paths he selects, the entirety of his behaviour, of the environment he has shaped, and of his usual repetitive, everyday conduct; *overt deliberate actions*, which represent specific volitional acts, deliberately designed for effect, with full awareness of all that they imply.

These individual findings will bring us at last to some conception of the patient's world, a conception of what he actually experiences as his reality. We can grasp directly the transformation that has taken place, a transformation that affects his world and his way of living in that world; that is, we can grasp the whole new configuration of this patient's world, the only thing that gives lucidity and meaning to the individual phenomena as they appear.

## § 1. ANALYSIS OF CONDUCT

### (a) Behaviour

Behaviour, especially in the minor things of everyday life, may be interpreted as a symptom of personality or of an emotional attitude, but usually such interpretation is not elaborated as it tends to be rather vague and indefinite. We describe the patients' 'habitus' instead and try to depict the behaviour. Behaviour as such is not particularly valuable as an objective symptom but in studying it we get a clue from the *idea of possible interpretation*.

Individual pieces of behaviour are easy enough to name: e.g. nail-biting, destructiveness (tearing up linen), etc. In the old texts we find descriptions of how patients behave when they get together on their own, at home, at work, out of doors, indoors and we find classifications such as: sociable, solitary, restless, immobile, pacing about, the collector, etc.

The description of the many odd kinds of behaviour met with in chronic states and acute psychoses is a task which falls to special psychiatry. What we need, therefore, is to find some *typical behaviour complexes* rather than strings of separate features. The following are a few examples:

Catatonic, and also hebephrenic, behaviour[1] is characterised by a dramatic quality and theatrical posing. Patients declaim and recite with vivid and absurd gesticulation. Trivialities are announced in a lofty manner as if the highest interest of mankind were concerned. A displaced preference for serious matters shows itself in a mannered, stereotyped fashion. Bearing and clothing become odd and strange. The prophet lets his hair grow and assumes the appearance of an ascetic.

*Hebephrenic* behaviour is illustrated by the following letter, written by a patient who was perfectly conscious and well oriented, after he had escaped from his father during a walk outside the hospital, though he had been quickly caught again. 'Dearest Dad . . . it was a pity you did not understand me . . . I am really not at all ill . . . you should have walked. I am now back in hospital because of your galloping after me . . . I hope you realise there is nothing wrong with me . . . you will understand I have to go back to my piano studies. I asked you again, please forgive me, chasing after me made you a little heated . . . don't be angry with me over this, greeting to you all, most sincerely your self-reproachful, because he couldn't—can't, can't couldn't (latest word!) escape from the hospital, Karl. Fetch me soon.'

During the examination of patients who consciously or unconsciously want to conceal something, there is often a very characteristic '*talking round the point*'. A patient when asked about his hallucinations, which he previously had disclosed, said: 'All the time one lives one hears voices; its only too easy for one to get the wrong idea; the expression "one hears voices" is really a legal phrase. In the beginning I did hear something, but after I had been in this hospital for half a year I got convinced that there could be no question of hearing voices in the popular sense

[1] Kahlbaum, *Die Katatonie* (Berlin, 1874), pp. 31 ff. Hecker, 'Die Hebephrenie', *Virchows Arch.*, vol.52.

of the word.' General remarks sometimes are all that one gets to hear: 'That not so much' . . . 'I can't say for certain . . .' 'I would like to tell you, something is not quite right . . .' . . . 'My enemy . . .? people say so . . .' 'I'll tell you, if I have to be so . . .'

In *acute states* we see any number of mannerisms and grimacings. Patients behave quite incomprehensibly (though sometimes the motive appears when later on some self-description is given). One patient may solemnly kiss the earth, again and again; others devote themselves to a military drill; others clench their fists, beat wildly on walls or furniture, assume strange postures.

At the *start of a psychosis* behaviour often shows restlessness, haste, irresponsibility. There is an apparent lack of feeling for everything, which is suddenly interrupted by an outbreak of strong feeling; uncertain, puzzled questions are asked of everyone, an exaggerated attraction or repulsion is shown to relatives; there are sudden, unexpected actions, journeys, long walks in the night. It is as if the adolescent years have returned. Attractions and interests change rapidly. Patients become devout, become indifferent to erotic interests or inhibited. They seem only interested in themselves and engrossed in themselves. People close to them notice their expression has changed, it is no longer natural. At first it is uncanny to see these subtle changes, the smile becoming more of a grin, etc.

The behaviour of the cheerful, excited (manic) patient and the sad, retarded (depressed) patient is directly self-evident.

In some reactive hysterical psychoses, *childish behaviour* is particularly characteristic. Patients behave as if they had become children again ('retour à l'enfance' —Janet). They cannot count, make gross mistakes, move helplessly like infants, put naïve questions, show their feelings like children, and generally give a 'silly' effect. They do not seem to know how to do anything, like to be spoiled and nursed, make childish boasts: 'I can drink such a big glass of beer, I can drink 70–80 glasses . . .' Such behaviour is an essential part of the Ganser-syndrome.

An example of *paralytic behaviour*: A capable and respectable business man in Vienna leaves his job when 33 years of age. A few days after that he is in Munich and steals a wallet with 60 Marks in it from his room-mate, as well as a watch and a waistcoat. Next day he buys a motor-bike for 860 Marks, and pays for it with a 1000-mark note. He has several such notes as well as a purse with 250 pfennig pieces. He does not know how to ride the bike and pushes it. Next day he has his motor-bike repaired in Nurnberg. Meanwhile he tells everyone that he wants to go to Karlsruhe where his business is. It is noticed however that he cannot ride the bike and the firm persuade him to go to Karlsruhe by train and they will send it after him. A few days later the motor-bike is returned to them, 'addressee unknown'. In Karlsruhe meanwhile the patient has perpetrated a few thefts at his hotel. He sells some stolen shoes to a shoemaker for 3 Marks. He introduces himself as the editor of the *Badisches Landeszeitung* and says he wants to go to the States. He buys three pairs of socks, and a camera but by evening he has been arrested and taken to the mental hospital at Heidelberg. The dilapidated man has no insight, comments on his thefts, 'everyone can slip up sometime'; otherwise he adjusts to his stay in hospital, satisfied and apathetic. He can be talked into any kind of notion; memory and power of registration are very poor; he talks all kinds of nonsense all day long. Soon the physical symptoms that had been noticed immediately began to increase and a severe paralytic dementia developed.

## (b) The shape given to the environment

Housing, clothing, and environment all feel our impact whether we are conscious of this or not, and they may be considered as the very emanation of human nature. Nowadays we see little of this in our patients. Mental hospitals do not afford much opportunity with their smooth walls, hygenic equipment and everything bare, cold, strange and impersonal. In some nursing homes, however, we see sometimes how characteristically and with what affection chronic patients will shape their environment, how they collect peculiar treasures and arrange them in strange patterns. We can also see how greatly attached some patients are to this private world of theirs and how all their happiness often depends on having possession of one small room they can call their own.

## (c) The whole way of life

A patient's whole way of life is built up of behaviour and actions that repeat themselves endlessly. They go to make up his general conduct in regard to others, his work and his family. From the patient's life history we can often see whether we are dealing with some development of an unchanging 'Anlage' or whether everything points to an alteration in the whole conduct from a given point in time.

Our destinies depend a good deal on the details and small circumstances which we have created for ourselves but rather more perhaps than we usually care to think on the type of our personality, and great good fortune is sometimes understandable as the direct result of a person's attitude in that he has taken quick advantage of an opportunity which others have let slide. It is in this sense that we try to understand a person's fate as in part at least the direct product of himself.

## (d) Overt actions

The mentally ill person can live outside hospital and not be primarily conspicuous for those symptoms which later strike us as important and basic features of the illness (e.g. subjective experiences). What makes him conspicuous is his *noticeable overt social conduct*. From the standpoint of psychological analysis, this is something 'peripheral', but individual actions are so striking that they often come into the centre of consideration as something ominous both for the community and the patient.

The ordinary environment always stresses the *content* of the activity and originally scientific psychiatry was no exception. *Different modes of action* were designated *according to characteristic content* and classified as different illnesses. Psychiatry thus built up a theory of *monomania*, which was soon discarded as it was only concerned with a description of externals; a few of the names still survive: kleptomania,[1] pyromania, dipsomania,[2] nymphomania, homicidal monomania, etc.

[1] G. Schmidt, *Zbl. Neurol.*, vol. 92 (1939).        [2] Gaupp, *Die Dipsomanie* (Jena, 1901).

Wandering, suicide, refusal of food and above all crime are the overt actions of patients that achieve most notoriety.

*Wandering*[1] is observed in paranoiacs who go from place to place hoping to escape persecution; also in demented patients who can no longer make any social adjustment but let fate drive them aimlessly up and down the country. It can also be observed in melancholic patients who will wander about in anxious distress but we come across it mostly in the form of particular states such as the so-called *fugue-states*.

Fugue-states imply wandering which begins *suddenly*, usually without any adequate understandable connection with the preceding psychic state; they do not appear as the sequelae of chronic disorder. The wandering has *no plan* and there is no *destination*. 'Fugue-states for the most part may be regarded as a morbid *reaction* of constitutionally degenerate individuals to *states of dysphoria*. These states of dysphoria may be *autochthonous* adverse moods. Insignificant factors in the environment may however *precipitate them*. The tendency to run away may become *habitual* and it can then be precipitated by smaller and smaller stimuli' (Heilbronner).

Suicide[2] when due to psychosis may be the result of extreme mental anguish in melancholia, an extreme weariness of living and utter despair or, in dementias, it may spring from a sudden impulse. A half-hearted attempt at suicide is not so uncommon. The individual sees to it that some lucky chance saves him at the right moment. Most suicides, however, are not committed by the mentally ill but by people who are abnormally disposed (psychopaths). The percentage of suicide in psychotic patients as against the total number of suicides varies with different authors from 3 per cent to 66 per cent. Gruhle assumes that some 10 per cent to 20 per cent of all suicides are due to genuine psychosis. Suicide in really mentally ill people is characterised by a particular cruelty and by the tenacity with which the attempt is repeated if it miscarried in any way. Often psychosis can be recognised by this one feature alone.

In acutely ill patients we sometimes come across brutal attempts at *self-mutilation*; they gouge out their own eyes, cut off the penis, etc.[3]

There are a number of psychic reasons for *the refusal to eat*:[4] conscious intention to commit suicide; total absence of appetite; disdain of food; fear of being poisoned; blocking when offered food (sometimes these patients will eat when unobserved); retardation of all psychic life to the extent of stupor. Other patients on the contrary will eat everything eatable and uneatable; everything they come across goes into their mouth; they will eat faeces, drink urine.

Sometimes patients will later give their reason for not eating: for instance, 'I have lost the feel of my body and think I have become a spirit which lives on air and love . . .' 'I don't need to eat any longer; I am waiting for paradise to feed on fruits' . . . 'Latterly food revolts me, I think it is human flesh or live animals which I can see moving' (Gruhle).

[1] Ludwig Mayer, *Der Wandertrieb*, Diss. (Würzburg, 1934). Stier, *Fahnenflucht u. unerlaubte Entfernung* (Halle, 1918). Heilbronner, 'Über Fugue u. fugueähnliche Zustände', *Jb. Psychiatr*, vol. 23 (1903), p. 107.

[2] H. W. Gruhle, *Selbstmord* (Leipzig, 1940) (excellent informative review). See my *Philosophie* (1932), vol. 2, pp. 300–14, for a philosophical discussion.

[3] Freymuth, *Allg. Z. Psychiatr.*, vol. 51, p. 260. Flägge, *Arch. Psychiatr.* (D), vol. 11, p. 184.

[4] Krüger, *Allg. Z. Psychiatr.*, vol. 69 (1912), p. 326.

The texts[1] on criminal psychology give good orientation in regard to the *crimes* committed by mental patients and people suffering from personality disorders (psychopaths).

*Persecuted paranoiacs* not only write to the papers, compose pamphlets, write to the Public Prosecutor, but take their own steps to murder; they not only write love-letters to famous people but will attack the supposed mistress in the street. The despairing *melancholic* kills his family as well as himself. Patients in *twilight states* may become violent as a result of sudden delusional notions or some accidental stimulus.

An especially alarming event is the *meaningless murder* committed in the *preceding or initial stages of schizophrenia.* Motivation appears lacking, the deed is carried out with an unfeeling callousness, there is no insight or regret. The person talks with an alien indifference of what he has done. These really sick people have not been recognised as such by those around them and often not by their own doctor. They consider themselves quite well but it is impossible really to understand what they have done. Only later on does diagnosis become certain.[2]


§ 2. Transformation of the Personal World

Every creature and hence every man lives in a world which surrounds him (*Umwelt*), that is, the world which the subject apperceives and makes his own, which becomes active in him and on which, he in his turn, acts. The *objective setting (objektive Umgebung)* is all that is there for the observer even if not there for the subject who characteristically lives as if it were not there. The *picture of the world (Weltbild)* is that part of the surrounding world of which the individual has become conscious and which has reality for him. The surrounding world and the objective setting both include more than the world-picture does: they include all that is unconsciously present in the surroundings, all that is actually effective and existent in feeling and mood, all that is simply the objective setting and all that has taken unknown effect.

The concrete world of the individual always develops *historically*. It stands within a tradition and always exists in society and community. Therefore any inquiry into how a human being lives in the world and how different he may find it must be of an historical and social nature. We are presented with a wealth of complicated structures which we may call after the particular human manifestation prevailing at the time: e.g. man as a creature of instinct, economic man, man in power, professional man, the worker, the peasant, etc. The world which objectively exists provides the space in which the individual

---

[1] v. Krafft-Ebing, *Gerichtliche Psychopathologie.* Cramer, *Gerichtliche Psychiatrie.* Hoche, *Handbuch der gerichtlichen Psychiatrie,* 3rd edn. Further: *Monatsschrift für Kriminalbiologie u. Strafrechtsreform,* Bisher, 32nd edn.
[2] Glaser, 'Tötungsdelikt als Symptom von beginnender Schizophrenie', *Z. Neur.,* vol. 150 (1934), p. 1. K. Wilmans, 'Über Morde im Prodromalstadium der Schizophrenie', *Z. Neur.,* vol. 170 (1940), p. 583. Bürger-Prinz, *Mschr. Krim.,* vol. 32 (1941), p. 149. Schottky, 'Über Brandstiftungen', *Z. Neur.,* vol. 173 (1941), p. 109.

takes his ways and byways and is the material from which he currently builds his personal world.

It is not the task of psychopathology to investigate all this but it is important for any psychopathologist to have some orientation here and be factually informed about the concrete worlds from which his patients come.

The question arises whether there may be transformations in a *psychopathological* sense, whether there are *specific 'private worlds'* in the case of psychotics and psychopaths (personality disorders). Or whether all 'abnormal' worlds are only a particular realisation of forms and components which are essentially universal and historical and have nothing to do with being sick or well. In this case it is only the mode of their realisation, and the singular way in which they are experienced, which could be called abnormal.

In every case it is most rewarding to try and grasp this abnormal world as such, whenever it may be open to our observation. Patients' conduct, actions, ways of thinking and knowing become connected meaningfully in all their detail once we have a comprehensive picture of their transformed world as a whole; then, given the over-all context, they become understandable even if the total structure has to remain incomprehensible to any form of genetic understanding.[1]

Two distinctions have to be made: there is the constant metamorphosis of all human worlds through the processes of culture, the *historical manifold*, and there is an *unhistorical variety* of psychopathological possibilities. L. Binswanger reminds us that Hegel's thesis still holds: 'Individuality is its own world'. But we can investigate it either as a cultural, historical phenomenon or as a psychological or psychopathological one. Whether and when psychopathological world-pictures, in themselves unhistorical, have had any relevance for history and culture is a matter for historical research but no unequivocal answers have yet been found.

*The fact of a 'personal world'* is both a *subjective* and *objective* phenomenon. Just as feelings give rise to thoughts which clarify the feelings and increase them by acting back on them, so the subject's total frame of reference grows up into a world, which manifests itself subjectively in emotional atmospheres, feelings, states of mind, and objectively in opinions, mental content, ideas and symbols.

When does a 'personal world' become abnormal? The normal world is characterised by objective human ties, a mutuality in which all men meet; it is a satisfying world, a world that brings increase and makes life unfold. We can speak of an abnormal personal world: (1) if it springs from a specific type of event, which can be empirically recognised, e.g. the schizophrenic process,

---

[1] von Gebsattel, E. Straus, von Bayer, L. Binswanger, Kunz, all make valuable contributions. Here we are dealing only with the descriptive aspect of such enquiries. What they try to achieve in the way of a 'constructive-genetic' psychology and anthropology is discussed later (p. 540). It sometimes may seem that these authors are only describing well-known findings in another way, but it is just in this fresh description that we find something essentially new, a concept of the whole that poses fresh questions.

even though the products of this world may be thoroughly positive. (2) if it divides people instead of bringing them together. (3) if it narrows down progressively, atrophies, no longer has any expanding or heightening effects; (4) if it dies away altogether, and the feeling vanishes of 'being in secure possession of spiritual and material goods, the firm ground in which the personality roots and from which it gains the heart to achieve its potentialities and enjoy its growth' (Ideler). Children who are uprooted from their own world at an early age fall prey to destructive nostalgia; so, at the beginning of psychoses, the transformation of the person's world may become an annihilating and ruinous catastrophe.

We cannot say how far this study of personal worlds will lead, we can only attempt it. Formulations of a comprehensive and general character may sound impressive but their use is limited. The chief thing is how successful can one be in presenting these concrete, private universes clearly and convincingly for purposes of observation. What sort of world is the patient's world, seen with his eyes? Here are a few reports:

## (a) *The worlds of schizophrenic patients*

Schizophrenic psychic life, particularly thinking and delusion, can be analysed as a particular phenomenon of experience (experience of primary delusion) and as a disturbance of the thought-process (schizophrenic thinking). In both cases attention has to be given to the form of the disturbance. We may rightly feel that this is an advance on the old classification of delusion according to content, but we should be wrong to neglect the question of the possible components of the disturbance, the enquiry into the specific schizophrenic nature of the patient's world-formation. There is without doubt a typical and common connection between content and psychosis: delusions of catastrophe, cosmic delusions, delusions of reprieve, rather less common but still very characteristic delusions of persecution, of jealousy, of marriage, etc. One effect of the change in personality already shows itself in connection with the primary experience of delusion, namely that the content is held to with the utmost conviction. von Bayer[1] quite rightly says the schizophrenic world discloses itself in the delusion more tangibly, vividly and in greater detail than in any other of the psychopathological phenomena. He finds that the formal changes in experience and function never by themselves define the nature of the schizophrenic psychic life satisfactorily. Rather it is an established fact that schizophrenia brings with it a transformation of *the content of experience*. It is not merely chance contents of a general human kind haphazardly interpreted into meaningless structures, but primary contents themselves that constitute the character of the disturbance.

Schizophrenics, however, are not surrounded by a single schizophrenic world, but by a number of such worlds. If there were a single, uniform world-formation schizophrenics would understand each other and form their own

[1] W. v. Bayer, 'Über konformen Wahn', *Z. Neur.*, vol. 140 (1932), p. 398.

community. But we find just the opposite. They hardly ever understand each other; if anything, a healthy person understands them better. There are, however, exceptions. These should be of the greatest interest. We can in this way obtain indirectly an objective picture of a typical schizophrenic world. A community of schizophrenics is certainly almost an impossibility, since in every case it has to grow artificially and is not there naturally, as with all communities of healthy people. In acute psychoses lack of awareness excludes any communal life anyway. In the chronic end states, however, it is the individual rigidity and the pervading egocentricity of the delusion that precludes any communal life, or almost so. A number of favourable conditions have to coincide for any schizophrenic community to arise and grow. We have found that it can happen and on occasion has actually existed. This is of some importance. v. Bayer observes:

A married couple fell ill simultaneously with a schizophrenic process, and this enabled their delusions to develop in common; it spread to the children (who were healthy and in them the illness was only 'induced'). A family delusion was elaborated with a common content and common behaviour resulted. They developed common ideas as to the origin and course of the persecution directed against them; 'people talk about them, newspapers allude to them; people are sent to spy on them; some machine hums and blows evil-smelling fumes into the house, and projects magic pictures and shapes on to the ceiling'. The husband tended to have visual, the wife acoustic hallucinations. The man reported thought-withdrawal, the wife had experiences of being bound. The community-aspect lies in the content not so much in the formal aspect of the disturbances. They achieved a form of understanding in a world they knew in common, in which the individual peculiarities of the separate experiences were absorbed into the common whole: 'we are persecuted; whenever we encounter the outside world, the persecution is there'. So these patients with their children lived as a group in a world of their own and mutually afflicted. Persecution and threats continually increased in their environment, the Authorities, the Republic, the Catholics, etc., were all acting against the family. Persecution came from all directions, from the whole of the world that surrounded them, near and far. The persecutors were always sly and secret, allusions always hidden, something caught in passing, showing that they were being controlled, talked about or mocked. Secret machinations assumed vast proportions. The patients were ringed round by a world of enemies, in a world which they understood in common, constantly nourished on new experiences. The result was common action, e.g. measures of defence against the 'machine', alterations to the house, plans to discover the persecutors, etc. The last result of all was the admission to hospital.

The *means* of communication were of course no different from those used by healthy people; logical constructions, the giving of reasons and information, systematising, with daily repetition and confirmation. The *content* of the communication, however, was the delusion that had risen from the springs of schizophrenic experience. Because of the actual proximity of the family members this became something which they all could share. We cannot unfortunately answer the question whether the patients understood among themselves something which we fail to understand. If this were so, we should be able to see at last the specific content of a schizophrenic world. The putting of the question is more important than the empirical answers so far obtained. In v. Bayer's case the delusional content was only one of personal persecution, a relatively trivial content. How would if be if one encountered the not very likely possibility of a schizophrenic community united in common delusions of a merciful cosmos, a content which they mutually elaborate as true by means of their common experience of it?

For the time being the question stays open: why is schizophrenia in its initial stages so often (though not in the majority of cases) a process of cosmic, religious or metaphysical revelation? It is an extremely impressive fact: this exhibition of fine and subtle understanding, this impossible, shattering piano-performance, this masterly creativity (van Gogh, Hölderlin), these peculiar experiences of the end of the world or the creation of fresh ones, these spiritual revelations and this grim daily struggle in the transitional periods between health and collapse. Such experiences cannot be grasped simply in terms of the psychosis which is sweeping the victim out of his familiar world, an objective symbol as it were of the radical, destructive event attacking him. Even if we speak of existence or the psyche as disintegrating, we are still only using analogies. We observe that a new world has come into being and so far that is the only fact we have.

## (b) The worlds of obsessional patients

The obsessional patient is pursued by ideas and images which not only seem to him alien but silly, and yet he has to keep to them as if they were true. If he does not do this he is overtaken by unbearable anxiety. The patient, for instance, finds he must do something or else someone will die, or something dreadful will happen. It is as if his doing and thinking can obstruct or influence events in a magical way. His thoughts become built into a system of meanings and his actions into a system of ceremonial rituals. But whatever he does or thinks, a doubt is always left behind whether his performance has been correct or complete. The doubt forces him to start all over again.

Straus[1] reports on the self-description of a 40-year-old obsessional patient, who was 'contaminated' with everything connected with death, corruption, graveyards, etc., and had constantly to defend herself against this 'contamination' and undo it. In her self-description she even had to leave out any words so related and there are therefore certain gaps:

In January 1931 . . . a very dear friend. His wife came to see us every Sunday after she had been to . . . At first this did not trouble me. After 4–6 months I felt uneasy about her gloves, then her coat, her shoes, etc. I saw to it these did not get too near me. As we lived close to . . . everyone who went there made me uneasy, and quite a number go. If any of these people touched me, I had to wash my clothing.

[1] E. Straus, 'Ein Beitrag zur Pathologie der Zwangserscheinungen', *Mschr. Psychiatr.*, vol. 98 (1938), p. 61.

Or if anyone who had been there came into my flat, I found my movements restricted. I got the feeling that the room was very small and that my dress was touching everything. I washed everything in Dettol to get some peace. Everything got large again and I felt I had room. If I wanted to go to the shops and there was someone in the shop, I couldn't go in because the person might come up against me; so I got no peace all day long and the thing persecuted me all the time. Sometimes I had to wipe something off, here or there, sometimes I had to wash. Pictures in the papers which showed such things troubled me. If my hand touched them, I had to wash. I cannot write it all down, there is too much that upsets me. Inside I am in a constant turmoil.

v. Gebsattel[1] gives an unusually impressive description of how these patients live in their own peculiar world, or rather how they lose their own life, world and all, in the trap of a magical mechanism:

Certain actions have to be repeated endlessly by the patients; they have to be endlessly controlling or making sure, they have to carry out something which is never completed until they are exhausted; all the time they are convinced of the nonsensical nature of their activity. The hand-washing, the rituals and ceremonies are a defence against disaster. They mean something different from what they mean to the beholder: everywhere contamination threatens, corruption and death—all kinds of disintegration. It is a magical world, though there is no belief in it; yet the obsessional patient has fallen into it; it is a pseudo-magical counter-world. It becomes restricted increasingly to negative meanings. The patient only responds to contents which symbolise loss or danger. The friendly, inviting forces of existence vanish, giving place to hostile and repellent ones. There is nothing that is harmless, natural or obvious. The world has narrowed to an artificial uniformity, a rigid, strictly regulated unchangeability. The patient is always in action but nothing is achieved. 'There is restless exertion without a break; he is always trying to cope with an enemy who is always behind him.' Existence becomes for him a move towards non-existence in the images of 'dirt or faeces, poison or fire, all that is ugly, impure or corpse-like'—and a futile defence against such a move. The countenance of the world has contracted to sheer hostility. But this world ceases to be a world as things undergo increasing derealisation. They no longer *are*, they only have meanings, and negative ones at that. There is a loss of solidity, richness and form, and hence of reality; the world is no more. The patient however is seized by a frightful feeling of being driven, because the whole apparatus of measures which must be taken if the patient is to do what he wants grows more and more complicated. The counter-compulsions and the auxiliary structures grow endlessly and increase the impossibility of reaching the desired goal. The patient is now never finished, but only stops through exhaustion. Since the patient knows the absurdity of what she does, but cannot stop doing it, she shies away from onlookers. 'Few doctors can have seen a patient like H. H., who goes through the most fantastic manipulations for hours when drying his limbs, or practices endless puppet-like compulsions. E. Sp. in the same way will lock herself in when she stands in the middle of her room in the evening, and carries on into the early morning with her repetitive compulsions, half senseless with exhaustion, gesticulating into the air and imitating the never-completed task of washing her stockings.'

[1] v. Gebsattel, 'Die Welt der Zwangskranken', *Mschr. Psychiatr.*, vol. 99 (1938), p. 10.

v. Gebsattel compares the world of the *anankasts* with that of the *paranoics*. Both live in worlds that have lost their candour, both see meanings everywhere in meaningless occurrences. No accident can be treated any more as mere chance. There are only intentions. Both show us indirectly how much we need a world that does not take any notice of us but to which we yet belong. The obsessional paitent however knows that the meanings that come to him are nonsensical. For the paranoic patient the meaning of the phenomena is integral with its reality. For the anankast there is still left a glimmer of former reality with its characteristics of harmless forthrightness. He cannot attain to this but he can still glimpse it through the 'Walpurgis' night of his magic meanings. The paranoic retains a measure of trust and naturalness in his delusional world, and a portion of certainty and conviction which has no analogue in the feverish restlessness of the anankast. Even that dreadful disorder, schizophrenia, with its delusions, might seem a respite in face of the restless chase of the wideawake mind, knowing otherwise yet helpless in the grip of its obsession. The obsessional patient in his small corner of compelling magical performance seems to see the whole world vanishing from him, with all his senses alive and intact to tell him so.

The world of the obsessional patient has two basic characteristics: It is a transformation of everything into threat, fear, formlessness, uncleanness, rot and death; and it is such a world only because of a magic meaning which supplies the content of the compulsive phenomena, but which is wholly negative: the magic is compelling, but the mind sees it as altogether absurd.

### (c) The worlds of patients with 'flight-of-ideas'

L. Binswanger has tried to understand these worlds as if they were meaningful wholes.[1]

There is a mood for a 'joyful existence', a basic attitude of 'bounding life' which makes the world look flat, not only this but it grows distant and faint for the patient and gives to his rapid, always distractible grasp of what is near and far, an absorption in the moment, a haste and confusion of movement, a ceaseless series of distractions. His world is pliant and variegated, bright and rosy. All that is left for curiosity and activity is a chatter of words and a play with speech. According to Binswanger there is, all the same, a specific pattern in this particular world that gives it a meaning as a whole. It has grown into a peculiar world of its own, conditioned by the spirit which illuminates it from within; this vital experience brings about immense vigour, the melting of boundaries, wholesale intrusions and the crowding together of things, an ineffective busyness, a general flitting, a press of talk and grandiloquent speech; in short, the whole behaviour of the manic state.

Let us *compare* these various attempts to understand the meaningful structure of such worlds. From this point of view the illumination of *the flight of ideas* seems only to catch at something quite superficial. Here we are not dealing with any real transformation of a person's world, but with an

[1] L. Binswanger, *Über Ideenflucht* (Zurich, 1933).

altered state, in which, it is true, a temporary transformation does take place; this transformation, however, does not contribute anything essential in respect of the whole it represents (which can only be grasped in the form of the subjective experience of the state, and as a change in the flow of the person's psychic life). Analysis of the world of the *obsessional patient* seems more productive; it has brought out very clearly an integration of a very peculiar kind. The enquiry into *the schizophrenic worlds* takes us furthest into fundamentals, but here it is only the problem that has grown in significance, the actual answers are sparse.

## SECTION THREE

## THE PSYCHE OBJECTIFIED IN KNOWLEDGE AND ACHIEVEMENT

### (PSYCHOLOGY OF CREATIVITY—WERKPSYCHOLOGIE)

Psychic life is perpetually engaged in the process of making itself objective. It externalises itself through the drive to activity, the drive to express, to represent and communicate. Finally comes the pure mental drive, the wish to see clearly what is, what I am and what these other basic drives have brought about. This final effort to objectify might also be expressed as follows: What has become objective should now be comprehended and patterned into a general objectivity. I want to know what I know and understand what it is I have understood.

The basic phenomenon of mind is that it arises on psychological ground but is not something psychic in itself; it is an objective meaning, a world which others share. The individual acquires a mind solely through sharing in the general mind which is historically transmitted and at any given moment is defined for him in a contemporary form. The general or objective mind is currently present in social habits, ideas and communal norms, in language and in the achievements of science, poetry and art. It is also present in all our institutions.

This objective mind is substantially valid and cannot fall sick. But the individual can fall sick in the way in which he partakes in it and reproduces it. Moreover almost all normal and abnormal psychic events imprint themselves somehow on the objective mind according to the way in which it appears to the individual. But if mind in itself cannot fall ill how is the individual seen to be sick in this respect? By reason of *deficiencies*, losses, distortions and inversions and everything contrary to normal in the realisation of his part in mind; also by reason of *a specific kind of productivity*, which indicates sickness not so much in its results but in its source (Van Gogh's pictures, Hölderlin's later hymns); lastly by reason of the *positive significance which patients give to these deficiencies and abnormalities*. The essence of being human and of being a sick human shows itself in the way in which the individual appropriates structures of the mind to his own use and modifies them.

A further basic phenomenon of mind is that only that exists for the psyche which acquires objective mental form, but whatever has acquired this form at once acquires a specific reality which impresses itself upon the psyche. Words, once formed, are like something insurmountable, and the psyche is at once confined by the mind through which it grows real.

Lastly, it is a basic phenomenon of mind that it can only become real if some psyche receives or reproduces it. The genuineness of this mental reality is inseparable from the authenticity of the psychic events that mediate it. But since it is through structure, modes of speech and diverse forms of activity and behaviour that mind becomes objective, automatisms of speech, conventional activity and gesture may substitute for the genuineness of authentic reproduction. Genuine symbols vanish into supposedly known contents of superstition; rationalisation supplants the authentic source. Both these factors play a significant part in psychic illness. On the one hand we find a maximum of mechanical and automatic behaviour and on the other a disturbing vigour of experience which overwhelms the psyche. The most extreme possibilities are realised in the illness.

We will now glance at the mental productivity of patients, which is a huge problem and we do no more than touch upon it briefly.

## § 1. Individual Instances of Creative Work

*(a) Speech (cp. pp.* 185 ff.).

Communication between rational beings and with their own selves is conducted by means of speech. Speech is a precondition for thinking (speechless thought only occurs as a passing phase within spoken thought, otherwise it remains as indistinct and broken as the thinking of apes).

Speech is the most universal of human 'works'. It is the very first and it is present everywhere and conditions everything. It exists in a great many forms as the given tongue of a particular human group or nation and it is always in the process of a constant slow transformation. The individual speaks by taking part in the common achievement.[1]

We have observed speech as performance and are now concerned with it as an achievement.

(1) *Speech as expression.* Where the speech apparatus is normal, speech apart from its content is psychic expression: as, for instance, shrieking, shouting, whispering in every possible nuance of tone, as we can observe in any disturbed ward; or it may be in the form of monotonous, expressionless speech or speech heightened in tone and lively. It may show itself in the rhythm, in nonsensical emphases, in normal syntax or in syntax that cuts across sense; or

---

[1] O. Jespersen, *Die Sprache, ihre Natur, Entwicklung u. Entstehung* (Heidelberg, 1925). An excellent book but there is an immense literature on this subject.

in the general manner, such as the imitation of infantile speech (agrammatism) in hysterical states, etc.[1]

(2) *The question of the autonomy of speech.* Disturbances in the speech-apparatus of a neurological character are to be distinguished from the transformations in speech due to psychic changes while the speech apparatus itself remains intact. A vast number of phenomena appear to lie between these two (psychotic speech-disturbances—see pp. 191 ff.), and belong properly to neither. They suggest that there is such a thing as autonomy of speech. In this connection we notice peculiar speech-structures and it is difficult to see their derivation; it is just as if speech developed a quality of independence, was producing on its own or having a disorder of its own. It is not an independence of the speech-apparatus but of mentation which appears in pure form in speech. The transformation of the individual and of his experience of mental productivity appears not as something secondary in his speech but primarily as speech. Speech may be called a tool and in this sense mind and tools are not in opposition but mutually shape each other; in the marginal case however they fuse into one; something purely linguistic. Later this becomes a factor in mental achievement which may leave an imprint on literature. The excellent work of Mette[2] draws our attention to this in a very fruitful way.

(3) *Formation of new words and private language.* The formation of new words[3] has long been noticed as an abnormality of speech. Some patients only produce one or two such words, but others produce so many that they seem to have produced a private language of their own, though it remains unintelligible to us. We can group these new word-formations according to how they originate: 1. New words are formed quite *intentionally* to describe feelings or things for which customary speech has not yet found words. These self-structured 'technical terms' (termini technici) are to some extent quite original and the etymology is incomprehensible. 2. New words are formed *unintentionally*, particularly in acute states, are then used secondarily to denote something and get taken over into the chronic state. A patient of Pfersdorff described certain of his hallucinatory phenomena as 'sensuous weapons' (sinnliche Gewehre). The patient is asked, 'What does this mean?' and he says, 'The words come to me like that, there is no explanation.' In acute psychoses we also find that recognised words have been given a different meaning:

A patient says: I used some words as I said before to express ideas quite different from what they customarily expressed—they had acquired a different meaning for me: for example, 'scabby', which I used quite comfortably for 'brave and plucky'; 'Gohn', the argot word for 'muck-raker', was used for a woman, rather like the student's 'char'. Ideas pressed thickly and I could not find exactly the right word for them, so I babbled inventively, like small children do, and created terms to my own taste such as 'Wuttas' for 'pigeons' (Forel).

[1] Isserlin, *Allg. Z. Psychiatr.*, vol. 75 (1919), p. 1.
[2] A. Mette, *Über Beziehungen zwischen Spracheigentümlichkeiten Schizophrener und dichterischer Produktion* (Dessau, 1928).
[3] Galant, *Arch. Psychiatr.* (D), vol. 61 (1919), p. 12.

3. Words of new formation come to the patient in the form of '*hallucinatory content*'. The patients themselves, as in the foregoing cases, are often surprised at these strange and alien words. Schreber heard in this way the whole 'basic language' of his 'rays'. He always emphasised that until he heard the words they had been quite unknown to him. 4. *Articulate sounds* are produced, to which the patients themselves probably attach no meaning. In fact there is no longer a speech-structure, as all meaning seems to have lapsed. An example would be the verbal remnants which one tries to catch in demented paralytics. One patient during his last few weeks of life could only produce the one word 'misabuck' on every occasion.

New word-formations are the main element in the private language of schizophrenics:[1]

Tuczek observed the development of such a language as a kind of game due to delight in translation and a certain facility for playing with words. It was done quite consciously without any need to express delusional experiences. Pride in this secret achievement and pleasure in success were the only motives: 'just listen how nicely it sounds!' Many different principles were involved in the word-formation but the words were then established and one could notice the not inconsiderable memory performance involved. There was undoubted creative ability. The syntax remained German and it was only the vocabulary that had been reconstructed.

### (b) Patients' written productions[2]

Patients who commit themselves to literary creation corresponding to their level of education often show us plenty of rational content mixed up with phenomena of expression, displayed in the language and writing. In rare cases there is a remarkable productivity of original speech. We can distinguish the following different types of writing: 1. Language and style are in good order and the writing shows normal sequence of thought. *Only the content* is abnormal; the patients report on their terrible experiences, try to clarify them and set forth their delusional ideas. Such writing in spite of the intense affect is sensible and controlled. The description by patients with insight after they have recovered from their psychoses also comes into this category. We find in this group a number of valuable self-descriptions. 2. The second group of writings comes from person suffering from *abnormal personality development* (querulants etc.). The writer elaborates his delusion-like ideas in a natural manner and in a thoroughly coherent way but extravagantly, fantastically, contentiously and fanatically. No self-description of morbid experiences occurs—and indeed such personalities have not had them—but they direct their attack upon mental hospitals, the authorities, doctors or they elaborate their ideas as inventors, explorers, etc. Most published writings of patients belong to this group. 3. More rarely we find writings, where the manner is very

---

[1] Tuczek, 'Analyse einer Katatonikersprache', *Z. Neur.*, vol. 72, p. 279. Jessner, 'Eine in der Psychose entstandene Kunstsprache', *Arch. Psychiatr.* (D), vol. 94 (1931), p. 382.

[2] A. Behr, *Schriftstellerische Tätigkeit in der Paranoia* (Leipzig, 1905). Sikorski, *Arch. Psychiatr.* (D), vol. 38, p. 259.

bizarre, and the style high-flown and striking, though for the most part we can understand them. The patients do not report their experiences, persecutions and other personal facts, but *develop theories*, new *cosmic systems*, new religions, new interpretations of the Bible, or of universal problems, etc. The form and the content indicate that they originate from patients suffering from a schizophrenic process. The presentation often will show the main delusion of the author (he is the Messiah, he is an inventor).[1] 4. Transitional types of writing develop from the above, and we get scripts that are thoroughly *confused*. Arrangement vanishes, the thoughts grow disconnected; there is a series of bizarre, unintelligible thought-formations.[2] In the end everything becomes incomprehensible: hieroglyphics are written, single syllables, there are ornamentations, and colours are used to characterise external events. 5. Finally we get the poetry of undoubted psychotics. Gaupp[3] published the case of a paranoic patient, who portrayed his own fate in a play concerning the sick King Ludwig of Bavaria; this dramatic work was an act of liberation for him and the only thing that had any value while he was in the hospital; he found his own nature again in the person of his dramatic subject. K. Schneider[4] published some verses of a young schizophrenic, which express the gruelling change taking place in his person and in his world. The most magnificent and the most disturbing examples are the later poems of Hölderlin.

### (c) *Drawing, Art and Handicraft*

We have grouped together defects in performance, the art of schizophrenics and the drawings of neurotic patients:

1. *Defects of performance.* These indicate organic neurological disturbance, poor education or insufficient training. As such they obstruct psychic expression and the communication of intention, but in themselves they have no positive significance as achievement. We encounter them as a lack of skill (the individual cannot draw a straight line), lack of education (the individual has not got the first elements of the technique of drawing); or as a disturbance of motor function and dexterity through some organic illness (signs of ataxia, tremor, etc.), or a disturbance of elementary psychic functions, such as registration, concentration, which leads to scribbles, fragmented shapes and lines rather than what could be called drawing (organic disorders, paralysis in particular). The same sort of defects appear in all the unsuccessful articles which patients make, and which can be seen in any clinical museum.[5]

2. *Schizophrenic art.*[6] We can only identify with certainty the cruder

---

[1] Swedenberg is an example; also Brandenberg, 'Und es ward Licht', in Behr, p. 381. Panucz, Tagebuchblätter eines Schizophrenen', *Z. Neur.*, vol. 123 (1930), p. 299.

[2] Example—Gehrmann, *Körper, Gehirn, Seele, Gott* (Berlin, 1893).

[3] Gaupp, *Z. Neur.*, vol. 69, p. 182.          [4] Schneider, *Z. Neur.*, vol. 48, p. 391.

[5] Lenz, 'Richtungsänderung der künstlerischen Leistung bei. Hirnstammerkrankungen', *Z. Neur.*, vol. 170 (1940), p. 98. (Defects of performance and change of performance.)

[6] Nearly all clinics and institutions have such a collection. Owing to Prinzhorn, the psychiatric clinic in Heidelberg has a number of schizophrenic productions of all kinds.

schizophrenic signs. They give the paintings and drawings a very characteristic appearance; meaningless repetition of the same line or of one and the same object, without any unity of construction, a scrawl that is all but 'methodical', a fine exactness which is no more than verbigeration in the pictorial field. It is all very similar to the involuntary 'doodling' normal people will do in moments of concentrated attention or during a lecture.

Schizophrenic art may be a real expression of the schizophrenic psyche and represent the world of schizophrenic thought that has developed in the patient, but we only get this when there is a certain level of technical skill and where the schizophrenic signs have not swamped the whole picture.[1] *Content* is characteristic; mythical figures, strange birds, grotesque and misshapen forms of people and animals, a bold and ruthless emphasis on sexual characteristics, usually the genitalia; in addition there is an urgency to present some universal whole, a world-picture, the essence of things. Occasionally complicated machines are designed depicting the source of the hallucinatory physical influences. Perhaps even more important is the *form* of the picture. Taking it as a whole we try to find out whether it has any meaning for the patient as a whole or whether it is only a collection of miscellaneous elements. Where in fact is his point of unity? The following are some characteristic signs: a certain pedantry, exactness, laboriousness; a striving for violent effects; stereotyped curves; making everything in a circle; or there are angular lines which give all the pictures an air of similarity. When we try to understand the effect of the drawings on their author and talk to him about it we find the simplest thing is symbolically important and a rich fantasy woven around it.

It cannot be denied that when the patients are gifted people suffering from process schizophrenia their drawings and paintings have a considerable impact on normal people, by reason of their primitive force, vivid expression, weird urgency and strange significance.

If patients are well off and not too ill to be restrained, they may really achieve the most remarkable productions such as those artistic efforts which Goethe saw belonging to Count Pallagonia and the Lodge at Lemgo.[2] The latter was a house where the owner who had been a lifetime building it had filled it to overflowing with carvings of his own and had covered everything with fantastic structures and countless repetitions so that there was not a single clear space or empty corner left.

[1] Prinzhorn, 'Das bildnerische Schaffen des Geisteskranken', *Z. Neur.*, vol. 52 (1919), p. 307. (A historical survey of psychotic art). Morgenthaler, *Ein Geisteskranker als Künstler* (Bern and Leipzig, 1921). Prinzhorn, *Bildnerei der Geisteskranken* (Berlin, Springer, 1922) (standard book on the subject, well illustrated). It also gives good summary of points for analysis: urge to make —drive to play—drive to decorate—tendency to make diagrams—tendency to arrange—desire to symbolise. A detailed report on ten schizophrenic pictures. Points of similarity, childhood drawings, unsophisticated drawings, drawings of primitives, of ancient cultures, folk-art, spiritualistic drawings. Jaspers, *Strindberg u. van Gogh* (Leipzig, Ernst Bircher, 1922; 2nd edn., Berlin, 1926).

[2] Fischer, 'Über die Plastiken des Ften. Pallagonia', *Z. Neur.*, vol. 78 (1922), p. 356. Weygandt, *Z. Neur.*, vol. 101 (1926), p. 857. Kreyenberg, 'Über das Junkerhaus', *Z. Neur.*, vol. 114 (1928), p. 152.

3. *Drawings of neurotic patients.* C. G. Jung introduced the method of letting patients draw and of giving particular attention to their 'psychic pictures', their plan of the cosmos or their basic conception of existence. He takes the Indian mandalas as an analogy.[1] These 'psychic pictures' should help us to penetrate into unconscious psychic life. Apart from the conscious use of symbolism and myth, psychoanalytic interpretation finds in them a way to elucidate the unconscious.

## § 2. The Total Mental Achievement—The Patients' General Outlook—'Weltanschauung'

We have tried to give as vivid a description as possible of the patient's existence in his own personal world. He himself cannot describe the shape of the world in which he lives, the factual whole of his world, and indeed he does not know it himself. Actions and behaviour all show what he thinks is the meaning of a situation and its effective possibilities or in what way it strikes him as obvious and unquestionable. We have to try and put everything together if we are to get even a partial glimpse of the patient's actual world. This is difficult because we can scarcely abandon our own limited worlds. Every step in understanding, however, increases our knowledge and also expands our own existence or suggests such an expansion. Object-awareness, the existing forms of which were described in the section on phenomenology, is always related in content to complex unities which give the momentary content of experience its meaning, function and significant living context. The content is, as it were, steeped in a number of worlds which perhaps are never fully known in their totality but only show themselves indirectly in the way the ideas move and form and the many images and thoughts emerge.

Under favourable circumstances an individual can *become aware of his personal world in a systematic way.* He makes a poem about it or a work of art; he may breed a philosophy or elaborate ideas about the universe. What the patient tells us and what he puts there for us to see is the foundation for any subsequent representation of how he regards the world that has grown in his consciousness. Instead of coming indirectly to the conclusion that we are investigating only the configuration of a world, we have to grasp at the totality of a mind as it objectifies itself in its own way. So far we have barely begun to do this:

From the point of view of method this field offers unlimited scope. But patients do not often offer us anything empirically objective to investigate. There have been certain important historical phenomena and by a lucky chance we may get something from our patients. The methods for knowledge in this field are only acquired through a training in the humanities. We will make two brief points:

Nietzsche conceived all knowledge of the world as 'interpretation' (Auslegen). Our understanding of the world is an interpretation and our understanding of some

[1] Heyer, *Der Organismus der Seele* (München, 1932).

alien world is an interpretation of an interpretation (cp. my book *Nietzsche*, Berlin, 1936, pp. 255 ff.). In understanding the world therefore we not only find an absolute objectivity of the true world but an element of movement for which (from the point of view of the observer of different worlds) the idea of the one, real, true world acts as a marginal concept of which he himself can never take possession.

Each man's world is already a special one. This special world which the individual knows as his own and has so far confronted is always something less than his real world, which remains obscure, all-embracing, an over-reaching whole (see my *Psychologie der Weltanschauungen*, Berlin, 1919, Aufl. 3, 1925).

Analysis of the patients' worlds as they have come to know them is only in its beginning and we group the few attempts that have been made as follows:

## (a) *Realisation of extremes*

There is a particular interest in those realisations of mental possibilities which can be called neither healthy nor sick in themselves and are certainly not psychological in character, though they are something that the patient experiences. Thus *nihilism* and *scepticism* are only complete in psychosis. Nihilistic delusion in melancholia gives us the prototype. The world does not exist any more, the patient himself does not exist; he only appears to live and he must live like this for ever. He has no feelings and he cares for nothing. At the beginning of a schizophrenic process, complete scepticism is not just blandly conceived but is experienced as a desperate affair.[1] There are also classic realisations of *mystical* experiences in hysteria and revelations of a meta-physical-mythical character in the initial stages of schizophrenia.[2]

## (b) *Patients' specific outlooks (Weltanschauungen)*

We may ask what is the special factor which allows a philosophic knowledge of Being to spring up from the schizophrenic base. We may also ask to what extent are these philosophic possibilities merely a caricature. The mind has its historical aspect and is tied to its culture; it has racial characteristics and is bound to tradition. As such it is no subject-matter for psychopathology but something intelligible in its own right, something eternal in time. As a reality of temporal existence, however, it is bound up with the empirical reality of the individual and as such can be explored. The conditions for mental productivity and the actual realisation of this are accessible to our investigation.

*Journeys of the soul* into the Other World, the transcendental geography of lands beyond our senses, form a universal lore. But it is only in patients that we find it all decisively confirmed in the form of a lively, vivid experience. Even today we can observe such events occurring in the psychoses with an impressive wealth of detail and intellectual depth.

The 'cosmic experience' is characteristic of schizophrenic experience. The

[1] Cp. my own work, 'Schicksal u. Psychose', *Z. Neur.*, vol. 14 (1913), pp. 213 ff., 253 ff.

[2] This is shown magnificently in the work of Hölderlin and van Gogh. Cf. my 'Strindberg und van Gogh' (Bern. 1922), 2nd. edn. (Berlin, 1926).

end of the world is here, the 'twilight of the gods'. A mighty revolution is at hand in which the patient plays the major role. He is the centre of all that is coming to pass. He has immense tasks to perform, vast powers. Fabulous distant influences, attractions and obstructions are at work. 'Everything' is always involved: all the peoples of the earth, all men, all the Gods, etc. The whole of human history is experienced at once. The patient lives through infinite millennia. The instant is an eternity to him. He sweeps through space with immense speed, to conduct mighty battles; he walks safely by the abyss. Here are a few examples from self-descriptions:

I have said that I had countless visions connected with my ideas of the end of the world. These were both horrible and magnificent. I will think of a few of them. In one I was going down in a lift into the depths of the earth, and I went down as it were back through the whole history of man and the earth. In the upper strata there were still woods in leaf; as I got lower it grew dark and black. On leaving the lift I came to a huge graveyard and found among others the place where the inhabitants of Leipzig lay and the grave of my wife. Sitting in the lift again I progressed to point 3. I was afraid to enter point 1, which marked the absolute origin of mankind. As I travelled back, the lift-shaft collapsed behind me endangering a 'sun-god' who lived in it. In this connection it seemed there were two lift-shafts, perhaps corresponding to the division of the realm of god into two (?), then the news came that the second shaft had collapsed; all was lost. Another time I traversed the whole earth from Lake Ladoga to Brazil and built there a sort of castle and a wall with the keeper's help for the protection of god's kingdom against the inflowing yellow tide. I related this to the danger of syphilitic infection. On yet another occasion I had the feeling that I was being pulled up to heaven and saw the whole earth under me, a picture of incomparable splendour and beauty stretched out under the blue dome.

Wetzel[1] gives an account of the experience of the end of the world as felt by schizophrenics:

The end of the world is experienced as a transition to something new, vaster, and is felt as a terrible annihilation. Despairing agony and blissful revelation occur in one and the same patient. At first everything seems queer, uncanny and significant. Catastrophe is impending; the deluge is here. A unique catastrophe approaches. It is Good Friday; something comes over the world; the last Judgment, the breaking of the seven seals of the Book of Revelation. God comes into the world. The time of the first Christians is here. Time wheels back. The last riddle of all is being solved. Patients are exposed to all these terrifying and magnificent experiences without showing it to anyone. The feeling of being quite alone is unspeakably frightening and patients implore not to be left to themselves, or alone in the desert, the frozen cold or in the snow (although it is the middle of summer).

In contrast to the experiences of delirium, these typical cases of schizophrenic experience display clear consciousness, a relatively sound memory and

[1] A. Wetzel, Z. Neur., vol. 78 (1922), p. 403.

good perception, if the attention can be attracted by something and is not entirely chained by the content of the experience. Patients can be doubly orientated, to the psychotic experience and to reality. However, such typical cases do not seem particularly common.

The schizophrenic world of acute psychosis with its double orientation is something quite different from the world of the chronic states. This can grow into a system of ideas which for the patients carry memories of unforgettable occurrences in the acute state, and take deep effect. However in the end the double orientation vanishes.

A delusional system with a typical world outlook of its own then develops on the basis of the transformed self, on the experience of superhuman powers and emanations, as well as of shattering dissolution, of hidden significance and altered mood. Hilfiker has described this as follows:[1]

The self is identified with the All. The patient is not just someone else (Christ, Napoleon, etc.) but simply the All. His own life is experienced as the life of the whole world, his strength is world-sustaining and world-vitalising. He is the seat of this supra-personal power. The patients talk of an automatic power, of primary substance, of seed, fertility, magnetic powers. Their death would be the death of the world; if they die, everyone else dies. Three different patients said: 'If you do not keep in touch with me, you will perish.'—'Once I am dead, you will all lose your minds.'—'If you can't find a substitute for me, everything is lost.' Patients feel they have a magic influence on nature: 'When my eyes are bright blue, the sky gets blue'—'all the clocks of the world feel my pulse'—'my eyes and the sun are the same.'

One of Hilfiker's patients said: 'Only one peasant in the whole of Europe can support himself, and that man is I . . . if I look at or walk over a piece of wasteland, it becomes good land . . . my body bears fruit . . . it is a world-body . . .' He, his wife and his son—three human lives . . . are the first seers and listeners; they are the three international peoples related to soil, water and sun, and correspond to the sun, moon and evening star . . . 'the warmer we are, the more productive the sun becomes . . . No state can support itself. If the world grows poor, they must come and fetch me; they have to have someone to support the world; the world must be represented or the world will disappear.'

### (c) Patients' own observations of a philosophical character

This group includes descriptions that note the modes in which the patients' general world-outlook appears and try to discover the particular modulation or colouring or even their identification with normal attitudes. Mayer-Gross tried to do this and showed how a remarkable form of jesting and joking, irony and humour appears in schizophrenic behaviour.[2] Gerhard Kloos took these observations further and deeper.[3] Many patients have shown powers of scientific reasoning and a certain freakish philosophy and efforts have been

[1] Hilfiker, 'Die schizophrene Ichauflösung im All', *Allg. Z. Psychiatr.*, vol. 87 (1927), p. 439.
[2] Mayer-Gross, *Z. Neur.*, vol. 69, p. 322.
[3] G. Kloos, 'Über den Witz der Schizophrenie', *Z. Neur.*, vol. 172 (1941), p. 536.

made to unravel them. For instance a patient devised a numerical system for 'solving life's problems'.[1]

Newspaper accounts of deaths, accidents, etc., were an occasion for him to prove that they had to happen. He devised combinations of figures from the names, circumstances, etc., which he said showed that what the papers reported as accident had in fact been inevitable. 'When everything is said and done the Trinity predetermines all that actually exists.' This unintentional parody of scientific method shows the mechanical nature of the reasoning; this was also to be seen in the other expressive phenomena, such as the pedantic arrangement of the material, the severely regulated handwriting, pointed and affected lettering, endless repetition and a general over-schematisation.

We can also find in the background of delusions of invention a philosophical attempt at preservation through the application of the reasoning powers; this is particularly seen in the repeated constructions of a 'perpetuum mobile'.[2]

[1] Pauncz, *Z. Neur.*, vol. 123 (1930), p. 299.
[2] Tramer, *Technisches Schaffen Geisteskranker* (München, 1926).

# PART II
# MEANINGFUL PSYCHIC CONNECTIONS

# PART II

## MEANINGFUL PSYCHIC CONNECTIONS
### (PSYCHOLOGY OF MEANING—VERSTEHENDE PSYCHOLOGIE)

In Part I we studied individual psychic phenomena. These were either patients' *subjective experiences*, which could be vividly represented by us (Phenomenology) or phenomena which could be grasped *objectively* in the form of observable performances, somatic symptoms, or meaningful phenomena found in expressive gesture and in personal worlds and creations (objective psychopathology). In Part I we were mainly interested in describing the facts as they presented themselves to us, but the question constantly intruded as to what might be the source of this or that phenomenon and with what else it might be connected. Up to now a great deal of our material has only allowed description, but in the following Parts II and III an attempt will be made to show what is our present knowledge in regard to connections.

In doing so we shall assume the same theoretical distinction as has been made between subjective psychopathology (phenomenology) and objective psychopathology. 1. We sink ourselves into the psychic situation and *understand genetically by empathy* how one psychic event emerges from another. 2. We find by repeated experience that a number of phenomena are regularly linked together, and on this basis *we explain causally*. Understanding the emergence of psychic events from each other has also been termed '*psychological explanation*', but this term is justifiably disliked by scientifically minded investigators, who are solely concerned with what can be perceived by the senses and with causal explanation, and who have reason to protest should 'psychological explanation' ever seem to be taken as a substitute for their own efforts. Meaningful psychic connections have also been called '*internal causality*', indicating the unbridgeable gulf between genuine connections of external causality and psychic connections which can only be called causal by analogy. These latter will be dealt with here in Part II; causal connections will be discussed in Part III. But first the main difference between the two and their mutual relation needs to be clarified from the viewpoint of our methodology.[1]

[1] 'Understanding is a fundamental human activity that from time immemorial has proceeded on its own methodical, conscious and scholarly way.' Cp. Joachim Wach, *Das Verstehen*, 3 vols. (Tübingen, 1926-33); Droysen distinguished the methods of natural science from those of history and called the one explanation and the other understanding respectively (*Historik*, 1867). Dilthey distinguished descriptive, analytical psychology from explanatory psychology. Spranger spoke of psychology as one of the humanities and I myself spoke of a *psychology of meaningful phenomena*. This last term has won the day. The work of Max Weber was mostly responsible for my deliberate use of understanding as a method which would be in keeping with our great cultural traditions. I was also influenced by *Roscher* and *Knies*, etc., in Schmöllers' *Jahrbüchern*, vols. 27, 29,

## (a) Understanding and explaining

We only try to grasp one kind of connection in the natural sciences, that is causal connection. By observation of events, by experiment and the collection of numerous examples, we attempt to formulate *rules*. At a higher level we establish *laws* and in physics and chemistry we have to a certain extent reached the ideal, which is the expression of causal laws in mathematical equations. We pursue a similar aim in psychopathology. We come across *particular causal connections*, though as yet we do not know how to generalise from them (the connection, for instance, between diseases of the eye and hallucination). We also find *general rules* (the rules, for instance, of constant heredity; disorders that belong to the group of manic-depressive psychoses appear in one family whereas disorders of the dementia-praecox group occur very rarely in such families and vice-versa). But it is rare for us to find any *laws* (as, for instance, there is no General Paralysis without syphilis), nor can we ever formulate causal equations in the manner of chemistry and physics. This would presuppose a complete quantification of the events observed and since these are psychic events, which by their very nature have to remain qualitative, such quantification would as a matter of principle remain impossible without losing the actual object of the enquiry.

In the natural sciences we find causal connections *only* but in psychology our bent for knowledge is satisfied with the comprehension of quite a different sort of connection. Psychic events 'emerge' out of each other in a way which we understand. Attacked people become angry and spring to the defence, cheated persons grow suspicious. The way in which such an emergence takes place is understood by us, *our understanding is genetic*. Thus we understand

30 (1903–6), reprinted in *Gesammelte Aufsätze zur Wissenschaftslehre* (Tübingen, 1922). My ideas were then carried further by Dilthey (*Ideen über eine beschreibende u. zergliedernde Psychologie*, Berliner Akademie, S. ber. 1894, together with Ebbinghaus' criticism in *Z. Psycholog.*, vol. 9) and by Simmel (*Probleme der Geschichtsphilosophie*).

My article of 1912 ('Kausale u. verständliche Zusammenhänge zwischen Schicksal u. Psychose bei der Dementia praecox', *Z. Neur.*, vol. 14, p. 158), and this present book (1913) were greeted as something radically new, although all I had done was to link psychiatric reality with the traditional humanities. Looking back now, it seems astonishing that these had been so forgotten and grown so alien to psychiatry. In this way within the confines of psychopathology there grew a methodical comprehension of something which had always been present, but which was fading out of existence and which appeared in striking reverse, 'through the looking-glass' as it were, in Freud's psychoanalysis—a misunderstanding of itself. The way was clear for scientific consciousness to lay hold on human reality and on man's mental estate, his psychoses included, but there was an immediate need to differentiate the *various modes of understanding*, clarify them and embody them in all *the factual content* available to us.

Since then, a whole literature has arisen on this topic in both psychology and psychopathology: L. Binswanger, *Internat. Z. Psychoanal.* (O), vol. 1 (1913) *Z. Neur.*, vol. 26, p. 107; Gruhle, *Z. Neur.*, vol. 28; Kretschmer, *Z. Neur.*, vol. 57; van der Hopp, *Z. Neur.*, vol. 68; Kurt Schneider, *Z. Neur.*, vol. 75; Isserlin, *Z. Neur.*, vol. 101; Stransky, *Mschr. Psychiatr.*, vol. 52; Bumke, *Zbl. Neurol*, vol. 41; Kronfeld, *Zbl. Neurol*, vol. 28; Störring, *Arch. Psychol.* (D), vol. 58; W. Blumenfeld, *Jb. Philol.* vol. 3 (1927); Walter Schweizer, *Erklären u. Verstehen in der Psychologie* (Bern, 1927); G. Roffenstein, *Das Problem des psychologischen Verstehens* (Stuttgart, 1926); finally, Kronfeld, *Das Wesen der psychiatrischen Erkenntnis* (Berlin, 1920); Binswanger, *Einführung in die Probleme der allgemeinen Psychologie* (Berlin, 1922).

psychic reactions to experience, we understand the development of passion, the growth of an error, the content of delusion and dream; we understand the effects of suggestion, an abnormal personality in its own context or the inner necessities of someone's life. Finally, we understand how the patient sees himself and how this mode of self-understanding becomes a factor in his psychic development.

*(b) Concrete reality and the self-evidence of understanding (Understanding and Interpretation)*

The evidence for genetic understanding is something ultimate. When Nietzsche shows how an awareness of one's weakness, wretchedness and suffering gives rise to moral demands and religions of redemption, because in this roundabout way the psyche can gratify its will to power in spite of its weakness, we experience the force of his argument and are convinced. It strikes us as something self-evident which cannot be broken down any further. The psychology of meaningful phenomena is built up entirely on this sort of convincing experience of impersonal, independent and understandable connections. Such conviction is gained *on the occasion* of confronting human personality; it is not acquired inductively *through repetition of experience*. It carries its own power of conviction and it is a precondition of the psychology of meaningful phenomena that we accept this kind of evidence just as acceptance of the reality of perception and of causality is the precondition of the natural sciences.

The self-evidence of a meaningful connection does not prove that in a particular case that connection is *really there* nor even that it occurs in reality at all. Nietzsche convincingly and comprehensibly connected weakness and morality and applied this to the particular event of the origin of Christianity, but the particular application could be wrong in spite of the correctness of the general (ideally typical) understanding of that connection. In any given case the judgment of whether a meaningful connection is real does not rest on its self-evident character alone. It depends primarily *on the tangible facts* (that is, on the verbal contents, cultural factors, people's acts, ways of life, and expressive gestures) in terms of which the connection is understood, and which provide the objective data. All such objective data, however, are always incomplete and our understanding of *any particular, real event* has to remain more or less an *interpretation* which only in a few cases reaches any relatively high degree of complete and convincing objectivity. We understand only so far as such understanding is suggested to us by the objective data of the individual case, that is, by the patients' expressive movements, acts, speech and self-description, etc. It is true that we can find immediate meaning in a psychic connection quite detached from concrete reality, but we can only assume the reality of such a connection to the extent that the objective data will allow. The fewer these are, the less forcefully do they compel our understanding; we interpret more and understand less. The position will be clarified if we compare these *immediately understood connections* with the *rules of causality* in respect of their differing relationship to *concrete reality*. The rules of causality are obtained inductively and culminate in theories about what lies at the root of the given reality. Particular cases are then subsumed under them. Genetically understandable connections, however, are ideal, typical connections; they are self-evident and not inductively obtained. They do not lead to theories but are a measure for any particular event, whereby it may be recognised as more or less meaningful. Because we note the *frequency* of a meaningful connection this does not mean that the meaningful connection becomes a rule. This would be a real mistake. Frequency in no way enlarges the evidence for the connection. Induction only establishes the frequency, not the reality of the connection itself. For example, the frequency of the connection between the high price of food and theft is both understandable and established statistically. But the frequency of the understandable connection between autumn and suicide is not confirmed by the suicide-curve, which shows a peak in the spring. This does not mean that the understandable connection is wrong since one actual case can furnish us with the occasion to establish such a connection. The fact of frequency adds nothing to the evidence thus gained and the establishment of frequency serves a different purpose. A poet, for instance, might present convincing connections that we understand immediately though they have never yet occurred. They have not been realised yet but contain their own evidence in the sense of being ideally typical. It is easy to fall into this trap of stating some meaningful connection as concretely real when it only offers evidence of this general kind. Jung, for example, says 'it is a well-known fact that it is easy to see where there is a connection and where there is not', but in the case of real people we know that the exact opposite may be the truth.

### (c) *Rational and empathic understanding*

Genetic understanding has many modes and certain essential distinctions need to be preserved. For instance, thoughts may be understandable because they emerge from each other according to the rules of logic and here the connections are understood rationally (that is, we understand what is said). But where we understand how certain thoughts rise from moods, wishes or fears, we are understanding the connections in the true psychological sense, that is by empathy (we understand the speaker). Rational understanding always leads to a statement that the psychic content was simply a rational connection, understandable without the help of any psychology. Empathic understanding, on the other hand, always leads directly into the psychic connection itself. Rational understanding is merely an aid to psychology, empathic understanding brings us to psychology itself. From this we can see how there are obvious differences in the modes of understanding and later on we shall have to make yet other indispensable distinctions. But for the present we shall continue to speak of psychological understanding as a whole.

*(d) Understanding is limited and explanation unlimited*

It is a mistake to suggest that the psyche is the field for understanding while the physical world is the field for causal explanation. Every concrete event—whether of a physical or psychic nature—is open to causal explanation in principle, and psychic processes too may be subjected to such explanation. There is no limit to the discovery of causes and with every psychic event we always look for cause and effect. *But with understanding there are limits everywhere.* The existence of special psychic dispositions (Anlagen), the rules governing the acquisition and loss of memory-traces, the total psychic constitution in its sequence of different age-levels and everything else that may be termed the substratum of the psyche, all constitute limits to our understanding. Each limitation is a fresh *stimulus* to formulate the problem of cause anew.

In thinking about causes in psychology we need *elements* which we can take as cause or effect, e.g. a bodily event as cause, an hallucination as an effect. Every concept in phenomenology and the psychology of meaningful phenomena becomes drawn into the domain of causal thinking to serve as an element of causal explanation. The units of phenomenology (e.g. hallucinations, modes of perception, etc.) are explained by bodily events. Complex meaningful connections in their turn are considered as units (e.g. a manic syndrome plus all its contents can be regarded as the effect of a cerebral process or of some emotional trauma such as the death of an intimate). Even that entirety of meaningful connections which we term the personality of an individual may be considered causally as a unit or element and its original causes investigated from the point of view of heredity, for example.

When searching for causes we are always forced to think of something *extra-conscious* that underlies the phenomenological elements or meaningful connections. We find ourselves constrained to use concepts such as extra-conscious disposition (Anlage), psychic constitution and extra-conscious mechanism. These concepts, however, cannot be expanded into comprehensive psychological theories and we can use them only as working hypotheses in so far as they prove themselves useful for our enquiries.

Every act of understanding in respect of *concrete* psychic events points to a *causal* connection as a matter of course. But this connection only becomes accessible to us in the first place through understanding. So long as there are no other data than those provided by the understanding to help us establish the empirical facts, it is useless to speculate further and construe the connection by extra-conscious facts (see the chapter on theories). If we had these other data, important causal connections could be discovered simply as the result of empirical research. On the other hand, we are wrong if we say that psychic causal connections can be fully *echoed* by empathy and that therefore we can discover causal mechanisms by such empathy. Speculative elaboration of extra-conscious mechanisms through empathic understanding is a sheer waste of time and the literature is far too full of such attempts. Understanding by itself does not lead to any causal explanation except in indirect fashion, when it happens to come up against *the ununderstandable.*

## (e) *Understanding and unconscious events*

*Extra-conscious mechanisms* therefore are construed as something additional to conscious psychic life. They are extra-conscious in principle and not verifiable. They remain purely theoretical constructs which we use to penetrate into the extra-conscious sphere, while phenomenology and the psychopathology of meaning remain concerned with *consciousness*. It is never wholly clear, however, where, from these latter points of view, the frontiers of consciousness are. Both continually expand beyond the immediate frontiers and penetrate deeper. Phenomenology finds itself describing hitherto unnoticed modes of psychic experience, while the psychology of meaningful phenomena grasps psychic connections that were previously unobserved (e.g. Nietzsche's conception of moral attitudes as reaction-formations against awareness of weakness and misery). Every psychologist experiences how his own psychic life is gradually illumined, how he grows more aware of what had previously gone unnoticed in himself, and also how his own last frontier is somehow never reached. This unawareness, which is turned into awareness by phenomenology and the psychology of meaningful phenomena, this unnoticed content which becomes conscious in this way, must not be confused with what is genuinely unconscious. This is in principle extra-conscious and something of which we can never become aware at all. We can actually experience something of which we are unaware, in the sense that we have so far not noticed or regarded it, but we cannot experience this in the sense that it is *extra-conscious*. It would be as well to keep the term *extra-conscious* for the latter type of unconscious event and speak *of what we are generally unaware* in respect of the former.

## (f) *Pseudo-understanding*

Psychology traditionally takes on the task of bringing into consciousness material of which we are unaware. Evidence for such insight has always rested on the fact that, circumstances being favourable, other people could notice the same things, provided they had undergone the same experiences. Certain events, however, cannot be understood in this way. They do not seem to be genuine experiences that have been subsequently brought to notice, yet we believe that in some sense they are understandable. For instance, Charcot and Möbius draw attention to the fact that the distribution of sensory-motor signs in hysteria coincided with the patient's crude and mistaken anatomical notions, and thus the signs became meaningful. But it could not be proved that such notions did in fact give rise to the disturbance, except when there had been direct suggestion. The signs were understood only *as if* some conscious event had determined them. It remains an open question whether in these cases such an event could be the source inasmuch as the actual, unnoticed psychic event is never demonstrated, or whether this is just an apt but fictitious characterisation of certain symptoms. Freud described these 'as-if-understood' phenomena in considerable number and compares his activity with that of an archaeologist who builds up his interpretations from fragments of human works. The great difference is that the archaeologist interprets what has once actually existed whereas in the case of this 'as if' or pseudo-understanding the real existence of what is said to be understood remains entirely undetermined.

The psychology of meaningful phenomena is thus faced with great possibilities of expansion in that it is bringing *unnoticed* material into consciousness. It has to remain doubtful whether this fiction of pseudo-understanding can also penetrate into *extra-conscious material*. We can make no general statement regarding the usefulness of characterising certain phenomena 'as if' they were understood; the matter can only be decided in the individual case.

*(g) Modes of comprehensive understanding (cultural, existential and metaphysical)*

We repeat the differentiations which we have made so far:

1. *Phenomenological understanding* and the *understanding of expression:* the former is our inner representation of patients' experiences, gained with the help of their self-description. The latter is our direct perception of meaning in an individual's movements, involuntary gestures and physical form. 2. *Static and genetic understanding:* the former grasps particular psychic qualities and states as individually experienced (phenomenology); the latter grasps the emergence of one psychic event from another, the whole moving psychic context of motive, contrasting effect and dialectical opposite (the psychology of meaningful phenomena). 3. *Genetic understanding and explanation:* The former is the inner, subjective, direct grasp of psychic connectedness, so far as it can ever be grasped in this way; the latter is objective demonstration of connections, effects and ruling principles, which cannot be understood by empathy and are only explicable in terms of cause and effect. 4. *Rational and empathic understanding:* the former is not really psychological understanding at all. It is a purely cognitive understanding of rational content, common to all (e.g.: we can understand the logical structure of a delusional system of a world in which an individual lies submerged). The latter—empathic understanding—is the proper psychological understanding of the psyche itself. 5. *Understanding and interpretation.* We speak of understanding when what has been understood has been fully expressed in some movement, utterance or act. We speak of interpretation when in a given case sparse clues allow us to apply with a reasonable degree of probability certain meaningful connections that we have come to understand from elsewhere.

The above differentiations are really sufficient for our present purpose, which is to clarify the perception of empirical facts. In practice, however, understanding is constantly in touch with *something more comprehensive in which all such acts of understanding lie embedded*. We will, therefore, indicate those main areas over which our understanding moves, over and beyond what has been discussed so far.

(a) *Cultural understanding.* It is not only the logical content which has to be understood in an objective, non-psychological sense, but all the other mental content, the pattern of ideas, the images, symbols, ideas of obligation, ideals, etc. We do not understand a person merely by isolating out a number of such contents, but the degree to which the psychologist is at home with them will limit and condition his psychological understanding. This kind of understanding is a cultural not a psychological understanding, but the psyche only becomes accessible to us if in this sense we understand the element in which it lives, the things that are visible to it, the things which it accepts and allows to take their effect.

(b) *Existential understanding.* In the act of understanding psychic connections, we come up against the limits set by the ununderstandable. *In one sense* we may see this as the extra-conscious, the limit of the understandable. As the body that carries us we have to accept it in all its causal connections, as matter we have to shape it and as material possibility we have to grasp it and where it fails this has simply to be endured. *In another sense* what cannot be understood is also the source of the understandable and it thus goes beyond the understandable; it is a self-illuminating process, something becoming understandable, if only we can lay hold of it out of the unconditioned absolute of Existence itself. Therefore, in relation to the ununderstandable, where this is a limiting factor that can be causally explored, psychological understanding becomes an *empirical psychology.* But in relation to the ununderstandable as a phenomenon of possible Existence, it becomes the philosophical illumination of Existence itself. Empirical psychology affirms how something is and how it happens; the illumination of Existence through what may be possible makes its appeal to Man himself. Both have radically different meanings, but psychological understanding contains them both, linked inseparably together. From this rises an almost insurmountable ambiguity. In both instances the act of understanding presupposes and implies something that cannot be understood; this baffling element, however, is twofold and heterogeneous. Without the one aspect (the 'givenness' of causality) the understandable would cease to exist and without the other (Existence being itself) there would be no content.

The ununderstandable discloses itself to *causal enquiry* as instinctual drives, biological somatic facts and supposed specific extra-conscious mechanisms. The ununderstandable is as much present in all normal life as it is in morbid states and processes, in a deviant form. The ununderstandable *from the existential aspect* presents itself as a freedom, which discloses itself in free decisions, in a grasp of absolute meanings, and in that basic experience where the marginal situation rises from the empirical situation—that marginal point where we are roused from ordinary existence into an autonomous self-hood.

The illumination of Existence itself brings concepts into being, which lose their meaning altogether if a misguided psychological opinion then treats them as available modes of concrete existence and therefore as relative. The field of empirical research has no freedom nor does it contain anything of that liberating challenge offered by the philosophical illumination of Existence proper: the challenge of validity, awareness of the absolute, of marginal situations, ultimate decisions, responsibility, and of oneself as an original source. Through the psychology of meaningful phenomena, existential illumination comes into contact with this something that goes beyond understanding, with the reality proper that lies in the possibilities of autonomous self-hood through the processes of memory, attention and revelation. If we treat this illumination as some kind of psychological theory of general application, we have confused and misstated its nature; so too, if actions, behavioural modes, instinctual drives and people themselves are classified in psychological categories of existential illumination, and treated for the once in this respect as natural facts.

(c) *Metaphysical understanding.* Psychological understanding is linked with empirical experience and free, existential achievement. Metaphysical understanding reaches after a meaning into which all the other limited meanings can be taken up and absorbed. Metaphysical understanding interprets the empirical facts and the free achievement as the language of unconditioned Being.

This interpretation is not a mere device of reason, something futile, but the illumination of fundamental experiences with the help of symbol and idea. As we look at the inanimate world, the cosmos, the landscape, we experience something we call 'soul' or 'psyche'. When faced with what is living, we proceed to grasp a number of purposeful connections and then advance from that to a vague perception of a Life that embraces all things and in the sequence of its forms realises itself as a fathomless meaning. As with nature, so it is with man—and we are confronted by him in all his actuality and freedom. He is not only an empirical reality to us but under the scrutiny of our metaphysical understanding, he, like everything else that is real, becomes a meaning we cannot verify. He is not only meaningful like a tree or a tiger but meaningful in his own unique way as a human being. This metaphysical experience of him is not a matter for the science of psychopathology but the latter can help in clarifying facts that will refine the experience: for instance, the fact that extreme psychotic states offer us a human parable, and that they seem to contain inverted and distorted attempts to realise and elaborate marginal situations, which are common to us all. There is also the fact that patients see into depths which do not so much belong to their illness as to themselves as individuals with their own historical truth. Finally there is the fact that in psychotic reality we find an abundance of content representing fundamental problems of philosophy: nothingness, total destruction, formlessness, death. Here the extremest of human possibilities actually breaks through the ordinary boundaries of our sheltered, calm, ordered and smooth existence. The philosopher in us cannot but be fascinated by this extraordinary reality and feel its challenge.

*Digression into understanding and appraisal:* all potential meaning implies an unresolved tension, in the intellectual field between truth and falsehood, in the field of existence between empirical event and freedom and in the metaphysical field between what inspires faith and what arouses dread (between the love and wrath of God). In understanding (and this includes psychological understanding) we experience this tension constantly through the basic phenomenon that our understanding is also an appraisal. Meaningful human activity is in itself an expression of values and everything understandable carries for us an immediate positive or negative colouring: everything understandable has a constituent potentiality of worth. In contrast we do not value the ununderstandable as such but only as the means and condition for our understanding; we disapprove of a memory disorder which we understand as a purposeful suppression but we simply assess the physiological mechanism of memory as a tool.

The scientific attitude suspends all value-judgment in order to arrive at knowledge. But though this is possible when attempting causal explanation it is not possible with empathic understanding, at least not exactly in the same sense. We can, however, make an analogous claim for impartiality when we try to know what we have understood. We may lay claim to impartiality when we have shown an understanding that is fair, many-sided, open and critically conscious of its limitations. Love and hate bring values which are indeed the pacemakers of understanding but their suspension brings us a clarity of understanding that amounts to knowledge.

In understanding a concrete case we inevitably appear to make an appraisal and to fail in scientific understanding because with human beings every meaningful connection as such is immediately judged negatively or positively. This is due to the fact that the understandable as such implies some evaluation. To understand correctly is to appraise; to appraise correctly is finally to understand. Hence in all understanding there lies on the one hand a finding of fact which can be free of appraisal and on the other a challenge to appraise which calls out value-judgments. Correct understanding is hard to come by and rare, so our appraisal of others is usually false and depends on chance and emotional impulse. Every man likes to be judged favourably so that a favourable appraisal tends to make him feel understood. Thus in everyday language understanding and positive appraisal have become identical. Where people have been negatively judged—particularly in situations that expose them—they will consider themselves particularly hard to understand and will nearly always see themselves as persons misunderstood.

It is true there is the idea of objective appraisal, that is, of understanding and correct appraisal compellingly linked together. The establishment of understanding would then be the final true appraisal. But this is only a theoretical coincidence. Understanding can be linked equally with contrary value-judgments (thus Nietzsche continued to understand Socrates but sometimes he evaluated him positively, sometimes negatively). So long as we merely understand, the understandable becomes contradictory in itself, ambiguous and a source of ambivalent behaviour, the more fully it is grasped.

*(h) How what can be understood psychologically moves midway between meaningful objectivity and what cannot be understood*

At the point where our psychological understanding comes to a halt, we find something which is not itself psychologically understandable but a precondition for such understanding. Let us summarise:

In depicting connections that can be understood genetically, we always find: (1) we have presupposed a *mental content* which is not a psychological matter and which can be understood without the help of psychology; (2) we have perceived an *expression*, which brings an inward meaning to light; and (3) we have represented a direct *experience* which phenomenologically is irreducible and can only be statically produced as a datum.

We can have no psychological understanding without empathy into the *content* (symbols, forms, images, ideas) and without seeing the *expression* and sharing the *experienced phenomena*. All these spheres of meaningful objective facts and subjective experience form the matter for understanding. Only in so far as they exist can understanding take place. They come into a context through the comprehension of our genetic understanding.

These subjective and objective findings are not, however, the only province of psychological understanding. On the contrary: (1) it is hardly possible to talk about contents without thinking of the psychological reality for which they exist; and (2) we can hardly scrutinise an expression without understanding the motive at work; and finally (3) we can hardly describe anything phenomenologically without immediately coming upon meaningful connections.

Psychological understanding operates where there is a totality of complex facts. It also meets with the *ununderstandable* in the form of extra-conscious mechanisms or of Existence itself. When understanding wishes to investigate causes, an extra-conscious bodily mechanism is inevitably implied and inversely it is impossible to talk of extra-conscious mechanisms without pre-supposing something that can be understood or has been understood and that evokes at its own limits the idea of some such mechanisms. When understanding wishes to grasp and illumine Existence as possibility and so call men back to themselves, it touches on a source of freedom in Existence itself without which everything understandable would lose its foundations, lack personal reference and become ineffective and void. Existence itself, however, can only manifest itself in an understandable phenomenon and only so can it attain its own self-realisation.

The understanding psychologist proceeds as follows: he starts from a comprehensive intuition of meaning. He then makes an analysis: expression, psychic content, phenomena on the one hand, extra-conscious mechanisms on the other, while existential potentialities are detected as an empirically un-explorable base. As a result of this analysis of facts and meanings he gains an enriched understanding of all the connections. In the given case the results will be scrutinised, the procedure repeated and insight steadily increased by the collection of objective data interwoven with fresh intuitions of the whole, which lead in their turn to a fresh analysis.

Thus our psychological understanding lies as it were *midway* between the objective facts, the phenomena of experience and the implied extra-conscious mechanisms on the one hand and the spontaneous freedom of Existence itself on the other. We might deny the object of psychological understanding alto-gether and maintain that phenomena, psychic contents, expression, extra-conscious mechanisms are all subjects for empirical research alone, while the possibilities of Existence itself are purely a matter for philosophy. But let us try to manage with such a division of the field! Most of our psychological seeing and thinking would disappear and it would become impossible to speak of the facts and fundamentals of the Human Being without bringing back the psychology of meaningful phenomena once more. But this meaningful psychology is always in balance between these two realms and we can never speak of it in isolation. It is related to them both and if there is to be a complete presentation they cannot be separated.

Thus the psychology of meaningful phenomena never comes to any point of rest within itself. If it does, it has either become an empirical psychology, busy on the comprehension of phenomena, expression, content and extra-conscious mechanisms, or it has become the philosophical illumination of Existence itself.

Psychological understanding only serves psychopathology in so far as it makes something visible to our experience and fosters our observation. As I understand, I find myself asking what are these facts I am looking at and what am I indicating? When do I reach the limit of my understanding? The midway status of psychological understanding has to be constantly re-established by objectifying the psychic phenomena and discovering the limit of this understanding.

This intermediate status of our understanding throws some light on the old question of the psyche in its relation to mind and body. We see the mind as meaningful material content, to which the psyche relates itself and by which it is itself moved. We see the body as the psyche's existence. We never seem to grasp the psyche itself but either explore it as something physical or try to understand it as content. But just as the whole realm of the corporeal cannot be exhausted by the various physical phenomena which are biologically explorable—indeed, this extends right up to the body–psyche unity of expressive phenomena—so too the reality of the mind is linked to the psyche, inextricably bound to it and carried along by it.

Our view of concrete reality would be unnecessarily limited if we simply conceived the psyche as bodily expression and grasped it thus exactly, finding it here whole and complete, the psyche itself, with nothing to mediate it. Expression is only one of the dimensions in which the psyche is apparent and it is not an enclosed unit but can be understood only in connection with what does not become expression.

We conceive the psyche as the objective correlate to the method of understanding. The psyche appears to recede and in its place we are occupied with its foreground (phenomena, expression, psychic content) and with conditioning factors (the body and Existence itself). What psychological understanding gives us is the bond that holds together all that we can understand and all that belongs to it which we cannot understand.

The midway position of the psyche makes it impossible for genetic understanding to be self-contained and round itself off in what is thought to be a decisive knowledge of the whole. Every act of understanding is a mode of apperception. It throws a beam of light into human reality. It is not the method which makes mankind accessible as individuals nor as a whole. All psychology of meaningful phenomena is therefore incomplete.

### (i) The function of understanding in psychopathology

There are two main undertakings. We try first to *extend our understanding* to unusual and remote connections which at first sight perhaps seem incomprehensible (for example, sexual perversion, instinctual cruelty, etc.). Secondly, we try to discover universal and in themselves understandable connections in those psychic states where *abnormal mechanisms* appear as the conditioning factor (for example, hysterical reactions). In the first instance, it is a matter of understanding something that is felt to be pathological or unique but in any case alien from everything understandable; the emphasis lies on the special nature of the understanding. In the second instance, it is a matter of recognising the abnormal realisation of connections which are for the most part quite understandable in themselves and by no means unusual. Here emphasis lies on the *abnormal extra-conscious mechanisms*. These, however, become accessible to us only when we set out to understand.

Two chapters have been devoted to the above. The one deals with the 'what' of meaningful connections. They themselves provide the main theme and here the abnormality lies in the nature of what needs to be understood. The other deals with the 'how' of meaningful connections and the way in which they reach realisation through extra-conscious mechanisms. Here the abnormality lies in the mechanisms themselves. They cannot be understood as such and form the ground of the peculiar manifestation of what in itself needs to be understood.

The subsequent chapters deal with the two basic properties of what is understandable. These are: (1) All that is understandable, understands itself; it is in particular an operation of self-reflection, for example the attitude of the patient to his illness; (2) Everything understandable has its own coherence within the individual. The *concrete total of meaningful or understandable connections* constitutes what we call the personality or character of a person. This forms the subject-matter of the final chapter.

To ensure clarity of discussion on the subject of the understandable, we will recapitulate as follows: In the psychology of meaningful phenomena, the application of directly perceived, understandable connections to an individual case never leads to deductive proof but only to probabilities. Psychological understanding cannot be used mechanically as a sort of generalised knowledge but a fresh, personal intuition is needed on every occasion. 'Interpretation is a science only in principle, in its application it is always an art' (Bleuler).

# CHAPTER V

# MEANINGFUL CONNECTIONS

§ 1. The Sources of Our Ability to Understand and the Task of the Psychopathology of Meaningful Connections

We all know a great many psychic connections which we have learnt from experience (not only through repetition but through having understood one real case which opened our eyes). We make use of these connections in our analysis of psychopathic personality and of those psychoses which are still open to partial 'psychological explanation'. The richer we are in such meaningful insights, the more subtle and correct will our analyses be when we apply 'psychological explanation' in a given case. Neither in normal psychology nor in psychopathology has there been any attempt to elaborate the psychology of meaningful phenomena in any systematic way, perhaps because it has been thought impossible or too difficult to do this. Such meaningful connections as we all know and as constantly conveyed by our language lose all their force if we try to give them a general formulation. Anything really meaningful tends to have a concrete form and generalisation destroys it. But we expect systematic knowledge in science and if we cannot systematise meaning we can at least order our methods according to *principles of understanding*. First, however, we should remind ourselves of those sources on which the richness, flexibility and depth of our understanding depend.

In the case of every investigator it is a matter of his human stature as to what he understands and how far this understanding reaches. Myths are works of creative understanding and they have been creatively understood by all great poets and artists. Only through a lifelong study of poets such as Shakespeare, Goethe, the ancient dramatists and such moderns as Dostoevsky, Balzac, etc., do we arrive at the required intuition, and gain a sufficient store of images and symbols and the ability to exercise an understanding imagination necessary to guide the concrete understanding of the moment. We are sensitised by reflection over the whole range of the humanities. If the investigator has the basic features clear this will ensure that he has some real measure of understanding and can frame certain possibilities. As an investigator into meaning I am conditioned by the sources of my understanding, by such confirmation as I find and by my own problems. These all decide whether I remain tied to banal simplifications and rational schemata or whether I endeavour to comprehend men in their most complex manifestations. It is fair to say to the investigator of meaning: 'Tell me where you got your psychology from, and I will tell you who you are'. Only a close association with poetry and human reality at its greatest will provide the horizons within which the most simple everyday occurrence can become interesting and vital. The levels reached by the one who would understand and by the object of his understanding will decide whether orientation is towards the ordinary or the extraordinary, the plain and uncomplicated or the complex and manifold.

Besides the world of meaningful myth and poetic image, there is a whole literature of intense thinking on the matter of understanding, based on *Plato*, *Aristotle* and later the *Stoics*. But it was *Augustine* who first elaborated psychological understanding for the Western world. After him there were a number of attempts in aphoristic form, mainly among the French: *Montaigne*, *La Bruyère*, *La-Rochefoucauld*, *Vauvenargues*, *Chamfort*. Magnificent and towering above them all was *Pascal*. Only *Hegel* produced a system: 'The Phenomenology of the Mind', while *Kierkegaard* and *Nietzsche*[1] stand out unique as the greatest of all psychologists interested in meaning.

*Basic patterns of human life* underlie all our understanding and at the back of our minds we are more or less clearly aware of what man is and can be. Every psychopathologist visualises these patterns to himself but does not give validity to any single one. He tries them all out and sees what his concrete observations are and how his potential experience can be widened.

Psychopathology is not called on to develop and present all manner of meaningful connections in their totality. The realm of meaning is unbounded and we are protected from any apparent subordination to rigidly schematised thinking, simple or complex, if we remain fully aware of this and fortify ourselves by interweaving the heritage of the past with our own life experiences. The true problem for psychopathology is that meaningful reality which specific extra-conscious mechanisms, normal or abnormal, have brought into being.

Psychopathology, however, is obviously called upon to give a searching presentation of *rare connections with abnormal meaning* as they appear in individual, concrete cases. This is something outside the natural sciences and causal explanation and as such is not often attempted, certainly not in any thoroughgoing way. The tendency to accept only the causal knowledge of the natural sciences has obscured the sovereignty of any such investigation and has falsified objective enquiry by the introduction of 'psychological explanation', much as, in the natural sciences, pure understanding tends to get falsified by the use of theoretical constructs. Valuable contributions have been made in the fields of sexual perversion by the expert examination of Court cases and by good psychiatric case-histories. In psychopathology it may well be the task of special psychiatry to describe personality disorders and make us aware of singular meaningful connections (in the instinctual life, in the scale of values and in behaviour), but there are also a number of *common* meaningful connections which are the subject of relatively frequent observation and form part of the ordinary equipment of everyday practical understanding.

[1] Cp. my lectures 'Vernunft u. Existenz' (Groningen, 1935). Re Nietzsche, see my book *Nietzsche, Einführung in das Verständnis seines Philosophierens* (Berlin, 1936).

*Note on the examples given of meaningful connections:* There is an infinite world of meaning and in this chapter we can only indicate a few possibilities. During the last decades certain basic modes of understanding have grown into our everyday practice in rather haphazard fashion. We do not need to select arbitrarily a number of meaningful connections from the valuable literature mentioned above, but in psychopathology we have to be aware of our methods and of the viewpoints that have general acceptance among the psychiatrists and psychotherapists of today. These current points of view indicate the ways of understanding that are most acceptable today. They may not be universally valid nor so for ever but they are appropriate for our own particular world. All understanding presupposes *some picture of the individual and his personal world* at the same time as it enlarges this, and so it is with our contemporary understanding. The following seem to me material among the presuppositions that underlie our present picture of man: the impoverishment of the possibilities of inner experience compared with earlier times; the determination to correct this poverty by adhering to tradition; a knowledge of radical conflicts; a frankness of basic attitude and irreligion, inducing a tendency to believe in systems of faith-healing and certain passionately adopted symbols.

In what follows we present some contemporary viewpoints but the principle remains that we need to be acquainted with the great historical traditions of understanding as a background for our everyday, practical understanding. These should never be forgotten as original sources and as standards of measurement when contemporary experiment tends to crowd into the foreground of our awareness.

We present examples of meaningful connections from three aspects: (1) *Meaningful content*—instinctual drives are the sources of a subject's movement, which takes place within *an individual relationship to the world*. This movement becomes meaningful to itself in life through the use of *symbols* (we discuss instinct-psychology, psychology of the real, the psychology of symbols); (2) *The basic forms of the meaningful*—the individual's movement takes shape as an *opposition of forces* with accompanying tensions, reversals, reconciliations and critical decisions. The movement is *reciprocal* (we discuss the psychology of opposites, the psychology of reciprocity); (3) *Self-reflection* as a basic phenomenon of all meaningfulness (we discuss the psychology of self-reflection).

These three aspects of understanding (content, form and self-reflection) converge into one coherent meaningful whole. They are not a set of mutually exclusive and diverse elements but each one illuminates the whole from its own point of view. Therefore our psychological understanding if it is to be complete is constrained by each one of them to include the rest.

## § 2. CONNECTIONS WITH A MEANINGFUL CONTENT

*(a) Instinctual drives, their psychic manifestations and transformations*

All experiencing contains an element of being driven. There is something instinctual in everything we do and suffer, in everything we would bring about, enjoy or angrily avoid; it is the same whether we pursue something, grasp it, hold on to it and affirm it or whether we fly from it, avoid, by-pass or destroy it.[1]

(1) *Concept of Drive*. The question 'what is a drive?' may be answered in several ways: drives are *instincts which we experience*, that is, functions carried out as the result of an urge without conscious awareness of content or aim but in such a way that complex purposeful activity finally reaches its end by being moved towards it. Drives are *physical wants*, e.g. hunger, thirst, need for sleep; that is, urges which reach their target directly provided the means are there. Drives are *a form of creative activity* shown, for example, in bodily movements that develop and manifest the bodily essence or in some way express and represent it (urge for expression, urge for representation); or they are shown in directed effort (urge for knowledge, creative urge). Drives are *motivated acts*, that is, impulses which are conscious of their aim and reach it intentionally using the available means to a purpose.

Any such dissection of the whole state of being driven, which is a unity in itself, always reflects some *attempt at interpretation*. We have then to ask which point of view governs the interpretation. Thus the above classification was according to the purposes objectively achieved (instincts); according to physical urges (drives); according to what is creatively produced (creative urges); according to the ideas, subjective goals and purposes present (motivated action). Such classification has only *relative* meaning. For instance the 'sexual drive' contains all these categories in itself: it is an instinct manifesting itself as an inborn function which fertilises without conscious awareness; it is a physical want or need (tumescence and detumescence); it shows erotic creativeness and motivates actions which will realise erotic ideas.

We can make a further differentiation of the whole state of 'being driven' from yet another point of view and ask whether *the motive of the urge is to gain pleasure* (by pleasure in this context we always mean physical pleasure) or whether the content provides the goal, to achieve which displeasure, pain and suffering are accepted, or whether displeasure itself can motivate the drive. *Pleasure* is an experience of harmonious biological function, of general wholesomeness and success, of a capacity to linger over things; pleasure also lies in psychic equilibrium and well-being. Drives, however, are not aiming just at such pleasure, but are *beyond pleasure and pain*. We cannot describe their essential nature except approximately through an attempt to classify them from a number of different aspects.

---

[1] Nietzsche: *Triebpsychologie*. See my *Nietzsche*, pp. 113–15.

There are still other points of view which we may follow, and we can differentiate according to certain broader aspects of meaningfulness which we are about to discuss. Thus we may take *the relationship of the individual to his environment*, in which case drives are conceived as stemming from the primary defencelessness of existence, in particular of man in his world. *In order to survive* he has the drive for power and self-assertion. He has gregarious drives (social feelings) for *the survival of the species*. If these two are mistakenly turned into absolutes, all drives become reduced to these basic drives and the highest aims are interpreted as merely devious ways whereby the basic drives achieve their elementary goals. Or we may take *symbols as meaningful content* and interpret them as a means, a language, a deception in the process of the self-realisation of the drive. Finally, we may take *the dialectical tension* which psychic movement creates. In this case we direct our attention to the conflicts that spring from resistance to a drive. We ask what resists and what is resisted. We understand the movement of self-control and discover what is irresistible and how it may grow to what is uncontrollable, always however for the time being, never absolutely so.

But, whatever our classification, there is a basic element of something given in all human drive. It cannot be understood as meaningful in any way, but from it all understanding of meaning has to start. At the same time there is a psychic impulse which drives towards definition through content. Understanding the drives and how they manifest themselves throws light on something which is itself a process of continuous self-illumination.

(2) *Classification of drives:* The contents of drives are as manifold as life itself. Every drive contains an urge and hence a movement which is moved on as it were by the force of something which is experienced (a symbol—according to Klages), something felt in the urge itself, unaccompanied by any specific idea or thought. Drives can therefore be distinguished from each other by their content, and enumeration of this would be as endless as that of the content of feelings. The important thing is whether classification can penetrate the elementary properties of drive and there have been repeated and various attempts to make some kind of catalogue.

Drives are polarised in some of the following possible ways: Drives arising out of a surplus of energy may be contrasted with those arising out of a deficit, e.g. the need to discharge energy as against the need to regain it. Then there are drives that can be aroused at any time as against drives which are essentially periodic, which are gratified and then arise anew. Some drives represent a continual need which can only be gratified repeatedly and are incapable of further development. They can be satisfied completely but only for the time being. In contrast, other drives change each time they are satisfied; they grow, develop and are never satisfied completely. The hunger does not diminish but increases with every gratification.

*Freud* distinguishes drives according to those opposites which he regards as the most profound—the drive to live and the drive to die. The *drive to die* is a drive to destroy which can be directed outwards (aggressive drive) or inwards against the self.

It is a drive to return to the inorganic. The drive for food has something in common with the drive to destroy because it destroys what is eaten. The *drive to live* (Eros) is differentiated into the *ego-drive* and the *sexual-drive*. The *ego-drives* are drives for self-preservation (drive for food, acquisitive drive, defensive drives and gregarious drives) and for self-expansion (drives for power and importance, the drive for knowledge and creative drives). The *sexual drive* includes the drive for the preservation of the species, care for the generations.[1]

In the following classification drives are divided into three levels of drive:

*Group 1. Somatic, sensory drives.* Sexual drive, hunger, thirst—need for sleep, drive for activity—pleasure in sucking, in taking food, in anal and urethral excretion.[2]

In this group the basic polarity is that of *need* and *satisfaction*. All the drives have some bodily correlate. The drives are positive only with no other positive drive opposing. The negative would be disgust or aversion.

*Group 2. Vital drives.* They have no definite localisation in the body but are directed out towards human existence as a whole. They are:

(*a*) *Vital drives for existence.* The will to power—will to submit; the urge to self-assertion—urge to surrender; self-will—social drive (herd instinct); courage—fear (aggressive anger—retreat for help); self-importance—urge to humility; love—hate.

In this group the drives fall into pairs, each drive with its counter-drive. The *preservation* and *intensification of life* seems to be of objective significance in them all but only at the price of conflict which makes at any time the exact opposite possible—the destruction of life, whether of oneself or another and ultimately perhaps the urge for universal destruction. The polarity of drive and counter-drive will often produce an amazing dialectic, bringing about conversion of the opposites, one into the other . . .

(*b*) *Vital psychic drives.* Curiosity, protection of the young, the drive to wander, to find ease and comfort, the will to possess.

In this group the drives are defined by their particular content at any time.

(*c*) *Vital creative drives.* The urge to express, to demonstrate, make tools, work and create.

*Group 3. Drives of the human spirit.* Drives to comprehend and give oneself to a state of being which manifests itself as an experience of absolute values, whether religious, aesthetic, ethical or pertaining to truth. Philosophy undertakes to examine this world of values and clarify it independently from subjective psychological experience. It is a psychological fact that there is a basic experience of this sort, qualitatively different from that of the two

---

[1] There are many other classifications: e.g. Klages (*Grundlagen der Charakterkunde* (8th edn., 1936); *Der Geist als Widersacher der Seele*, vol. 2, pp. 566 ff.). Macdougall, *Aufbaukräfte der Seele* (D), (Leipzig, 1937), pp. 76 ff.

[2] Investigation of this group can only be through physiological examination, e.g. D. Katz, 'Psychologische Probleme des Hungers u. Appetits', *Nervenarzt.*, vol. 1 (1928), p. 345. *Hunger u. Appetit* (Leipzig, 1932).

previous groups and extremely complex and rich and derived from a dedication to these values. It is an instinctive longing for them when they are absent and a sense of delight incomparable to any other pleasure when the longing is fulfilled. It is decisive for any picture we form of people that we should know how this whole group of phenomena affects their lives. Although as a group these drives may sometimes recede to vanishing point they are never quite absent in any man.

The common factor in this group is the *drive for immortality*, not in terms of temporal duration but in the sense of participating in some temporal form in a pattern of Being that cuts across Time.[1]

The material of these three groupings is of such heterogeneous meaning that we may well hesitate to talk in terms of drive in every case. And yet any such grouping has to separate what in reality is linked. Taking this classification as a *hierarchy of drives* we see that each preceding group can realise itself without the others but not vice-versa. It is characteristic for man alone that his whole instinctual life is pervaded by the drives of the last group. Nothing in man is simply identical with what we find in animals, nothing can be carried out simply and naïvely (Man, says Aristotle, can only be more or less than an animal). Inversely, however, man cannot, as it were, participate in nothing but purely intellectual or spiritual drives. A tinge of sensory-somatic drive is always present but to deduce from this that higher drives are nothing but a veiled form of basic ones would be a mistake. 'To be involved' is not 'to be origin'. The universality of the effects of sexual drive does not mean that this is always the determining, let alone the only, power of the psyche. Suppose we propose the more modest thesis that the mind is powerless, all power comes from the lower levels, or in other words that our deepest experiences and strongest impulses always originate at the lowest levels of our existence—this thesis of Schiller (hunger and love (sexuality) preserve humanity so that only those ideas can realise themselves that win the support of the natural drives) is by no means unequivocal. Such a thesis may perhaps hold for the mass-events of history but by no means certainly so for all times. It may help us, it is true, to understand how spiritual, or ethical, motives are often advanced or kept in the foreground of consciousness when essential and vital drives are *de facto* in sole charge. But this does not exclude authentic spiritual and intellectual drives from ruling the lower levels of drive, utilising them as tools and as a source of energy. We cannot doubt the primary quality of every movement of our impulses but their interaction and collision presents us with a fundamental problem of human existence. Once we see that this is so, we can no longer believe in any final and unequivocal classification of drives within a single and uniform hierarchy.

(3) *Abnormal drives*. There is a countless host of these. We find perverse tastes, like the pica of pregnant and hysterical women who develop cravings

---

[1] See Münsterberg, Scheler, Rickert, etc., for Values and their classification. Recent work: S. Behn, *Philosophie der Werte als Grundwissenschaft der pädagogischen Zieltheorie* (München, 1930).

for sand or vinegar, etc. We also find insatiable hunger, or an abnormally increased thirst which can become an addiction.[1] There is the drive for any kind of emotion at any cost, for excessive gesture and expression, the desire for inactivity, countless persistent drives to wander, get drunk, etc. All require particular analysis, which is the province of special psychiatry. Perverse sexual and other instinctual activities, usually correlated with the type of sexuality, are one of the main topics for investigation. We find an urge to suffer and pleasure found in pain, suffered or inflicted. The drive to be cruel is so wide-spread that it might almost pass for normal. Nietzsche saw it so and took orgies of cruelty as a basic factor in human affairs. When related to sexuality, such drives are called sadism (infliction of pain on others) and masochism (suffering pain) where the inflicted pain is the condition for sexual pleasure. But sexual frigidity is also linked with a drive to torture and with a lust for power, showing itself as a delight in inflicting pain. Moralistic attitudes towards others may often be a manifestation of the drive for power and the drive to torture ('right' sounds very like 'racked', said Nietzsche). Those who have gained importance in the history of culture are markedly surrounded by the specific atmosphere of abnormal instinctual states, of passionate hate, sado-masochistic pleasure, sexually frigid cruelty and a craving for domination in love, etc. It is important to know of the many and limitless transformations of these abnormal instinctual states if we are to understand some of the cultural movements of history, for instance, the link between asceticism, lust for mastery, cruelty (particularly in the Middle Ages) and fanaticism in almost all its forms. History obscures all this. It is not something which is talked about and handed on. Often it can be inferred only from concrete experiences accessible to the doctor but now and again accidentally preserved documents and records may give us a powerful illustration. But understanding will also show us the effects of healthy instinctual states and can trace the clear atmosphere of passions free from perversions and cultural transformations of this sort. Of the two, it almost seems that the healthy passion is the rarer.[2]

We can observe the power these instinctual perversions exercise over the whole of a person's life. If we try to understand, we are always faced with ambiguity: is a particular abnormal instinctual disposition the origin of a personality change or is an abnormal personality the condition of the possible abnormal manifestations? From the point of view of psychological understanding both seem to be the case. In outstanding personalities a most abnormal

[1] H. Marx, *Innere Sekretion*, pp. 420 ff. (*Handbuch der inneren Medizin*, von Bergmann, Staeholin, Salle ((Berlin, 1941), vol. 6, part I).

[2] The literature on abnormal sexuality is immense. For nineteenth-century description see v. Krafft-Ebing, *Psychopathia sexualis* (Stuttgart, 1886), 14th edn., 1912. Havelock Ellis, H. Rohleder, *Vorlesungen über Geschlechtstrieb u. Geschlechtsleben der Menschen* (Berlin, 1900), 2nd edn., 1907. I. Bloch, *Das sexualleben unserer Zeit* (Berlin, 1906). A. Moll, *Handbuch der Sexualwissenschaften*. Recent psychological enquiry, e.g. v. Gebsattel, 'Über Fetischismus', *Nervenarzt*, vol. 2, p. 8. Kronfeld, 'Über psychische Impotenz', *Nervenarzt*, vol. 2, p. 521. Hans Binder, 'Das Verlangen nach Geschlechtsumwandlungen', *Z. Neur.*, vol. 143 (1932), p. 83. A. Paunez, 'Der Learkomplex, die Kehrseits des Oedipus-complexes', *Z. Neur.*, vol. 143 (1932), p. 294.

instinctual disposition may be balanced by humane qualities which render it factually ineffective (as with Wilhelm von Humboldt). In other cases we have the impression that abnormal drives retain their power and perhaps originate in the personality, which is therefore defenceless against them. Ruinous consequences thus appear—instinctual disposition and personality are equally involved—so that the individual is unable to build a life with others. Or we find a number of intermediary stages where as a result of perverted drives a person is in ceaseless struggle with himself and stands tortured by an unsurmountable division in his existence. In the last resort the decisive thing is the personality into which the abnormality is absorbed and from which it springs, either evaporating, as it were, in the personality's pure ether or stamping itself indelibly upon it.

The following is a classification of the ways in which abnormal drives can be understood:

(*aa*) *As disintegration of the higher levels of drive.* As the higher levels vanish, drives at the lower levels gain uninhibited outlet and increase in importance within the psychic life as a whole. We may observe, for instance, the ravenous hunger of dements. In terms of *personality* this is a devastation of the psyche.

(*bb*) *As dissociation between the levels of drive.* Different levels of drive split away instead of cohering and mutually limiting each other as clearly differentiated parts of one whole. Drives at each level are realised to the exclusion of the others, the sensual purely sensually, ideal ones purely ideally. The ravenous eating of certain neurotics is of this kind. More common is a splitting-off of sexuality and the isolation of this essential drive without any integration of it into the whole psychic destiny. Heyer speaks of those who 'forget the loving surrender to Eros by reducing it to banal sexual gratification'. All natural drives have something of the psyche in them, but the isolated drive is characterised by violence and soullessness. In terms of *personality* the effect is recklessness, heartlessness and malice.

(*cc*) *As inversion of the relation between lower and higher levels of drive.* Lower-level drives fulfil themselves in their own appropriate way by being free to lend themselves to some deep and indivisible unity, e.g. the sexual drive in love. Love manifests itself in the sexual drive as one of its forms. But the lower-level drives may realise themselves in the shape of higher-level drives by perversion so that the higher drives are not really there, except as a mask, as, for example, when religious feelings are experienced as sensual gratification or dedication to God as lust.

If we call this higher-level mask a 'symbol' and state that the sexual drive finds realisation in such 'symbols' we have to admit that such 'symbolic' gratification does exist. But it is not universal and when it occurs it is always the sign of an abnormal psyche. It is the direct inclusion of sensual drive in a non-corporeal form (the drive, so to speak, empties the form as it takes possession) instead of a sublimation in which the drive is there but transformed into a part of the whole. This direct inclusion of the sensual element changes the very nature of the non-corporeal, turns it into a means, into dead matter, disguise and deception. In terms of *personality* the effect is that of dishonesty and hypocrisy.

(*dd*) *As fixation of drive.* Perversion rises through the accidents of our first experiences. Gratification remains tied to the form and object once experienced, but this does not happen simply through the force of simultaneous association with that former experience. If so, such phenomena would have to belong to human experience in general. The conditioning factor is rather something else, which we believe to have found when we suppose a hypothetical 'arrest at an infantile level' of the psyche as a whole.

For example: Fetichism is a perversion in which the objects of sexual attraction may be shoes, fur coats, underwear, girls' pigtails, etc. v. Gebsattel studied shoe-fetichism. The shoe for the patient was not just an object, but a living thing which he addressed, cuddled, as a child cuddles a doll. The fetish formation corresponds to an auto-erotic state of development arrested at an infantile level. The shoe-fetichist is 'incapable of letting his love and sexuality reach beyond himself. He cannot bring them together into any real consonance with the realisation of another living "Thou". Created in flight from other personalities and the other sex, the fetish becomes a substitute for the other "Thou" as well as for the other's body. The fetichist in the course of his development becomes fixed in the maternal/paternal love relationship and never grows out of it.'
Psychoanalysts interpret neurotic attention to food and digestion as an infantile attitude, coprophilia as well and other manifestations of anal-eroticism. They understand scrupulous cleanliness and anxious orderliness and other features of the 'anal-erotic' person in the same terms.

The *personality* reveals the effect of these fixations as an inner lack of freedom, as inhibition and a general impoverishment of feeling.

(*ee*) *Transformation of drive into craving.* Drives are not yet cravings. Craving as compared with drive is not only stronger and more difficult to overcome but it is experienced as something alien and compelling. Craving springs from an abnormal and intolerable state which it is supposed will be alleviated by satisfaction of the craving. Drives can turn into cravings. How does a craving arise? Firstly, through knowing. Reflection on sexuality can itself create a craving even though the drives themselves are not particularly strong. Secondly, a chance intake of intoxicants may lead to withdrawal phenomena (addictive cravings in the narrower sense are those due to intoxicants). Thirdly, there is a certain peculiar and increased sense of emptiness into which people may fall repeatedly through disposition or situation, and in order to escape from it they surrender to a craving. Thus v. Gebsattel remarks 'every sort of human interest can degenerate into a craving' in that it may be put into the service of this emptiness, whether it be work, collecting things, striving for power, indulging in sentimental feelings, making a cult of beauty, etc. Instead of a growing personal life, all that happens is a repetitive craving for the same thing. The dissatisfaction felt is only gratified for the moment, it is never removed. It returns at once and demands unreflecting repetition without any growing continuity of content.

All perversions are cravings (v. Gebsattel). They are more compelling than normal drives. The urgent desire for intoxicants is a craving. In this case there is a physiological emptiness produced in the person, for instance when morphine has been given for medical reasons and its effects cease. It needs a certain self-discipline to overcome this state. If however this whole sense of emptiness is an integral part of the personality and precedes the craving altogether, both factors combine, the physiological state and the urge to banish the emptiness in intoxication. We may say that all alcoholics, morphinists, etc., who are addicts, carry with them a basic, psychic readiness and that they can replace one craving with another but can never become radically free from any because the cause of the craving cannot be abolished.

(4) *Psychic developments due to transformation of drive.* Not all impulses arise from a basic drive. On the contrary we have to differentiate between primary drives and those drives which are only disguises, substitute activities or only apparent instinctual drives. In this case the meaningful connection is as follows: our real environment often impairs the gratification of instinct and this will happen sometimes to every one. Every instinctual gratification brings some kind of pleasure, and every impediment arouses displeasure. Where reality denies true instinctual gratification, the psyche will seek such gratification by a number of devious and unnoticed ways, although in principle we are always capable of noticing when this moment arises. Since real gratification is impossible, success is obtained through a deception. From this arise the host of our illusionary gratifications, the unnoticed dishonesty of human nature. Here are a few examples from this really inexhaustible field:

(*aa*) One possibility is that we simply exclude *concrete reality* from our consciousness. We believe that what we wish is real and what we do not wish is unreal. The majority of human judgments are distorted in this way. With one group of psychoses—the so-called reactive psychoses—we gain the impression that the psychosis achieves *a flight from reality*—a reality that has become unbearable.

(*bb*) Another possibility is that the *ungratified drive takes another object as a symbol* and gains a different, slighter but nevertheless acceptable gratification. The objects of the above third group of drives are very often turned into symbols by ungratified drives belonging to the first and second group. The drives of the third group are then not really experienced, but only apparently so. This becomes obvious in the different character of the subjective experience and also by the fact that as soon as a possibility for real instinctual gratification arises the false enthusiasm for the other values vanishes.

(*cc*) Similarly, there can be a translation of values, a '*falsification of value-scales*' (Nietzsche) whereby underprivileged people make their reality bearable. Poor, weak, impotent individuals turn weakness into a strength, e.g. in the formation of certain moral values, to make their existence tolerable. Nietzsche understood such a shift in values as the product of *resentment* at the positive values of others who were rich, privileged and strong. Scheler[1] has made an excellent analysis of the relevant connections and shows the deceptiveness of these changes in values.

Another falsification which is the direct opposite of that springing from resentment is the *attachment of value to social status* (Legitimitätswertung). The individual for whom things go well, who is fortunate in his birth and belongs to the ruling classes, tends not to ascribe this to luck but to his own innate superiority and natural merit. The privileged position is not seen in the first place as a challenge but simply as the individual's due. In addition to everything else underprivileged people have to bear, he maintains that their suppression is right because they are inferiors. Full of self-regard, he takes affluence, power and superiority as a sign of aristocratic nobility, and health, strength and good spirits as a sign of his ultimate worth. He does not let himself see the accidental nature of his own position and the roots of ruin in all this. He cannot stand modesty, humility or any knowledge of the realities which bought him all his advantages. He wants to avoid any threat of fall and decline and to escape the responsibilities of his position. He therefore makes use of the rightness of his status as a protective screen so that he can be free of his obligations and enjoy his possessions in peace. Thus suppressor and suppressed alike may both falsify their scales of value in a complementary manner, just as a sense of the realities, truthfulness and openmindedness are possible for them both.

### (b) The Individual in the World

The basic human situation is that each one stands in the world as an individual, a finite being, dependent but always with a possibility for activity within certain changing but none the less constricting bounds. Living is an encounter with a world which we call concrete reality. To live involves struggle, impact, creation. It means breaking against the world, adapting to it, learning and getting to know it.

1. *The concept of situation.* All life takes place in its own particular surroundings. In abstract physiological terms we say stimulus causes reaction. In real life, the situation releases activity, and gives birth to performance and experience; it may evoke them in some way or put them forward as something that has to be done. Social studies investigate the human situation as it derives from the objective relationships of social life. The psychology of meaningful phenomena investigates individual attitudes to typical situations. It objectifies the way in which coincidence, opportunity and destiny come to us through the situation itself and how we grasp or lose them. Situations have urgency, their sequence is changeable and unfixed, and mankind can contrive them. We use

[1] Max Scheler, 'Über Ressentiment u. moralischen Werturteil', *Z. Pathopsychol.*, vol. 1 (1912), p. 268.

the term 'marginal situations' for the ultimate situations like death, guilt, and inevitable struggle, which determine the whole of life unavoidably, though they go hidden and unheeded in our everyday existence. The human experience, appropriation and conquest of these marginal situations remain the final sources of what we really are and of what we can become.

2. *Concrete reality.* What concrete reality is cannot be maintained with any objective certainty but it depends to a certain degree on *beliefs which the community generally accept.* In trying to understand someone, we have to keep apart what he accepts as concrete reality and what we ourselves know it to be. Hence because concrete reality has no absolutes all understanding exists, as it were, in suspense.

Concrete reality is *nature,* in particular our body and our physical and mental abilities. Concrete reality is the *social order* which indicates what the individual must expect in any social situation from certain acts or modes of behaviour. *Other individuals* are also concrete reality and communication with them creates the familiar, supporting foundations of our life.

Man is driven towards concrete reality to fulfil his existence in bodily soundness and skilful performance or in social privilege and responsibility or perhaps in the only way in which he can truly realise himself, in the bond of close and genuine relationships. But such fulfilment does not just come automatically to him on its own.

3. *Self-sufficiency and dependency.* As humans, we tend to imagine some sort of ideal being that is self-contained and self-sufficient and content in itself without needing to receive anything from without because there are endless riches to be derived from itself. But if we want to become such a being we have first to learn the drastic lesson that in everything we are dependent. As vital beings we have needs that can only be satisfied from without. We have to live in society, and play a part there in order to get our share of the goods necessary for life. We have to live with others, surrendering to them while preserving ourselves, giving and taking in mutual relationship. We have to live, loving and hating, or we will grow empty and void in our solitude. We have to live in exchange with each other, and continually create afresh from what we learn, hear, understand and appropriate, if we are to partake in the human spirit to which we would have no access without our fellows.

There are limitations, inhibitions and collisions in all our external contacts, whether with nature or with man, with society or with the individual. Life is realisation through the processes of creation and adaptation, through struggles and resignations, compromise and fresh efforts at integration. In such realisation the polarities between preserving our own space and surrendering it to others become a unified whole and there is no dispersal into mutually exclusive opposites.

But we cannot avoid *conflict,* conflict with society, other individuals and with oneself. Conflicts may be sources of defeat, lost life and a limitation of our potentiality but they may also lead to greater depth of living and the birth of more far-reaching unities, which flourish in the tensions that engender them.

All finite life has a double character. It *reacts* to situations, facts and people and in its reactions it also becomes *active and creative* in the concrete reality of the confronting situation. Action and reaction are wrongly conceived as opposed and it is a mistake to imagine the possibility of an absolute creativity engaged in objectless activity. It is equally wrong to take reaction as the fundamental feature of life.

In the course of time the modes of activity and reactivity and of their admixture (with one or other pole predominating) take up a certain pattern of distribution in any one individual as with others, and thus a group-type is formed. As extreme examples we find: a *contemplative, closed inwardness* that devotes itself to quiet being and passes its life untested, unproven, in a continuity of looking and remembering. On the other hand there is the *activity of the extravert*, that accepts no finality of being but always wants to make a change, and prove itself in so doing, passing its days in conquest, creation and organisation.

4. *Typical basic relationships of the individual to reality.* The above-described ways of existence in concrete reality are never pursued without meeting resistance. Success is never complete. There is a constantly moving relationship between activity and reactivity and this can be meaningfully construed in terms of typical contrasts:

(*aa*) Kretschmer[1] confined the relationships between the self and outer world—that is the individual's style of life—to the following possibilities:

1. A *simple* sthenic or asthenic relationship

   *Sthenic:* feelings of superiority over the world, of strength and power to act. Tendencies to excessive self-assurance, recklessness and aggressiveness.

   *Asthenic:* feelings of inferiority, weakness, passivity. Tendencies to underestimate the self, give way and be uncertain in one's behaviour.

2. An *internally contradictory*, expansive or sensitive relationship.

   *Expansive:* Sthenic/asthenic polarity. Hence hidden feelings of insufficiency, overcompensation, touchy self-consciousness, readiness to take offence or feel injured. Tendencies to paranoid and querulant behaviour.

   *Sensitive:* Asthenic/sthenic polarity. Hence ambitiousness, vulnerable self-esteem, sudden strong feelings of insufficiency, uncertainty about life, self-torture, scrupulous conscience with little cause, feelings of moral reproach. Tendencies to ideas of reference.

3. *Intermediate life-styles:* conciliatory, practical and adaptable, in harmony with one's milieu. No contrast felt between the self and the outer world.

[1] Bumke's *Handbuch der Geisteskrankheiten*, vol. 1, pp. 686 ff.

(*bb*) To complement this typology of temperament, the content of the person's life-style can be classified according to his attitude to reality, and the meaning this acquires for him in the course of time. The contrasting polarities are as follows: Either his work, performance and life in general draw validity for him from *some continuing whole* or he finds every activity a game, an *adventure, an experiment.* In the former case we find the following of some task or calling, carried on historically by successive generations. The work of the past is a tangible whole which comes to life again daily in the individual's own activity. The farmer is such a type and knows himself to be a disappearing link in the service of his farm and acts accordingly. But in the latter case, we have the game of the adventurer, where everything is in pieces. There is no meaningful sequence of activity, the moment is supreme. His world is without plan, completeness or grace. The adventurer in his reality gives us a symbol of the impossibility of perfect fulfilment.

Both these contrasting polarities express a basic attitude to reality and in each case the reality is felt as radically different. For the one, reality signifies an enduring existence in an historical sequence of work, family and further development; for the other, reality has no foundation and signifies an eternal gamble and defeat.

5. *Denial of reality through self-deception.* It is difficult to expose ourselves fully to reality. Reality exacts constant self-denials, continuous effort and painful experiences and insights. There is therefore a strong urge to withdraw from reality. Life always finds a possible way to circumvent it, screen it off or find some substitute and this is accompanied by the momentary pleasure of easy gratification but it is always at the price of loss of health or life. In a host of individual situations, as indeed throughout his whole life, man is constantly faced with this choice of either penetrating or denying reality. The following are some of the ways in which withdrawal from reality seems to offer substitutes, gratification and satisfaction.

(*aa*) *In place of the denied reality,* the object of gratification becomes one's own *self-created contents.* Montaigne wrote: 'Plutarch says of people who waste their feelings on guinea-pigs and pet dogs, that the love element in all of us, if deprived of any adequate object, will seek out something trivial and false rather than let itself stay unengaged. So the psyche in its passions prefers to deceive itself or even in spite of itself invent some nonsensical object rather than give up all drive or aim. . . . What would we not hold on to, rightly or wrongly, so as to have something on which to vent our wrath?' Objects are then not taken as such but as symbols for something else.

We escape from reality with the help of *fantasies.* These conjure up easily and lavishly all that in reality would be so hardly and sparsely achieved. Fantasies are related to wishes which arise from the inhibitions and deprivations of individual existence and they bring us relief though they have no concrete reality. Bleuler calls this self-incapsulation in an isolated world 'autistic thinking'. The contents of fantasy longing may be, for example, one's lost childhood, foreign lands, spiritual homelands, but the crucial point is the tendency to turn away from present conflicts and obligations. It is an aspect of metaphysics and poetry that they rob man of his real personal part in Existence itself in favour of a dissipation of his powers in fantasy, and this was most profoundly comprehended by Kierkegaard.

(*bb*) At first these modes of unreal subjective gratification are only a sort of game we play, but they can lead to a *subjective realisation of their contents*. A transformation occurs which must be due to some underlying abnormal mechanism which we no longer understand. Here belong the hysterical realisations (in all kinds of bodily and physical phenomena), elaborate lying in which the person convinces himself (pseudologia phantastica) and the construction of delusion-like worlds in schizophrenic processes.

(*cc*) Transformations of this sort do not often occur in normal, understandable psychic life, but once the game of fancy has started, it frequently leads to *self-deception*. The self-deception can be corrected but we see it at work in the understandable forgetting of painful things or obligations, the subsconcious relief of illusionary misinterpretations, of which we are certainly subjectively aware, and in temporary excursions into hysterical behaviour. The contrast to such behaviour is the striving for reality, truthfulness and authenticity. The person wants to have a transparent vision of what he really is in his concrete reality. Such an effort returns him to the world if defiance has not led him to the utter clarity of negation and isolation.

The behaviour of neurotics and psychotics, criminals[1] and eccentrics has been understood as a form of self-deception, a self-surrender to a fictitious existence, which has arisen from an urge to get away from reality. Seclusion of the self comes to mean falsity because self-deception and self-constriction inevitably follow. Seclusion from reality as given is indeed a seclusion from the very basis of being which manifests itself through reality. And 'sin is separation from God'. Falsity of this sort has been thought to be a universal human trait; like Ibsen, we look for the 'life-lie' which everyone needs and acknowledge Goethe's saying that no one ever reaches such insight into truth and reality as would take away the conditions of his own existence. Others limit this world of radical self-deception to a particular group of persons who suffer from personality disorders (psychopaths) and define personality-disorder (psychopathy) as 'a suffering from self-deceptions necessary for life' (Klages). Any reasonable psychologist will guard against generalising in either direction. We try to understand our problems but we do not expect any final answers.

The struggle is real. We see that we are threatened, that the situation makes demands. Flight, attack or defence are all weapons we can use. But the whole procedure may become obscure. Unbearable reality tends to get veiled. We do not accept the threat nor the demand that we should fight or endure it. Our defence becomes an avoidance in self-deception. We have no clear intention

[1] Andreas Bjerre, *Zur Psychologie des Mordes* (Heidelberg, 1925).

but make an instinctive arrangement to get away from the demands of the situation, perhaps through illness or some misfortune or suffering. Both the situation and its demands and the meaning of our own attitude are hidden from conscious scrutiny. In addition to the deliberate deception of others or substituting for it, we find self-deception and a distortion of reality. The person's consciousness can no longer accord with his unconscious.

6. *Marginal situations.* Man is always in one situation or another, and all these situations are finally resolved into marginal situations, that is, certain impassable, unchangeable situations that belong to our human existence as such. In these situations mere human existence founders and awakens to Existence itself.[1] Empirical psychology can throw no light on these marginal frontiers nor on what an individual can become when confronted with them, whether he conceals them from himself or lays himself open to them. But the psychopathologist interested in meaning must be aware of all this because the personality disorders (the psychopathies and neuroses) and the psychoses are veritable sources of human possibility, not only deviations from a healthy norm. The abnormal happening and experience is very often a manifestation of something that is a strictly human concern. The psychopathologist who confines himself to mere observation and objective phenomena cannot perceive this; he can only do this within the bond of human fellowship where one person shares his destiny with another.

Neurosis (personality disorder) has been conceived as failure in the marginal situations of life. The goal of therapy has then been visualised as a self-realisation or as a self-transformation of the individual through the marginal situation, in which he is revealed to himself and affirms himself in the world as it is.[2] This conception is valid so far as its philosophical truth is also valid for the neurotic person. The practical philosophy of becoming truthful also has a therapeutic effect. But we should remember that avoidance of marginal situations does not in itself create illness. We see it carried out quite successfully in a perfectly healthy dishonesty and cowardice, without any abnormal phenomena.

### (c) *Symbols as the content of ultimate knowledge*

To understand the individual, we need to understand what he knows, what objective contents exist in his consciousness. The crucial point, however, is not so much what he knows but what this means to him, that is, how was his knowledge acquired and what are its necessary effects? The nature of an individual is determined by what he experiences, sees and is confronted with as his own concrete reality. Most of all it is determined by his concrete certainty of this reality. What sort of God he has sums up the man.

1. *Ultimate knowledge.* The knowledge which belongs solely to the indi-

---

[1] 'Über Grenzsituationen', see my *Philosophie*, vol. 2, pp. 201 ff.

[2] Johanna Dürck, 'Die Existenzformen von Bemächtigung u. Verneidung', *Zbl. Psychother.*, vol. 12, p. 223.

vidual and which *conditions* the certainty of his knowledge or is the *precondition* of any other knowledge he may gain, we have termed ultimate knowledge. Another term is the 'a priori'. As such, it is the *general* 'a priori' of universal consciousness in the categories of understanding. As regards ideas, it is the 'a priori' of the intellect; as regards practical drives and forms of reaction, it is the 'a priori' of human existence. *Historically* it is the 'a priori' of the person, present in his own world as part of his tradition, as a momentary figure in time, as an incarnation of the universal, which has meaning and import, not as a universal but as an infinite particular.

Ultimate knowledge resides in the prevailing types of intuition, in the types of seeing and conceiving primary phenomena and facts, in the modes of individual and group existence, in the various tasks and callings and the dominant values and tendencies. Symbols play an important part within it and are all-pervasive.

2. *Concept of the symbol and its significance in real life.* Kant states: 'every object must be concrete before we can grasp it. Symbols help us to grasp things by analogy. For example, monarchy may be represented as a body with a soul and dictatorship as a machine. There is no similarity between actual object and image but they have the common principle of making us think about both and their inner causality. Now if "reflection on an object of direct apperception is transferred to an entirely different concept which can never be directly apperceived", then we have the symbol. In symbols we behold all that our reason thinks without there being any corresponding concrete apperception for the thought. What is beheld in the symbol proper is *only* accessible in symbolic form; the object of the symbol never shows itself directly as concrete experience. "Thus knowledge of God is purely symbolic." To take the symbols, for example, of God's will, love and might in a direct fashion, only lands us in anthropomorphism, and if we ignore the intuition in the symbols we shall slide into Deism.'[1]

Symbols that do not contain a concrete reality become non-committal aesthetic contents. They are only fully symbols if they express reality. Human thinking is prone to take this symbolic reality as if it were the reality of direct apperception, so that symbols tend either to become objects of superstition (where their concreteness is mistaken for reality) or to pass as unreal (mere metaphors or symbols when measured by concrete reality itself). To live deeply rooted in symbols is to live in a reality which as yet we do not know but can appreciate in its symbolic form. Symbols therefore are infinite, accessible to infinite interpretation and inexhaustible, but they are never reality itself as an object which we could know and possess.[2]

It is true that ultimate knowledge has categories to *structure* it and ideas that form *complex unities* but the *reality* that lays hold of us in it takes a

---

[1] Kant, *Kritik der Urteilskraft*, Section 59.
[2] Fr. Th. Vischer, *Das Symbol in 'Kritischen Gängen'*. His conception is an aesthetic one, and the reality-content vanishes.

symbolic form. This means that ultimate knowledge is not a well-developed intellectual knowledge but lies in apperceptions and images that carry infinite meanings and bring to us the language of reality. Their presence, as it were, protects us, helps us to reassure ourselves and brings us peace. Even the logically systematised knowledge of the philosophically educated person comes at last to the determining symbol. Even systems of ideas are like symbols in their complex unities and when they carry a real awareness mean more than is seen in them by reason. All basic philosophic concepts are, not so much definitions, but rather comprehensive symbolic apperceptions, which not even the most detailed of rational systems can fully explain.

Symbols are an historical 'a priori' but their truth impresses us as something eternal in time. They order themselves in an infinite succession. They come to light in myths, philosophy and theology. They appear in the play of the imagination, flourish uncommitted in aesthetics, compel with absolute power in extreme situations and are the hidden guide of every full-bodied, meaningful life.

Everything in the world can become a symbol. The basic forms of life, the universe and of all that happens, the elements, the basic facts of our existence, types of real things, human ideals and counter-ideals. Every one of them can be turned into a symbol according to what we value. If seen simply as objects, they cease to be symbols, even when one signifies the other (e.g. the machine signifying the dictatorship) provided both are seen on equal terms, explaining each other as ends in themselves. Where symbols become carriers of infinite meaning, of something inaccessible except through the symbol, they become as it were 'creatures with souls', attracting us to themselves, inspiring us, delighting us, making us shrink but always absorbing us. They leave their imprint on us in so far as they leave us free, but should they become lasting objects of superstition they keep us fettered.

*In common usage* the word 'symbol' has many meanings. In its widest sense it is used merely as a sign, as a metaphor or simile, as some schematic abbreviation for what we see in the world, as anything significant. We must always ask 'a symbol of what?'. If the answer refers to some other concrete object then we are not dealing with a genuine symbol. The genuine symbol contains the 'of what' within itself and there is no actual object referred to, except perhaps in the form of some transcendental philosophic concept.

In the psychology of meaningful phenomena we need to differentiate carefully between a symbol as a *carrier of meanings that have a personal validity*, springing from the person's life-history, a kind of surrogate structure as it were, and a symbol as a *carrier of a comprehensive meaning, the bearer of an immanent transcendence.* Jung conceived the first as arising from the personal unconscious, and the latter as from the collective unconscious.

3. *The possibility of understanding symbols.* Can one understand symbols? Other people's symbols, not one's own, can only be seen as they appear from without. We cannot understand them from within, from the very heart of their

reality. The symbol must incorporate one's own life if the meaning is to be fully understood. Our own symbols can be illumined, and translated into metaphysical ideas and in the process much is brought out of the dark into a rich unfolding. While they remain part of our life and we live in them they can be understood. Formal understanding of symbols, on the other hand, can only reach as far as an aesthetic appreciation, the special excitation of feeling by a tentative play with exotic material, while the true seriousness of reality is lacking. Symbolic knowledge amounts to more than thinking in images.

Psychological understanding of symbols moves among perilous *ambiguities*. We study symbols in myths and religions, dreams and psychoses, in daydreams and in the personality-disorders (psychopathic states). We get to know about them but only from without and our own beliefs are not involved. On the other hand, in the course of such scientific study we get bent on the truth of the symbols themselves; we would like to heal through communicating our knowledge of symbols; we want to bring them to life ourselves, and invite participation in them. There is a confusing interweaving between knowledge of symbols as historical and psychological facts—seen from outside even when we have some inner representation of them in ourselves—and knowledge of symbolic truth. The two meanings get inextricably mixed.

4. *The historical study of symbols.* The exploration of symbols is usually confined to myths, fairy-tales and sagas. Research into Greek mythology seems to have been the main source especially since the Romantic period (Creuser). The most productive authors have been O. Müller, Welcker, Nägelsbach, Rohde.[1] Schelling's[2] imposing and comprehensive study still has interest in spite of gross mistakes in detail, but among all these interpreters, Bachofen[3] remains the one who had inspiration, as it were, in spite of his collector's zeal and solid approach.

Nowadays it is Klages[4] and Jung[5] who have become known as the interpreters of symbols. What Burckhardt termed 'archaic images' ('urtümliche Bilder'), Klages termed 'images' and Jung 'archetypes'. But there are certain essential differences between Klages and Jung. Klages' interpretation has a fascinating vividness. His presentation of the symbols of poetry and art remains as perhaps the really lasting contribution in all his great work, in

[1] Otfried Müller, *Prolegomena zu einer wissenschaftlichen Mythologie* (Göttingen, 1825) *Die Dorier* (Breslau, 1844); F. G. Welcker, *Grieshische Götterlehre* (Göttingen, 1857); C. F. Nägelsbach, *Homerische Theologie* (Nürnberg, 1840); *Nachhomerische Theologie* (Nürnberg, 1857). Erwin Rohde, *Psyche* (1893), 4th edn., 1907.

[2] Schelling, *Philosophie der Mythologie u. Offenbarung* (Werke, 2 Abt., Stuttgart, pp. 1856 ff.). In particular vol. 1 of the *Vorlesungen*, pp. 1–10—'Über die Geschichte der Mythologie'.

[3] J. J. Bachofen, *Die Auswahl 'Der Mythus von Orient u. Occident'* (München, 1926). Historical introduction by A. Baeumler. Selection by Rud. Marx in Kroner's *Taschenausgabe*.

[4] Ludwig Klages, *Der Geist als Widersacher der Seele* (Leipzig, 1929).

[5] C. G. Jung, *Wandlungen u. Symbole der Libido* (Leipzig and Vienna, 1912). *Seelenprobleme der Gegenwart* (Zürich, 1931). Über die Archetypen des kollektiven Unbewussten, *Eranosjahrbuch* (Zürich, 1935). On Jung himself: Die kulturelle Bedeutung der komplexen Psychologie, *Festschrift zum 60 Geburtstag* (Berlin, 1935).

which he brings forward rather doubtful evidence for the development of a strange, precritical philosophy through a synthesis of rationalism and gnosticism. Jung on the contrary lacks the impressive vividness of Klages and his work has nothing like the same weight. He is the deft master of all the means of interpretation but the inspiration is missing. Klages has inspiration, in as much as he is the true successor of Bachofen, whose work he rediscovered. Jung's expositions become tiring and irritating because of many undialectical contradictions. As the reader emerges from many of Klages' pages, he is struck by a winged quality which is lacking from the work of Jung who favours a worldly scepticism. The present day is poor in symbols and both these men are anxious to discover primary reality. Jung's efforts strike me as a fruitless new start through the exploitation of what is old, while Klages' attempt, as he appears to have felt himself, seems a rather hopeless recollection of the lost depths of history.

Jung's theories have gained esteem among psychotherapists, and even outside these circles there has been some enthusiastic agreement. The eminent Indologist, H. Zimmer, speaks of 'the magical, soul-guiding function of Jung's teaching'. 'It has discovered in the underworld of our being the eternal source, the ancient murmurings. The Myth which peoples and their poets have spun for our understanding is thus restored to its home in these unplumbed depths from which all its forms arise.' 'C. J. Jung's art of dream interpretation throws a remarkable light upon the dark world of myth and fairy-tale'. Each should look for himself and see what he can find. But for myself, I cannot be convinced that such judgments are correct.

5. *The possible function of symbol-exploration.* Symbols have a certain role in modern public life but they tend to be few. Compared with earlier times, life nowadays is extraordinarily poor in symbols. Yet it is a fact that symbols appear in great number in dreams, daydreams, psychoses and personality disorders (psychopathic states); whether they do so as by-play or in all seriousness cannot be determined. In psychopathology, symbols have become a favourite object of attention for psychotherapists because in psychotherapy symbols become important. There are three reasons for this: firstly, they give us an insight into what are the dominating preoccupations of the individual; secondly, unnoticed symbols can be evoked, fostered and brought into consciousness; and thirdly, symbols can be used to give indirect guidance to the patient. This at least appears to be so, although all these three procedures have been doubted by some. But if symbols do have this importance—hard to overestimate—then their exploration becomes of extreme consequence.

(*aa*) *Recognition of symbolic material.* Psychotherapists began by letting patients tell their dreams. Similar contents were also found in psychotic experiences, fantasies and delusions. Lastly it was discovered that an otherwise unregarded world emerged in the dreams of everyone. These findings became significant, in as much as parallels could be drawn between them and universal myths, in the same way as ethnologists had already found parallels between myths all over the globe, giving rise to the hypothesis of 'elemental human ideas' (Elementargedanken—Bastian).[1] These were thought to arise spontaneously everywhere without any spread of ideas through communication. Similarly psychotherapists assumed something universal to humanity and not only could it be discovered by ethnologists and mythologists but it could be found in dreams, personality disorders (neuroses) and psychoses. It was necessary, therefore, to have some general acquaintance with the myths of the world as they appeared in religion, in fairy-tale and legend and in the poetic imagination.

(*bb*) *Recognition of symbolic connections.* Symbols may be analysed from three different aspects: *philosophically* as to their truth (Plato, Plotinus, Schelling); *historically*, as to their development in concrete reality; *psychologically*, as to their origin in the individual psyche and their effect upon it, in accordance with the general rule or as a variation. These three approaches involve questions of very different significance. All three equally demand an understanding of the content, it is true, but questions regarding *the eternal truth* of the symbols pursue a goal independent from those regarding the *universality of symbols as concrete historical phenomena*, and both sets of questions are quite independent from the question of symbols as *cause and effect*, even though all three sets of questions are found constantly intertwined in any exploration of the symbols themselves.

1. *Systematisation of symbols.* We now comprehend that the human being lives in symbols all the time. They are his dominating reality and since this symbolic existence is part of the basic structure of human life, our aim is to grasp these symbols in all their particularity, collect them in all their diversity, survey them carefully and bring them into some kind of order. We have two different standpoints at our disposal. We may either approach them as strange, exotic forms which, even if we cannot understand them, we would at least like to know from the outside. Or we may see them as a unique world of symbolic truth from which, to our detriment, we have grown alienated to a great extent but which we might recapture. This would give us a vast world of constantly moving images which represent the truth of primary types. We should then seek for the basic elements as unchanging elements in our human awareness of reality. The systematisation of symbols will not then appear to us as a classification of certain peculiar fantasies but a ground-plan of truth. The development of possible symbolic content means that a space is opened up in which the individual can become a substantial self. Bereft of symbols, his impoverished psyche would, as it were, freeze into nothing, and, left with reason alone, he would make but a futile bustle in a world that has somehow grown empty.

When the collection and classification of symbols from the purely external point of view (morphology of symbols) has been distinguished from the inward construction of symbolic truth as a whole (philosophy of symbols), we find that both can serve each other though the one does not complement the other. If we confuse the two, we discredit them both.

[1] Richard Andrée, *Ethnographische Parallele u. Vergleiche*, p. 1878. N.D. 1889.

Heyer undertook a classification of symbols.[1] We may follow him (see p. 245) as he presents his 'circle of life', moving through the different psychic levels from vegetative through the animal to the spirit, and we may see how they are rooted in myth and symbol. We may feel convinced that his classification provides a stimulating picture though from a very special point of view which both philosophy and psychology would find extremely questionable. But we must not let ourselves be misled by Heyer's first-class writing and the heady atmosphere of ideas that stem from the world of Goethe and others and have very little to do with the matter in hand.

2. *The laws of symbols.* When observing *subjective visual images* we cannot but be astonished by the way figures, landscapes, people we have never seen, suddenly emerge out of nothing. The same thing happens in dreams. In a way we cannot really measure, our unconscious life gives form to something that is presented to consciousness later as finished and complete. This final product is a content and has meaning. In so far as we find no meaningful connections and see only an aggregate of random, meaningless fragments, we talk of chance but the demand for meaningful understanding always spurs us on to look for some rule or connection.

We should indeed find such a connection provided we are not dealing with irrelevant fragments and chance groupings but with contents that emerge from unconsciousness with at least the partial significance of symbols. In attempting to interpret any factually experienced content symbolically we make two basic discoveries: *firstly*, interpretation is unlimited, there is no end to it and the ramifications of meaning go on for ever.

Jung writes: 'Once we examine the types in relation to other archetypal forms, there are so many far-reaching symbolic-historical connections that we are driven to the conclusion that the multiformity and opalesence of the basic psychic elements defeat our ordinary human powers of imagination.'

*Secondly*, interpretation becomes itself an experience, a continuation of a symbolism in which there is a continually growing content which throws light upon itself, a productive process. In the translation of symbols, we reach no terra firma.

In the course of interpretation it becomes clear whether the symbols of the dream or fantasy stand in any kind of relation to waking life, that is, whether their meaning has any influence on waking life or dominates it altogether. We can hardly doubt that symbols play a leading role in all waking life. They display themselves with effect; they not only play around life but determine its course and this fact has been explained by Jung who calls upon 'living dispositions and systems of reaction' that rule our lives unseen, unregarded and for this reason, all the more powerful. 'There are no inborn images but there are inborn possibilities of images, and these set limits to even the most daring imagination.' The philosophical 'a priori' becomes here, speaking psychologically, the effective structure of the archetypes. 'On the one hand they pro-

[1] G. R. Heyer, *Organismus der Seele* (München, 1932).

vide a powerful, instinctive bias, and on the other we may conceive them as the most effective help for instinctive adjustment.'

The archetypes of Jung have multiple meaning and as such they are not true symbols. For Jung they are universal and stand for all those forces which bring into being the specific forms, images, ideas and modes of apprehension in which the world and mankind appear to me, in which I fantasy and dream, in which I build my beliefs and in which I find the certainty of my Being. Thus among the archetypes we also find authentic symbols, and that is when transcendent contents of Being itself define for me the meaning and significance of people and things in the world; that is, when my attitude to these is decided not by any particular purpose or interest, vital antipathy or sympathy, but by something in them which transcends them. Symbols may either be the clear voices of Being itself, transcendence objectified, or they may simply be products of the human psyche (mere images or ideas), and it is in this latter sense that they tend to be of importance in psychological discussions. This leads to a confusing ambiguity: Do symbols offer us an *ultimate truth* or should we see through them and treat them simply as semblances? It is the same if we try to clarify the basic principle that *in symbols I am confronted with something that also contains myself.* Is the process of becoming one's true self a self-illumination, whereby in understanding symbols we understand the real truth? Or is this commerce with symbols just a struggle with our own shadows and it is precisely in understanding the symbols as semblance only that we become our true selves?

In Jung's work the following basic phenomenon plays an important part: Throughout life there is a constant division within us. Our relationship with objects is a relationship with ourselves, especially when we think we are dealing with something that is certainly not us. I hate and love my own possibilities present in the other, in criminals, adventurers, heroes and saints, gods and devils. I ascribe to the object what lies dormant in myself. I master this or become its victim by fighting it outside myself or making it my own by hating or loving it. The same circumstances prevail in the individual psyche as Hegel saw in the universe. I become what my opponent is. I am more or less transformed into that which I fight against.

Jung argues: The system of adaptation, through which at any one time we keep contact with the world, is the 'persona'. We either retain control of these systems, which are formed by the archetypes, or we fall captive to them by identifying with them or becoming obsessed by them. The 'shadow' on the other hand is the sum total of the inferior functions, which are always with us, just as no one can ever be in the light without throwing a shadow. The shadow draws its form from the archetypes. The man who is possessed by his shadow, that is, who lives beneath himself, stands in his own shadow. He gets unconsciously caught in a trap of his own devising when there is nothing in reality to make him stumble. The archetypes form his world into successive situations of failure, misfortune and lack of achievement.

3. *The origin of symbols.* From the empirical study of symbols we learn of the *parallels* that exist in the symbols of different peoples. We have to conclude

that there is something which is universally human, something which humanity shares. We also find *definite types of symbols*, which are limited to a number of parallel cultures and are not universal. Finally we come across *certain unique, historical symbols*, which belong to particular peoples. Thus symbols expressing the most general polarities are to be found everywhere (male and female, waxing and waning, rhythm and recurrence, elementary natural phenomena), and in this way we can discover the basic symbols of the human race, existing timelessly in the unconscious, quite apart from human history and tradition. But we never discover Apollo and Artemis, for instance, in this way. They belong to history, and are unique and irreplaceable. They cannot be found even in the depths of the unconscious and are accessible through cultural tradition alone. Between these two extremes lie those special symbolic forms which are not universal but belong to a wide range of cultures. In conclusion, there are a number of peculiar contents, not found everywhere but yet in so many places that they cannot be strictly historical and in spite of their oddity seem of a general character: for example, the cephalopods (Kopffüssler).

Symbols only affect life in their particular, historically unique, form. They have universality of structure and content, it is true, but in itself this is ineffective. There is however another view which holds to the contrary, that effectiveness lies *just in* that *universal* characteristic which disguises itself under the many historical variations.

Schelling held to the first view. He had a magnificent vision of the peoples of the earth and their myths coinciding in origin. The Babylonian Tower of Babel bore witness to the dispersion of the unified human race into peoples, who as they groped their way were at the mercy of their myths. There were as many myths as there were peoples. Every myth creates its people, just as all peoples create their myths. 'The general principles of myth-formation took on specific shapes from the very start.'

Jung takes the opposite view: He distinguishes a collective unconscious from the personal unconscious that grows out of the life-history. The collective unconscious is the universal biological and psychological basis of human life. It exerts its influence on everyone, though it is deeply hidden. Yet he conceives this universal element as 'the mighty cultural heritage of human development' and again as 'the residue of all human experience right back to its most obscure beginnings'.

Jung construes the collective unconscious as a domain of archaic images which are the truest thoughts of mankind. This again does not avoid ambiguity. On the one hand the construct implies an objective knowledge, based on research, of earlier times and of the hidden dispositions of men (Anlagen); on the other hand it calls for participation in these substantial truths for one's own good.

He writes as follows: 'The most archaic images are the oldest, most universal and profoundest thoughts of mankind. They are as much feelings as ideas and indeed they even have something like their own independent life, something perhaps like their own particular soul, as may be seen clearly in all those gnostic systems which accept as a basic tenet the existence of a perceiving unconscious as a source of know-ledge. St. Paul's image of the angels, archangels, principalities and powers, the Gnostic's archons and aeons, the heavenly hierarchies of Dionysius Areopagitica, all stem from the relative sovereignty of the archetypes.' These contain all that man could think of as most beautiful and magnificent as well as all the wickedness and devilry of which he is capable.

These historical-cum-psychological theses are very questionable, quite apart from their supposed bearing on truth. At first glance there are surprising analogies to be drawn between the myths of almost all races and between these myths and the contents of dream and psychosis. But they are insufficient to provide us with a convincing construct of a universal and fundamental human unconscious, fully stored with content. Looking at these analogies more closely we find they are superficial and confined to general categories. It is precisely their effective content which is missing. For example, the point of similarity in dying and rising gods (Osiris is killed, Dionysius torn to pieces, Christ crucified) does not constitute their essential nature. The analogy throws light on what is inessential.

(*cc*) *Awakening of latent contents.* The psychotherapist in his exploration of symbols is impelled by a wish to find the symbolic truth and participate in it. He runs a considerable risk here of being confused and deceived.

1. The occurence of symbols in dreams, fantasies and psychoses is a psycholo-gical phenomenon which needs to be differentiated as such from the existential sig-nificance of symbols in the sensible, waking state. If we take dream-experience as a starting-point for *interpretations of human life which are to be existentially effective,* are truth and well-being thereby enhanced? Perhaps so, but can it not easily happen that what matters in earnest is then deflected on to a shifting play of feeling and supposed statements of what is only supposedly so?

2. Self-fulfilment comes from the success or failure of some particular, historical solution of the great problems of the human order. For the person who loses this capacity for self-fulfilment in the course of his life, myths and poetic images lose their meaning also. If he becomes aware of this deficit, the withering seed of human possi-bility may reach out for the air in which it may breathe and grow. In this case *breath-ing space may be given* through *some idea of the basic human possibilities* from Homer to Shakespeare and Goethe and as the old, eternal myths preserve them. The individual may not be untouched by these yet they still do not represent *his own original reality.*

3. Where historical and psychological knowledge is treated as if it could provide effective symbols for suffering people, *superstition* may be the result, a credulous belief which attempts in a limited fashion to fixate symbols that are themselves in-definite, constantly in motion and not to be grasped objectively. Deeply rooted traditions are turned inside out in the process and misused for therapeutic purposes (they become a sort of measuring-rod for happiness and health). Where this is so, the symbols are symbols no longer.

4. The individual may find in symbols a language for something which would otherwise never be objective to him or have any influence on him. Once these sym-bols are evoked from his unconscious, the question arises as to *what historical factor*

needs to be added to give form to the awakening symbol and bring it to self-aware-ness. Whoever tries to answer this question can only *prophesy*. He cannot be didactic, he can only proclaim. He cannot hold up any helping mirror nor ask helpful questions, but he can proffer something material. The scientist and philosopher may think this goes beyond human power and possibility. We stay confronting the symbols with wondering respect as a whole world of hidden truth. Science and philosophy carry us only so far as the frontier where our understanding tries to approach the symbols, not in a general way but in their individual and historically concrete form; here we listen for the echo in ourselves which may help us to understand whatever comes to meet us in the other person.

5. Over against *this whole world of symbols* we have within ourselves a primary resource whereby this whole world is made *relative*. We are liberated from our bondage to symbols by self-reflection. This protects us from credulity, which is a constant threat to us, and carries us through and beyond all symbols, making it pos-sible for us to form a new and deeper bond, that of Existence itself now linked with an imageless transcendence that speaks to us in the absolute of goodness and in the miracle of receiving oneself as a gift in the spontaneity of freedom. It shows itself in the uncommitted certainty with which we find our way through inward acts and out-ward behaviour, once the directness of reason has discovered for us the choices and decisions of Existence itself.

## § 3. Basic Patterns of Meaning

### (a) Opposing tendencies in the psyche and the dialectic of its movement

Psychic life and its contents are polarised in opposites. It is through the opposites, however, that everything is once more re-connected. Image calls forth counter-image, tendencies call forth counter-tendencies and feelings other feelings in contrast. At some point sadness turns spontaneously, or with but little provocation, into cheerfulness. An unacknowledged inclination leads to exaggerated emphasis on an opposite one. Meaningful understanding must always be guided by such opposites, and were we to enumerate them all we should be surveying the whole field of psychology.

1. *Logical, biological, psychological and intellectual opposites.* In order to consider the various opposites we need some general standpoint: we may regard them as the diverse categories of *logic*, as biological and psychological *realities* and *intellectually*, as spiritual possibilities which might realise themselves.

We have to differentiate *the logical categories of mere otherness* or difference (e.g. of colour and tone) frc_n *oppositeness*. Within the latter we have again to differentiate *polarity* (red and green) from *contradiction* (true and false). We are concerned here with a universal form of thinking which cannot proceed with-out there being 'the one' and 'the other', that is without differentiation and without at least two points of reference. We are also concerned with a form of universal Being as it appears for us (since reason cannot think anything which has not something else external to itself; all Being therefore is polarised for reason as it operates; otherwise it would be unthinkable).

*In biology* we observe real polarities: inspiration and expiration, the systole and diastole of the heart, assimilation and dissimilation of metabolism, antagonistic functions with their opposing rhythms, wakefulness which finally compels sleep and sleep which in its turn compels waking. In the functional cycles in which inner secretion plays a part, there are polarities in the latter also. (Thyrotoxicosis and myxoedema contrast as opposites and seem to contain something that makes them diverge in opposite directions.) One basic polarity of all living things is the division into male and female and their reunification.

*In psychology* the polarity of opposites is all-pervasive. We find activity and passivity, consciousness and unconsciousness, pleasure and displeasure, love and hate, self-surrender and self-assertion, all polarities of the psychic states and drives. We find also a will to power and an urge to submit, self-will and social sense (I and We), an urge towards the light, towards self-direction, responsibility, activity, life; and an urge towards the dark, towards safety, irresponsibility, peace and death. There is also an urge to disrupt order and an urge to conform. There are an infinite number of opposites and polarities which can be developed in this way. In their rich and varied transformations they dominate the psychology of meaningful phenomena and its written productions. All such psychology has to deal with polarities.

Intellectually, polarity leads to *the establishment* of opposing evaluations: true–false, beautiful–ugly, good–bad, positive–negative. Our mind lays hold on all the blind and accidental polarities, recognises their significance and views them as symbols from the spatial levels of up and down, left and right, for example, up through darkness and light, the biological poles of male and female to the psychological antagonisms of pleasure–displeasure, joy–sadness, upward rise and downward fall. For the mind itself, however, the movements it carries out upon itself are essential. As it makes its way from one pole to the other, it cannot tolerate contradiction and endeavours to overcome all contradictions, unify the polarities and contain them within tensions of ever-widening range.

The mind grows conscious of the fact that all these opposites belong together and it becomes aware of the manner of their connectedness, and all this becomes an immense work of its own doing. Our intellect identifies the infinite transformations of the basic phenomenon wherever it appears, and grasps it, bringing it into being within itself. Opposites do not merely exist but all Being is moved by them. Opposites are bound to each other and thus become the source of constant *movement*. This movement is termed a *dialectic*. In the face of such movement, there arises the dissatisfaction, or rather the revolt, of reason, which desires to establish things and know what it is presented with in terms of facts. So, too, wherever reality is dialectical in character, terms of definition become universally inappropriate.

2. *Dialectical modes.* In concrete psychic reality, the movement of opposites takes place in three ways: 1. *Reversal* through time without consciousness taking part—inspiration changes into expiration, grief into cheerfulness,

enthusiasm into boredom, love into hate and vice versa. 2. A *battle* of opposites, both opposites are present in the psyche, the one hurling itself against the other. 3. *The self decides* between the opposites, excluding one in favour of the other. Where there is reversal of opposites we are concerned with an *impersonal event*; where there is battle between opposites, we are concerned with *an inner activity* and in the decision between them with a *final choice*. The two latter modes lead to radically different dialectical movements; in the one case there is a *synthesis* of 'this as well as that', in the other a *choice*—'either–or'.

In *synthesis* the opposites are locked in a constructive tension, at any moment there is the possibility of harmonious resolution into some whole which, it is true, must immediately dissolve into fresh movement. As this proceeds, however, it builds up, by holding the opposing polarities together in an increasing complexity and to an ever-widening extent. The whole as a unity of opposites serves as origin and goal and by this movement through the opposites comes to its full realisation. Here the dialectical mode leads to the whole.

With *choice* the matter is quite different. The person faces the 'either–or' and has to decide what he is and what he wants. The ground of validity and responsibility is won with the absoluteness of a decision that excludes all other possibilities. The contradictions of human existence and of what is possible in our world have a final character. We are not honest if we try to escape them by hiding them from oneself even if the most admirable harmony is achieved thereby. There is the moment of truth where one's action is good or bad and where a total, all-embracing attitude which excludes all opposites, becomes impossible. This dialectical mode leads to the frontiers of decision.

Both modes carry a special risk for the psyche. Aiming at *the whole*, looking only at this and feeling only this, the psyche may without noticing lose its ground, be enticed into pleasing generalities and, using the dialectic of 'this as well as that' grow characterless, unreliable and sophisticated. On the other hand where the psyche endeavours to reach *the sure ground of decision* through the sacrifice of one of the opposites, it may become unnatural, psychically impoverished, enjoying a lifeless one-sided quiet. It may moreover become a victim of what has been sacrificed or excluded (in short, repressed) which returns unnoticed as it were and overpowers the psyche from the rear.

These two dialectical modes have *positive* aspects. To see 'this as well as that' offers *a middle way* where opposites may be linked together for the construction of further wholes. The 'either–or' *alternatives of decision* offer an absolute validity. These two modes also have *negative* aspects. We find featurelessness in the one and restrictiveness in the other, each having a certain falsity of its own. In considering these aspects we discover that we cannot set the positive aspect of the one against the negative aspect of the other but keep both the positives in mutual contradiction.

What then is the psyche to do in the face of these two basic dialectical possibilities? Does it have to support the one against the other? Or is there some further possible synthesis of the synthesis and antithesis (of maintaining the whole and of choosing alternatives)?

It is fundamentally characteristic of our temporal human situation that we cannot accomplish such a synthesis. This means that in life we select and realise our destiny from among the chances and risks of historical events, while all correct resolutions disappear at the frontiers of tragedy and in the presence of other transcending possibilities.

Dialectical transformation is a universal and basic form of thought, and is in contrast with rational understanding, which it uses and surpasses. It is indispensable for the understanding of the psyche and bestows a satisfactory quality of its own on our conception of human situations, human facts and movements.[1]

3. *Application of the dialectic of opposites to psychopathological understanding*.[2] We formulate the following as a measure for psychically healthy people: There is normally a full integration of the opposites that arise in the psyche, either through a clear, decisive *choice* or through some comprehensive *synthesis*. In abnormal circumstances one of these tendencies becomes independent without the other ever asserting itself, or else integration just does not occur. Or it is just the counter-tendency that gains a special independence. Measures such as these can be applied to the analysis of meaning in the neuroses and psychoses.

(aa) In *schizophrenia* we can find examples of the *drastic realisation of one tendency without its counter-tendency*: automatic response to a command, echolalia and echopraxia, patients put out their tongue when asked, even though they know they are going to be pricked. They imitate senseless movements and repeat parrot-fashion. We also find examples of *the failure to unify*: a simultaneous positive and negative affect in relation to the same object, which Bleuler called 'ambivalence'.[3] In normal life this will lead either to direct choice or some kind of constructive synthesis. Schizophrenic patients, however, can love and hate simultaneously in an undifferentiated and unconnected way, or consider something both right and wrong so that, for instance, though they are correctly orientated, they will continue to adhere to a delusion-like orientation with the utmost conviction. We further find examples of *an independence of the counter-tendency*: negativism, where the patients oppose everything or do the direct opposite of what is asked. They go to the lavatory but use the floor. When supposed to eat they refuse, but gladly take other patients' food away from them. In classical cases the patient goes backward when asked

---

[1] The philosophy of Hegel and of his learned followers (in diluted form) expands the complexity of such 'dialectical' possibilities, going far beyond psychology though including it. Hegel's 'Phänomenologie des Geistes' is almost inexhaustible.

[2] Re the psychology of opposites, examples are given by Th. Lipps: *Vom Fühlen. Wollen u. Denken* (Leipzig, 1907), 2nd edn. For psychopathology see Bleuler, Gross, Freud, *Psychiatr. neur. Wschr.*, 1903, I; 1906, II; 1910, I. *Jb. Psychoanal.*, vol. 2, p. 3. Bleuler, *Dementia Praecox oder Gruppe der Schizophrenien* (1911), pp. 43, 158 ff., 405.

[3] E. Roenau, 'Ambivalenz u. Entgegnung von E. Bleuler', *Z. Neur.*, vol. 157 (1936), pp. 153, 166.

to go forward. One patient, when out in the garden in pouring rain, asserted that a hot sun was shining. Kraepelin interpreted certain stuporous states in this way. He observed the beginning of movements and retardation caused by these counter-drives which he distinguished from the simple inhibition of psychic events with accompanying motor manifestation. Sometimes voices tell the patient the opposite of what is intended. They call 'Bravo' for instance, signifying that the patient should not have done this or that.

(*bb*) In the neuroses, we interpret the inability to stop or finish as a failure to unify and choose; for example, the incapacity to decide. Psychotherapy in particular will show this dialectic of *tension and release*, which is found at all levels, from the biological to the psychological and intellectual, from the muscles via the will up to the person's basic philosophy. What in the physiological sphere leads naturally and rhymically to equilibrium, becomes in the psychic sphere a change from a mere event to a definite undertaking. The undertaking, it is true, is only discharged when vital events successfully carry the necessary movement, but the struggling, self-driving human effort is also a necessary part, that inner activity through which alone the individual becomes what he is. Physiologically, we find spasm and flaccidity, with health being neither. In the psyche we find rigidity and flabbiness, wilfulness and irresolution, and clear, candid purpose which is not a party to either. The polarities of tension and release, inevitable for the mastery of every kind of opposite, give rise to movements which either deviate into rigidity or flabbiness, or change over from tension through release into a temporarily successful synthesis which creates further new tensions.

4. *Fixation of psychopathological concepts as opposing absolutes.* On studying the efforts of characterology and meaningful psychology we cannot but notice the prevailing importance of opposites. Even the most modest contrast, once it has become conscious, gains a compelling force. Almost unavoidably one keeps yielding to the temptation of taking it as an essential with which the deepest energies are allied. But if we use this to help us comprehend psychic life in its entirety, we only rob the contrast of its distinctness and increase its ambiguity. Apparently it may throw light in all sorts of directions but it tends to grow commonplace and in the end, in spite of its continual applicability, it comes to denote nothing more than some generalised opposition.

A number of diverse opposites that have been generalised in this way offer us an analogy: for instance, the contrast between object-cathexis and narcissism (Freud), extraversion and intraversion (Jung), objectivity and subjectivity (Künkel).

Basically, in generalising a contrast, we do one of two things. We either perceive *two possibilities of equal worth but polarised* (intraversion–extraversion) usually with a recognised connectedness between the two poles, or we contrast *something valued with something that devalues it* (life-bestowing and life-destroying) as in the case of sensual drives and the repressing morality of the mind (Freud) or Klages' psyche and spirit (which he sees as an adversary of the psyche). Again, a *universal, reconciling, pandaemonic point of view* stands in contrast with a *daemonic dualism of God and Devil.*

We believe we can detect the error which occurs when opposites are made absolutes. Hence it seems to us that our understanding may make use of every opposite in one way or another, if we take it in its own proper polarity and that some serviceable meaning may be given to it, however limited this may be. But we cannot map out opposites in their totality so as to understand the whole range of human existence. Understandable meaning is tied to the polarity of opposites, but the deeper we grasp this the more we are pointed on into the non-understandable, extra-conscious ground of life and the non-understandable, historical absolute of Existence itself.

### (b) The reciprocity of Life and Meaning

Dialectic is the form in which a basic aspect of meaningful connections becomes accessible to us, namely, that these connections are not a simple sequence of events but show a constant reciprocity, a repercussion on motivation, a progression of expanding or diminishing cycles of movement.

Affect is expressed in gesture and bearing. Both these have repercussion on the affect, increase it, differentiate it and let it develop. An obscure drive may come to light in action, productivity or idea. Only in this way does it gather in strength and definition and reach its realisation. The individual defends himself against inner impulses which he rejects. They thereby grow stronger. Or he ignores them and gives them little rein and they weaken.

Such reciprocal movements as these appear not only in *the psyche by itself* but also as it *develops in its own milieu.* The resistance of things evokes the human will. As man lays his impress on things, they in turn mould him. So events in their course bring quantitative increase and qualitative change.

Authentic becoming, living and acting all need to form a whole, to round themselves as they build. Mere sequences of events, mere willing and persisting in one direction only, bring limitation, rigidity and end destructively. If we wish to understand, we must be able to stay suspended and learn to leave the firm grounds of unequivocal definition. At the same time we must take our leap into the reciprocity of life. We have mistaken its meaning if we forgo any risk and insist on one and not the other, insist on having and not losing, asserting and not submitting, and will only live not die. Indeed we must always accept the opposite, risk it, let it become a thorn of distress and include it as a factor in all our movements. Anything that merely is without an opposite means fixation, loss of all otherness and soon an end to all that has already become lifelessly fixated. But when we expose ourselves to the reciprocal dialectic of movement and risk, life expands its meaning. Any intention that moves in one direction only, any fixation of reason, is only an instant—an indispensable instant—in the whole system of circling movements. From these it derives its meaning, and by these it is measured and they are also the condition for its realisation. Our ideas, everything that is comprehensive, human life, intellect and Existence itself all take this circular course and as the moving cycles are broken asunder, fresh ones form.

We may compare *meaningful human existence* with *biological existence*. Even in biological events we need to grasp this reciprocity. For example, there is the reciprocity of endocrinal–neurological relationships (H. Marx). The simple antagonism of endocrines with opposing effects is insufficient. It is the totality of the reciprocity that takes living effect. Purposeful intensification of one isolated factor introduces something that takes different effect according to the various reciprocities, as constituted in any one individual. Hence room for the unpredictable is quite extensive. Prediction depends on how far one knows the whole set of reciprocities. Another example: the functions of neuro-muscular and sensory events only become comprehensible within the total internal and external situation of the living organism (the Gestalt-kreis: v. Weizäcker). Meaningful life also fulfils itself in reciprocal movement in a comparable way but there is one difference. We are dealing with conscious and unconscious events. Unconscious events may be carriers of the complementary part of the reciprocal event or take effect as a primary source of freedom, which, though it never becomes a conscious intention or an object for empirical investigation, is itself a determining factor. The specific inner tension, the recoil back on itself again, the mutual reinforcement or release—the 'mysterious paths of the inner reversals' (Nietzsche)—are the incalculable elements within the meaningful totality of psychic movements.

They are the acts which determine our life from early childhood onwards. A small boy who had only just started to speak saw his baby brother on his mother's lap where he felt he ought to be. He was startled, hesitated, his eyes filled with tears. Suddenly he went to his mother, stroked her and said: 'I do love him too'. He remained after that a reliable and loving brother.

Biological events only provide an analogy for what is meaningful. In the field of the meaningful, we discover risk, fear of making the inescapable leap (always into the reciprocity of the whole), choice and creation. In the biological sphere on the other hand there only is the cycle of reciprocal events which, though perhaps not mechanical, is nonetheless automatic and unfree.

Cycles of meaning are *static* when they are configurations of complex expression, personality and achievement taken as a whole. The cycles which we are now discussing are *movements*. These meaningful reciprocal movements are of two opposing kinds, those that drive life upwards or those that drive it to destruction. All meaningful life, it is true, remains within their confines but it can either develop within them or use them to annihilate itself. An individual can thus try to overcome resistances by means which can also defeat him. He can fight against something in such a way that he only strengthens his opponent. He may want to gain in status but so long as he concentrates on this alone and not on the actual matters which he must deal with if his goal is to be reached, his behaviour is likely to lose him his own self-respect and that of others. His isolated wish for status will then grow and he will prod it on into new, futile and even more disastrous behaviour. For this sort of circular behaviour psychotherapists tend to use the term 'circles of bedevilment' (Teufelskreise)—Künkel. A 'vicious circle' is formed instead of one of the genuine, constructive cycles of life. The meaningful behaviour then becomes a kind of thrashing about which only forces the victim down into the quick-sand of his own devising. Thus we may pair the creative cycle with the destructive one, and liberating and expanding cycles with those that inhibit and restrict.

There are a number of cycles in which disturbances are self-aggravated. Fear adds to fear and grows out of fear until it reaches an extreme pitch. Excitement is fought and increases. An affect overflows as it is surrendered to and verbalised. Anger grows in raving; obstinacy grows more and more obstinate. Inversely, a suppressed drive will grow and man, by suppressing his sexuality, sexualises himself.

Such cycles grow into something neurotic because of *mechanisms* that *split apart* what normally remains integrated and isolate what normally has its place in the whole. In this way the unconscious becomes inaccessible to consciousness. What is repressed gains increasing independence from the repressing impulse, and the self experiences defeat by something else which is still at the same time a part of itself.

## § 4. SELF-REFLECTION

We can say: all that an individual does, knows, desires, and produces will indicate how he understands himself in the world. What we have termed the 'psychology of meaningful connections' is then an understanding of *his* under-standing. But it is a basic human characteristic that man as man understands his own understanding and gains a knowledge of himself. Self-reflection is an inseparable element in the understandable human psyche. It was therefore already implied in the connections we discussed above, which were under-standable in content and form. Self-reflection may be halted at the start: action in the world and knowledge of things may then be largely unconscious, and carried out without any self-reflection. But it is only the stirrings and possi-bility of self-reflection that make psychic activity human.

The psychology of meaningful connections must understand self-reflection, which it practices itself. As practitioners of this psychology we either achieve for another what he has not yet achieved by his own self-reflection or else we understand his self-reflection, share and expand it.

### (a) *Reflection and the unconscious*

Self-reflection has its place in the comprehensive relationship of the conscious and the unconscious. We will first consider all that is included in the term '*Reflection*'. Reflection means growing illumination, which comes about from the separation of what is related.

The *clarification* of psychic life begins with a *separation of subject and object* (Self and Object). The things we feel, experience, and strive for, grow clear to us as *ideas* or *images*. We can only expect illumination when there is an object, a form, something thinkable, in short when there is some objectivisation. Separation gives rise to further reflection: I turn back again on myself by directing reflection upon myself (self-reflection); I reflect on each content, each image and symbol to which as mere objects I have been bound in the first place without any full awareness, and I ask *what are they?* From this point awareness grows unchecked up to the final awareness of awareness itself. Lastly, *I reflect on the division into subject and object as it takes place within the whole*, that is, by a philosophical transcendence, I make myself aware of what this division means to me in terms of a manifestation of Being.

Each act of reflection throws light on something which up to then had been unconscious and obscure and with this comes *release*; release from the obscure bondage of the undifferentiated, from the given thus-ness of the self (Sosein), from the power of uncritically accepted symbols and from the absolute reality of the objective world. Each release 'from something' begs the question 're-lease for what?'. When I grasp an object, I win freedom from an obscure bondage to the undifferentiated. It is a relief that at last I know what up to then I have only felt. If I know what happens to me, I have taken the first step to freedom in contrast to being blindly overpowered. Out of the given thus-ness of the self, as I might conceive it if I turn myself into an object, I emerge freed by self-reflection for the task of becoming myself. Instead of a determined finality, I gain potentiality. Instead of bondage to symbols I gain through knowledge of them the freedom to transform them. Imprisoned as I am in the supposed absoluteness of existing objects, my awareness of existence as mere appearance enables me to transcend them into objectless Being itself, but there is no illumination except by way of the totality of objective possibilities.

Each liberation implies *risk*. Each release brought by reflection cuts *the ground from our feet*, takes away substance, earth and world, unless with every step towards freedom there remains an ever-changing bond that extends with the extending freedom. In all the objectification one must also feel the all-embracing darkness at its source, and in the course of one's own individuation accept and incorporate everything one finds oneself to be in one's given existence. So, too, in our conquest of the imprisoning symbols, our life must be borne along by the symbolic nature of the whole and in the very act of trans-cendence we must also merge ourselves deliberately into the world as it exists. The hovering flight of freedom loses touch with its ground completely unless we confine it somehow. Wings need the wind's resistance.

In psychological terms, this losing touch with the ground can be formu-lated as the *extinction of the unconscious*, upon which, after all is said and done, I live my life in all its varying stages of consciousness. The drives of life, its matter and content, come to me continually from the unconscious. I meet the unconscious constantly in everything that enables my performance, from my everyday automatic activities to my creative and original thinking and to the decisions which form the very substance of my freedom. Illumination at its highest rests on the darkness of the unconscious. All clarification implies a *something* that grows clear.

Our life is not a simple bi-polarity of intention (reason, will) and that which is unconscious. There is rather a complex *hierarchy of changing relationships* between consciousness and what is unconscious, and this pervades the whole of our psychic and intellectual existence. There is never the one without the other or else there follows psychic catastrophe, destruction or decline. The bright power of the Will which operates in the clarity of knowledge is still unconscious in its core. In so far as it is continuous realisation, it is a step forward in the never-ending illumination of man. It does not abolish the kingdom of the unconscious but rather uses its own consciousness to give such a kingdom infinite extent.

### (b) Self-reflection as a spur to the psychic dialectic

If we give the term '*mere happening*' to whatever occurs to us without our being aware of its significance, and keep the term '*experience*' for what is felt to be a significant happening, self-reflection then becomes an indispensable element in experience, since there is no awareness of significance without self-reflection.

Yet self-reflection is something essentially different from knowledge. 'To know that one knows' is not the same thing as knowledge itself. Knowledge requires an object which will continue to exist and be available. But self-reflection is that kind of knowing which makes itself the object and changes itself at the same time. It never reaches, therefore, the quiet stability of a knowledge of something which continues to be as it is, that something 'which I am' but remains with us as a continually prodding spur.

To change our metaphor, self-reflection acts like a ferment, whereby something merely given is turned into something accepted, mere happening into history, and the sequence of a life into a biography. If we are to understand self-reflection, it means we must try to grasp its nature in its structure.

### (c) The structure of self-reflection

The structure of self-reflection is hierarchical. Isolated, wholly unequivocal self-reflection does not exist.[1]

1. *Self-observation.* I notice events in myself which are my modes of perceiving, remembering, feeling, etc. I track down what is there in all the fleeting, elusive phenomena. There is a distance between myself and what I observe as an external object in myself, and this I take into account. My attitude is neutral as with any datum.

2. *Self-understanding.* I ascribe what happens in me to motives and connections and try to throw some light on this. In so far as this self-review is no more than observation, it can indicate a host of possibilities. But meaningful

[1] Cp. my *Nietzsche*, pp. 111–13, 335–8, for the attitude of the self to the self.

interpretation of myself is also endless and always relative. In the last resort I neither know what I am nor what moves me nor which motives are the decisive ones. Everything at all possible I can recognise within myself somewhere, hidden perhaps, but still a possibility. The mere wanting to know robs all self-understanding of its ground.

3. *Self-revelation.* Passive self-understanding provides the medium for actual self-revelation. This occurs through profound involvement with an activity which philosophy descries as a form of inner behaviour, the absoluteness of decision; in psychology such activity eludes definition though the crises of self-understanding with all their obscurities and inversions are accessible enough. Kierkegaard remains unsurpassed in the art of making this revelation tangible through the use of conceptual constructs in the medium of understanding.[1] The following are a few points of interest to the psychopathologist.

If we are mere spectators, revelation does not come to us. I am only revealed to myself by an inner activity which also transforms me. Apparent revelation, unembarrassed exposures of the inward self, lavish self-confessions, endless introspection and self-description, revelling in the observation of inner events, usually cover a lurking attempt at concealment with no intention to reveal the self. Revelation is not an objective event, like a scientific finding, but rather a form of inward behaviour, a grasp of the self, a self-election, a self-appropriation. Uninhibited expressions of what is supposed to be the brutal truth are only pseudo-honesty; the fixed nature of the assertion already carries falsity. The honesty of revelation is as humble as it is deep and it is simple as well as effective.

Revelation comes in being oneself. Being oneself is never the same as being an object. What I myself actually am is never anything that can be unambiguously recognised and defined as an object. The basic relationship in being an object is the causal relationship. The basic relationship in being oneself is the relationship of the self to the self, the process of absorption, inner activity and self-determination.

If we desire final knowledge in the field of self-understanding, we have made a completely wrong start. The absoluteness of existential decision manifests itself in the midst of the unlimited flow of possible interpretation. What is existentially in order is only in the balance for knowledge. It may be that whatever is done is certain for the moment but it then becomes open for further interpretation. The unifying source and the line of its direction, which emerges through the phenomena and carries them further, is unknown to us, and we cannot know it because it is precisely this directing source which mobilises and furthers all our knowledge. It manifests itself in our knowledge and not on its behalf.

[1] Cp. my *Psychologie der Weltanschauungen* (pp. 419–32) 3rd edn.—where I refer to passages in Kierkegaard's works.

*(d) Examples of the effect of self-reflection*[1]

From the philosophical point of view self-reflection takes a variety of paths and has many contents; we will not follow these up here but merely give a few illustrative examples of interest to psychopathology:

1. *The connection between intended and unintended events.* One of the major polarities in the psyche is that of intentional act and unintentional becoming, intention (activity) and occurrence (passivity). Intention is the purposefulness that springs from reflection. But the whole wealth and variety of psychic life and content depend on dispositions (Anlagen) that lie outside intention (talent, drive, affectivity, impressionability, etc.). Intention can only delimit, select, mobilise or inhibit. Without intention, the psyche would grow and develop in an aimless and unconscious manner just like non-psychic life. Intention, without all that wealth of content to mobilise or restrain, can achieve nothing. It would, as it were, only tick over like an idle machine.[2]

Intention spreads its influence far beyond conscious events, though there are great differences in individuals. For instance, a person can wake up or fall asleep at a given time intentionally.

The will may intentionally influence the body in three ways: (1) by the direct influence of intention: e.g. movements to restrain the expression of pain or the simulation of a paralysis; (2) by the indirect influence of intention: e.g. we put ourselves into a sorry state so that we cry or have palpitations; (3) by the influence of intention without any conscious awareness of how this happens: e.g. through simple imagination or the affective toning of vividly evoked images and attitudes. Here the suggestive effect goes much further than that of direct intention. But it is an autosuggestive operation in itself and needs the intention to evoke and guide it.

Where the reciprocal relationship of intention and occurrence is unbroken, it is a sign of healthy psychic life. As unintentional events begin to gain in autonomy and the will to lose its influence, we begin to be interested in what causes this phenomenon, which is often thought to be a morbid one. Where intention exerts its influence but the psychic dispositions which it seeks to mobilise or restrain are only slight, we talk of an individual who is psychically impoverished. Therefore, that psychic influence on the body which we term 'hysterical' cannot justifiably be called morbid, so long as it is wholly due to intention.

We once had an opportunity to observe a village family engaged in spiritualism: One of the sons introduced the subject of spiritualism from elsewhere. The incredulous members tried it out. Soon one person, then another, found that they could 'do automatic writing'. In the end all of them, except the mother, managed to do

---

[1] Reflective phenomena are discussed in the section on Phenomenology (pp. 109 ff.), the section on expression (p. 213), and on character (pp. 370 ff.).

[2] Klages recognised and gave a good description of this psychological polarity. But we cannot follow him in identifying will with intention and purpose. At its greatest, the will is full of content and is itself an original source.

something. They now thought they were in contact with dead friends and relatives and held seances in a room reserved for this purpose. In one such seance we could observe trances in which people danced, seizures where there were broken utterances —sometimes meaningless—and automatic writing. These people thought everything was evoked by the dead. The cries of someone in a seizure were cries of spirits. The phenomena were the same as hysterical phenomena but only appeared when wanted, when people came into the room with the intention of holding a seance. They thought themselves quite healthy since they had no such hysterical phenomena in their ordinary life. Just as intentional falling asleep succeeds more or less according to the individual disposition, so the 'phenomena' in these seances were sometimes more, sometimes less, successful. However, later on several members of this family actually did fall ill with hysteria.

There are two ways in which the reciprocal relationship between intended and unintended events may be disturbed:

(1) Intention feels overpowered or powerless in the face of the unintended occurrence. The healthy person surrenders to the unintended possibilities of his inner life, as they arise. But even if this should amount to ecstasy, he only loses his own influence momentarily. *Domination by what is unintended* is experienced in the numerous morbid phenomena which are conditioned by the original constitution or by the start of a process. Unintended events—automatic instinctual forces—elude intentional control and in spite of changes in situation and intention continue on their own course uninterrupted.

(2) Intention has some influence on the unintended events but fails to steer them in accordance with the intention. Instead it *interferes disturbingly* with their spontaneously purposeful and orderly flow. For instance, it fosters insomnia instead of bringing sleep. Full concentration on a performance hampers its success. If it were unintended and automatic, it would go much better. In such a case people will suffer particularly from 'an agonising apperception of the moment'. Wherever they are, whatever they do, no sooner do they allow their conscious attention to intrude than they get confused and can do nothing that they intend; if they will only let themselves go, they are at their best.

*Drives and instincts* are not bound simultaneously to the motor reaction, like reflexes. The instinctual certainty shows itself rather in an unconscious choice of the right way to gratify the drive according to the situation. The instinctual drive is disturbed if the natural control of the mechanism fails or if no unequivocal goal is found. Conscious reflection may be responsible in either case. (The same thing may occur even more radically through inversion of the instincts themselves, through associative links or through fixation in infantile attitudes such as we have discussed above.) If conscious reflection should then want to improve things, it only increases the disturbance. Once the *mechanisms of transmission* fail, intention has to carry out what can no longer be instinctually performed: there are intentional movements of expression, forced speech, and torturous gestures and behaviour. Where the half-conscious instinctual goal is no longer unambiguous, conscious intention can establish the goal but neither instinct nor the transmitting mechanism obey.

Drives and instincts follow a complex course without any help from consciousness and in humans they are under a controlling force which can use intention to set them in motion or restrain them. Moreover, through learning and conscious practice man continually enlarges the realm of automatic events. All our co-ordinated motor activity—and later activities such as writing, riding a bicycle, etc.—is carried out consciously at first and then becomes automatic, and we only reach the peak of our potential performance through a host of automatisms. Complex thought-processes and techniques of observation become automatic in this way and provide us with tools for every occasion. What was once a lengthy performance is now shortened to a moment through the possession of a function that can be completed almost instantaneously. Everything that is instinctive, impulsive or automatic—the whole manifold of unconscious happenings—penetrates right up into the most highly conscious performance. The carrier is always something unconscious. Health consists in a continuing interplay at all levels from reflexes up to clear-cut volitional acts. The healthy person can rely on his instincts. They neither dominate him nor elude him, they are under his control and they themselves direct the impulse to control through a sweeping certainty which can never be sufficiently explained by plain intention or by simply having an idea. Hence they have mobility and plasticity; they are not mechanical and there is nothing fixed or determined about them.

2. *Awareness of personality*. Reflection produces an awareness of the self as a person. It modulates and colours this awareness and is the source of its self-deceptions.

Fully developed awareness of personality, where the individual is aware of himself as a whole, of his persisting drives, motives and values, is an intermittent awareness and in the last resort is nothing but an idea. Indeed we distinguish if from that *immediate awareness* which can be partly understood as a reaction to the environment of the moment. We have thus an *'impressional-self'*—a particular, momentary shift of personality-awareness, which falls back on the self proper through the impression made on others. Or in a quite general sense there is a *'situational-self'* which will come more or less strongly to the fore according to the individual disposition. Then, if we are thinking of the response to the environment as a response to a lasting milieu, not just a momentary response, we can contrast a *'social-self'* with the personal self proper. But in all these instances awareness of personality is always composed of two inseparable constituents: a *feeling of self-valuation* and the plain awareness of one's own particular *being*.

At all times man not only has to be but has to adopt some *attitude*. Not only does he communicate himself but he also presents himself; that is, *he plays a role* and not always the same one, since this depends on his function, position and situation. The role is not purely formal. The external attitude begets an inner one, which may be tentative and can become a reality. This playing of roles is a natural gift and so is the capacity to take up some attitude and change it, if necessary.

Psychology cannot answer the question as to *what the individual person really is*. We understand how almost all roles can be separated from the person himself. He stands outside them, they are not he, himself. But what this self then is remains inaccessible to us, a mere point outside. Or else it is—something which cannot be grasped psychologically—his innermost nature which never presents itself, the inward element which never becomes the outer and therefore empirically does not exist. In comparison with this, all awareness of personality is mere foreground.

The situation is different when a person *identifies himself* with his actuality in the world in some finalised act or attitude. Human life is then embedded in an historical record which can either be a matter for psychological observation, in which case it becomes something restricted, fixed and immobile, or it is an instance of truly being one's self, in which case there is a transcendence of everything observable and of all reflection. It is pure, unreflected self-being at the summit of infinite reflection. This does not exist for empirical knowledge, and when there is an instance of it, it becomes apparent through the language of history, not through the language of universals. We are left, therefore, with the ambiguity of all the phenomena through which the individual in the world becomes identical with his empirical reality, that is, they may either signify his decay and decline or his moment of personal fulfilment.

From the psychological point of view, we are impressed by the fact that awareness of the self is linked inextricably with *awareness of one's own body*. The human being is his body and at the same time, in reflecting upon his body, he stands outside it. The fact that he is his body leads to the objective problem of the relationship of body and psyche. The fact that through reflection he is aware of his body as his own and yet as something outside himself is an integral event of his existence. His body is a reality of which he can say: I am it and it is also my instrument. The ambiguity of the physical awareness of the self derives from this double activity of identifying the self with the body—since empirically no separation is possible—and of standing outside it as an unfamiliar object, in no way belonging to the self.

3. *Ultimate (basic) knowledge.* We use the term 'ultimate knowledge' for all the presuppositions that invest whatever else we know and give it firm foundation. Ultimate knowledge resides in ideas and images rather than in concepts. It is the awareness of reality as against mere being. Everyone develops in accordance with his ultimate knowledge. The direction he takes in the formation of his self is determined by what he himself knows.

Once there is reflection on this knowledge, it becomes *conceptualised in consciousness*. There are then two possibilities: Either it grows more certain, more logical and more reliably present at any moment, as well as more conclusive. Whereas the effective symbols were inconclusive, free but sure, the

conceptualised knowledge is fixed, firm and dogmatic. Or it becomes a possibility of thought, a potential question. Effective symbols then become its
refuge while the conceptualised knowledge loses all hold and pitches over into
emptiness.

If we want to understand an individual, it is indispensable that we *participate in this ultimate knowledge of his*, which is hard to glean, hidden as it is
behind a confusing mass of words and foreground phenomena. Understanding someone's ideas and trains of thought teaches us to see the fastnesses of his
nature which cannot be invaded, his inner sanctuaries and absolutes. It also
shows us the real danger of losing hold altogether, when the individual openly
and unreservedly asserts his absolute freedom in an historical concreteness that
has no general application.

This is the sphere in which it becomes clearly apparent how an individual
sees himself and his world. In the last resort he can never know himself but
he draws up schemata of himself that depend on what his ideas are at the
time. In the ideal case this would include all that is known of psychology and
psychopathology. Alternatively he may keep his own Being open and remain
exposed to the world of meaning in all its width and depth and possible
interpretation.

## § 5. The Basic Laws of Psychological Understanding and of Meaningfulness

As long as our understanding is limited by the framework of the natural
sciences, we find we are involved in contradictions, uncertainties and irritating
irrelevancies. This inclines us to push the whole procedure aside as unscientific. But the understanding of meaning demands other methods than
those of the natural sciences. What is meaningful has quite different modes of
Being from the objects of those sciences. The methods of understanding are
governed by certain general basic principles which need explicit formulation
if we are to know what goes on in understanding, what cannot be expected
from it and where the peculiar satisfaction of knowledge can lie in this field.

Where we follow the method of understanding, what is meaningful
possesses *properties* and certain *basic principles* will apply to them. (*a*) What is
meaningful only has empirical reality in so far as it appears in perceivable
facts. It is related to this that all *empirical* understanding is an *interpretation*.
(*b*) What is meaningful in the particular instance is part of a connected whole.
This whole, the character or personality, determines its meaning and lends it
colour. A related principle is that all understanding takes place within 'the
hermeneutic round'—that is, we may only understand the particular from the
whole but the whole may only be understood via the particular. (*c*) Everything that is meaningful moves in opposites, and it is related to this that,
methodologically, *opposites are equally meaningful*. (*d*) What is meaningful is
bound, as a reality, to extra-conscious mechanisms and rooted in freedom. It

is related to this that all understanding remains *inconclusive*. Although it goes beyond every level so far reached, it comes up finally against the two marginal limits of Nature and Existence itself. Meaning is self-generating and there is an infinite recession of what can be understood. Therefore the understanding related to it is equally inconclusive. (*e*) The particular, whether an objective fact, an expression, intended content or act or indeed any single psychic phenomenon, loses meaning when isolated but gains meaning in context. It is related to this that all phenomena are open to *unlimited interpretation and reinterpretation*, just at the point where understanding stops. (*f*) What is meaningful can reveal itself through phenomena or hide itself in them. It is related to this that the process of understanding is either *illumination* or *exposure*.

### (*a*) *Empirical understanding is an interpretation*

'The understood' attains empirical reality only so far as it is manifested in objective, meaningful phenomena of expression, action and creation. The criteria of reality for all meaningful connections lies in these demonstrable phenomena and in those experiences which can be phenomenologically observed. Meaningful connections, it is true, are self-evident. Our psychological imagination—a most desirable precondition in psychopathology—continually designs for us what seem to be convincing patterns as such, yet in the face of psychological reality these are no more than hypotheses that need to be tested. The *scientific* practice of the psychology of meaning is marked by its careful, critical approach, which keeps distinct what is understood empirically from what is understood as a self-evident possibility. Every step in understanding is then linked to objective phenomena, but it is recognised that all understanding nevertheless remains interpretation, however much the certainty of understanding increases with the extent to which phenomena are concordantly interpreted. Another possible way of understanding is always at hand.

The statement—inner and outer are the same (what never becomes external, does not exist internally either)—is valid only for the aspects of the psyche that can be known empirically. Those marginal facts, which existentially might become real as pure inwardness, elude understanding. The inner without the outer manifestation is not a fact that we can demonstrate empirically. But empirical existence is not an absolute. The understandable is an interpreted connection between meaningful facts and as an empirical fact it is only in the foreground of human selfhood.

### (*b*) *Understanding follows 'the hermeneutic round'*

We understand the content of a particular thought or the flinching of the body in fear of a blow. But such isolated understanding is meagre and unspecific. Moreover, the whole nature of an individual pervades even the most isolated outpost of his being, giving it objective context and the complexity of psychic motivation. Understanding therefore will push on from the isolated particular to the whole and it is only in the light of the whole that the isolated particular reveals its wealth of concrete implications. What is meaningful cannot in fact be isolated: There is no end, therefore, to the collection of our objective facts which provide the starting-point for all understanding. Any one particular starting-point may gain an entirely new meaning through the addition of fresh meaningful facts. We achieve understanding within a *circular movement from particular facts to the whole* that includes them and *back again from the whole* thus reached to the particular significant facts. The circle continually expands itself and tests and changes itself meaningfully in all its parts. A final 'terra firma' is never reached. There is only the whole as it is attained at any time, which bears itself along in the mutual opposition of its parts.

## (c) Opposites are equally meaningful

We can perhaps understand how a person who is feeling weak and wretched must feel spiteful, hateful, perhaps envious and revengeful, towards people who are better endowed, happy and strong, since psychic poverty is linked with bitterness. But the opposite is just as understandable. The person who feels weak and wretched can be frank about himself, can be unassuming and love what he himself is not, and in the uprush of this love create what he can within his limited possibilities and thus purge his soul in the school of need and pain. We understand how weakness of will may be obstinacy and how the rake may also be a bigot, but the opposite is equally understandable. Therefore when only single elements of such understandable connections appear, we cannot jump to the reality of the rest. We should always look out for possible ambiguities.

The most radical mistakes spring from conclusions drawn as to the reality of what has been understood, whenever these conclusions have been based on the self-evidence of some one-sided understanding. The exclusion of the opposite, without any attempt to follow it up and understand it, means that we manipulate reality in favour of an 'a priori' understanding that makes an arbitrary selection of the facts, since understanding is achieved but not within any empirical whole. It follows that we shall soon find it possible to understand the exact opposite. These arbitrary reversals of understanding, this sophistry of psychological understanding, is rooted in some confusion over the equal meaningfulness of opposites and thus the necessity arises, if we are to understand the real person, of linking our understanding exactly with the totality of the meaningful objective facts.

## (d) Understanding is inconclusive

*That which is meaningful* is itself inconclusive because it borders on the ununderstandable, on what is given, on human existence and on the freedom of Existence itself. *Understanding* must be related to the nature of the meaningful and therefore must itself be inconclusive. (Furthermore it always remains an interpretation, since even with the fullest possible number of objective meanings, empirical finality is never reached.)

That which is meaningful is *rooted in extra-conscious mechanisms and dispositions*, for instance, in instinctual drives. It has to start, therefore, from something which is not understandable. But the starting-point is a flexible one. With the self-development of what is meaningful, there is an accompanying change in the starting position, so that even when understanding borders on the meaningless, this is not final because once meaning is understood it moves within its own precincts and changes them as it expands them.

Understanding *founds itself on existential freedom*, though freedom cannot be grasped in itself, only in its meaningful effects. Understanding, therefore, in its turn is inconclusive, related as it must be to the inconclusiveness of everything that can be understood in time. Where the freedom of Existence itself is accomplished in time as something historically concrete, the accomplishment cannot be made objective. Hence we cannot get to know it as a fact but it is itself infinite, because as an existential conclusion it is eternity in time. It is no longer any object for psychological understanding.

If understanding is inconclusive, then our predictions of what someone will do or how he will behave are equally so. Yet in fact we make such predictions with considerable certainty. This certainty, however, does not mean that it is necessarily derived from understanding. What has already happened repeatedly is expected to happen again in the future, either it results from the frequency of experience or it is rooted in the existential certainty of communication, the reliance we place on our companions in fate. Such complete certainty is not knowledge. Perhaps it is greater than the certainty that any knowledge can give but it is of a radically different character. It lies beyond all calculation and is not subject to any objective laws nor is it lifeless matter of which knowledge can dispose.

*(e) Unlimited interpretation*

Myths, dream contents or psychotic contents are all subject to unlimited interpretation. As soon as we believe we can make some definite interpretation, another presents itself. Antiquity was well aware of this endless quality of all symbolic interpretation, and in mythology it has been a principal matter for discussion since the seventeenth century when Bayle emphasised it as a basic fact. It was also noticeable later in the dream-interpretation and psychoanalyses of modern times. This is not by chance nor are we mistaken about it. It lies in the very essence of meaningfulness. The understanding and what is understandable are in constant motion. Even in the self-interpretation of one's own life, though superficially the facts may not seem to change, their meaning changes for us or moves on to other levels and from this viewpoint our earlier understanding may be preserved as something with a preliminary, partial and foreground quality. The same applies to the understanding of myths, dreams and delusional contents. Understanding, therefore, in defining the knowledge it is aiming at, must not adopt the orientation of the natural sciences nor use their criteria nor must it take over the formal logic of mathematics. The truth which understanding seeks has other criteria, such as vividness, connectedness, depth and complexity. Understanding stays inside the sphere of possibility. It offers itself in a tentative way and remains mere proposition within the cool atmosphere of knowledge that comes from understanding. It does, however, structure the objective meaningful facts, so far as they can be defined as facts, when meaning lies open to unlimited possibilities of interpretation. On the other hand, as empirically accessible material grows, understanding becomes more decisive. Multiplicity does not necessarily imply haphazard uncertainty but can mean a flexible movement within the range of possibility that leads to an increasing certainty of vision.

## (f) To understand is to illuminate and expose

In practice the psychology of meaningful connections develops a remarkable double function. It may often appear malicious in its exposure of deceptions and beneficial in its affirmations when it throws light on essentials. Both activities belong to it. The malicious aspect often seems to predominate in actual fact. In a mood of scepticism or dislike we think we are always 'seeing through it'. The intended truth of this understanding is the penetration of general dishonesty. There is a mischievous psychology of opposites in which opposites are used simply to turn all that an individual does, says or wants into the opposite of what seems to be his real meaning. Symbolic interpretation is brought into use in order to find the meaning of every drive in some unconscious baseness that has been repressed. The psychology of 'being in the world' narrows the individual down and confines him to his particular environment and, according to this psychology, he knows no escape from it. The psychology of instinct exposes all higher impulses as manifestations of more elementary phenomena hidden within them. The individual who would understand himself gets into a desperate situation within himself—'a self reflected in a hundred mirrors'—and in the end seems to find nothing that is the self. In contrast to this, understanding which illuminates and does not expose involves an attitude which is basically positive. It approaches human nature sympathetically. It tries to visualise, it deepens its observations and watches the living substance grow before its eyes. The psychology which exposes acts reductively and finds 'this is nothing but . . .' The psychology which illuminates makes us positively conscious of that which is. The psychology which exposes is an unavoidable purgatory in which man has to test and try himself, refine and transform himself. The psychology which illuminates is a mirror in which positive self-awareness and sympathetic observation of the 'other' become a possibility.

## Excursus into psychoanalysis

Freud's psychoanalysis is, in the first place, a confusing mixture of psychological theories (see p. 537). In the second place it is a philosophical movement or a creed which has become a vital part of certain people's lives (see p. 773). In the third place it is a psychology of meaningful connections and, as such, we will give it a brief characterisation as follows:

1. *As a cultural, historical phenomenon,* psychoanalysis is a *popular* psychology. What Kierkegaard and Nietzsche had achieved at the highest cultural level was again achieved at a lower level and crudely reversed to correspond with the lowest level of the common man and metropolitan civilisation. Compared with the valid study of psychology it appears as a mass-phenomenon and lends itself, correspondingly, to a massive literature. Practically all the basic ideas and observations stem from Freud himself, and his successors, though they form the bulk of the movement, have hardly added a thing.

It is not correct to say that Freud had 'for the first time and without question introduced the meaningfulness of psychic deviations into medicine ... as compared with a psychology and psychiatry which had become devoid of psychology . . .' In the first place meaningful understanding of this sort was already in existence, though by 1900 it had retreated into the background. In the second place, psychoanalysis made use of it in a misleading way and this blocked the direct influence on psychopathology of great people such as Kierkegaard and Nietzsche. Psychoanalysis therefore is partly responsible for the general lowering of the cultural level in psychopathology as a whole.

It can be said that psychoanalysis appeared with shattering truthfulness in a hypocritical age. This is only partly correct and again only at a lower cultural level. It unmasked a bourgeois world which lived without faith within the conventions of a society that had definitely relinquished religion and morality 'with "sexus" as its secret god'. But the exposure was no less false than that which it unmasked. Both were bound to sexuality as their supposed absolute.

2. With regard to psychopathology, psychoanalysis has the merit of having intensified *the observation of meaningful connections.* The attention that was paid to small and minute signs and to phenomena which hitherto had been unnoticed or thought unimportant, taught our consciousness to apprehend countless expressive phenomena. Such apprehension expressed itself as interpretation. Gestures, actions, mistakes, modes of speech, forgetting, as well as neurotic symptoms, dream-contents and delusions, all came to mean something other than what they appeared to do at first or what was at first intended. Almost everything became a symbol for something else—according to Freud's teaching a symbol for sexuality.

Here are some examples from Kielholz[1] to illustrate this symbolic understanding of behaviour: a single woman of advanced years stole from the village councillor a young bull and a pair of uniform trousers—symbols for her sexual desires. A soldier steals from his room-mate at night a purse with keys which he kept in his trouser-

[1] Kielholz: 'Symbolische Diebstähle', *Z. Neur.,* vol. 55, p. 304.

pocket. This was after he had competed unsuccessfully with him for a barmaid's favours on the previous evening—a symbol for his wish to rob his comrade of his potency.

The following self-description shows how such 'significant meanings' may be experienced in hashish intoxication: a woman proband tore up a cigarette which was offered her. This act could be interpreted as a mere wilful act but it had a deep significance for her. The cigarette embodied for her the essence of a 'role' which she had to play but resented strongly. 'The cigarette made me become the officer's wife, so I tore it up.' 'The cigarette was not a symbol for the officer's wife but the whole affair itself' (Fränkel and Joel).

Interpretation brings with it a basic feeling of 'getting behind the scenes'. One uncovers, exposes and displays, as it were, the art of cross-examination, a police-technique. Almost the whole of psychoanalytic understanding is dominated by this fundamental, negative attitude of unmasking. With C. G. Jung it grows a little less obvious and in the case of Heyer has almost vanished. With him, it was not there initially and it intruded so little he did not seem to notice it in others.

3. Psychoanalysis caused new and vigorous attention to be paid to *the inner life history* of individuals. A person becomes what he is because of his earliest experiences. Childhood, infancy, even intra-uterine life, are thought to be decisive for an individual's basic attitudes, drives and essential characteristics. Much of our understanding of what a person has become stems in fact from what has befallen him, from his experiences and disasters. So too we come to understand how he is what he is, how his body and its psychosomatic functions work, what he wants and what is important for him. But here also psychoanalysis made use of certain individually valid observations as a point from which to start its journey into the sphere of early personal histories, which were deductive only and to the uninitiated appeared quite unfounded. To some extent the method is analogous to that of archaeology, where one tries to find some connection between the prehistoric fragments and so rebuild the ancient world. With the psychoanalytic method—as Freud himself knew—there is linked a reduction in scientific requirements. 'If,' said Freud on one occasion 'we can temper the severity of the requirements of historical-psychological investigation, we may be able to clarify problems which have always seemed to merit our attention'. We are thus led into a world of hypotheses which are not only unproven but unprovable. They remain pure speculation and leave any meaningful phenomena far behind. This can be seen particularly in the contents as understood.

4. The *content* of understanding is of very great interest and actually enriches it. The individual's personal contents are thought to become meaningful in terms of what happens to mankind generally, and this is meaningful in its turn in terms of history. Psychoanalysis was wanting to master the whole human realm of original meaningful content by an interpretation of cultural history, the early history of the 'collective unconscious' in particular (Jung),

which was thought to have its effect on man from the dawn of time onwards. Here is an example taken from Freud:

In *Totem und Tabu* (1912) Freud developed a theory of history which he further elaborated towards the end of his life. The following picture emerges: Mankind lived originally in small groups, each under the power of an older male who appropriated the females and punished all younger males, including his own sons, or killed them. This patriarchal system ended in a revolt of the sons, who united against their father, overpowered him and mutually devoured him. The totemistic brother-clan thus replaced the father-clan. In order to live in peace the victorious brothers gave up their claim to the females for whose sake they had killed the father in the first place and imposed exogamy on themselves. Families were then instituted with matriarchal rights.

But ambivalent emotional attitudes on the part of the sons towards the fathers remained in force all through the later development. The father was replaced by a certain animal as totem. This was regarded as an ancestor and protector and was not to be killed. However, once a year all the men in the community gathered for a feast during which the totem animal though venerated on all other occasions was now torn to bits and communally eaten . . . this ritualistic repetition of the father-murder became the beginning of social order, custom and religion.

Following the institution of brother clan, matriarchal rights, exogamy and totemism, a development began, signifying the return of the repressed (analogous to the repressed in the individual human psyche). It is a valid assumption that the psychic precipitation from this early period has become a heritage which only needs to be evoked with every new generation and which is not in any way a new acquisition. The return of the repressed goes through a number of stages. The father once again becomes head of the family though his power is not unlimited as in the original horde. The totem animal is replaced by God. Ideas of a supreme deity appear. The only God is the return of the father of the original horde. The first effect of encounter with what had long been missed and desired was an overpowering one. There was admiration, awe and gratitude. The intoxication of devotion to God is a reaction to the return of the great father, but ancient feelings of hostility also return and are experienced as feelings of guilt. In St. Paul we can see how an understanding of this breaks through —we have slain God the Father and therefore are we wretched. The same thought was concealed in the teaching of original sin. But at the same time there came good tidings. Since one of us has sacrificed his life, our guilt is all absolved. What had to be atoned for by a sacrificial death could only have been murder—that is, the murder of the father. But in the sequel Christianity evolved from a father-religion to a son-religion. However it did not escape the fate of having in some way to put the father aside.

This account shows how Freud himself evolves a rationalistic, psychological 'myth' analogous to the formation of imaginative myths. His myth contains less empirical reality than these old myths. It is a product of the ostensible modern loss of faith and, moreover, has the disadvantage that although the content is poor enough and nothing but **rational** platitude, the empirical scientific value of its absurdity is stressed. But by evoking these ancient myths Freud breathes round his platitudes an air of lost memories, mysterious and pregnant with foreboding. Thus in an age without faith such thoughts may well have a certain charm for some. One thing only is right in all this, namely, that in prehistory and in the individual's own history inner events probably play a part which continuously eludes empirical research and which external factors alone can never satisfactorily explain.

5. The *limits* of every psychology of meaningful connections must necessarily remain the same for psychoanalysis in so far as the latter is meaningful. Understanding halts first before the reality of the *innateness of empirical characteristics*. These, it is true, are neither finally knowable nor can they be firmly established. But meaningfulness comes to a halt before them, as something impenetrable and inalterable. Individuals are not born equal but rare and ordinary in their degree through the most manifold dimensions. Secondly, understanding halts before the reality of *organic illness and psychosis*, before the elementary nature of these facts. This is the decisive reality though many of the phenomena show much particular content that in one aspect at least seems meaningful. Thirdly, understanding halts before the reality of *Existence itself*, that which the individual really is in himself. The illumination of psychoanalysis proves here to be a pseudo-illumination. Though Existence itself is not directly there for psychological understanding, its influence is felt in the limits it sets for psychological understanding at the very point where something is which only shows itself in the inconclusiveness of the meaningful. Psychoanalysis has always *shut its eyes* to these limitations and has *wanted to understand everything*.

# CHAPTER VI

# MEANINGFUL CONNECTIONS AND THEIR
# SPECIFIC MECHANISMS

*(a) The concept of the extra-conscious mechanism*

Normally we do not give a thought to those extra-conscious mechanisms which are the understructure of our psychic life and without the intact functioning of which no meaningful connection can ever be realised. We live wholly by a genetic understanding of psychic events and, since we have no direct knowledge of extra-conscious mechanisms, there is all the less reason to bring them to mind. We only come to think of changes in them when in the course of some illness meaningful connections dwindle away or appear in some abnormal fashion, e.g. as physical sequelae (perhaps the psychogenic paralysis of an arm). We then add an hypothesis of abnormal mechanisms to give some temporary explanation for the existence of such abnormal meaningful connections. It is an important function of psychopathology to try and find out all it can about meaningful connections arising on the basis of extra-conscious mechanisms and the present chapter is concerned with this. The mechanisms themselves are inaccessible to investigation. Our understanding of the meaningful connection is the only way in which the facts can be grasped at all and this can only be done indirectly.

It is fundamentally important for the comprehension of abnormal psychic life that we clarify the concept of *psychic mechanism* as an extra-conscious precondition of psychic phenomena and of their effects on bodily function. As yet there has been no successful description of these mechanisms in more exact bodily or physiological terms. They remain purely a theoretical, psychological concept to help us bring some order into the phenomena (hysterical phenomena, for example), the true existence of which has sometimes been denied both by physicians with a purely somatic orientation and even by psychiatrists, who intellectualise. Investigation of mechanisms from their point of view is impossible. We can only describe the *different ways in which meaningful connections come about in actuality*. Any detailed theoretical construct which tries to go beyond the use of extra-conscious mechanisms as a general auxiliary concept would be untestable and, so far as I know, has never been fruitful. The Freudian investigations, in so far as they are constructions of extra-conscious events—and they are that to a large extent, particularly in dream-interpretation—are wide open to criticism. But sometimes they provide us with surprising insights when they evidently describe actual meaningful connections (a number of symbolisations, repressions, etc.). Hence we will leave the *general concept* of extra-conscious mechanisms and move on to a *construction of them in detail*, in the exceptional cases where we can make convincing use of such a construction for the ordering of the phenomena (cp., for example, the concept of dissociation).

Our present subject-matter, therefore, is not meaningful contents as such but how they come to appear through the mechanisms that give them their form. We would like to recognise the abnormal mechanisms. But the presentation of extra-conscious mechanisms, as shown by the meaningful content, only brings order into phenomena, and does not provide us with any theory. The following grouping, therefore, is not in the nature of a logical deduction, and the individual paragraphs tend to overlap. Our aim is to demonstrate the large variety of the phenomena in question, rather than the narrow confines of a theory, which in the last resort can never be true.

### (b) *Meaningful content and mechanisms*

In dreams and psychosis there arise contents which can only appear through given mechanisms of this sort, but have nothing to do with the mechanism itself in so far as it is there and brought into action. On the other hand meaningful psychic content—along with physical illness, fatigue and exhaustion—can often be a factor in setting these mechanisms in motion. Psychic drives and attitudes even play a part in falling asleep and frequently turn the inner attention in a certain direction in dreams: I want to go on dreaming this or I do not want to do this but want to wake up. A person can only be hypnotised if he is willing. In all psychogenic reactions (Erlebnis-reaktionen), it is the meaning of the experience which is the decisive factor in precipitating the state.

### (c) *Mechanisms that are universal and constantly in action and those that are specifically evoked by psychic experiences*

Whenever meaningful connections are taking effect, then extra-conscious mechanisms are invariably active, such as habituation, memory, after-effect, fatigue, etc. There are in addition still other mechanisms which are set in motion by meaningful psychic traumata; they can be grasped only through understanding the meaning and in themselves retain a glimmer of meaning, even though we ourselves are still vague. Nietzsche's insights into such mechanisms offer us an example:

*Instinctual drives* will simply realise themselves wherever possible, where there is no resistance. *Resistances* arise countering this realisation. 'If instincts have no outward discharge, they will turn inwards . . . our whole inner world, originally confined between two membranes, has gained extension and grown, acquired depth, width and height, pari passu with the fact that the individual power of outward discharge has suffered inhibition.' This *inhibition* arises either from the reality situation or from active suppression. The inhibited instincts in either case take effect in a changed form, namely:

1. A search for inadequate and in any case different contents, *a disguised or symbolic gratification*. 'The majority of drives—hunger is an exception—can be gratified "with imaginary supplies".'

2. *An inadequate discharge* of existing tensions or moods. 'Even the psyche needs

certain cloaca for the discharge of its excreta, and for this purpose it makes use of people, relationships, status, its country or the world at large.' 'Malicious remarks made about us by others are often not intended for us but express anger or a mood brought on by quite different reasons.' 'The individual who is dissatisfied with himself is always ready to wreak this dissatisfaction on others' ... 'Gifted, but lazy, people always appear irritated when one of their friends has finished a good piece of work.' 'It is only envy that is stirring and they are ashamed of their own laziness.' 'In this mood they criticise the new work and their criticism turns into a revenge which deeply alienates the author.' *Confession* is a special kind of discharge. The individual 'who communicates himself' gets free of himself and the person 'who acknowledges something, can forget'.

3. A process which Nietzsche termed '*sublimation*'. There is 'strictly speaking, no selfless way of acting and no point of view is entirely disinterested. In each case there are only sublimations, in which the basic element appears volatile and only reveals itself to the sharpest observation.' Nietzsche speaks of 'people with a sublimated sexuality'. 'Some drives—the sexual drive, for instance—can be much refined through the intellect (into human love, prayers to the Virgin and the Saints, artistic enthusiasm. Plato considered the love of knowledge and philosophy to be a sublimated sexual drive). Yet with this the drives retain their old direct effect.' 'The quantity and quality of an individual's sexuality extend to the highest reaches of his mind.'

(Freud has popularised these ideas in cruder form. He took over the term 'sublimation' for the transformation of sexual drives into artistic, scientific and ethical activity, etc. He used the term 'conversion' for the appearance of physical phenomena due to psychic causes and 'transformation' for the appearance of different psychic phenomena, anxiety, for instance, in place of the sexual drive.)

We can easily understand that where real satisfaction is lacking, a substitute is looked for and mentally conceived. But if an *actual* substitute-gratification is to be experienced or an *actual* sublimation is to take place, some extra-conscious mechanism is called for. Sublimation in particular and the real relief brought by confession both have to be attributed to something completely unconscious. It is through the meaningful connection itself that such mechanisms are set in motion.

In kleptomania the theft can be literally experienced as an act of sexual gratification. Sensuous pleasure in the phenomenon accompanies many neurotic phenomena. So with the drive to self-inflicted pain the struggle with the symptom is also enjoyed and through this cycle of pseudo-gratification there comes about a destructive increase of the symptoms.

## (d) Normal and abnormal mechanisms

All meaningful psychic life comes to realisation by means of *normal* extra-conscious mechanisms. We speak of *abnormal* mechanisms when psychic experiences lead to an *exaggerated* or *entirely new* kind of transformation. Here margins are fluid. We take as our norm the ideal type: that in the meaningful personality connectedness remains intact, there is always a possibility of full illumination through self-reflection and the link with consciousness and the state of consciousness continues sensible and subject to control.

## SECTION ONE
## NORMAL MECHANISMS

(a) *Psychogenic reactions* (*Erlebnisreaktionen*)

This is not the place to remind ourselves of all the infinite world of human experiences. We would only observe the basic fact that the individual in his temporal course passes by fate and change through a number of situations and events and comes upon fundamental experiences that shake him to his roots and form his subsequent nature.

We must distinguish between violent emotional shocks such as terror, horror, rage (arising, for example, from sexual assault, earthquake, death, etc.), which are due to *sudden* catastrophe and those deep emotional changes which grow slowly out of the *fixities of fate* (the wasting of hope with increasing age, lifelong captivity, the crumbling of self-deceptions which had helped one to evade reality, restricted living through poverty and lack of opportunity, a lack of positive experiences). 'Each generation, class or individual collects cultural wounds of their own in the areas of nature and external circumstance, and every one has a different point at which he is most vulnerable, a different quarter from which he is most likely to receive his most violent shocks, for one it is his money, for another his reputation, for a third his feelings, religion, knowledge or family' (Griesinger). In the order of frequency the chief role seems to be played by: sexuality and eroticism, fears for life and health, worry over money, material existence and domestic life; then come motives related to success in one's calling and in one's human relationships; finally there is religion and politics. Where we want to analyse the meaningful connections we must apply ourselves to the particular contents of each individual case.

Traumatic experiences can bring a person into a state and afford him experiences which may well appear to him abnormal compared to his everyday life. We consider these experiences normal in the first place so long as they remain under that person's control and, in the second place, so long as they have no obscure, disturbing sequelae; thirdly, so long as they are more or less possible for anyone to have. (Man has an extraordinary capacity for extreme endurance.)

Terror by itself, without any other precondition (psychic attrition, physical weakness), is hardly likely to precipitate a psychosis. Such effects of terror in the 1914–18 war were always linked with other causes. The explosion at Oppau[1] (where 657 workers out of 6,000 were killed and 1,977 were wounded) did not cause a single acute reactive psychosis.

But acute traumatic experiences may lead to very remarkable phenomena:

1. In the most vehement emotional upsets when there is desperate fear of death a *complete loss of adequate emotional response* has sometimes been observed—a marked

[1] Kreiss, *Arch. Psychiatr.* (D), vol. 74, p. 39.

apathy appears, a rootedness to one's place, with unfeeling, quite objective observations of events as if one were merely registering them. This has been noted particularly among the survivors of earthquakes and conflagrations. They seem indifferent to everything. These states may sometimes be difficult to distinguish from a vigorous self-control in a taxing situation. Occasionally this stunning through pain has been described subsequently as a subjective calm.

Baelz[1] describes his own experience of a Japanese *earthquake*: 'There was a sudden, lightning change in me. All my better feelings were extinguished, all sympathy and possible participation in others' misfortunes, even interest in my threatened relatives and my own life disappeared, while mentally I remained quite clear and I seemed to be thinking much more easily, freely and quicker than ever. Some earlier inhibition seemed to have been suddenly removed and I felt responsible for no one, like Nietzsche's superman. I was beyond good and evil . . . I stood there and looked on at all the ghastly events around me with the same detached attention with which one follows an interesting experiment . . . then, just as suddenly as it came, the abnormal state vanished and gave way to my old self. As I came to, I found my driver tugging at my sleeve and begging me to get out of the danger from the nearby buildings.'

From the description of a South American *earthquake* (Kehrer, Bumke's *Handbach*, vol. 1, p. 337) . . . 'Nobody tried to save their relations. I was told it was always like this. The first shock paralysed all the instincts save that of self-preservation. Once real misfortune happens, many regain their senses and one sees miracles of self-sacrifice.'

2. *Experiences occurring seconds before an apparently certain death* (during a fall from a height or during drowning) are rarely reported but often discussed. Albert Heim[2] gives the following account: 'As soon as I began to fall I saw I was bound to be dashed on the rocks and waited for the impact. I dug my fingers into the snow to try and break my fall and tore my fingertips without feeling any pain. I heard my head bump on the rocky corners and then I heard the thud when I finally hit bottom . . . I only began to feel pain after an hour. It would take me ten times as many minutes to tell all that I thought and felt during the 5–10 seconds of the fall. First I saw my possible fate . . . the results for those I would leave behind . . . then I saw my past life rolling off as countless pictures on a faraway stage . . . it all looked translated, as it were—beautiful without pain or fear or anguish . . . atoning thoughts pervaded everything and sudden peace flooded me like magnificent music . . . I grew more and more enveloped in a marvellous blue sky of small clouds, rose and faintly violet . . . I floated quietly and tranquilly away among them . . . observation, thought and feeling went on side by side . . . then I heard a thud and the fall was over . . .' Heim was unconscious for half an hour after this as a result of the impact, though he himself did not notice it.

3. Here is one illustration from the descriptions of *front-line experiences* in the first World War: Ludwig Scholz[3]—'We were reduced to having to "wait and see" although we were in immediate danger. Our minds froze, grew numb, empty and dead. Every soldier knows such an experience if he has had to lie still under heavy barrage. One gets so tired, so utterly weary. Thoughts crawl, to think is such a

[1] Baelz, *Allg. Z. Psychiatr.*, vol. 58, p. 717.
[2] A. Heim, 'Über den Tod durch Absturz', *Jb. schweiz.Alpenclub*, 1891 (quoted by Birnbaum).
[3] Ludwig Scholz, *Seelenleben des Soldaten an der Front* (quoted by Gaupp).

labour, and even the smallest voluntary act becomes painful to perform. Even talking, having to reply, get one's thoughts together, jars on the nerves and it is felt as a sheer relief to doze and not have to think of anything or do anything. This numbness may indeed grow into a dreamlike state, time and space disappear, reality moves off infinitely far, and while one's consciousness obediently registers every detail like a photographic plate, feelings waste away and the individual loses all touch with himself. Is it you who sees, hears and perceives, or is it only your shadow?' This is an experience common to men 'who are condemned to inactivity and at the same time are exposed to grave and immediate danger'. Scholz goes on: 'Feeling is frozen. As the firing gets louder and never ceases, it blends with a sense of fatalistic calm. The threatened man becomes numb, cool, objective—the senses slowly grow enveloped with a merciful stupefaction, become clouded and conceal the worst from him . . . the monotony of uninterrupted droning noise narcotises him . . . the eyes slowly close and right in the middle of the deadly uproar he falls asleep.'

4. Experiences *while being severely wounded*. Scheel[1] describes his experiences as follows: 'In 1917 I sustained two shot-wounds in my jaw with damage to my tongue, two right-sided shots in the arm and a shot in the seat . . . I immediately collapsed though consciousness was preserved. At first I felt no pain . . . on the contrary I felt almost quite comfortable and well, the running blood gave me the feeling of a warm bath . . . my thinking, though preserved, was retarded. I could hear grenades exploding near me and the cries of the wounded but I had no idea of the danger of my situation . . . I understood everything said and I can still hear my battalion commander rallying those who were calling out though not so badly hurt: "grit your teeth—what are you shouting about? Here's Lieutenant Scheel—so badly hit but not a word out of him" . . . My silence was interpreted as sheer heroism, but if it had been known it was only the effect of shock which robbed me of the pain the others were suffering . . . I lost all power of movement once I was hit . . . I never felt uncomfortable nor the bump on the ground when I fell.'

5. In the period *immediately after traumatic experiences* there may be the most vivid dreams (e.g. battle-dreams of the wounded). There is a compulsion to see, hear and think the same thing over and over again. It haunts the individual's mind and he gets depressed, feels changed, cries, is tense and restless.

Grief, it seems, is often not immediate but takes time to grow. After the first period of calm, there is violent reaction. We speak of a time-lag in the affect.

6. People *differ enormously in their psychogenic reactions*. Baelz writes: 'In an earthquake, some are terrified by the slightest tremor, while others keep comparatively calm even when the quake is severe. People who have given proof of their courage in combat or elsewhere may grow deathly pale at the smallest tremor, while a sensitive woman who might be terrified by a mouse will remain relatively calm'. From these and similar remarks we can see the wide extent of what is normal.

## (b) After-effects of previous experience

Everything we experience and do leaves its trace and slowly changes our disposition. People with the same disposition at birth may eventually find themselves in entirely different grooves, simply through their life-history and experiences and the effects of their upbringing as well as of their own efforts at

---

[1] Scheel, *Münch. med. Wschr.*, vol. II (1926) (quoted by Kehrer).

self-education. Once such development has taken place there is no point of return. In this lies the personal responsibility involved in every single experience.

The course of psychic events leaves diverse after-effects: 1. *Memory-traces*: which make the recall of events possible. 2. The facilitation of psychic events through repetition (*practice*). 3. Abbreviation of the same events, so the same result is achieved with fewer conscious phenomena (*automatisation or mechanisation*). In learning to ride a bicycle most movements are first learnt consciously and one does not rely on one's instincts. But as we learn we gradually give up conscious guidance of our movements until the decisive moment is reached when we dare to trust the learned mechanism (acquired instinct). Finally automatisation has gone so far that only the expressed intention of wanting to ride the bicycle needs to be in consciousness. Everything else happens automatically while consciousness can be concerned entirely with other matters. 4. A general tendency for the same psychic experience to recur (*habit*). 5. Lastly there are *unnoticed influences* often at work in emotionally-toned experiences, and they have an effect on other psychic events, on feelings, values, actions and the general conduct of life (*effect of complexes*). Memory, practice and mechanisation have already been dealt with in our discussions on the objective psychology of performance, so here we shall only deal with habits and the effects of complexes which have a meaningful aspect for us. They are to be encountered in practically every psychological analysis.

I. *Habits* dominate our life to a degree which we only rarely admit. Traditional customs and accidentally acquired habits affect most of our actions and feelings. Habits grow on us and become needs. Even bad actions to which one has been forced soon grow bearable through the strength of habit. Habits are responsible for the constancy of our attitudes and are an effect of discipline. They become our 'second nature'. What we have grown used to—even if it is criminal—becomes entirely unremarkable to us. Spontaneity of the psyche retires in the face of it. To try and analyse or sort out the diversity of our habits would present us with an endless task.

II. *After-effects of emotionally-toned experiences*, particularly *unpleasantly-toned* ones. These normally fall into the following types: (*a*) affects, like habits, once they have run their course *can be fully roused again through association* as soon as one element of the original experience reappears. Moods may thus appear which at first seem quite groundless to the person concerned until the associative link has been recognised. (*b*) *Affects can displace themselves* in that objects which were associated with an unpleasant or pleasant experience may take over the same feeling-tone. Hence emerge the countless subjective emotional values which objects acquire for people as a consequence of chance, coincident experience. This displacement can also take place when affects are simply aroused associatively, without any fresh reason or fresh object, so that the subjective feeling-tone which the object acquires for the person may originate in something which can no longer be disentangled either by the individual concerned or his analyst. If, however, there is patient evocation of associations, in some cases it is possible to arrive at a meaningful clarification. (*c*) Unpleasant experiences are *worked out*. Either we give free rein to our affects in tears or acts, in irony, defence reactions or creative activity, utterances or confession so that they exhaust themselves in this way (*abreaction*) or free discharge is inhibited and the whole experience is therefore *worked out intellectually*. The experience is summed up as a whole, the connections are weighed up, conduct evaluated and action decided upon as seems necessary. This is an emotionally-toned, intellectual task and in so far as it is a true and genuine effort, character traits for the future become engraved and basic principles formed as a result of this impassioned yet reflective intellectual labour. (*d*) When unpleasant experiences are blocked from outlet and 'swallowed direct', denied, deliberately pushed aside and forgotten, '*repressed*' without any such intellectual elaboration, they tend to show exceptionally strong after-effects. In this case the associative re-awakening and the emotional displacement—which always occur as after-effects—tend to be even more intensive and widespread. Repression, however, can occur without any such consequences, particularly when the personality is stolid and dull.

Attempts have been made to *demonstrate the normal after-effects of emotionally-toned experiences*, particularly through the use of *association-tests*.[1] The investigator examines the effects of certain facts known to him. He compares the reactions to a series of stimuli of people who are and are not involved in these same facts. A number of differences can be detected (e.g. prolongation of reaction-time, forgetting the reaction, meaningless or absent reaction, exaggerated gesture or other accompanying phenomena on the part of those involved) and these can be explained partly as simple after-effects of the experience and partly by a tendency to conceal. However, such reactions occur not only when something has really been experienced or done but also when the proband merely imagines he is suspected to have experienced or done something like that.

The disposition, which is the residual result of the experience or type of experience and which uniformly influences the later psychic life in a way that is meaningful in terms of the original experience, is called a *complex* (Jung). All complexes have it in common that they are supposed to characterise a particular, irrational after-effect arising from some experience in the past. This leads to feelings, judgments and actions which do not have their source in objective values or in objective truth or purpose but in these personal after-effects themselves. It is always implied that if the individual concerned only had good self-observation and would exercise self-criticism he would not attribute any objective validity to the content of such after-effects. Complexes have a tendency to dominate the personality to such an extent that the individual

---

[1] A critical summary with full bibliography is given by O. Lipmann, *Die Spuren interessebetönter Erlebnisse u. ihre Symptome* (Leipzig, 1911). He also indicates the symptoms shown in other tests (e.g. experiments on evidence). Ritterhaus, *Z. Neur.*, vol. 8, p. 273. Jung, 'Diagnostische Associationsstudien', *J. Psychiatr.*, vols. 3, 4, 5—a basic study.

no longer has complexes but the complexes have him. The concept of the complex carries various shades of meaning:

1. *Projection of a single experience on to the world as perceived:* After an experience which has made one despise oneself one feels—and one's whole demeanour betrays it—highly embarrassed as if people were noticing. One instinctively believes that the change in oneself will be conspicuous to every-one else. A 'delusion-like' state develops from over-valued ideas. Goethe describes this in Gretchen's experience: 'The most casual of glances troubled me; it was no longer mine to be happy and unaware, and go about unknown, of good repute and not imagine the silent watcher in the crowd.'

2. The *disposition* which remains on as the trace left by an experience: When certain elements bring back the experience, it recalls the other elements through association and this leads to *affectively-toned reactions that are personal to the individual* (e.g. antipathy to a place or to some phrase, etc.).

3. The disposition which as a result of prolonged experience of *certain situations* leads to particular affectively-toned reactions. For example, a man becomes afraid whenever he has anything to do with the military. He accumulates hatred and resentment against superiors or preferred persons and on some trivial occasion there is an explosion of rage. One person has an antipathy towards every party-opponent or a liking for the 'outsider' as such. Another finds those types attractive which remind him of some loved person. Another has an irreversible servant/master attitude which rests on long habit and tradition, and with which, should the external circumstances change, he will have to wrestle as if with an uncontrollable inner force.

### (c) Dream-contents

The decisive step in the mastery of reality is the making of a clear distinction between dream and waking life and between the meaning of both experiences. The dream, however, remains a universal human phenomenon. It may be regarded as an indifferent pseudo-experience or as a symbolic or prophetic experience, the interpretation of which is an affair of some importance. The psychic life is so changed in dreams that it could be called abnormal were it not tied to the sleeping state and were it not so common a human experience. It is, so to speak, an abnormal event which is normal and comparisons between psychoses and dreams are an old matter.

In the first place sleep and dream can both be investigated as to what objective *somatic factors* are involved. We can thus consider the dream's richness of content and its frequency in relationship to the factor of ageing (more in the young than in the old), or to the depth of sleep (more frequent when sleep is light), etc.

Secondly, one can investigate *the psychic existence of the dream-experience phenomenologically*, the modes in which objects present themselves, the levels of dream-consciousness, the shifting contents, their infinite variability and interchangeability.

Lastly, we can try to understand the *contents of the dream-experience, what they mean.* The question *whether dreams have meaning* has been debated down the ages.

1. Dream contents can be regarded as *being of cultural interest in themselves,* in so far as they are *an experience.* It is as if deep meanings for humanity come to light in dreams. We look then for typical dream-contents—characteristic anxiety dreams, dreams in which one experiences a longing for something unattainable. The dreamer feels harshly abandoned in a desert place while all that he strives for vanishes into the infinite distance. He wanders through a labyrinth of rooms. There are dreams of flying and falling.

2. We either dismiss the infinite variety of dream as chance and impenetrable chaos or we can try to answer the question why particular contents occurred in this situation to this individual and not to others. In answering this question, we *'interpret'* the dream. We practise the psychology of meaningful connections and enquire into experiences, conscious or unconscious aims and wishes, into the personality and life-history, the situations and special experiences of the dreamer and into tendencies common to everyone. In opposition to the concept of dreams as *accidental and chaotic events,* Freud put forward the proposition of their *complete determination* and meaningfulness. Perhaps both these extremes are wrong. Some dream-contents do perhaps have a meaning other than their relationship to trivial, insignificant experiences of the previous day or two. Perhaps they can be understood in a much more fundamental way.[1]

Let us set out possible interpretations briefly in the form of question and answer:

*What does symbol-formation mean?* One dreams that one is in the street naked—the bedclothes have fallen off. One dreams one is at a drinking-party— the dreamer is actually thirsty. One dreams one is flying—obstacles, frustrated wishes, difficulties, are thus overcome. The dream images are—at least in part—objectifications of something else which appears in them symbolically and which can be interpreted as their 'meaning'.

*What is it that is symbolised?* Silberer suggests the following grouping: 1. Bodily stimuli (somatic phenomena). 2. Functional phenomena: the ease of the psychic state, how heavily it is burdened, how retarded. 3. Material

---

[1] 'Dream-interpretation' is extremely ancient (cp. the famous classic: Artemidor, trs. Fr. Krauss, *Symbolik der Träume* (Vienna, 1881), but this nearly always meant interpretation of dreams as prophetic signs, revelation of metaphysical meaning, divine commands. *Modern dream-interpretation* understands dream-content as stemming from wishes, repressions, symbol-formation, as a pictured representation of the dreamer's situation, state, and of the prognosis in relation to his own somatic and psychic happenings. Scherner (*Das Leben des Traums* (Berlin, 1861)) found symbolic portrayal of bodily events—physical stimuli such as restricted respiration, pressure sensations, etc., in great numbers. Wundt (*Physiologische Psychologie,* 5th edn., pp. 652 ff.) accepted this in principle with some individual interpretations. But Freud's work was the first to offer a fresh interpretation of great importance: *Die Traumdeutung* (Vienna, 1900), 1st edn.—containing an historical survey. H. Silberer, *Der Traum* (Stuttgart, Enke, 1919) is a short book giving an introduction to Freud's theorising. For a historical presentation see L. Binswanger, *Wandlungen in der Auffassung und Deutung des Traumes* (Berlin, 1928).

phenomena: the content of wishes, the desired goals. Freud differentiates different levels of wish, as it were: those that are the unfulfilled, inoffensive ones of every day; those which have cropped up during the day but have been dismissed and repressed; and, at the deepest level of all, unconscious wishes which are hardly ever related to daily life but stem from the world of infancy, as for example the incest-wish.

*What are the ways of symbol-formation and of moulding the dream-content?* Symbol-formation may take place directly and openly as the mere pictorial representation of a thought, something self-evident and scarcely to be doubted. But this type plays the smallest part in Freud's dream-interpretation. Far more important are the wishes dismissed by consciousness as objectionable and disguising themselves in images that are difficult to recognise on the face of it, in order to reach symbolic fulfilment in the dream. Many tendencies to symbol-formation combine within the single image (over-determination), the 'censor' transforms the symbol till it becomes unrecognisable to consciousness. Thus and in many other ways, according to Freud's point of view, does the dream-content proceed to structure itself.

Instead of discussion, an example, abstracted from Silberer and condensed, will illustrate better what is meant:

*Paula's dream.* In an Egyptian temple, altar of sacrifice. Many men present but not in ceremonial dress. Emma and I stand near the altar . . . I put an old yellowed manuscript on the altar and say to Emma . . . just watch . . . if what they say is true, sacrificial blood should appear on the paper. Emma smiles incredulously. We stand there a fairly long time . . . suddenly a red-brown spot appears on the paper in the form of a drop. Emma trembles all over. Suddenly I am in an open field and see a magnificent rainbow . . . I call the lady of the house (for whom Paula worked as companion) to show her but she will not come. Then I come to a narrow path enclosed by high walls on both sides. I become terribly frightened because the narrow path with its high walls seems endless. I scream, no one comes. Suddenly the wall gets lower on one side; I look over it and see close to it a wide river which again blocks the way. I walk on and see an uprooted rose-bush. I decide to plant it back as a memorial in case I die there and start to dig with a stone from the wall. It is pure black garden earth. I plant the bush and looking up from the work I see the wall quite low and beyond it beautiful fields and sunlight.

Silberer interprets the dream as follows: Paula, who had not had sexual intercourse for some considerable time, must have taken it up again. Without using contraceptives she was anxious about the consequences because her period was delayed. She had ideas of death as if faced by a great danger. Paula communicated her dream by letter and after a few weeks she confirmed the interpretation. Some time after the dream she had given herself to a man but at the time of the dream it was only the thought of doing so that had occupied her mind. The dream did not reflect an actual event but the intention and the fantasies linked with it. As to the details: The altar stands for the marriage altar. The apparently irrelevant emphasis on 'not in ceremonial dress' together with the other details may be seen to refer to the absence of contraceptives (which Paula called 'covers'—Ueberzieher). The unfolded manuscript stood for the vagina where blood is expected to appear. Several times people are called but do not come—the 'good lady' of the house does not come—the menstrual periods are not so 'good' as to start. The frightening passage between the walls refers to a phantasy about the lower bodily passages and to birth . . . Silberer deals in more detailed fashion with the blood and the rose-bush. The anxiously awaited bloodstain is in the first instance the menstrual blood supposed to appear in the vagina (the folded manuscript). The manuscript is yellowed, Paula is worried that she is growing old. Hence the second interpretation of the blood, defloration blood—Paula wishes she was 'virgo intacta' (a clean page) so that defloration was still possible. The rose-bush is a symbol of sexuality and fertility. Paula thinks of the possibility of becoming pregnant. She has in fact played with the idea that if she becomes pregnant she would rather die but she would like the child to live. The walls are the walls of inhibition. As she breaks these down, she makes her own grave, giving the child life. Silberer, whom I have only quoted in a fragmentary way, concludes: 'This by no means exhausts all the dream connections, which are extremely complex and it would fill a whole book to go through them every one.'

*What criteria are there for correct interpretation?* Any interpretation can be made to sound plausible if we pursue the path of associations, which leads from everything to everything else, and if we follow the line of reasonable connection, especially as in dreams platitudes are common and contradictions a matter of course and usually there are a host of over-determinations, transformations of meaning and heterogeneous identifications, of oneself with the content and so on. We can recognise the content but because of the unlimited possibilities of its interpretation, we need some special criteria for preferring one interpretation to another, or for declaring one particular interpretation as the correct one. Initially it is a question of probability—should we accept the coincidence of comprehensible contents of experience with comprehensible dream-contents as accidental or significant (for instance, in Paula's dream, the Egyptian temple allows the reminder that the man with whom she wanted to have intercourse used to call her 'sphinx'). But that does not get one very far because it is obvious that all dream material is rooted in some experience or other. Interpretation presents the problem of finding out what factor is decisive for the content and what is just accidental. In the last resort it is the subjective evidence of the dreamer that will be decisive, when he is awake and interprets the dream or has it interpreted for him. Only the dreamer can give validity to the colouring, feeling and emotional tone attaching to the dream-content, and this validity is essential if the interpretation is not to be just an unending game of logical associations. We certainly come across the most illuminating instances but usually the particular case presents endless problems and verification becomes an impossibility.

Instead of correctness (in the sense of making an empirical statement of a meaning that is already effective in fact) interpretation may have a certain truth, in that it brings the given dream-material into some relation to reality, to an actual train of thought which can now become effective in life through an act of self-understanding. Here the process of dream-interpretation is not the process of getting some empirical knowledge, but a productive activity, a form of communication between the interpreter of the dream and the dreamer himself, a communication which influences his whole outlook, something which indirectly educates him for better or worse, but capable at any stage of deviating into nothing but an entertaining game. In every case the analysand is open to the analyst's suggestions and theories, and success depends on the degree to which he accepts them.

*What is the scientific significance of dream-interpretation?* In the first place it may discover *universal mechanisms* and determine their presence or absence. But, as far as Freud's theory is concerned, I find it to be largely a construct from extra-conscious material, with no scientific interest since verification is impossible. On the other hand, much of it strikes one as particularly apt, for instance, all that refers to the psychology of association, but this soon becomes a rather boring performance, an endless process of analysing contents according to the conventional procedure. In the second place, it is thought that by dream-interpretation we can penetrate into *the depths of a particular personality*, with the idea that we can get a better history in this way than by taking note of accounts given when consciousness is clear. This may be quite true in certain rare cases but the proof of correctness can only be furnished by further data from experience. In the third place, there is the question whether we get a *broader understanding of meaning, a widening of the intellectual field* in respect of dream-interpretation and through its use. So far our understanding has been almost wholly of an elementary, primitive and platitudinous kind and to this has been added our re-discovery of folk-myths in the content. But the result in this third respect seems to me almost zero. In the fourth place, we might conceive of the biological significance of dreaming in general. Freud explains the dream as the *'guardian of sleep'*. Sleep-disturbing wishes are hushed through dreamed-of wish fulfilments. This basic idea cannot be dismissed lightly and a small proportion of our dreams may possibly be of this sort.

Taking it all in all, I think that some truth is to be found in the principles of dream-interpretation. My objection is not raised against its correctness (though it provides an endless field for fantasy and mock-performance) but rather against the importance attached to it. Once the main principles are learnt, and tested out on certain cases, there is little else to learn. The dream is a remarkable phenomenon, but after the first flush of enthusiasm to investigate it we are soon disillusioned. So far as any knowledge of psychic life is concerned, the information we gain in this way is of the slightest.

## (d) Suggestion

On the appearance in an individual of a wish, a feeling, a judgment of something, an attitude, or alternatively when he acts, we usually 'understand' the content in terms of his previous traits, his basic nature and the presenting situation. Moreover if, in spite of the fact that we know him extremely well, our understanding fails us, we look to see whether the phenomena might not constitute the 'ununderstandable' part of a morbid symptom. There are a large number of psychic events which fall into neither category. We call them the phenomena of suggestion. Their content can of course *be understood* but not in terms of the person's character nor in terms of a logical or other adequate motive. It can only be understood in terms of a specific psychic effect which other persons have exercised on the individual, or which he has exercised on himself in an almost mechanical way without the aid of his own personality or any motive that strikes us objectively as sensible or comprehensible. 'Realisation' sets in *without counter-ideas,* counter-motives or counter-evaluations. Judgments, feelings, attitudes achieve their realisation without any question or criticism, without act of will or personal decision. Under cover of the hypothesis that there are mechanisms of suggestion which are ununderstandable and cannot be further explored, the resultant phenomena unfold themselves in a series of understandable connections, in so far as the content of the psychic operation and the content of the phenomena that ensue have some correspondence with each other.

In the widest sense *involuntary imitation* belongs to the phenomena of suggestion. (This is not so with voluntary imitation which in each case can be understood in terms of the individual's motives and goals.) In a crowd the single person loses his self-control not because he himself is enthused but because the crowd infect him.[1] Thus passions spread and it is in such imitation that fashions and customs have their source. We imitate the movements, phrases and ways of others without noticing it or intending it. So far as we are not dealing with an understandable development of our personality, the forces of suggestion are at work.[2] Every kind of psychic experience can be aroused in this way, feelings, points of view, judgments. Most striking of all are the involuntary imitations of physical phenomena, appearing without any influence of the conscious will. Somebody, for instance, feels acute pain in that part of the body where someone nearby has sustained a fracture of the bone, or someone has paralysis or cramp because the sight of others so suffering has alarmed him. It is possible to speak of an imitative-reflex. It is one of the basic characteristics of human nature.

A type of suggestion is that of *judgments and values.* We exercise judgments, affirm values and take up attitudes which we have simply taken over from others without intending or knowing that we have done so. It is not our judgment, evaluation or attitude yet we feel *it is ours.* This acceptance of others' judgment as our own along with the semblance of its being our own all the same has been termed 'suggested judgment'.

All the kinds of suggestion we have discussed so far may operate unintentionally and involuntarily. There is no intentional suggestion and the victim himself does not notice it. But suggestion may also be *intended* and in that case

[1] Gustav Le Bon, *Psychologie der Massen* (German trans.) (Leipzig, 1912), 2nd edn.
[2] *Tarde (Les Lois de l'imitation)* described imitation and enlarged the concept considerably. He wanted to make it the basis of sociology, as a result of the common procedure of turning one particular mode of understanding into an absolute. Involuntary imitation is only one among many other factors that give a distinctive character to particular social circles, strata, callings, etc.

the concept of suggestion grows more circumscribed and is of more superficial application. It then signifies only the intentional influence of people on each other (which in its intensified form becomes hypnosis). Finally a suggestion may be realised *with the knowledge of the person affected.* I want something and I expect it, or I am afraid, in spite of what I know, that I cannot defend myself, or rather it is just my knowing that prompts the suggestion. But knowledge of this sort is already self-suggested; it is the knowledge of a believer, the expectation of the unavoidable.

Experiments have shown that in human beings the effects of suggestion are universally drastic. For instance, at the end of a dark passage a light-coloured bead is suspended and the task is to say when it first becomes visible as one approaches it. It is seen by two-thirds of all the probands, even when it has been removed. A professor tells his audience to turn away and pours distilled water from a well-wrapped bottle on to a wad of cotton wool, ostensibly to test how quickly a smell will spread in a room. At the same time he sets a stop-watch. Two-thirds of his audience, those in the front bench first, give the sign that they have perceived the smell. In the same way one can achieve mass-hypnosis and other forms of suggestion but in all these cases we find a minority who do not respond. They exercise natural powers of criticism, perceive nothing, experience nothing and find themselves surprised.

*Autosuggestion* has a special role and may be contrasted with suggestion from others. For one reason or other, and it may be quite understandable, an individual is struck with some idea, some expectation or conjecture and the content is immediately realised within his psychic life . . . He expects to smell something and at once he smells it. He supposes something to be so and immediately there is conviction. He expects a blow to paralyse him and at that moment his arm is paralysed. Here is a mechanism which only produces worthwhile results when a conscious will is at work. We intend to wake up at a certain time and succeed in waking up punctually. We want to banish a particular pain and in fact it disappears. We want to go to sleep, and in fact we do.

### (e) Hypnosis

With most people, provided they are willing and believe in the power of the person in authority and have confidence in him, one can in the first place suggest that they are feeling tired, are tranquil, are surrendering to the words of the suggestor, and should concentrate on these words alone. One can then induce a state varying from the mildest sleepiness to the deepest degree of hypnosis with exclusive rapport with the suggestor. Such a state provides the most suitable condition for the realisation of further suggestions. How successful this is depends on the depth of the hypnotic state. Insensibility of the skin, different postures, immobility, specific sensations, hallucinations, can all be evoked. Once the hypnotist has ordered it, the hypnotised individual cannot move, or a potato tastes to him like a luscious pear. While deeply hypnotised he carries out a theft, etc. During the deepest stages of hypnosis, the eyes are again open, the individual starts up, walks about and moves as if he were awake but all his movements and experiences are conditioned exclusively by rapport and suggestion (somnambulism). These states are subsequently covered by complete amnesia. We do not *differentiate* hypnotic states solely by their depth but according to the kinds to which individuals are prone in varying degree. Somnambulism is a kind of partial wakening, which remains tied to specific conditions. There are certain remarkable *post-hypnotic* effects (Termin-suggestion). The hypnotised individual will carry out an order days or weeks after it was given under hypnosis, he will pay a visit perhaps. At a certain time, in a way which he himself cannot understand, he will experience an urge to do something and he will give in to this unless some overwhelming inhibition, rooted in his personality, makes him resist. He will often fabricate a motive which suits him and which he will consider as the real reason for his action. Finally, physical phenomena can be suggested under hypnosis and so brought about though voluntarily this would be impossible, e.g.: determining the menses to a particular day, reduction of bleeding, blister formation on the skin (suggesting that a piece of paper is a mustard-plaster).

Hypnosis resembles *sleep* yet is something quite different. The difference lies in the *rapport*, in the 'island of wakefulness' in the otherwise sleeping psychic life.

Hypnosis is also something different from *hysteria*. The phenomena of hypnosis and hysteria are identical so far as their mechanism goes, but the difference lies in the fact that with hypnotic phenomena the mechanism is brought into action by specific conditions which are transitory while with hysterical phenomena it is maintained as a lasting peculiarity of the psychic constitution of certain individuals.

However, there is some relationship between *hysteria* and the *capacity to be hypnotised*. The latter is common to all humans but it varies in type and degree. The deepest degree of hypnosis is achieved most commonly by those who are inclined to spontaneous hysterical mechanisms and by children (whose psychic life is normally much closer to the hysterical psychic life). On the other hand some patients *cannot be hypnotised at all*, for instance, the dementia praecox group and other patients who can only be put into the lightest of artificial sleeps which one can hardly call hypnosis, e.g.: psychasthenics.

Hypnosis is a human phenomenon and presupposes self-reflection and the adoption of an attitude to the self, and hence it is not possible in very young children. There is no hypnosis of animals. What is referred to by that name refers to reflexes which are physiologically quite different and in nature essentially quite another matter from human hypnosis.[1]

There is in addition *autohypnosis*. Here it is not another person but I myself who put myself into a hypnotic state intentionally through auto-suggestion. In this state I can achieve far more wide-reaching physical and

[1] Hypnotic phenomena were closely studied in the last decade of the nineteenth century and descriptions are largely concordant. Explanations and theories are numerous and of changing nature but not of particular interest here. The most important are Bernheim, *Die Suggestion* (German), from Freud (Vienna, 1888); Forel, *Der Hypnotismus* (Stuttgart, 1902), 4th edn.; Moll. *Der Hypnotismus* (1907), 4th edn. Of the psychologists Lipps, *Suggestion u. Hypnose* (*Abbr. Bayr. Akad.*, 1897); Wundt, *Hypnotismus u. Suggestion* (Leipzig, 1892).

psychological effects than in the waking state. This control of physical events and this sort of awareness derives from very ancient practices and still survives in the Yoga techniques in India. In the Occident it has almost been forgotten. Levy was the first to use it in the field of medical therapeutics[1] but it was J. H. Schultz who elaborated every aspect methodically, tested it, made observations and gave it a physiological and psychological interpretation.[2]

Everyone can through the exercise of his own will bring suitable conditions about whereby a switchover into the hypnotic state occurs without any external suggestion. This calls for relaxation—the most comfortable position for the body, reduction of outside stimuli—a co-operative readiness and concentration (fixing on some point, monotony). According to Schultz, the switchover is a vital event that occurs without any suggestion only when concentrated relaxation is present. We are dealing with a basic vital reaction, analogous to the release of falling asleep. Autohypnosis is a 'concentrative alteration of set', commonly of course the effect of suggestion but not strictly tied to this. It is rather an automatism that requires certain conditions for its appearance.

The experiences in this state are typical. At first, feelings of heaviness, warmth, sense-phenomena, phantom limbs, heart-regulation. As the state deepens, a wealth of experience becomes possible, productive picture-worlds, automatisms such as medium-writing, etc. In rare cases performances in such a state reach a fantastic level.

It is essential that the switchover establishes itself slowly at first and not too effectively, but gradually improves with practice. Repetition brings it on more quickly and finally it can be brought on at once by an act of will. It is possible to link the switchover with partial relaxation of the muscles of the neck-shoulder region. As training progresses, the switchover takes place immediately this local relaxation occurs. 'The well-trained person, therefore, should he want to arrest an emotional state that has unexpectedly arisen, only needs to carry out the above-described sliding and lowering of the shoulder-girdle. This can be done whatever the posture and so inconspicuously that only those who know will notice the postural change.'

Thus the switchover is a technique that can be learned. It takes 6–8 weeks to acquire it in the first place. 'Usually only after 3–4 months this self-directed switch-over is so well learned that a considerable performance becomes possible.'

In India this procedure has been developed for thousands of years to a degree that to us seems almost unbelievable. Schultz has investigated this procedure under the conditions of occidental culture and looked at it purely physiologically, apart from the original contents of philosophy and faith. He secured the facts as a whole but in so doing he robbed the procedure of its philosophical weight. He separated empirical reality from metaphysical reality. Once the content was lost, there only remained a technical method. The effects of this method are limited if we measure them by those achieved

[1] Levy, *Die natürliche Willensbildung* (D) (Leipzig, 1909).
[2] J. H. Schultz, *Das autogene Training* (Leipzig, 1932).

in India where the exercises are the operation of a life-time and the individual throws his whole existence into them. In psychotherapy the procedure becomes a way of obtaining a period of recreation, refreshment and repose. It enables a certain control over bodily events which, analogous to the control of the muscles, are then, so to speak, appropriated through the vasomotor, cardiac and vegetative systems. The aim is to bring about a regulation of sleep, suspension of pain and a relaxation of the self.

## SECTION TWO
## ABNORMAL MECHANISMS

Abnormal extra-conscious mechanisms are defined not as a single type but from a number of standpoints:

1. We speak of abnormal phenomena when in their amount, degree and duration these go beyond what is usual. From this standpoint we find temporary transitions occurring everywhere between phenomena, that can be called average, and those that are pathological. Excitement becomes *overexcitement*, inhibition becomes *paralysis*.

2. Associations that have become mechanical habits turn into despotic and *binding ties*, into *fixations*. A normally mobile psychic life becomes immobile. As a result it is directed by complexes, fetichisms and inescapable images and is trapped finally in a cul-de-sac. Here too we find all sorts of transitions from the normal to the manifestly abnormal.

3. Since all psychic life is a continual synthesis of what has been separated, a holding together of what tends to fall apart, final and complete *dissociation* (splitting-off) is something abnormal. Consciousness, the momentary crest of our psychic life, is linked normally with the unconscious in a mutual reciprocity. Nowhere is the latter closed to consciousness, but it can be grasped, acquired and sustained by consciousness at every point. From consciousness itself over the borders of what is unnoticed to what is unconscious there stretches an entirely accessible expanse where everything is potentially linked with consciousness. All that happens and is experienced, even if for the moment it may become almost independent, will presently find its return-link with the personality, be accepted, defined and shaped into the context of the psychic life as it is led in its entirety. *Radical dissociation* (splitting-off) is abnormal in every case and so is its inaccessibility for consciousness, its failure to integrate into the personality and the disruption of continuity with the individual life as a whole. This dissociation (splitting-off) is to be *sharply demarcated* from those divisions of normal life that commonly reunite again into context. Dissociation (splitting-off)—like the crossing of a Rubicon—demarcates anarchy from unified experience. *Interpretation according to the category of dissociation* occurs with numerous modifications: neurotic symptoms, organ-complaints, come to be regarded as phenomena torn away from their meaningful life-source. Independence of apparatus leads, for example, to uninhibited isolation

of the sensory fields. The term dissociation (splitting-off) is given to the inability to remember experiences which remain effective none the less. A lack of relationship in psychic development, the disintegration of integrated wholes, unconnected double-meanings, double-interpretations and similar phenomena in dementia praecox have led to the use of the term dissociation-insanity (schizophrenia). Experiences of a double-self are called dissociation of the self. The continual problem is *what is it* that produces this *tearing apart* and *by what means* can *re-integration* take place and with it the restoration of meaning, definition and proportion.

Dissociation (splitting-off) itself, however, has not been clarified as a concept methodologically or systematically. It is a descriptive concept for something factually experienced as well as a theory for what happens in the particular state of dissociation and it provides the hypothesis for an occurrence which eventuates in this dissociated state. As a basic idea we encounter it everywhere in psychopathological thinking. It certainly does not describe anything uniform but in every case it touches upon modes of extra-conscious mechanism.

4. There is a mechanism that *switches over* the state of consciousness. J. H. Schultz distinguishes the switchover that takes place in hypnosis and his autohypnosis from that which takes place in suggestion. In hypnosis the switchover is usually achieved by means of suggestion but favourable circumstances and appropriate actions can also bring it about automatically. A similar switchover happens daily in the experience of falling asleep; this may partly be due to the will to sleep acting autosuggestively but it can happen without this, simply through tiredness, habit or conditions that induce sleep. Schultz differentiates the switching-over process, the state of consciousness induced by the switch-over and the phenomena and effects possible in this state. All this is really indivisible but these three aspects can be separated out for consideration.

All changes of consciousness and general alterations of a person's state can be considered as switchovers analogous to the switchover into sleep or hypnosis. In abnormal psychogenic reactions, hysterical phenomena, and psychotic states, however different they are in meaning and implication, we always find the same, sudden jolt into an entirely different psychic state which becomes the condition for new abnormal phenomena to appear. The switchover can obviously be of very different kinds, if only we had more exact knowledge and did not have to apply a somewhat crude analogy. A switchover is something specific but we can only grasp this specific element in a crude way, principally by an analogy with normal extra-conscious mechanisms.

Reviewing the various ways in which we have characterised abnormal extra-conscious mechanisms we see that we neither know nor understand any one of them. *Our formulations only represent various ways in which we try to grapple with the puzzle.* We have factual knowledge of the phenomena possible on the basis of these hypothetical mechanisms and to a limited extent we know what has set these mechanisms in motion. Where these abnormal mechanisms come from remains problematical, even if they are called into action by stimuli in which psychic excitation plays a contributory part. We attribute them to special abnormal dispositions (constitution), to cerebral processes or to other somatic morbid processes. Or we speak of psychic causes in the narrower sense, when the formation of the mechanism derives from some unwonted psychic shock, though even here we have to make the additional hypothesis of some predisposition which would not have manifested itself without that particular trauma. Or we have to suppose that anyone may be brought into the power of abnormal extra-conscious mechanisms by certain situations and experiences, which is a view favoured by some investigators on the basis of individual observations and probably without sufficient ground. In any case there are quite specific mechanisms, such as those effective in schizophrenia, which certainly cannot appear in everybody, and it is likely that there are many others also, such as those in gross hysteria.

Where some understandable experience triggers off the extra-conscious mechanism we think we have understood the transformation as much as the content but we are mistaken. The everyday occurrence of such mechanisms leads to familiarity with them but not to any understanding of them. What is understandably abnormal in extra-conscious mechanisms is not their meaninglessness, which applies to all mechanisms as such, but the extraordinary character of the mechanisms that occur. There are most unusual realisations of meaningful connections, based on abnormal mechanisms for which the meaningful element itself—due to preconditions usually unknown—has become a causal factor.

The switchover into altered consciousness occurs understandably and intentionally through suggestion and autosuggestion. The same thing happens understandably but unintentionally through psychogenic reaction (Erlebnisreaktion). It may also occur understandably in illness, poisoning, extreme fatigue, all of which enforce the switchover, whereas suggestion and experience, if they are to operate as causes, call for some kind of 'co-operation', and this remains as the one factor in the causal chain which is psychologically understandable.

## § 1. PATHOLOGICAL PSYCHOGENIC REACTIONS

The term 'reaction' has a number of different meanings. We speak of the reaction of the physical organism to the influences and conditions of the external world; of the reaction of an organ, for instance the brain, to events within the organism; of a reaction of the individual psyche to a psychotic disease process and finally of a reaction of the psyche to an experience. In the following we shall deal only with this last type of reaction.

The meaning which certain events have for the psyche, their value as experience, the psychic commotion which accompanies them, all evoke a reaction which in some measure is 'understandable'. For instance, in the reaction to prison, there are the psychological effects of knowing the significance of what has happened, and the possible consequences; then there is the whole atmosphere of the situation, the loneliness, darkness, cold walls, the hard bed, harsh treatment and the tension and uncertainty as to what will happen. Perhaps there are other factors too, such as lack of nourishment, owing to poor appetite or bad food, and exhaustion through sleeplessness. Such physical effects prepare the ground in part for the specific type of reaction that follows and contribute to the establishment of the whole clinical picture of prison psychosis. The pathological reactive state does not often occur after *one single* experience but after the summation of many effects. Psychic and physical exhaustion were often observed to be the basis in reactive war psychoses, where the onset was sometimes triggered off by a relatively trivial experience following long resistance to severe trauma.

However well we understand the experience, its shattering significance and the content of the reactive state, the *actual translation* into what is pathological remains nevertheless psychologically incomprehensible. Additional extra-conscious mechanisms have to be construed. We explain these by means of special predispositions (Anlagen) or a somatic disease process, or we suppose that psychic shock as such may cause a transient alteration in the underlying structures of our normal psychic life. Psychic distress is immediately followed by a host of bodily accompaniments and similarly it can effect an alteration in the psychic mechanisms which in their turn condition the abnormal state of consciousness and the manner in which the meaningful connections are realised (clouding of consciousness, dissociation, delusional ideas, etc.). This alteration in the extra-conscious foundations is a theoretical construct; we have to conceive of it as causally conditioned and analogous in some way with the manifest somatic sequelae of an emotional upset.

### (a) *Reaction as distinct from phase and thrust*

Pathological reactions are to be differentiated in principle as follows: 1. *Pure precipitation of psychosis*—where the content has no meaningful connection with the experience. For instance, a bereavement may precipitate a catatonic illness or a circular depression. The type of psychosis need not correspond to the experience at all. The psychic upset is only the last and possibly quite dispensable provocation upon which an illness breaks out either as a transient phase or as the thrust of some process which would finally have emerged without this provocation, and which now takes its own course following its own independent laws. From this we must differentiate 2. *Reaction proper*—where the *content* is meaningfully connected with the experience. The reaction would *never* have occurred *without* the experience and throughout its entire course remains dependent on the experience and what is connected with it. The psychosis remains linked to the central experience. Where the psychosis is simply precipitated or rises spontaneously we can observe a primary growth of the illness which can only be explained in physical terms and is unrelated to the patient's life-history and experiences. It has content as every psychic illness must have, but this is only accidental and carries none of the effective weight of previous experience. Where there are recoverable phases, we find a subsequent tendency to recognise the experience clearly as an illness and to look at it in a detached way as something completely alien. In reactive psychoses we observe either an immediate reaction to some incisive experience or some kind of explosion following a long period of unnoticed growth and meaningfully connected with the life-history and recurrent impressions of every day. When the psychosis is over the patient may be able to assess the psychosis unreservedly as an illness. However, the psychotic contents which have grown out of the life-history tend to have lasting effect on the subsequent life so that the patient, in spite of his intellectually correct attitude, is apt to stay attached to the morbid contents in his emotional and instinctual life.

The concept of pathological reaction has an aspect of *meaningfulness* (experience and content), a *causal* aspect (a change in what is extra-conscious) and a *prognostic* aspect (this change is transient). Even though the immediate translation into an abnormal state is reversible, and particularly when there is rapid recovery after the cessation of traumatic events, after-effects will persist owing to the close link between the experience and the personality, and where there is repetition and summation of the experience will lead finally to a reactive, abnormal development of personality. After every reaction, it is true, there is return to the 'status quo ante' as regards the specific psychic mechanisms and functions, the capacity to perform, etc. But the various contents may continue to exert an influence.

It is only in the obvious borderline case that *reactions proper* need to be radically differentiated from 'thrusts' (Schuben). On the one hand we have psychoses materially conditioned by psychic trauma and showing convincing meaningful connections between the psychotic content and experience (the reactive psychoses proper). On the other hand we have psychoses which are the result of processes. Here the psychotic content has no meaningful connection with the life-history though of course what content there is must be drawn from the former life but its value as experience, as part of the context of the patient's life, is not the decisive reason why it has merged into the psychotic content (genuine phases or thrusts).

(b) *The three different ways in which reactions become meaningful*

We understand the *extent of a trauma* to be adequate cause for breakdown. We understand *a meaning*, which the reactive psychosis subserves. We understand the *contents* of reactive psychosis in particular.

1. Psychic experiences as we have seen are always accompanied by bodily changes. They set in motion extra-conscious mechanisms which indeed we cannot describe in detail but which are a necessary theoretical postulate that provides the ground for abnormal reactions with a meaningful content. In

some cases, however, psychic traumata will lead to somatic or psychic disturbances which have no meaningful connection with the content of the experience. The experience is itself the 'psychic source' for an event entirely alien to it. Extreme psychic excitements give rise directly to drastic effects. How this comes about usually remains hypothetical. But generally speaking we know that affects influence the circulation, that they bring about somatic sequelae by acting via the vegetative sympathetic/parasympathetic nervous system and the endocrine glands, and that the somatic changes in their turn have an effect on the brain and the psyche. It is possible that affects bring about seizures in epileptic patients via some such chain of somatic events. Through the media of circulatory changes and rise in blood pressure, an affect may possibly bring about the bursting of blood-vessels in the brain and strokes. The following effects of psychic events are particularly worth noting:

(*aa*) Abnormal psychic states are *cured* by psychic shock. The best-known example is the way in which even heavily intoxicated persons are suddenly sobered up by some important situation which makes severe demands on them. It is surprising how the undoubted physical effect of alcohol can suddenly be annulled in these cases.

Apart from this group and belonging to the field of meaningful connections are the cases where the contents of abnormal personalities are changed by the impress of psychic experiences. Morbid jealousy in an abnormal personality ceases as soon as some serious illness absorbs the attention, or neurotic complaints fade away as soon as the individual has to exert himself strongly.

(*bb*) Severe psychic traumata (catastrophes, earthquakes, etc.) may *change the entire psycho-physical constitution*. The signs and manifestations of this sometimes lack all meaningful connection with the experience itself. There appear changes in the circulatory system, anxiety states, sleep-disturbances, reduction in performance and numerous psychic and neurasthenic phenomena which tenaciously remain over long periods.

(*cc*) Very severe psychic excitements seem to produce *effects similar to those of head-injuries*. Cases have been observed which after delirium ended fatally and others also which showed a Korsakow syndrome (Stierlin). It is still uncertain[1] to what extent we are dealing here with a disorder which can only be due to an existing arteriosclerosis and therefore must be regarded as organic and to what extent a psychic experience can bring about such organic sequelae where the blood vessels are healthy.

(*dd*) It is possible—though rare—for some *pleasant experience* to produce a *somatic illness* by upsetting the equilibrium. Psychasthenic patients for instance often tell of an increase in their discomforts after delightful experiences and in that context will speak of some 'set-back'.

2. We understand a *meaning in the reactive psychosis*: The abnormal psychic ftate as a whole serves a certain purpose for the patient and the individual seatures of the illness are all more or less adapted to this end. The patient

---

[1] See Bonhoeffer: To what extent are there psychogenic illnesses and morbid processes other than hysteria? *Arch Z. Psychiatr.*, vol. 68, p. 371. Bonhoeffer does not differentiate between meaningful connections and causal effects.

wants to be irresponsible and develops a prison-psychosis. He wants to get compensation and develops a 'compensation-neurosis'. He wants to be cared for in some institution and develops the varied complaints of the haunter of hospitals. Thus patients strive instinctively for the gratification of their wishes and these reach fulfilment in the psychosis or in the neurosis (purposive psychosis, purposive neurosis). In rare cases the illness can be laid on more or less consciously. In the first place the illness is fostered by an initial, possibly conscious simulation. Subsequently the patient finds himself confronted by it without being able to help himself. Or a psycho-neurotic affective upset arises extraneously in the first place and only becomes hysteria in due course, inasmuch as the illness serves a purpose (release from the Services, compensation, etc.).

Kohnstamm gave us the phrase 'failure in *the duty to keep well*' (Gesundheitgewissen). The healthy individual who naturally wishes to be and keep healthy will gloss over many complaints and bodily discomforts. A number of immediate phenomena are thus made to disappear because he does not pay any attention to them. Even when somatic illness impairs performance and calls for sensible treatment, healthy people will inwardly detach themselves from it.[1] It is not easy to determine anyone's limits of endurance (it is perhaps easier to decide where continuing effects may do harm, may bring about a worsening of the illness or be the cause of death). In extreme situations, where an individual is utterly exhausted, he is overcome by feelings of real powerlessness, the whole vital tone falls to indifference and the simple statement that one can do no more rings true and credible. If nevertheless the question is pressed, whether one did not want to do more, and was there not a wish to give in to the existing weakness and helplessness, there is often no possible answer. But with hysterical and hypochondriacal reactions in the form of physical illness, the absence of any sense of obligation to keep healthy is usually only too obvious.

3. We understand the slide into psychosis or into physical illness from *the contents*. It is like a *flight into illness* in order to escape from reality and relieve oneself of responsibility in particular. What needs to be endured inwardly, worked through or integrated is replaced by a physical illness for which one appears to have no responsibility, or by a wish-fulfilment in psychosis, an actuality that not only obstructs but masks the empirical reality. The flight into psychosis allows one to experience as apparently real what reality itself refuses, though usually not without ambiguity. The psychosis manifests all the individual's fears and needs as well as his hopes and wishes in a motley procession of delusion-like ideas and hallucinations.

[1] Kant (writing on the power of the mind to be master of its own morbid feelings through the exercise of sheer determination) says: 'a rational person will ask himself when he is worried whether there is any real ground for it. If he does not find any, or even if there is one and he cannot do anything about it, he will tell himself this and return to his daily routine. That is, he leaves his apprehension where he found it as if it were no concern of his and turns his attention to what he has to do.'

There are some unusual cases which are reactions in certain extreme situations created by the individual's own actions (infanticide, murder). A development changes the person's entire life and leads to delusion-like *conversion experiences in the course of an acute psychosis*. The contents are then tenaciously maintained as a basis for the individual's whole life.[1] There was a patient who was a farmer's daughter, and who up to then had seemed robust and psychologically healthy. She was pregnant by a Russian prisoner of war and killed the child immediately after birth. Another case was that of a borderline defective who committed murder through the influence of another person. Weil summarises as follows: In both cases—the infanticide and the murder—the psychoses started as a matter of fact after confinement in prison. Both wrestled in prayer and this led the child-murderess to the certainty that God wanted it like that and the murderer further than that to a false memory, that he had once offered himself to God as a sacrifice so that God would use him to show that bad deeds too came from God. Both had visions from the same sphere. The one found her 'peace of soul' and the other his 'peace of heart'. Both accepted the reality of the phenomena and their significance, that is they were tokens of redemption and grace. Through the psychosis both were absolved from remorse. She became 'God's child' and he became 'the preferred child of God'. Both were converted and had feelings of elation. Neither persons were alike in constitution, personality or character, so that their analogous psychoses of wish-fulfilment were all the more remarkable.

These cases differ from schizophrenia (the early stages of which are often marked by baseless conversion experiences) through the absence of primary symptoms, the centering of the psychosis on delusional content which was almost wholly meaningful, the purposiveness of the delusional content as a unique meaningful revolution of the individual's essential attitude and the absence of any chaotic, haphazard or non-sensical symptoms.

It is noteworthy how in such a context even feeble-minded persons may have meaningful and magnificent experiences. Weil's case described his ecstasy on Xmas morning, after his wrestle in prayer with the desperate question of his misdeeds: 'As I looked at the wall it grew clear as glass. I seemed high in the air like the sun . . . then it got rather dark like night, then red . . . I saw a frightening, great fire coming from far away, closer and closer . . . as if the world and the earth was on fire . . . I saw millions of people on the bare fields, no houses, or trees, nothing but horribly disfigured faces, most of them praying in fear, turning their eyes up and lifting their hands as if they still hoped they would be saved . . . there was some red light from the great fire and I saw the devil chasing about in it . . . then it got dark but not for long . . . then for a minute I saw the mighty world of heaven above this one . . . I can't really say how lovely and wonderful everything was . . . I saw the souls so wonderful and beautiful . . . everything suddenly went . . . and it got pitch dark . . . and the thought came back that I was in prison . . .'

It is really doubtful whether we can conceive of such cases as being healthy and not hysterical. There must be some quite specific predisposition or gift for such a transformation (if indeed these cases did not turn out in the end to be schizophrenic).

---

[1] Villinger, 'Do psychogenic, not hysterical, psychoses spring up on normal psychological ground?', *Z. Neur.*, vol. 57. Weil, 'Ein Bekehrungserlebnis als Inhalt der Haftpsychose eines oligophrenen Mörders', *Z. Neur.*, vol. 140 (1932), p. 152.

*Let us now summarise:* The psychosis has a meaning, either as a whole or in its individual details. It serves as a defence, a refuge, an escape, as a wish-fulfilment. It springs from a conflict with reality which has become intolerable. But we should not over-rate the significance of such understanding. In the first place the actual mechanism of the transformation can never be understood. In the second place, there are almost always more abnormal phenomena present than could ever be accommodated wholly within a single, meaningful context; and in the third place even where traumatic experience plays its part as a causal factor, it is hard to assess the extent of its causal significance.

*(c) Classification of reactive states*

For purposes of review, we classify reactive states as follows:

1. *According to what precipitates* the reaction. 2. According to *the particular psychic structure* of the reactive state. 3. According to the type of *psychic constitution* that determines the reactivity.

1. *According to the precipitating factors:* First we distinguish the *prison-psychoses* which have been investigated very thoroughly[1] and on which the whole teaching on the matter of reactive psychoses has been built. Next there are the *compensation-neuroses* after accidents,[2] the psychoses due to *earthquakes* and catastrophes,[3] the *reactions of homesickness*,[4] battle-psychoses,[5] the *psychoses of isolation,* whether due to linguistic barriers or deafness.[6] Vischer[7] has described reactive states which occur when there is isolation along with a few comrades as in the prisoner-of-war camps:

The situation: loss of freedom for an indefinite period. Communal life with a

---

[1] Siefert, *Über die Geistesstörungen der Strafhaft* (Halle, 1907). Wilmanns, *Über Gefängnis-psychosen* (Halle, 1908). Homburger, *Lebensschicksale geisteskranker Strafgefangener* (Berlin, 1912). Nitsche u. Wilmanns, Referat in *Z. Neur.,* Ref. u. Erg. 3 (1911). Straüssler, *Z.·Neur.,* vol. 18 (1913), p. 547. 'Über den Begnädigungswahn der lebenslänglich Verurteilten.' Rüdin, *Über die klinischen Formen der Seelenstörungen bei zu lebenslanglichem Zuchthaus Verurteilten* (München, 1910).

[2] Wetzel, 'Ein Beitrag zu den Problemen der Unfallneurose', *Arch. Sozialwiss.,* vol. 37 (1913), p. 535.

[3] Stierlin, *Über die medizinischen Folgenzustände der Katastrophe von Courrières* (Berlin, 1909). Cp. *Dtsch. med. Wschr.,* vol. 2 (1911). Zangger, 'Erfahrungen bei einer Zelluloid-Katastrophe', *Mschr. Psychiatr.,* vol. 40, p. 196. Die Wirkung der Fliegerangriffe auf die Bevölkerung in Freiburg.' Hoche, 'Beobachtungen bei Fliegerangriffen', *Med. Klin.* vol. 2 (1917). Air attack did not cause a single psychiatric admission. But there were individuals who got into a state of sleeplessness and perpetual fear which only stopped when the weather was bad and air attack impossible. There was also over-sensitivity to acoustic stimuli. Those able to leave town did so. The overwhelming majority got accustomed and some neurotics got into a state of pleasant excitement during attacks. Victims of direct explosion fell into the type of apathy described by Bälz.

[4] Author's dissertation on Heimweh u. Verbrechen, *Arch. Kriminalanthrop.,* vol. 35.

[5] Wetzel, 'Über Shockpsychosen', *Z. Neur.,* vol. 65, p. 288. Kleist, 'Schreckpsychosen', *Allg. Z. Psychiatr.,* vol. 74. Bonhoeffer, 'Zur Frage der Schreckpsychosen', *Mschr. Psychiatr.,* vol. 46 (1919), p. 143. *Handbuch der ärztlichen Erfahrungen im Weltkriege* (1914–18), pub. by O. v. Schjerning, vol. 4. Bonhoeffer, *Über die Bedeutung der Kriegserfahrungen für die allgemeine Psychopathologie.* Gaupp, *Schreckneurosen u. Neurasthenie.*

[6] Allers, 'Über psychogene Störungen in sprachfremder Umgebung', *Z. Neur.,* vol. 60.

[7] Vischer, *Die Stacheldrahtkrankheit* (Zürich. Rascher & Co., 1918). Cp. *Zur Psychologie der Übergangezeit* (Basel, 1919).

limited number of comrades, always the same, no privacy. Cropping up of violent antipathies. Increased irritability. People cannot bear the least contradiction. Craving to discuss things. Petty in one's relationships. Each interested only in himself. Foul language. No concentration. Restlessness and irregular habits. Complaints about excessive fatigue (e.g. when reading). Frequent jumping up, inability to sit still. Loss of memory. Greyness of mood. Distrust. Frequent sexual impotence. Few remain free of such a state if they have been prisoners for longer than six months. There are many subtle variations of the symptoms.

*Vischer:* recalls Dostoevski—*Memoirs from the House of the Dead.* He also recalls the experiences of a few people living isolated from the world for a long time, white people living in the Tropics (jungle-madness); ships' crews (particularly in the old sailing vessels), monastic life (*Siemer, H., Meine fünf Klosterjahre*, Hamburg, 1913), polar exploration (Nansen's description, Payer, Ross).

2. *According to the type of psychic structure of the reactive states:* A whole series of types could be characterised. Clear demarcation would only be possible if we could distinguish the different extra-conscious mechanisms and so recognise the specific hysterical or paranoid reactions, the reactions of altered consciousness, etc. At present this is impossible. We have to be satisfied with enumerating a number of types:

(*a*) All experiences, particularly the less important ones, are reacted to with feelings that are qualitatively understandable but are excessively *strong, linger on abnormally*, and *quickly create fatigue and paralysis* (psychasthenic reaction). States of *reactive depression* are very common, but reactive manias are extremely rare. Sadness tends to grow naturally, cheerfulness may exceed all bounds and become unmanageable but it is volatile and dissipates itself. Abnormality, apart from lying in the strength of the reaction, may also lie in the *intensity of the after-effects*. It is a common experience for our mood in the morning to be influenced by the dreams of the preceding night even if traces are slight and only susceptible to introspection. Some people are greatly affected by their dreams which may dominate their whole day. Similarly the duration of after-effects may be abnormally long, a melancholy feeling is slow to creep away; all the affects run a long-drawn-out and curving course.

(*b*) There may be an *explosion* in the form of fits, tantrums, rages, disjointed movements, blind acts of violence, threats and abuse. There is a working-up of the self into a state of narrowed consciousness (prison-outbreaks, frenzies, short-circuit reactions, are some of the terms used). Kretschmer calls this whole group 'primitive reactions'. They quickly rise to full height and as quickly disappear again.

(*c*) Strong affects, anger, despair, fright, bring with them a certain *clouding of consciousness*, even within the normal limits of intensity. Memory *afterwards* is incomplete. In the abnormal situation there are twilight states with disorientation, senseless acts and false perceptions, also theatrical repetitions of certain acts which are rooted in the original experience rather than in the present reality. We call such states hysterical. In the state of clouded consciousness the original experience is usually not in mind and it can be completely repressed during the brief psychosis. Afterwards it can be completely forgotten. Wetzel observed shock-psychosis in the Front Line, in cases where the patients had repressed the death of their comrades who had been mortally wounded. They showed theatrical behaviour and woke up suddenly when 'the return from theatrical gesturing to the behaviour of the disciplined soldier was extremely impressive'. Such cases contradict the view that such 'theatrical, hysterical' behaviour must always be to a great extent rooted in the total personality.—This clouding of consciousness, however, does also occur in individuals who remain aware of the original event for a long time. They even realise that they are ill and their subsequent memory is largely unimpaired.[1]

(*d*) If a dreamy state dominates the picture, and there is a kind of behaviour which strikes one as contrived and childish (puerilism), a talking past the point (e.g. how many legs has the cow—five) or, in a word, a state of 'pseudodementia' and if, in addition, one finds physical signs of hysteria (analgesia, etc.) then one is dealing with *the Ganser syndrome*.[2] If while consciousness is still clouded, with disorientation, there is theatrical repetition of the content of the precipitating experience (sexual assault, accident, etc.) and there are 'attitudes passionelles', emotional expressions and gestures, we term the state a *hysterical delirium*. *Stuporous* pictures may also be observed (stupor of fright), fantastic delusions while orientation is clear as to place and time. During the course of long imprisonment *elaborate ideas of persecution* may grow out of normal mistrust and understandable suspicion, and querulant tendencies may develop from the notion that the whole conviction was unjust. None of these states can be sharply differentiated but we find them combined with one another in the most varied ways.

(*e*) *Reactions with hallucinations and delusions.* These have been observed in the prison-psychoses and arise from the persisting influences of the unpleasant situation. Patients are anxious and tense and do not feel in control of their own thoughts. They want to get some result, see something happening, take up an attitude. They long for something unattainable. They hear suspicious noises. People have malicious views about them. They hear suspicious footsteps along the corridor and suddenly a voice says: 'Today we shall finish him off'. The voices multiply and one of them calls the patient by name. Now he see figures as well, he is in a dream-like daze, tears at his mattress in fear, attempts suicide. States such as these are fairly common. The contents are later easily elaborated into delusion-like ideas and the patient is convinced he is really being persecuted and is to be killed. Kurt Schneider[3] has reported some rare and interesting cases of *acute paranoid reactions*.

3. Finally we can classify reactive states *according to the type of psychic constitution* which determines the reaction. In wartime we can sometimes observe reactive psychotic states. They are of brief duration and occur in personalities who show nothing psychopathic either before or after the event.[4] The idea might well be held that everyone has his 'limits' at which point he falls ill. Yet even if no predisposition can be demonstrated objectively in such cases, and even if robust personalities are found who fall ill on rare occasions though their psychic health appears particularly good, we still have to retain the view that in such cases there is a specific 'Anlage', nevertheless, since many

---

[1] Sträussler, *Z. Neur.*, vol. 16 (1913), p. 441.

[2] Ganser, *Arch. Psychiatr.* (D), vol. 30 (1898), p. 633. Hey, *Das Gansersche Syndrom* (Berlin, 1904). Raecke, *Allg. Z. Psychiatr.*, vol. 58, p. 115.

[3] K. Schneider, 'Über primitiven Beziehungswahn', *Z. Neur.*, vol. 127 (1930), p. 725. Knigge, *Z. Neur.*, vol. 153 (1935), p. 622.

[4] Cp. Wetzel, 'Über Schockpsychosen', *Z. Neur.*, vol. 65, p. 288.

people can be physically wrecked, suffer from cerebral disease and utter exhaustion and still show no reactive psychotic state. In most cases, however, the preconditioning factor is clearly visible in the constitution as a whole, quite apart from the reaction. This constitutional factor is either innate and persistent (personality disorder—psychopathy) or it fluctuates (phases) or it is acquired and transient (exhaustion). So it is with the observed characteristics of increased reactivity (excitability, irascibility) and the hysterical, psychasthenic reactions. But these may all appear in certain people and at certain times that to the superficial observer seem quite unremarkable. We see the same people who at other times appear quite normal display excessive affectivity and an inability to absorb experience on the occasion of some relatively trivial provocation. The unfavourable times may be conditioned by pure endogenous phases or by psychic or physical exhaustion, head injury or long-lasting emotional stress, insomnia etc.

Organic disease processes may, like the constitution, be the basis for abnormal reactions. In *schizophrenics* we find reactive psychoses based on the advancing disease process. These differ from the thrusts of the process itself because the patient returns approximately to his former state, whereas the thrusts of the process bring about a lasting change even though the florid manifestations may subside.[1] Content in the thrust is general and derived from any past event; content in reactions is well defined and derived from single or several experiences from which the psychosis emerges as a continuum. Thrusts occur spontaneously, reactions are linked temporally with experience. Obviously there are reactive aspects in all illnesses in so far as there is still some connectedness in the psychic life, but so far as the course of the illness is concerned they are almost always inessential.[2]

In conclusion let us once more summarise the factors common to all *genuine reactions*: There is a *precipitating factor*, which stands in a close time-relationship with the reactive state and has to be one which we can accept as adequate. There is a meaningful connection between the *contents* of the experience and those of the abnormal reaction. As we are concerned with a reaction to an experience, any abnormality will lapse with the course of time. In particular, the abnormal reaction comes to an end when the primary cause for the reaction is removed (regaining one's freedom, the return of the homesick girl to her people). Reactive abnormalities are therefore a complete contrast to all morbid processes which appear spontaneously.

However, causal and meaningful connections are so interwoven and the imposition of the one on the other so complex that in the individual case we

---

[1] Bleuler first formulated the concept of *a reactive psychosis in schizophrenia* (*Schizophrenie*, 1911). On the problem of reactive states in schizophrenics, see my paper, *Z. Neur.*, vol. 14. Also Bornstein, *Z. Neur.*, vol. 36, p. 86. Van der Torren, *Z. Neur.*, vol. 39, p. 364. K. Schneider, *Z. Neur.*, vol. 50 (1919), p. 49. Schizophrenic reactions without process (schizoid reactions) affirmed by Popper, *Z. Neur.*, vol. 62, p. 194. Kahn, *Z. Neur.*, vol. 66, p. 273. Critique of the above views: Mayer-Gross, *Z. Neur.*, vol. 76, p. 584.

[2] Schilder, *Z. Neur.*, vol. 74, p. 1, shows this in certain cases of delusions of grandeur in G.P.I.

cannot draw any sharp distinction between reaction proper and phase or thrust. A lack of meaningful content can be misleading in cases of psychogenic reaction, and the wealth of such content be equally so where there are disease processes. On the one hand we may find abnormal psychic states actually caused by psychic trauma (e.g. catastrophe psychoses, primitive reactions with raving and fits), where there seem to be few meaningful connections between content and cause and, on the other hand, we find extra-conscious processes effecting changes in psychic constitution where the individual phase or thrust exhibits an abundance of meaningful connections with the person's life-history.

*(d) The curative effect of emotional trauma*

It is an interesting fact that experiences may precipitate a psychosis but can also have a favourable—although not a curative—effect on a psychosis already in existence. It has been observed, relatively frequently, that paranoid patients suffering from a schizophrenic process lose all their symptoms on being admitted to hospital (symptoms such as hallucinations, persecutory ideas, etc.).[1] It has also been reported that patients in states presenting a marked catatonic picture have been aroused by strong affect as if 'from a deep sleep' and have progressed to recovery from the acute state. Bertschinger,[2] for example, reports the following case:

A young woman who had behaved immodestly for weeks and who enjoyed showing herself in the nude, was surprised in a very indecent situation by someone in the institution whom she had known before. She blushed and was embarrassed and for the first time in weeks was able to go to bed. From then on she remained quiet and could soon be discharged.

There are many subjective reports by patients that this or that experience exerted a particularly favourable influence on them as they were recovering from acute psychoses. A striking objective improvement can also be observed; a patient, for instance, who has been stuporous for long periods, becomes accessible when relatives visit (if they do so infrequently). But after a few hours the old state has reasserted itself and the course of the illness goes on unaffected.

We may wonder to what extent the heroic treatments of a hundred years ago and the modern therapies of insulin and cardiazol shock effect the change which we call 'cure' through providing a traumatic death-experience, through a repeated reduction of the patient to extremities, and to what extent there are somatic causal factors at work in these endeavours.

[1] Riklin, 'Über Versetzungsbesserungen', *Psychiatr.-neur. Wschr.* (1905).
[2] Bertschinger, 'Heilungsvorgänge bei Schizophrenen', *Allg. Z. Psychiatr.*, vol. 68 (1911), p. 209. Cp. Oberholzer, *Z. Neur.*, vol. 22 (1914), p. 113.

## § 2. ABNORMAL AFTER-EFFECTS OF PREVIOUS EXPERIENCE

### (a) *Abnormal habits*

We will give a few striking manifestations of habit: once someone with a personality-disorder (a psychopath) gets caught up in a situation while he is in a certain mood, he finds he can no longer abandon it. For instance, an unpleasant word at the start of a meeting spoils the whole evening. A querulant attitude towards the hospital where he is cannot be laid aside. In another hospital, where conditions may be worse, he has no complaints.

Criminal acts tend to be repeated. There are some striking examples offered by women poisoners (Marquise de Brinvilliers, Margarethe Zwanziger, Gesche Margarethe Gottfried and others) who did not seem to consider their murders anything out of the ordinary. There was no particular purpose but they murdered out of pure craving for power and finally simply for pleasure. Feuerbach (*Merkwürdige Kriminalfälle*, Bd. I, p. 51) describes a case: 'Making poisons and administering them rapidly became an ordinary enough business for her, whether done in joke or in earnest. Finally it became something which she pursued with passion not for its consequences but for its own sake . . . poison appeared as her last, most faithful friend. She felt drawn to it irresistibly and could not abandon it. It became her constant companion, and when caught by the police she had poison in her handbag . . . when the arsenic found on her was shown to her after many months in prison, she appeared to tremble with joy, her eyes shone entranced as she stared at the white powder. However, she always talked of her deeds as mere "minor offences" . . . there is nothing remarkable about what we have become accustomed to.'

Abnormal movements and abnormal expression will linger on some time after acute psychotic states as a matter of habit, though there is no longer any actual cause for them to do so.

Once a strong normal or abnormal reaction has been experienced after some trauma, this produces an effect which varies in degree according to the individual. The same reaction returns with the same strength after lesser stimuli that lie in the same direction as the original experience, or it recurs after stimuli which are merely reminiscent of it and finally after all kinds of emotionally toned events, where the connection with the original experience can only be understood with difficulty or not at all. Someone who has experienced lightning at close quarters is put into a state of extreme panic by every thunderstorm. Someone who has seen a beast slaughtered may never be able to eat meat again (not for any theoretical reason but simply because of the inner resistance). Hysterics develop their first morbid symptoms after severe trauma. At this stage the contents of the symptoms are understandable in terms of the experience (paralysis of an arm, aphonia). But later the same symptoms are brought on again by other—sometimes quite trivial—experiences. They have become habitual, abnormal types of reaction. The tendency to form insurmountable habits is universal and with personality disorders this is stronger than in normal circumstances. There is every gradation from habits which could in certain circumstances be dealt with as 'bad habits' to unalterable acquired forms of reaction. In the case of sexual perversions, it is well known that these spring from chance events, particularly those of childhood, and may then continue to conduct themselves like primary instincts.[1]

A case of Gebsattel's may serve as an example of the after-effects of experience (*Gegenwartsprobleme der psychiatrisch-neurologischen Forschung*, p.60, Stuttgart, 1939). —A 40-year-old man was flung against the roof during a car accident. For a moment things went black and for a second he lost consciousness. Shortly after that he went to work in his office. Subsequently, among other symptoms, he could not go out in the dark without an anxiety attack. He could not look out of the window at night nor enter a dark room from a lit corridor. He always sat with his back to the window and entered a room backwards until he could switch on the light (cathartic hypnosis removed the symptom). It turned out that darkness recalled the moment of the accident—blackness before the eyes—along with the fear of the black door of death.

In *schizophrenic psychic life* we meet with *habits* which in an excessive form dominate the whole psychic life. These are termed *stereotypies*.

Every kind of event that can be possibly linked with the psyche—from the simplest of movements to the most complex actions, chains of thought and experiences—may be repeated perhaps thousands of times in such a monotonously regular way that anyone would be forced to compare such an individual with an automaton. Patients walk round the garden in exactly the same circle, take up one and the same place, make the same sequence of arbitrary movements, lie for weeks in bed in the same position, always have the same mask-like facial expression (stereotypes of movement and posture). They will repeat the same words and sentences, the same lines and shapes when they draw. Their thoughts move in the same circle. For instance, a patient wrote the same letter for years to the Paris Police, Petersburg, which she often handed over to the Doctor in batches without ever bothering about what happened to them afterwards. One often observes in old cases turns of phrase recurring over the years as the only verbal utterance. A patient greeted everyone with 'For, for or against, against'. He was satisfied with the answer 'For, for' and never said anything else.

## (b) The effects of complexes

These become abnormal when they get out of the individual's control split-off (dissociated) and operate from the unconscious.

1. A patient could not return to the place where he had become bankrupt without getting into a severe depressive-paranoid state and showing symptoms

---

[1] In regard to sexual perversions (homosexuality in particular) views are opposed. There are those who explain them as inborn instinctual tendencies, the content of which is determined from the start and those who regard them as accidents of the life-history, a fixation of the first experience of waking sexuality directed to inappropriate objects and so acquired. As usual with such opposite opinions, both parties can be right, depending on the case. Cp. Stier, 'Zur Aetiologie des konträren Sexualgefühls', *Mschr. Psychiatr.*, vol. 32 (1912). Also Naecke, *Z. Neur.*, vol. 15 (1913), p. 537. Some workers think that in many cases homosexuality is due to a predetermined Anlage of the sexual feelings, while the perversions (e.g. fetishism, exhibitionism) are acquired through experience and rest on sexual fixations that can be partly reversed.

of a neurasthenic complex. When facing a situation where something terrifying has once been experienced, one undergoes an access of fear; for instance, after a railway accident, there may be a fear of travelling in trains, and after an air attack, or earthquake, the same thing happens. At the slightest sign that such a situation is imminent, or indeed when there is the very smallest resemblance, anxiety will appear.

Further, in cases where the experience seems to be a source of complex-effects, usually these have understandable roots reaching beyond this one experience into the past. An experience which in itself is not so significant—and inadequate for understanding—may become the source of a neurotic state, because the ground was already prepared by previous experience. For instance, the individual with erotic problems is much more hurt by upsets in other fields than someone whose erotic life is happy and whom the same event may leave quite untouched. Lastly, the roots of abnormal psychic states and symptoms ramify into the whole past history, and if one is patient one can tease out a whole nexus of meaningful connections, the threads of which all happen to cross at this one point. Freud brought this situation to light with his concept of 'over-determination'.

2. In all the cases we have mentioned so far the complex in question can become conscious, though hitherto it has been disregarded. With the help of some self-criticism, the individual can make himself aware of it. But the complex becomes the source of certain morbid bodily and psychic symptoms, which can be traced back to an experience it is true, but while the morbid state is in being, the experience is forgotten, truly unconscious and not something that is merely disregarded: *split-off (dissociated)* complexes or repressed complexes (e.g. some prison psychoses, where the patient is no longer conscious of his crime but when an attempt is made to evoke the memory of what he has done, develops florid symptoms). In order to comprehend these phenomena we need the theoretical concept of dissociation (splitting-off) of psychic events.

### (c) Compensation

Inner defects, defects in experience, psychic losses take effect through *compensation*, a utilisation, as it were, of the total possibilities of the person concerned.

The analogy is drawn from physiology, in particular from neurophysiology, where the direct morbid phenomena are differentiated from the compensatory phenomena.[1] The living organism usually reacts to all disturbances and destructions with alterations in function which serve the continuance of life under the changed conditions. When such events take place, we speak of substitute phenomena, of self-regulation. These matters have been studied in detail in the case of neurological phenomena which have only secondary interest for psychopathology.

Ewald's experiment is most striking. Disturbances in posture and movement

[1] Anton, 'Über den Wiederersatz der Funktion bei Erkrankungen des Gehirns', *Mschr. Psychiatr.*, vol. 19, p. 1.

appear after extirpation of one labyrinth in a dog. Within a week the disturbances disappear. If the other labyrinth is then extirpated, disturbances appear once more, only more severely. After some months, everything is again all right. One then begins to ablate the leg-area in the cortex. The usual disturbances disappear after some weeks. If then the other leg-area is ablated, all the other previous symptoms reappear floridly and do not disappear. If the eyes are occluded by a bandage, the few remaining capacities for movement disappear completely. Here we see how the second labyrinth, the cortical areas for movement and posture and the visual sensations which subserve stance and movement all take over from each other until every possibility for compensation is exhausted.

Good compensation often occurs in organic cerebral diseases. For instance, after hemiplegia and aphasia. But that this is only a compensation and that the defects remain latent is proven by the immediate, severe disturbances created when big demands are made or when there are strong affects, and by the rapid fatigue and slowing down of function.

When there is restitution of disturbed function, there is either a kind of new creation, in that areas which up to then have been resting now develop the relevant function (in the lower animals there can be a morphologically recognisable regeneration), or there is compensation, in that other functions which before had been only ancillary now take over all the work.

Comparable with this are the psychic compensations that arise when whole sense areas are missing. Helen Keller in spite of her total blindness and deafness was able to acquire the culture of a modern individual by using the sense material of touch alone. Perhaps some contrast-phenomena also belong to the field of psychic compensation (colour-brightness in the visual sphere; and, in the sphere of affects, incomprehensible good spirits following deep pain, etc.).

However, when we come to 'meaningful' psychic connections we are dealing with something quite different. 'There is such a thing as a neurotic cowardice which is really deep-rooted self-defence. Where the individual should be mastering his anger, he shows lassitude and apathy. When compassion threatens to upset him, he works himself into a blasé and detached attitude. He avoids all thought-complexes that are affectively toned, he evades the matter in hand, the thing that is important, and deflects himself to what is peripheral' (Anton).

We can understand the psychological development of these connections, which indeed are self-evident, but if we conceive them as 'compensation' for some 'weakness' this can only be in a metaphorical sense. Such connections do not have much in common with the compensations we have been recounting above. It is, moreover, doubtful whether they can be said to be at all purposeful in the biological sense. There is no replacement of this or that missing function but there is an effort to bring about a subjective reduction of displeasure which biologically may even be harmful.

(d) Disintegrating and integrating tendencies

Experience has constructive as well as destructive effects. If we look at life and the psyche in a vague and general way, everything that happens may be seen as a 'dying and becoming'. Life is a constant re-emergence from dying, that is from dissolution, a physical dissolution into mere chemical-physical processes, a psychic dissolution into mere mechanical-automatic events. Psyche and mind are the constant holding-together of opposites and polarities into which at every moment they tend to fall apart. If we call these integrating tendencies, plasticity, then disintegration may be seen as an increasing rigidity. Life may thus be measured by the level of plasticity, and a process of recovery become a progress towards plasticity.

This vague, general view of life can be analysed further: from the *biological aspect* life is a constant integration of the body in its environment. From the *aspect of the mind*, life is a synthesis of all the facts of mental experience through the dialectical process of negation, preservation and integration. From the *existential aspect* it is the discovery of the ultimate origins of one's own being.

In no one case can we comprehend these events in their entirety and so control them. Everything rests on the unconscious which at the decisive moment creates something fresh whereby disintegration is overcome. Failure in this creative effort of the living whole is death itself and all its preparatory stages. Our knowledge and practice can advance only so far as those limits where we encounter the decisive act of the living event in its entirety. As an object of knowledge, we only circle round it, and in our therapeutics we only deal with it through the use of stimulus, set task and persuasive appeal. It is the act of life itself, the act of creating, the act of being oneself. We are not in control of these acts but they are the prime source of every potentiality. Our knowledge and our practice deriving from this knowledge may be capable of psychoanalysis but not of psychosynthesis. The latter always has to emerge from the unconscious element in life, in mind and in Existence itself. We can prepare the way, foster, inhibit and endanger it but we cannot achieve it through any kind of arrangement, power of persuasion or goodness of intent. There always remains the all-embracing precondition which we call the vitality of life, idea, creativity, the initiative of Existence itself. We can call it Grace, or the Gift of oneself, but none of these names say anything of what it properly is.

There is above all no finality. Dying, growing rigid, failing to appear, are but instances of Life. Life in its entirety can never be attained by humanity. Man travels along the path of ever-recurring death and renewal until his finite existence in time is extinguished in death.

Even in *severe pathological states*, as long as the person remains alive, we find *tendencies towards some restitution of a whole*. These may range from compensations for particular defects to the recreation of personality in schizophrenics. In the case of demented patients, integrated worlds come about somehow. There is always something that moves into a new context, into direction and control under new conditions, that arise perhaps from tendencies that have themselves become abnormal. Certain efforts at order oppose the distractions, the derailments, the disintegration and the tendency to split off. But all these generalisations only give broad expression to the over-all aspect, which only becomes of scientific relevance when there can be empirical demonstration in some definite context.

## § 3. ABNORMAL DREAMS

### (a) Dreams during physical illness

Sometimes the beginning of a physical illness will show itself in an individual's dreams or when he is dozing. Abnormal body-sensations and general feelings of abnormality, as yet unnoticed in the waking state, now penetrate into consciousness. In febrile illnesses there are troubling dreams with compulsion-like phenomena as if one were spinning round. Then after various haemorrhages there are vivid dreams that leave strong impressions behind.

### (b) Abnormal psychotic dreams

Epileptics, just before a seizure, often have frightening and troubling dreams. After the seizure these are pleasant and easy, and on the night of the seizure there are never any dreams.[1] Similarly with catatonic illness of brief duration. The brief periods of sleep during the thrust are usually dreamless. (On the other hand hysterics always dream during their attacks.)[2]

In acute psychoses, particularly in early schizophrenia, the mode of dreaming often alters.

Kandinsky gives the following description: 'During the sense-delirium my dreams (so far as visual images and the feeling of moving in space were concerned) were *unusually vivid*. It was *hallucinating during sleep*. In an hallucinating patient the waking and sleeping states generally are not so sharply differentiated. In the dream the images are so vivid that the patient is, as it were, awake while he sleeps, and in the waking state the hallucinations are so strange and various that we might say the patient is dreaming while he is awake. During my illness the dreams were often no less vivid than something experienced in reality. When certain dream-images came into my mind, I sometimes had to weigh things up carefully and it took me some time to recognise whether I had really experienced them or only dreamed them.'

Schreber thinks: 'The fact that someone who sleeps restlessly believes he sees dream-images that have been conjured up, so to speak, by his nerves is such an everyday occurrence, it needs no talking about. But the dream-images of the previous night and similar earlier visions went beyond anything I had ever experienced, at least when I was well, so far as their *plastic clarity and photographic truth* were concerned.' Another patient recounted that her dreams were so remarkable that she often did not know *whether it was reality or dream*. 'Last night she had the feeling of flying. The moon moved above her head as she floated, two faces appeared between a small cloud. Another time the angel Gabriel appeared, then she saw two crosses, Christ on one, herself on the other. Such dreams made her happy. On waking she

---

[1] Göttke, *Arch. Psychiatr.* (D), vol. 101 (1934).

[2] Boss, 'Psychopathologie des Traumes bei schizophrenen u. organischen Psychosen', *Z. Neur.*, vol. 162 (1938), p. 459.

was blessedly content.' Patients often take such dreams as reality. They experience persecutions, bodily influences; sometimes it seems as if the sensory base for delusional ideas may well lie in abnormal dream experiences of this kind.

Boss describes *two modes of dream experience* which are only found in schizo-phrenics. They are not easy to elicit because the patients 'themselves detect the work of the psychosis in the dreams and are guarded about them':

The '*dream-bustle*'. The dream-scenes flit past the dream-consciousness with an unpleasant and uncanny rapidity. The scenes are pale and fleeting and appear to chase along and vanish. The patients try vainly to hold on to something in the dream. Quite intentionally they will keep themselves lightly asleep from the fear of losing hold of reality entirely in these troubling dreams.

*Dream-actuality*. The content of the dream is quite trivial but the patient awakes trembling in extreme terror and screams for help. She had dreamt she was in bed in hospital and a nurse came and propped her pillow up. This schizophrenic patient was so frightened because the outside world had long grown shadowy to her and she experienced the dream-scene in all its long-forgotten actuality and warmth of feeling. 'These patients cannot bear it when in their dreams their affects try once more to establish a profounder relationship with their objects.'

### (c) *The content of abnormal dreams*

Herschmann and Schilder[1] believed they had found that melancholics frequently had happy and joyous dreams, and that generally speaking just those symptoms of melancholia which are not specially prominent in the waking state will make their appearance in dream.

Boss investigated series of dreams in schizophrenics, starting at the time when they were well and following them through their illness. He found an increase in brutality and raw crudity, 'a reduction in the dream-censorship'. The Ego lost its powers of repression. When remission occurs, the dreams change but never return to the same degree of normality as does the waking personality.

Boss writes:

'We found poorly censored dreams with little symbolisation. The obvious con-tent stands in stark contrast to the patients' own moral attitudes. In spite of this *they arouse no anxiety or very little* and so with the other affective defence-reactions of the Ego. Such dreams are *an early and important symptom* for the diagnosis of schizo-phrenia.' He says crude sexual dreams occur in hebephrenic patients, aggressive dreams in catatonic ones and homosexual dreams in paranoid patients.

The following is an example of a dream of a schizophrenic patient in the sixth year of his illness: 'I was going across a moor with my mother and Anna. Suddenly a furious anger rose in me against my mother and I deliberately pushed her into the bog, cut off her legs and pulled her skin off. I then watched how she drowned in the bog and felt a certain satisfaction. As we were about to walk on, a big man with a knife in his hand ran after us. He took Anna first and then me, got us down on the ground

[1] Herschmann and Schilder, 'Traüme der Melancholiker', *Z. Neur.*, vol. 53, p. 130.

and had sexual intercourse with us. In all this I was not at all afraid and was suddenly able to fly over a beautiful landscape.'

We may question whether there are 'prognostic dreams', any anticipation of the future in the dream, the dream-images being a symbolic representation of one's own life and illness. Boss describes as 'endoscopic dreams' the representation in the patient's Ego of the past, present and anticipated psychotic happenings and believes he has found instances of this in neurotics, schizophrenics and in organic disorders, as well as certain prophetic dreams before the onset of an illness.

A patient dreams she sees the onset of an eclipse. There was a faint twilight. Then she saw herself standing in the middle of a busy street. A crowd of people and motor cars came towards her in reverse. The minute they arrived close to her they always avoided her and slid by her with ever-increasing speed. Everything passed her by and she became giddy and sank down in a faint. She found herself again in a homely farmhouse room where an oil-lamp gave a warm light. A fortnight after this striking dream, the patient passed through a mild schizophrenic delusional state which lasted two days. She was, however, soon able to regain a hold on herself and after the attack she was if anything rather more released and emotionally warmer than before, just as she had anticipated in her dream.

## § 4. HYSTERIA

When the will purposefully controls the play of the mechanism of suggestion, a mental force is in operation that rules our own unconscious psychic and bodily life and it is not a case of illness. But if mechanism of suggestion functions without *our knowledge or volition* and *against our will* then something most unhealthy happens which we describe as hysterical.

In hysterical phenomena every kind of suggestion is developed in exaggerated fashion. All sorts of tendencies are stimulated and reach realisation without any inhibition from critical attitudes in the personality as a whole or from previous experiences. Quite often there is a meaningful choice of the phenomena which are realised, meaningful in terms of the wishes and drives of the personality which are thus displayed. During inoculations we may observe involuntary imitation, when after someone has fainted, all the others faint one after the other. Only a few decades ago hysterical fits were spreading in girls' schools, for instance, as they used to do in convents. The effects of suggestion on the judgment is shown in the hysterical gullibility. The mechanism operates as auto-suggestion when falsehoods, which were initially conscious, develop into self-believed fantasies (pseudologia phantastica). The mere play-acting of a mental illness may develop into an actual psychic change. A patient relates how in her childhood she became frightened and gave up playing at madness when she noticed this tendency for its realisation. In people of hysterical predisposition prison-psychoses frequently represent actual psychic changes, which have arisen in the first place from simulation and from the desire to be ill. Out of the role which is merely played develops real delusion, the 'wild fellow' gives place to the autonomy of irresistible excitement. Half-simulated physical complaints turn into compensation-hysteria which then becomes an actual, self-established illness. An hysteric in prison developed involuntary and insistent pseudo-hallucinations of sexual scenes between the public-prosecutor and his fiancée, due to his anxious fancy that they were having an affair and he came to believe in the reality of these relationships. The essential suggestibility of hysterics can be seen in their adaptability to any and every environment. They are influenced so easily that they do not seem to have a personality of their own. They take on their environment as it is at the time, they are criminal, devout, industrious, enthusiastic for suggested ideas which they will adopt with as much intensity as their originator and just as readily drop in the face of some other influence. They intend to give only one inter-pretation to a situation and to exhaust the possibilities of this. A patient re-ceived 250 Reichmarks from his Accident Insurance. He felt enormously rich and thought of nothing else, became engaged, bought rings, furniture, clothes on hire-purchase, and then took to theft and got two years in prison. He felt subsequently that his condition had been like an illness.

The *concept of hysteria* has been the subject-matter of many discussions. The net result has been that the concept increasingly moved away from the early concept of a disease-entity towards a general psychopathological characterisation of certain phen-omena which occur in all sorts of illnesses, though most commonly there is also a predisposition present. We differentiate *hysterical character* (p. 443) from *hysterical attack* (accidents mentaux) and these in turn from *hysterical stigmata* (physical symptoms—p. 241). In all these three, we distinguish the tendency or rather the wish to be ill—as we do all other contents and tendencies—from the mechanism which is connected in some way with the dissociation.[1]

We have got to know certain peculiar amnesias either restricted to a single experience or covering the entire past which do not prevent the patient all the same from moving and acting unconsciously as if he remembered everything quite well. We also know the disturbances in sensation which we may find in hysterics and which never involve the consequences of any real loss of sensation. Janet has described all these peculiar facts in a metaphorical way as 'the dissociation of psychic material'.[2] In normal life we find a true forgetting, a genuine loss of psychic dispositions or else the continuously maintained unity of psychic life, that is, the lasting ability to endure passively the after-effects of past experience as well as to be actively aware of them. In abnormal states, however, we find dissociations of entire psychic areas. Sensibilities, memories, have effects which can be objectively described but which do not become conscious. Feelings, actions, performances appear which are con-ditioned by this dissociated psychic life. The dissociated and conscious psychic

[1] 'Über die Psychopathologie der Hysteria', Janet, *L'état mental des Hysteriques*, 2nd edn. (Paris, 1911).
[2] Janet, *L'automatisme psychologique*, 6th edn. (Paris, 1910).

life are in some way connected, in that what is dissociated exerts an influence on conscious operations and reaches up, as it were, into what is conscious. The clearest example is that of the post-hypnotic time-suggestion. A girl pays a visit at twelve noon as she had been ordered to do under hypnosis on the previous day, though she does not know anything about this order. She feels she is driven to pay this visit but she finds quite a different motivation for it subsequently. When these time-suggestions concern the performance of certain foolish acts—to put a chair, for instance, on the top of a table—the urge do so is felt subsequently most keenly but it may perhaps be so erroneously motivated or regarded as so stupid that it is suppressed. In these cases the connection between the original experience (the hypnosis) and the emergence of the urge from the unconscious can no longer be doubted. The 'dissociation of psychic complexes' is a good metaphorical expression for these phenomena, which, should they appear *spontaneously*, we call hysterical. It is of course only a metaphor, a theoretical construct which Janet developed very clearly, in order to cover certain cases and it is not necessarily applicable to psychic life in general. Following Janet rather freely we may illustrate the situation in the accompanying diagram (Fig. 3):

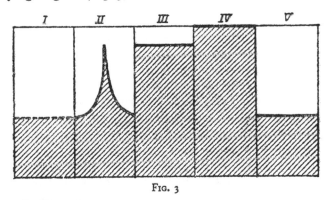

FIG. 3

  *I*  Normal
 *II*  Appearance of a hysterical symptom
*III*  Hypnoid state
*IV*  Twilight state or 'double personality'
  *V*  Chronic hysterical state without manifest symptoms

The shaded parts indicate the unconscious. The blank parts indicate the conscious psychic life. In column I the healthy state of the shifting border between what is unnoticed and what is extra-conscious is indicated by a dotted line. In the other sections a full line is drawn to denote the sharp separation, the dissociation. In column V we find the chronic hysterical state, for the moment without any manifest symptoms. The dissociated elements are quiescent. In column II the appearance of a hysterical symptom (nausea, vomiting, false perceptions, etc.) is indicated. In column III a hypnoid state of day-dreaming is shown and in column IV there is a twilight state excluding normal consciousness. These latter cases have been strikingly described as *double personalities*[1] or as *alternating consciousness*, because the dissociated psychic life appears so richly developed that it feels as if one is dealing with another personality. When however the state comes to an end, the normal personality has no memory of it.

It is rare to find cases where Janet's experiments are successfully demonstrated and there is proof of the existence of a dissociated consciousness. Post-hypnotic suggestions are also rare and alternating consciousness particularly rare. None the less the *same underlying mechanism is assumed for a great number of hysterical phenomena*. The chief justification for this assumption lies in the observations made by Breuer and Freud,[2] concerning the origin of particular symptoms, which were found to lie in upsetting experiences (*psychic traumata*). While Janet had conceived the dissociation to be spontaneous and to arise solely from the Anlage, these authors recognised that dissociation could also be brought about, given the Anlage, by certain experiences. This is not only so after physical accidents (hysterical paralysis of an arm after a fall from a carriage in one of Charcot's famous cases) but after all kinds of affects as well (fright, anxiety, etc.). 'Thus a painful affect which arises during a meal may be repressed and later cause nausea and vomiting which continue as hysterical vomiting for a month.' 'In other cases the connection is not so simple. The relationship between the cause and the pathological phenomena is only a symbolic one, as it were, when, for instance, neuralgia is added to psychic distress or vomiting to the affect of moral contempt.' The experiences that underlie the morbid symptoms are not remembered by the patients in their ordinary state but they can be brought out under hypnosis. Memories are split off or dissociated, the patient has no access to them, yet he suffers from their effects without knowing it. Once the memories are made accessible to the waking consciousness (psychoanalysis) and the patient simultaneously lives through the original affects once more (abreaction) a cathartic effect sets in: the symptoms in question have vanished. During the traumatic experience there is a hypnoid state and this along with intentional repression of affect or unintentional 'damming up' of it, all play a part as factors which facilitate the dissociation.

The whole process of *repression* and its effects may be illustrated by some examples from Pfister[3] who has set them out in a table which we reproduce in a modified way below. The factual correctness of the examples is not so

---

[1] Azam, *Annal. méd-psychol.* (July, 1876). Summary: Binet, *Les altérations de la personnalité* (Paris, 1891), 2nd edn., 1902. Classic case: Morton Prince, *The Dissociation of a Personality* (New York, 1906). Cp. Flourney, *Die Seherin von Genf.* (Leipzig, 1914). Hallervorden, *Z. Neur.*, vol. 24 (1914), p. 378.

[2] Breuer and Freud, *Studien über Hysterie* (Vienna, 1895). Freud later developed very different views. The original views on these traumatic connections were followed up chiefly by Frank, *Über Affektstörungen* (Berlin, 1913), theoretically and therapeutically.

[3] Pfister, *Die psychoanalytische Methode* (Leipzig, 1913).

important as the way they show us how **repression** and **dissociation** are to be conceived:

| Experience | Conflicting wishes and drives producing repression of one side | | Understandable result in a dissociated image of real gratification of a wish or of escape (dissociated realisation) | Resulting understandable content of an objective manifestation |
|---|---|---|---|---|
| | (a) | (b) | | |
| 15-year-old girl; student wants to kiss her; she manages to resist | wish to be kissed | shy of forbidden sexuality | 'I have been kissed too much' | Swollen lips |
| A boy masturbated and stole from his mother | need to confess the sexual misdeed and the theft | shy to confess such things | He intends to confess one evening but shame prevents. The thought then comes: 'I can't talk any more as I want to; it's all dark ahead'. | At that time he showed hysterical mutism and dim vision. He knows nothing of his previous monologue which comes to light only in analysis |
| 16-year-old girl is in love with a priest whom she has seen once | feelings of desire | feelings of something forbidden and unattainable | 'The priest assaults me sexually' | Spreads malicious accusations: The priest molests her with obscene remarks. She knows she is lying but cannot help it. Reproaches herself bitterly |

Repression does not always depend on direct action by the personality but it is much more often due to the hardly noticed conflict between opposing drives and wishes and to the final 'damming back' of the one or the other. Repression as such does not produce hysteria. Normal people can repress successfully without any such disturbance but in some individuals repression discovers hysterical mechanisms which transform the repressed material. This conversion into symptoms is what is pathological and could not come about without the dissociation. The conversion issues in bodily symptoms and in psychic ones. It appears both as affect and as lack of affect, and as disturbance of function, etc.

In order to try and grasp the relationship between the experience and the symptom, we either have to take the meaningful, symbolic connections which we previously discussed, the transference of affects, etc., over into the dissociated psychic life as we conceive it, or we have to turn to yet another analogy: that of the *energy of affects* which can be transformed into other forms of energy. When repression prevents discharge in a natural reaction, the suppressed energy will show itself in changed form elsewhere. Janet constructed the concept of 'dérivation'. The diverted energy discharges itself through motor attacks, pains, through other uncalled-for affects. The affect is converted, e.g.: repressed sexual libido converts into fear and vice versa. The affect reactivates old pathways (e.g. evokes rheumatic pains that were there before, or heart-pains and so on). This analogy undoubtedly holds for a few cases; we only have to be cautious with any general theoretical elaboration. The use of these analogies of dissociation and of transformation of affect-energy led to findings which, as Breuer and Freud were able to show, vividly illuminate the 'contradiction that lies between the statement that "hysteria is a psychosis" and the fact that a number of clear-headed, strong-willed and critical people of good personality are to be found among hysterics. The waking, thinking individual may well be thus, but in the hypnoid state, he is changed as we all are in dreams. But while our dreams do not influence our waking-state, the products of the hypnoid state extend far into the waking life in the form of hysterical phenomena.' The incomprehensible excess of feeling, the excessive enthusiasm for things which objectively do not seem to justify such enthusiasm, becomes explicable through the analogy of an influx of affect-energy from the drives, the content of which (as symbol, or through similarity, etc.) has a meaningful connection with the content of the enthusiasm. Inversely, the incomprehensible coldness becomes explicable through the concentration of all affect-energy in one single area of drive and a fixation on the contents of this. Thus in hysteria, if we presuppose mechanisms of dissociation and transformation, this allows us to bring the notable contradictions of affective excess and insufficiency into some meaningful connection with the patient's experiences.

Dissociation is a fairly obvious theoretical help in clarifying the *ambivalence* of hysterics. The person clearly has the conscious intention to get well and this is perfectly credible; there is the wish to get rid of the paralyses and other disturbances. He also has another intention—not connected with the first—which strives with all its might against it once recovery comes on in earnest. The conscious will of the personality will only regain its normal power and the other intention will only vanish, at least in this particular form, if there is a remarkable switchover which has often been seen to take place, through suggestion-therapy, or through some severe and painful shock or through some of the chances of the life-situation.[1]

We may ask what are the criteria whereby we can legitimately assume in any particular case that the source of a phenomenon is psychic dissociation (i.e., there is a repressed, 'encapsulated' affect which has now become a 'foreign body' that operates with an alien power)? (1) the precipitating psychic experience must be objectively established; (2) there must be a relationship between the symptom and the experience which is understandable in the context; (3) the lost memory should return during the hypnotic state together with other concrete phenomena of the experience when emotionally re-lived (abreaction) and there should be subsequent recovery from the symptom in question; (4) all kinds of expressive phenomena accompanying the appearance

[1] Kretschmer vividly described hysterical volition. 'Die Willensapparate der Hysterischen', *Z. Neur.*, vol. 54, p. 251.

of the symptom should do so in a way which is understandable in the first place and which points to content other than that which is present in consciousness (for instance, sexual movements during an investigation into the refusal of food).

The relationship between the content of the repressed experience and the content of the illness can be seen particularly clearly in some hysterical deliria where the precipitating experience (accident, sexual assault, etc.) is repeatedly relived in a hallucinatory way though it is no longer remembered in the normal consciousness. We also see the same thing in some Ganser twilight-states during captivity where the crime is now forgotten but every wish is felt to be gratified (innocence, liberty, etc.).

Suggestions become all the more effective, the more they are directed towards the patient's *wishes* (the enormous effect of auto-suggestion in neurotic patients who are receiving compensation for some traumatic event), and the more they *arouse fear* (the immediate realisation of hypochondriacal complaints which initially were only suspected). Timid people can be made ill by relevant suggestion as in the same way one can make them well again.

*Everything connected with suggestion and hysteria is obscure and misleading to the investigator.*

In every field of psychic life it is extremely common but always surprising to observe a *deficiency in the conscious psychic events* which, when looked at from another angle, proves to be *not a true deficiency at all*. The missing element continues to exist in the unconscious, as we say, and to spread its influence from there. It can be brought back into consciousness by psychic means (suggestion, affect). A large number of disturbances are of this order: total amnesia for circumscribed periods, for particular objects or for the entire past; total disturbance of registration, loss of sensation, paralyses, loss of volition, alterations in consciousness, etc. Just as astonishing as the deficiency itself is the way in which in some sense it is 'not there'. A patient who has forgotten her entire previous life behaves as if she still knew everything. The blind person never stumbles over anything as she walks about. The paralysed person can walk when situation and impulse force her to it. It is always possible to discover conditions under which the deficiency appears to be corrected. *All tests*, therefore, which try to make some clear distinction between *hysterical phenomena and simulation come to grief*. With *hysterical* phenomena we are *never dealing with events which allow us to study certain psychic functions more precisely in the defect-state*. In hysteria psychic functions are always disturbed in one and the same way, a way which we cannot characterise precisely and the unity of which in many cases we can only guess at rather than know and to which we give the name of the hysterical mechanism. The study of this hysterical mechanism teaches us about one side of psychic life that is as puzzling as it is important. The mechanism we are dealing with, once we have recognised it, reveals itself as something we can also trace in ourselves and in everyone to a slight degree. But the phenomena which are conditioned by it only lead to the study of the mechanism itself. It is *an old mistake to make use of hysterical phenomena for the analysis and interpretation of psychic and somatic phenomena in general*. Hysterical disturbances of memory, for instance, are wholly unsuitable for us to learn from when it comes to the particular functions of memory, just as hysterical somatic disturbances can teach us nothing about the normal physiology of the organs. We have to admit, however, that all psychic events take on a new aspect once the hysterical mechanism is in charge.

Once suggestion and hysteria play a part, there is no chance to investigate any laws or necessities of a physiological or psychological kind. *Everything*, it seems, *is possible*. All these phenomena, therefore, can only be used to illustrate hysterical mechanisms and nothing more of physiological or psychological relevance. Cases in which they play a part must be omitted from any material evidence offered in support of any psychological theory or thesis. Exact experiment is not really possible, and nothing can be properly verified or determined. Just as it can be said that the most experienced psychiatrist can be tripped up by hysterics, so it may be said that even the most critical of investigators in the psychological and somatic field will continue to be caught by the phenomena of suggestion. It is however annoying to find some authors who make use of what are obviously phenomena of suggestion and hysteria as supportive evidence for a general insight into psychology and physiology.

The phenomenon of so-called *induced insanity* (psychic epidemics)[1] is a particularly striking kind of suggestion-phenomenon to which many, though not only hysterical, persons are prone. There is a wide spread of hysterical fits, attempts at suicide and delusion-like convictions. It is of course out of the question that any disease process can be transmitted psychically. Dissemination comes about through a mass consciousness, a group feeling, which plays all the greater part—sometimes to an uncanny degree—the greater the number of persons involved. There is the particularly interesting case where someone suffering from a paranoid process infects a number of healthy people with his ideas so that he becomes the centre of a movement which quickly dies down again when once he is removed from it. Inversely, as paranoid persons are beyond any influence, these cases have produced the proverbial remark: 'It is easier for one madman to convince a hundred sound people than for a hundred sound people to convince him'.

## § 5. MEANINGFUL CONTENT IN THE PSYCHOSES

Much has been explained as meaningful which in fact was nothing of the kind.

Thus attempts have been made to make *feelings* the explanation for all abnormal phenomena. If we use the term 'feeling' to denote everything for which common usage permits us to use the word, there is always some truth in this, but it then comes to very little if we go on to derive delusions, for instance, from feelings. Ideas of senselessness, sinfulness, impoverishment, can be understandably said to arise from depressive affects and it was generally supposed that the depressed patient concluded

---

[1] Wollenberg, *Arch. Psychiatr.* (D), vol. 20, p. 62. Schönfeldt, *Arch. Psychiatr.* (D)., vol. 26, p. 202. Weygandt, *Beitrag zur Lehre von den psychischen Epidemien* (Halle, 1905). Hellpach, 'Die psychischen Epidemien' (in der Sammlung, *Die Gesellschaft*), Schoenhals, *Mschr. Psychiatr.*, vol. 33, p. 40 ('Literatur'). Riebeth, *Z. Neur.*, vol. 22 (1914), p. 606. Peretti, *Allg. Z. Psychiatr.*, vol. 74, p. 54 ff. W. Dix, *Über hysterische Epidemien an deutschen Schulen* (Langensalza, H. Beyer and Söhne, 1907). Nyiro and Petrovich, *Z. Neur.*, vol. 114 (1928), p. 38.

there must be something which made him so miserable. People also wanted to explain delusions of persecution by the affect of distrust, and delusions of grandeur by euphoric moods, but they did not realise that, though one may understand ordinary mistakes and over-valued ideas in this way, one can never do this with delusions. Frightening hallucinations in sleep during fever or a psychosis have been attributed to some kind of anxiety, otherwise conditioned. In all these cases we can, it is true, find meaningful connections, and they teach us something about the relationship of delusional content and previous experiences but nothing at all of how the delusions, false perceptions, etc. could have come about in the first place.

For delusions to develop a new factor has to be added. If one calls the new element 'the paranoid mechanism' this is only a name and one which includes very heterogeneous material such as the formation of delusion-like ideas as well as of delusions proper.

## (a) Delusion-like ideas

There is nothing new in the circumstance that the contents of delusion-like ideas have 'meaning' in terms of the patients' life-experiences, wishes and hopes, fears and anxieties. Friedmann[1] has described peculiar cases of 'mild paranoia' where the content of the delusion confines itself to the connection with some specific experience. Birnbaum[2] has described the frequent occurrence of delusion-formation in prison, where the delusions are changeable, can be influenced and tend to disappear on discharge. He therefore termed them 'delusion-like fancies' rather than delusional ideas. The content was to a large extent meaningful in terms of wishes and the situation in general.

This is also the place, perhaps, for the 'sensitive delusion of reference',[3] found in the psychasthenic individual who is tender, thin-skinned but full of self-conscious ambition and obstinacy. They become ill because of some experience of humiliating insufficiency, in particular defeats of a sexual–moral nature, for instance, the late love of middle-aged single women, which cannot find any free outlet. Paranoia comes instead with depressive self-reproach, fears of pregnancy and delusions of reference. The patient knows she is observed and spited by family and friends, the public and the newspapers. She fears pursuit by police and Courts. There are transient, acute psychoses with excitement and severe neurasthenic symptoms and so many delusions that the clinical picture may well look like some progressive incurable disorder but content and affect remain centred round the originating experience.

[1] Friedmann, Mschr. Psychiatr., vol. 17.

[2] Birnbaum, Psychosen mit Wahnbildung u. wahnhafte Einbildungen bei Degeneration (Halle, 1908).

[3] Kretschmer is responsible for the description. Der sensitive Beziehungswahn; ein Beitrag zur Paranoiafrage u. zur psychiatrischen Charakterlehre (Berlin, 1918). These processes may only be special types of paranoid schizophrenia in personalities which have remained intact and natural. Similar cases may be seen where no decisive experience precedes the psychosis, as K. Schneider demonstrated in his own patients (Z. Neur., vol. 59, p. 51). But the clear delineation of such types and the tracking down of all the meaningful connections brings knowledge of a kind with a value of its own in as much as it reduces what are otherwise chaotic phenomena into some sort of order and form.

## (b) Delusions in schizophrenia

From time to time and incidentally attempts have been made to understand the contents of delusion as well as other psychotic symptoms in terms of the individuals' wishes and longings. This approach has been extended to schizophrenia by the Zürich school (*Bleuler* and *Jung*). However, they did not stop at the obviously meaningful contents but followed in Freud's footsteps and treated them as symbols. They have thus come to 'understand' almost all the contents of these psychoses by applying a procedure which as the results show only leads on into endlessness. In the most literal sense they have rediscovered the 'meaning of madness' or at least they believe they have. Their results cannot be summarised briefly nor are they ready for an objective formulation. We therefore refer to some of the publications of this school for an orientation on the problem.[1] The following is a crude example: Voices accuse the patient of sexual intercourse; to have perpetrated this would correspond with his repressed wishes.

Bleuler and Jung conceived that schizophrenic psychoses, the contents of delusions, of catatonic behaviour and of false perceptions become meaningful in terms of repressed complexes of a *dissociated* kind. This 'interpretation' of symptoms is doubtful but can be discussed. It is noteworthy that according to Bleuler these complexes need not be repressed. They can have remained in consciousness and yet dominate the schizophrenic deliria. From this angle there is sometimes a surprising analogy to be drawn between hysteria and schizophrenia and Jung draws attention to this. The whole interpretation is a *translation to schizophrenia of concepts which have been arrived at during the analysis of hysteria.* We should, however, never forget the radical differences which exist between hysteria and a schizophrenic process and which show themselves for example in the fact that schizophrenics as opposed to hysterics cannot be hypnotised and are not at all easily suggestible.

Meaningful contents are to be found in every kind of objective phenomena. Even the *contents of hallucinations*, for example, need to be looked at in this way. They are not completely accidental but to some extent have meaningful connections, and are significant of experience in the form of commands, wish-fulfilments, teasing and ridicule, agonies and revelations. Freud called hallucinations thoughts turned into images.[2]

## (c) Incorrigibility

In countless cases the mistakes of healthy people cannot actually be corrected but usually the mistakes are shared in common with others and this adds confirmation. Conviction comes not from 'insight' but from the sense of 'all

[1] Jung, *Über die Psychologie der Dementia praecox* (Halle, 1907). Bleuler, *Die Schizophrenie* (Vienna, 1911). Maeder, 'Psychologische Untersuchungen an Dementia praecoxkranken', *Jb. psychoanal. u. psychother. Forsch.*, vol. 2, p. 185. Circumspect interpretations are given by Hans W. Maier, 'Über katathyme Wahnbildung u. Paranoia', *Z. Neur.*, vol. 13, p. 555.
[2] Jung, *Der Inhalt der Psychose*, 2nd edn. (Leipzig, 1914).

of us together'. The mistake which is delusion is peculiar to the solitary individual. In that respect delusion has been referred to as an illness of the social self (Kehrer). But the *truth* of an individual may also assert itself against the majority and it may hardly be possible to differentiate this from delusion so far as the social behaviour is concerned. In trying to understand the incorrigibility we may find what interest it serves: the delusional content is of vital necessity for the deluded person and without it he would inwardly collapse. Indeed no one, even the healthy, can be expected to appreciate a truth which makes utter nonsense of his existence, but the *incorrigibility of delusion has something over and above the incorrigibility of healthy people's mistakes.* So far, however, we have not succeeded in defining what this is. We may speak of a *stability of affect* (Bleuler) or emphasise the tendency of delusion to spread or progress, or talk of the logical reasoning which serves the delusion and can never turn and refute it but in so doing we simply give a name to something which we can neither see nor comprehend. And yet it is precisely this problem that gives us no peace. Delusion, particularly the delusional system, presents itself as a whole coherent world of appropriate behaviour apparent in a personality that is quite sensible and by common standards not otherwise to be considered ill. This constitutes what is called 'being unhinged or mad', and is all the more alarming in that quite often others in the environment may take over the delusion. In principle, but not perhaps in practice, untruth can always be overcome by the great process of human reason which amongst a welter of mistakes, falsifications, obscurities, sophisms and bad intentions pursues truth. In the case of delusion, however, we may see someone irretrievably lost in untruth—an extreme situation which we may not be able to correct yet would much like to comprehend.

### (d) Classification of delusional content

From very early on we have collected the contents of delusion and classified them. They are of striking variety, imaginativeness and eccentricity. The initial folly was committed of considering every single delusional content as a special illness and giving it a name (Guislain) without noticing that nomenclature of this sort has no end. But the contents do have a number of general, common characteristics that recur repeatedly and give a peculiarly uniform character to the multiplicity of the contents. We are not wanting to extend the wealth of contents but only to discover basic types. In this respect we can look at the material from several angles:

1. *Delusions that are objective and delusions centred on the person.* Human drives and wishes, hopes and fears, are universal so that most delusional formations may be regarded as in the closest relationship to the individual's particular weal or woe. The patient is almost always the centre of his delusion but on rarer occasions the delusional formations are objective in content, the delusion is about the meaning of the world, is connected with some philosophical problem or historical event not related to the person of the patient. The patients

have made a magnificent invention and work at it all the time; they have squared the circle, trisected an angle, etc. or by the use of numerical symbols they have prophetically grasped the basic laws of events. The patient feels his personal importance as a discoverer, the content has no particular significance for himself. He fills his time with hard mental work that is meaningful to him. He has an interest in being right, since if he were not life would lose all meaning for him, but what he has thought out is objective. These constructions, however, which in themselves are interesting, do not occur nearly so often as those which are egocentric.

2. *Actual delusional content.* The following are frequent contents which relate to the patient's well-being or otherwise:

(a) *Delusions of grandeur:* relating to origin (aristocratic stock, royal birth, brought up as a foster-child), to possessions (owning large estates, castles, etc., which are withheld by intrigue), to abilities (great inventors, discoverers, artists, possessors of special wisdom, gifted with inspiration), status (adviser to leading diplomats, the real director of political destinies). (b) *Delusions of diminished status:* relating to property (delusions of poverty), to abilities (demented, ineffective), to moral status (delusions of sin, self-accusation). (c) *Delusions of persecution.* The patient feels noticed, observed, put at a disadvantage, despised, ridiculed, poisoned, bewitched. He is persecuted by authorities or by the public prosecutor for crimes of which he is falsely accused, by gangs, Jesuits, Freemasons, etc. There are also delusions of physical persecution on the basis of bodily influences (false perceptions) and 'made' phenomena (passivity feelings), and querulant delusions about injustices, plots and treacherous manipulations. (d) *Hypochondriacal delusions.* In contrast with neurasthenic complaints of palpitations, headache, weakness and pain, there are delusional contents such as, the bones have softened, the heart is not right, the bodily substance has altered, there is a hole in the body, etc. There are delusions of being changed; the patient is changed into an animal and so on. (e) *Erotic delusions.* Erotomania is the term for the delusion that one is loved by another person though there is not the slightest sign of this and the person concerned declares the contrary (delusions of love and marriage-delusion). (f) *Religious delusions.* These may appear as delusions of grandeur or of diminished status: the patient is a prophet, mother of God, bride of Jesus, or the patient is the devil, is damned, or the anti-Christ.

The description of delusional formations as characteristic for particular diseases is the province of special psychiatry. For illustration's sake we would simply remark here that it is characteristic for certain paranoid processes to have delusional contents about great world events of which the patient is the centre. He is 'in touch with the whole world', the 'whole history of the world depends on him' or he is the centre of cosmic revolutions in which he plays a very special if passive role. A patient who was already quite deluded said, 'Every spark of well-being has been quenched, and so I have wandered about for thousands of years, always unwittingly reborn. The reason for this must be attributed to the creation of the world.'

3. *The binding of opposites.* All delusion is understandably rooted in the tension between opposites. Friedmann saw the basic conflict in every delu-

sional formation as lying in the patient's experience of having his own will overpowered by the whole will of the community. What is visible in the delusion is the conflict between reality and the individual's own desires, between compelling demands and private wishes, between being honoured or humiliated. Delusion always *encompasses both poles*, so that honour and humiliation of the self, delusions of grandeur and delusions of persecution go together. Gaupp[1] described the mutual relationship between delusions of persecution and of grandeur as a meaningful whole, which he based on the sensitive personality disposition (accompanied by pride, shame, fear), presupposing that the form of the delusion as such cannot be understood. Kehrer[2] described delusions of persecution and grandeur as similar meaningful wholes. Whether we are dealing with a schizophrenic process or a personality development in which the individual reacts to life's conflicts in a delusion-like way, the meaningful element remains no different. There is a difference only in the course taken, in the form of the experience and in the psychic phenomena in their totality.

4. *Forms of paranoid attitude to the environment.* Kretschmer differentiated *wishful, combative* and *sensitive paranoics.* The delusion may be a reactive gratification of illusionary wishes, or an active affirmation of its own truth to the world around, or it may suffer its ideas of reference and persecution with little outward action but content itself with the inner pride of delusions of grandeur. Whichever it is, essential differences of content result in fact. On these lines, prison-paranoia with its delusion-like imaginings is a type of wishful paranoia, querulant delusion is a type of combative paranoia and delusions of reference and grandeur are a type of sensitive paranoia.

[1] Gaupp, *Z. Neur.*, vol. 69, p. 182.
[2] Kehrer, 'Der Fall Arnold', *Z. Neur.*, vol. 74, p. 155.

# CHAPTER VII

# THE PATIENT'S ATTITUDE TO HIS ILLNESS

An individual can face himself reflectively and in the same way a patient can face his own illness. Psychic illness looks different to the medical observer from what it looks like to the patient who is reflecting on himself. Thus it happens that someone, who regards himself as quite healthy, may be analysed as mentally ill or that someone may consider himself to be ill in a way that has no objective validity and is in itself a morbid symptom, or that someone through his own contriving may influence morbid processes for good or bad.

The concept of 'the patient's attitude' embraces a number of different phenomena. What unites them is that through them we try to *understand* the patient's attitude to the symptoms of his illness. We may observe how the vast majority of normal personalities will react to illness with the healthy part of themselves, as it were. But in understanding the particular attitude adopted we come up against the *limits of insight which a person has into himself*. These limits provide one of the most important criteria for personality type and in particular for the change which the personality has undergone as a whole through the illness.

*(a) Understandable attitudes to the sudden onset of acute psychosis (perplexity, awareness of change)*

Perplexity is one of the most understandable reactions in normal people to the onset of an acute psychosis. It is therefore a frequent observation and in some psychoses this perplexity pervades the most severe confusional states as a sign of what has been preserved of the normal personality, otherwise masked. Retardation, difficulties in comprehension, incoherence, inability to collect one's thoughts (Unbesinnlichkeit), all evoke the same reaction, which shows itself objectively in the puzzled expression, the searching about, a certain marked restlessness, a marked amazement and distractedness, and in such remarks as:

'What is it? Where on earth am I? Am I really Mrs. S. L.? I don't know what is wanted of me . . . What am I supposed to do here? . . . I don't understand any of it . . .' In addition there may be the questioning of the psychotic content: 'Surely I haven't killed anyone? Surely my children are not dead?' etc.

A schizophrenic wrote the following, which illustrates the perplexity felt in relation to the psychotic situation while the sensorium was still clear:

'I understand my situation less every day and so I make more mistakes every day. I simply cannot act in any considered way but just act instinctively because I cannot reach any real conclusion. What are the brown blankets on my bed? Do they represent people? How am I supposed to move if my mouth has to be closed? What am I supposed to do with my hands and my feet if my nails are so white? Am I supposed to scratch? What on? My environment changes every minute as the nurses move about. I don't understand them and therefore cannot respond. How can I do anything right if I don't know what is right? I think as simply as I thought when I was Leonora B. and cannot grasp this queer situation. I understand it daily less and less.' (Gruhle).

From this purely reactive and understandable perplexity which comes from an inability to orientate oneself to the situation and grasp the new experiences we must differentiate other forms of perplexity, which is often difficult to do in the individual case.

There is (1) *Paranoid perplexity:* with a clear sensorium. The patient is driven into a painful restlessness by the delusional experience and the still vague contents of his consciousness. He feels something is afoot and goes round searching; he asks questions and cannot make things out: 'If you would only tell me what it is, there is something I know' a patient asked her husband. (2) *Melancholic perplexity:* The utterances are reminiscent of the reactive type. The patients are in the grip of their delusions of poverty, diminished status and nihilism and view everything in an anxious, questioning way: 'Why are there so many persons? All these doctors— what is to happen? Why are there so many towels?'

At the beginning of a mental illness some persons undergo an *uncanny feeling of change* (as if they had been bewitched, enchanted or there may be an increase in sexuality, etc.). All of this adds to the awareness of impending madness. It is difficult to say what this awareness really is. It is the outcome of numerous, individual feelings, not a mere judgment but a real experience.

A woman who suffered from periodic insanity described how this feeling arose even when the psychosis itself was not at all unpleasant. 'The illness itself does not frighten me but only the moment when I begin the experience again and do not know how it will turn out.' Another patient who suffered from brief, florid psychoses wrote: 'The most frightening moments of my life are when I pass from my conscious state into confusion and the anxiety which goes with it.' Referring to prodromal phenomena, the same patient said: 'The uncanny aspect of the illness is that its victim cannot control the passage from healthy to morbid activity . . .'

We often learn of *individual instances*, noted at the start of an illness: an isolated false perception, a conspicuous change in affectivity, an unfamiliar and uncontrollable tendency to rhyme, verses come to mind unwittingly and so on. But here we are not dealing with some feeling of over-all change but with post-hoc statements of what it was like at the beginning. The *fear of going mad* is sometimes found in the early stages of a process, particularly among better-educated people. They become terribly restless and try to reassure themselves by testing out their environment. A patient put a woman friend's finger into his mouth to see if she would show signs of fear. If not, he would bite it. He took this as a sign that she thought him quite well and for a short time this reassured him.

Further, the fear of becoming mentally ill and feelings of impending madness are common but baseless symptoms which are found particularly in people suffering from personality disorders (psychopaths) and mild cyclothymics who do not as a matter of fact fall ill.

## (b) Working through the effects of acute psychoses

Individuals have a complex-laden attitude to everything which has once been a significant experience for them. For example, someone cannot think of his terrifying war-experiences without lapsing into uncontrollable gloom. Another may resist seeing again the object of an old passion or revisiting a place or environment where there has been unresolved suffering. Thus we find psychoses which introduce new significance in themselves, others which are linked in content with the personality and yet others which always remain entirely alien to the personality and bring no added burdens or significance to the psyche. Here the patient often will show an obvious embarrassment when talking about things except to the private ear of his doctor.

Mayer-Gross[1] studied the forms which after-effects took following acute schizophrenic psychoses and analysed them according to their meaningful connections. He distinguished: despair, 'renewal of life', shutting out (as if nothing had happened), conversion (the psychosis offered something fresh by means of a revelation) and integration.

## (c) Working through the illness in chronic states

Relatively sensible patients, particularly in chronic states, offer us a great variety of reactions to the individual phenomena of their illness. The patient *works through his symptoms* somehow. Laboriously he develops a delusional system out of his delusional experiences. He assumes an attitude to the contents of his experience; for example, he remarks on the increasing stupidity of the originator of the voices, who repeats trivial phrases endlessly or meaningless fragmented sentences. Awareness of physical illness and psychic change is often ascribed to painful influences of all kinds. The patient thinks of means of defence against these, particularly against the feelings of physical influences and various kinds of 'made' phenomena (passivity phenomena). Various methods of distraction are used and are sometimes helpful (saying a paternoster, working). In other cases patients will pass their time with the contents of their false perceptions. They evoke their visual pseudo-hallucinations intentionally and enjoy them. They annoy the voices by changing the rhythm of their step which the voices follow and this change puzzles and silences them. A number of unpleasant phenomena can be countered by self-control, such

[1] Mayer-Gross, 'Über die Stellungnahme zur akuten abgelaufenen Psychosen', *Z. Neur.* vol. 60 (1920), p. 160.

as the above-mentioned distractions, or by some active effort of will; for instance, an effort directed against the 'made' (passivity) movements or against 'made' (passivity) feelings of anger. Self-control also will help many in respect of the physical complaints in psychic illness and the agonising feelings which abnormal psychic life brings along.

In the cases so far mentioned the patients' attitude is on the whole understandable. As it becomes less so and the attitude to the illness becomes stranger, this in itself becomes a sign of the change in total personality which the illness has wrought. Thus in many cases it is remarkable how the patient gets used to his symptoms (for instance, to painful false perceptions and other experiences which are passively accepted), how he grows to look at them indifferently in spite of alarming content, and how apparently he does not notice fundamental delusional contents of utmost importance to him or else forgets them again rapidly. On the other hand we may be equally surprised by the overpowering strength of some hallucinations and delusions which seem to dominate the patient as by some physical compulsion. It is striking how some contents appear to captivate the patient's attention and how he is moved profoundly by matters that seem quite trivial. In the acute, florid psychoses we may observe how patients simply submit to feelings of loss of will, and bear the most agonising things passively. This helpless state, which they often characteristically describe, links up with their feelings of indifference as to what will come. Even where mighty cosmic revolutions are concerned, the patients nevertheless go on with their accustomed jokes or make frivolous remarks.

Much can be learnt from *patients' own interpretations*, when they are *trying to understand themselves*. A schizophrenic patient explained the specific contents of what he saw as follows:

'The figures seem exaggerated personifications of little, unimportant mistakes I have made; for instance, when I have enjoyed a meal, there might follow on the same evening—like an echo of the sensation—a demon who showed himself in the shape of a ravenous, gluttonous man-beast with enormous mouth, luscious thick red lips, fat belly of enormous size. I felt this monster near me until for a time (perhaps 2 to 3 meals) I had refrained from enjoying the food which seemed to be the source that fed him.' 'In everyone around me I saw their smallest failings as ugly, menacing figures that stepped out of them and attacked me' (Schwab).

The same patient *interpreted his illness as a whole:* He unified into a single meaning everything that the psychiatrist saw as the sequence of the process:

'I believe I caused the illness myself. In my attempt to penetrate the other world I met its natural guardians, the embodiment of my own weaknesses and faults. I first thought these demons were lowly inhabitants of the other world who could play me like a ball because I went into these regions unprepared and lost my way. Later I thought they were split-off parts of my own mind (passions) which existed near me in free space and thrived on my feelings. I believed everyone else had these too but did not perceive them, thanks to the protective and successful deceit of the feeling of personal existence. I thought the latter was an artefact of memory, thought-complexes, etc., a doll that was nice enough to look at from outside but nothing real inside it.

In my case the personal self had grown porous because of my dimmed consciousness. Through it I wanted to bring myself closer to the higher sources of life. I should have prepared myself for this over a long period by invoking in me a higher, impersonal self, since "nectar" is not for mortal lips. It acted destructively on the animal–human self, split it up into its parts. These gradually disintegrated, the doll was really broken and the body damaged. I had forced untimely access to the "source of life", the curse of the "gods" descended on me. I recognised too late that murky elements had taken a hand. I got to know them after they had already too much power. There was no way back. I now had the world of spirits I had wanted to see. The demons came up from the abyss, as guardian Cerberi, denying admission to the unauthorised. I decided to take up the life-and-death struggle. This meant for me in the end a decision to die, since I had to put aside everything that maintained the enemy, but this was also everything that maintained life. I wanted to enter death without going mad and stood before the Sphinx: either thou into the abyss or I!

Then came illumination. I fasted and so penetrated into the true nature of my seducers. They were pimps and deceivers of my dear personal self which seemed as much a thing of naught as they. A larger and more comprehensive self emerged and I could abandon the previous personality with its entire entourage. I saw this earlier personality could never enter transcendental realms. I felt as a result a terrible pain, like an annihilating blow, but I was rescued, the demons shrivelled, vanished and perished. A new life began for me and from now on I felt different from other people. A self that consisted of conventional lies, shams, self-deceptions, memory-images, a self just like that of other people, grew in me again but behind and above it stood a greater and more comprehensive self which impressed me with something of what is eternal, unchanging, immortal and inviolable and which ever since that time has been my protector and refuge. I believe it would be good for many if they were acquainted with such a higher self and that there are people who have attained this goal in fact by kinder means.'

Such self-interpretations are obviously made under the influence of delusion-like tendencies and deep psychic forces. They originate from profound experiences and the wealth of such schizophrenic experience calls on the observer as well as on the reflective patient not to take all this merely as a chaotic jumble of contents. Mind and spirit are present in the morbid psychic life as well as in the healthy. But interpretations of this sort must be divested of any causal importance. All they can do is to throw light on content and bring it into some sort of context.

*Every chronic illness confronts the patient with a task*, whether he is a cripple who has lost limbs but is otherwise quite healthy, whether he suffers from a somatic illness which affects him as a whole or whether he has a somatic illness accompanied with psychic disturbances. What can be achieved by people who are legless, armless or blind has been described often enough and it testifies to the energy, persistence and skilfulness of such individuals. But physically they were healthy. The situation is entirely different when the disturbance is not limited to an auxiliary member but strikes at the vital powers of an individual and affects his entire somatic and psychic state.

We may take an example from behaviour in chronic states following encephalitis epidemica (Dörer).[1] His cases show what different possibilities there are. The patients have to find their way about in a new situation. They suffer from the consequences of their illness at every moment. Their environment is changed, their occupation gone, the whole world alters in relationship to the patient. Isolation follows almost of necessity. Dörer describes the over-sensitive individuals who retreat into themselves, think only of themselves and demand the attention of the environment for their sufferings. They despond, become egotistical and complaining. Then there are those who 'in spite of everything' make greater displays of energy, want salvation at any price, undertake the most impossible things, and appear hunted and harried and turn into self-conscious outsiders. There are also those who remain spectators of life and so on. He wants to illustrate the saying: In the last resort it is a person's character that determines what the illness makes of him. The character shows itself to be modified by the particular culture with which it is interwoven and by relationship to the human community and the latter's response.

### (d) The patient's judgment of his illness

We can properly speak of attitudes only where the personality observes and passes judgment on the experience with which it is faced. When the judgment is a psychological one the patient makes himself aware of his experience and the manner of it. The ideal of a 'correct' attitude to experience is achieved by patients when they 'have insight into their illness'. Up to now we have got to know some features in patients' attitudes when faced with the content of morbid phenomena. We did this by looking at the *reaction* to the changed psychic life and at *the way patients work through* the contents. We will now describe features in patients' attitudes which appear when they turn away from content to their own selves and the experience they are having, and ask the reason for what is happening. They are in short passing a judgment on their illness either in its individual aspects or as a whole. We are concerned here with everything that can be collectively called awareness of illness or insight into the illness.[2]

The term *'awareness of illness'* is applied to the patient's attitude when he expresses a feeling of being ill and changed, but there is no extension of this awareness to all his symptoms nor to the illness as a whole. It does not involve any objectively correct estimate of the severity of the illness nor any objectively correct judgment of its particular type. Only when all this is present and there has been a correct judgment of all the symptoms and the illness as a whole according to type and severity, can we speak of *insight*, with the reservation that the judgment can only be expected to reach that degree of accuracy attainable

---

[1] Dörer, *Charakter u. Krankheit*, 'Ein Beitrag zur Psychologie der Encephalitis epidemica'.
[2] Pick, *Arch. Psychiatr.* (D), vol. 13, p. 518. Mercklin, *Allg. Z. Psychiatr.*, vol. 57, p. 579. Heilbronner, *Allg. Z. Psychiatr.*, vol. 58, p. 608. Arndt. *Zbl. Nervenkh.*, vol. 28, p. 773.

by the average, normal individual who comes from the same cultural background as the patient. Clearly the attitude of the personality to the illness will be well defined, well formulated and individualistic according to the intelligence and educational level of the patient. Someone steeped in the natural sciences and psychopathology will have a different attitude from someone with a background of theology or the humanities. We must always take the patient's milieu into account when attempting to evaluate his attitude as a *morbid* one. The same opinion might signify nothing but superstition in a simple peasant but betray a profound personality change, tending towards dementia, in an educated person.

1. *Self-observation and awareness of one's own state.* The patient's observations and judgment can encompass the phenomenological elements, the disturbances in psychic performance, the symptoms in all their complex unity, and the entire personality; in short, it can encompass everything that becomes the subject-matter for psychopathology.[1]

Patients' self-observation is one of the most important sources of knowledge in regard to morbid psychic life; so is their attentiveness to their abnormal experience and the elaboration of their observations in the form of a *psychological judgment* so that they can communicate to us something of their inner life. Self-observation depends on interest, on some psychological aptitude, on powers of discrimination and on the sick person's intelligence. Under certain circumstances, however, *self-observation* may appear as a *painful symptom of illness*. Patients are compelled to spend their time analysing their experiences. All their other activities are disturbed and interrupted by this self-observation and the results may be very poor indeed. Reflection on one's own psychic life has here become compulsive and torturing. Such cases have quite unjustifiably given rise to the assertion that self-observation can be harmful. Kant had already warned against it as leading to rumination and madness. Self-observation does not cause illness but some morbid conditions do produce an abnormal kind of self-observation.

There is an *awareness of one's awareness*. We may feel 'torpid', 'dozy' or especially alert. This latter seems to occur sometimes to an abnormal degree. Vision is felt to be extremely clear—as happens in schizophrenia—and this may have some connection. Again there is something quite different in encephalitis lethargica, as in the case of a patient who wrote:

'I have the feeling that I was never so wideawake and aware before the illness. Perhaps it is a result of my constant self-observation and immediately making myself aware of my smallest thought or slightest movement. Every bodily event, such as sneezing, coughing, thinking, fills me with a burning curiosity as to how it comes about. I then try to feel myself into it as far as possible.' The patient described what she called 'registering', i.e. drawing into awareness every physical and psychic event . . . 'this registering spoils enjoyment and anticipation, because I have always to keep telling myself: now you are enjoying yourself; now you have expectations' (Mayer-Gross and Steiner).

[1] See *Z. Neur.*, vol. 6, p. 460, for my analysis of reality-judgment in false perception.

Below a certain level of psychic differentiation, individuals seem to live purely in their environment and lack all knowledge of themselves. In the case of idiocy, the fully developed acute psychoses and deep dementia, the problem does not even arise as to what attitude the personality adopts. It would be better here not to speak of the absence of any awareness of illness but to talk of a loss of personality, which embraces the missing awareness of illness automatically as a part-element. To some extent those remarkable cases of organic dementia that are *quite unware of the most severe bodily defects* can be said to belong to this category.

In organic cerebral illnesses (tumour, softening, etc.) where paralysis, blindness, deafness or other such severe defects have occurred, we sometimes find an absence of awareness.[1] The completely blind patient says he can see perfectly well, reacts to examination with grumbling resentment, gets indignant and finally helps himself out by creating phrases of his own, like a patient with a Korsakow syndrome. When asked 'what is this?' (a watch held in front of him) he says as he gropes in the air 'you see it there, there it is'. 'What is it you want?' . . . He describes anything possible, the examiner for instance, goes around gesticulating as if he saw everything, swears, maintains it is dark, etc. Redlich and Bonvicini have shown how a general psychic change (torpor, apathy, euphoria, severe disturbance in registration) can make such failure in awareness understandable. Related to this is the fact that some patients can be brought to a certain insight into their blindness for short periods but they immediately forget it again. However, there seem to be particular defects in performance which are difficult to detect by their very nature, where defective insight does not necessarily appear as disintegration of personality. Thus Pick[2] describes: 'the amnestic aphasic individual who gropes for the missing word and has continuously a feeling of the inadequacy of his speech, whereas the aphasic who talks in telegrammatic style or uses infinitives never hesitates for a single moment when speaking. He does not feel that anything is missing which he should look for (even when the patient is aware of his speech defect).' In the same way we can observe the paraphasic flow of talk in patients with sensory aphasia who do not seem to grasp that no one understands them, whereas the patient with motor aphasia hardly utters a word; he makes attempts to speak but gets held fast in his own awareness of disability and gives up the effort.

2. *Attitudes in acute psychoses.* In psychosis there is no lasting or complete insight. Where insight persists we do not speak of psychosis but personality disorder (psychopathy). Individual phenomena may be judged correctly but, apart from that, the innumerable manifestations of the illness are not recognised as such and inversely there are morbid feelings where the content is a false one and is itself a symptom. For instance, a melancholic patient considers she is rotting away physically or a paranoid patient thinks his thought-processes are being interfered with by external machinations. Patients will say,

---

[1] Redlich and Bonvicini, 'Über das Fehlen der Wahrnehmung der eigenen Blindheit bei Hirnkrankheiten', *Jb. Psychiatr.*, vol. 29. Bychowski, *Neur. Zbl.*, vol. 39, p. 354. Stertz, *Z. Neur.*, vol. 55, p. 327. Pick, *Arch. Augenhk.*, vol. 86 (1920), p. 98. Pötzl, *Z. Neur.*, vol. 93, p. 117.

[2] Pick, *Agrammatische Sprachstörungen*, p. 54.

'I don't know . . . am I mad or what?' . . . 'I see something but I don't know what, am I imagining it?' . . . 'I don't know what all this means, am I bewitched or what?' In acute psychoses there are transient states of far-reaching insight. The patient returns from his fantastic experiences for a moment and finds he is in hospital; he may even try to expedite his committal to a mental hospital. Sometimes at the beginning of a process we find considerable insight, the correction of delusions, the proper assessment of voices, etc., which one might well consider as recovery and a benign psychopathic state, but insight of this sort is quite transient. We can occasionally observe how it comes and goes within a few hours or days. Sometimes clear consciousness will arise in the very middle of the schizophrenic experiences. The patients will say afterwards 'for a moment I was again aware that I was disturbed', or 'Suddenly I was quite aware that the whole thing was nonsense'. Thus the momentary insight which emerges is more far-reaching than the content of most of the verbal utterances suggest:

Miss B. explained she was not ill but pregnant. It was not a delusion, it was terrible that it had happened and the future was frightening. She didn't know what to do for worry. However, after a few minutes she explained quite spontaneously how situations like this had always passed before (she had had several similar phases from which she had always recovered).

In *states of personality disorder* (psychopathic states) where the patient is almost overcome, insight is still always there. Von Gebsattel described the insight of an anankastic patient as follows:

'She can distinguish between what is morbid and healthy. She feels she is "double" and thinks one day the whole compulsive system will have to "collapse like a house of cards" or "vanish like a ghost". At times the "scales fall from her eyes". She then "sees everything clearly and naturally" and feels very happy, but only for a moment. It is as if one had just left the theatre and "got rid of the scenery". She feels one day she will be able to step out of her illness or wake up from it as if from a dream.'

3. *Attitude to psychosis after recovery.* In order not to be deceived regarding the total picture of the illness, it is more important to penetrate beyond the content of the judgments as expressed (which can so easily mislead us) into the real attitude of the patient to the psychosis from which he has recovered rather than to the acute psychosis while it lasts. We get a clear picture of complete insight, it is true, in patients who recover from deliria, alcoholic hallucinosis or mania. They will say without reservation, and in respect of any one of their symptoms, that they have been ill. They will speak freely and frankly about the psychotic contents which are now quite alien to them and a matter of indifference. They can talk about them simply and detachedly and even laugh about them as if they did not belong to them. The consequences they draw from this insight are entirely understandable; they worry about relapse, the odium of certification, etc.

In contrast with this, cases are not so rare with other psychoses, and in particular the schizophrenias, where subjectively honest judgments seem to show full insight, but when examined more closely it is clear they do not. Patients will assert they have passed through a mental illness, they are convinced of the unreality of past contents and feel quite well again but they do not talk quite freely about all the contents and even if they want to one notices an inappropriate excitement when they are asked to talk about them. They will blush, grow pale, perspire, give evasive answers and say they do not want to be reminded of the matter because it is upsetting. There is every gradation from cases such as these to others where the patients refuse to answer point-blank. Occasionally we can notice that individual details (persecutions, etc.) are still maintained as real and remarks are dropped such as 'theoretically speaking, I am a bit doubtful whether it was really so or not; but in fact I cover it up or I should be locked up for ever', etc. In cases such as these we cannot talk of full insight. The patient's personality has been lastingly affected by the content of the psychosis—often without his realising it. He is not in a position to look at it at all objectively as something detached from him. He can only deal with it as something troublesome that has to be dismissed. In other cases patients do not remember the acute psychosis as unpleasant. They are even sorry their memory of it is slowly disappearing. They do not like missing the rich experiences which the psychosis brought into their life. Gerard de Nerval began his description of his illness as follows:

'I shall try to record the impression of a long illness that took place in the mysterious recesses of my mind. I do not know why I use the expression "illness" because, as far as I am concerned, I never felt better in my life. Sometimes I took my powers and abilities as twice as great. I seemed to know and understand everything and my imagination gave me immense delight. Should one regret the loss of all this when one has regained once more what men call reason?'

4. *Attitudes in chronic psychoses.* The verbal contents in chronic psychotic states often mislead one into thinking that a great deal of insight is present:

Patients with incurable paranoid disorders of the dementia praecox group may for instance make remarks such as the following: Miss S.: 'my trouble is secondary paranoia'; 'I am suffering from hallucinatory-paranoia of the Krafft-Ebing type; I seem turned upside down'. 'I am suffering from paranoia-sexualis, doctor, my textbook is dated 1893 and there was no dementia praecox then.'—Mr. B., a workman, is asked whether he is ill and replies, 'I have nothing to say on that; I come up against an iron curtain—disbelief. The world takes it as delusion, the world wants reality. I can't prove anything. I keep it to myself, otherwise I shall get shut up in hospital' . . . After an excited period the same patient said: 'It is all absolutely nothing, a fata morgana; I only believe what I see. That is the right principle for nowadays.' Another patient when reproached said: 'I can do that, you see I am mad'.

Although such utterances lead one to expect a far-reaching insight, the patients in fact have none. They are convinced of the reality of their delusional contents and at the same time draw no consequences from their apparent insight. They have merely learnt what psychiatrists and other people think and turn out appropriate phrases which to them are quite meaningless.

### (e) *The determination to fall ill*

Through self-reflection an individual can *see* himself, *judge* himself and *mould* himself. But there are forces which work in the other direction. The individual would like to be transparent, and *not see* himself, he would like to deceive himself and veil reality. In the morbid sphere we find a determination to be ill, *an instinctive drive towards illness* and in opposition to this the *inner obligation to keep well*. The will *can interfere* with the psyche which it may darken or illumine, inhibit or yield to, inflate in some respect or repress in another.

When the individual is ill, there are all these various possibilities open to him in so far as a state of illness is not only an objective biological condition but a subjective state as well, in the form of an awareness of illness. This latter is not merely something that happens alongside the illness, the mere reflection of it in consciousness, but it is an effective factor which is an actual link in the morbid state itself.

Objective physical illnesses run a typical course: there is a feeling of discomfort or of general disturbance not yet accepted as an illness. The judgment 'I am ill' arises in the setting of a radical reorientation of the vital self-awareness. This is due to the collapse of the patient's capacity to perform which forces him to stop work or seek medical opinion. What up to then had only been something irksome and did not really count now becomes an important symptom and a justified object of attention. The individual tends to the 'either-or'. Is he well or sick? If he decides he is well, then he should not worry over his irksome symptom, but if he thinks he is ill his discomforts and failing performance justify him in expecting to be treated with consideration, nursed and cured. When there are not only manifest physical illnesses but also a rich interplay of somatic and psychic symptoms and phenomena, the patient's basic attitude can sometimes be of decisive importance for the whole course which the morbid somatic phenomena take.

An attitude of 'not bothering about it' and of 'self-control' in the maintenance of normal life is the direct opposite of *being overpowered* by somatic illness and of that *completely unnoticed surrender* to illness, which appears almost as a *purposive determination to be ill*. Patients want sympathy, want to create a sensation or evade some obligation, want to get a pension or enjoy certain fantasy pleasures. Determination and surrender of this sort play a great part in neurotic illnesses as well as in the development of pseudologia phantastica (self-credited, fantastic lying, linked with apparently consequential behaviour) and other hysterical phenomena. After an initial phase of deliberate behaviour such patients are rapidly mastered by the illness against their will. The illness takes its own course (prison-psychoses, for example). One can also give in to manic excitement, one can foster it or manage to control it to a moderate degree.

We find people who have a need to be ill. When anything morbid appears, they will foster it and instinctively say 'yes' to it, though consciously they ask for medical treatment and cure. Their illness becomes the main content of their life, a means of playing a part, calling on others' services, gaining advantage or evading the demands of reality. Generally formulated, we may say that these people are *determined that events for which they are accountable and in which they are understandably concerned shall be taken as mere casual happenings, for which they themselves are entirely irresponsible.* For other people there is the necessity to be healthy at all costs and to be regarded as healthy. They would rather try to blame themselves than feel they are in the grip of some illness. They do not allow nervous phenomena to develop, for instance, because they are continually clearing these up for themselves. They do not want to accept predetermined causal relationships and will try to transform most situations into something understandable, undetermined and something for which they themselves can be held accountable. In abnormal states, if this attitude is taken too far, it may be a relief for them to have to accept something at last as a 'morbid' event.

Where the tendency to be ill has played a part in the development of morbid physical states, a remark of Charcot's becomes most applicable: 'There is a particular *moment between health and sickness* when everything depends on the patient.'

Psychic behaviour undoubtedly influences physical disturbance. Someone receives a distressing telephone message. On putting the receiver down, his hand and arm feel tired. He gets writer's cramp when writing. He ignores it while at work and after sleep, the disturbance vanishes, but it may be preserved and return at the slightest stimulus. A patient feels 'the sensation of something shooting down his arm' whenever he faces some depressing or disadvantageous situation. Möbius reports on a patient with *akinesia algera*, who 'tried to divert his attention forcibly on to something else, as he supposed thinking about his own state would be bad for him. He only failed when going off to sleep and on waking up. He then felt his thoughts rushing into his limbs, as it were, and how these became more sensitive.'

Kretschmer tried to clarify how a more or less definite determination to do so could maintain and develop a transformation into bodily phenomena.[1] We ourselves can see how the same patellar reflex can be strong or weak depending on whether we determine to reinforce it or not. This normal event can again be seen with hysterical phenomena. In the first place there is an acute affective reflex (e.g. trembling all over). At its initial peak it can hardly be suppressed. The intensity of the reflex then recedes and at this point it is readily accessible to voluntary reinforcement. Through habit, it becomes more resistive again and progressively stronger, and finally it cannot be suppressed even with all the will in the world. Volition can strengthen the reflex for the moment and then silently install itself within the reflex through repetition.

*(f) The attitude to one's own illness: its meaning and possible implications*

Kierkegaard wrote the following from his own experience: 'The worst affliction of all is, and continues to be, that one does not know whether one's suffering is an illness of the mind or a sin.'

---

[1] Kretschmer, 'Die Gesetze der willkürlichen Reflexverstärkung in ihrer Bedeutung für des Hysterie- u. Simulationsproblem', *Z. Neur.*, vol. 40. p. 354. Kretschmer works out a connection very well but we do not have to make it an absolute and deny the existence of hysteria.

The crude psychopathological categories which we use to classify and apprehend our subject-matter do not penetrate to human fundamentals. The individual has an original source from which he takes his start and which enables him to detach himself from all that happens to him or overcomes him, or that, in so far as he detaches himself from it, is not he. His 'Anlage', sex, race, age, illness—even if it be schizophrenia—are all in some way he himself, in so far as he is inextricably tied to them all. But he can also confront every one of them; he can adopt an attitude in face of them and instead of identifying with them ('this is just how I am'), he can make them his business and by so doing for the first time fulfil what he actually is in himself. He then has to understand this reality of his, interpret it, get to know its content by bringing out the meaning of the given facts. He must question what Nature has added and what comes from him, he must ask what is meaningless and what may be meaningful and what are the actual functions he is given to fulfil. This interpretation that understands and appropriates meaning can never end. The knowledge which we have that is objective and compelling has only limited extent and beyond this the individual's comprehension and attitude towards himself make endless progression. Those categories and images of human existence which are derived from the human world put the individual on the track but the mode of his behaviour goes beyond the explicit knowledge of the moment. It is linked with his essence in a way that cannot be objectified and is the whole that arises from what is given, understood and created, and the manner of its rising is something that no observer can unearth: there may be refusal or self-limitation, love or hatred for one's own foundations, methodical self-discipline bent only on giving form and shape or an inner behaviour whereby man meets himself at last through his own contriving.

If we keep this brief sketch of the basic situation of human life before us, we have to accept the possibility—only rare cases show it clearly—of extremely meaningful behaviour, produced by the vicissitudes of an individual's historical existence, being exhibited by cases which we have initially taken as schizophrenics; this is all our science was able to see and we discover we have reached the limits of our knowledge. What we have called the attitude of the patient to his illness contains a polarity: *objective knowledge* on the one hand, relating to the morbid process, and on the other a *comprehending appropriation of it*, related to the foundations of the patient's own true existence. The objective knowledge is identical in meaning with medical knowledge. The patient may read books or be a psychiatrist himself and apply scientific concepts. But the '*appropriation*' is by contrast an act which is meaningful only in the midst of an in-between existence, which unfolds all the more plainly the more complete the knowledge happens to be. As scientists we should guard against making the average our measure for everyone. The possibilities that are universal in man as man lie hidden and hardly appreciable and only seek expression in rare cases. Existence itself provides the limits for human knowledge and from it arises that element in the individual which confronts each illness as something other than itself but yet identifies itself simultaneously with what we commonly call the 'morbid' contents. The constant search for meaning, interpretation and inclusion, in respect of everything that seems objectively founded in the disease process, does not immediately signify lack of insight into the illness. Kierkegaard went to the doctor 'as a gesture to human institutions' and presumably also out of the urge to be fully and compellingly persuaded that he could accept as an illness what he had considered to be his sins. He was of course deeply disappointed. Presumably medical categories were as much related to what he was experiencing as the speech of Hottentots to platonic philosophy. It would have been no different in principle if he had been confronted with a psychopathology of the highest conceptual level. The secret contact with God, experienced in all seriousness and in clear conscious- ness, and in a way in which there could be no knowledge of what God said or intended, is not something to be juggled away in the form of a scientific know- ledge of some natural event.

The psychopathologist, however, is always left with knowledge of this marginal nature. He is acting counter to reason should he postulate a funda- mental change in Existence itself rather than some disease process which he could confirm empirically. Existence itself cannot be touched by the know- ledge or experience of psychopathology.[1]

---

[1] It would be extremely interesting to have a thorough knowledge of the phenomena in cases where there is self-interpretation and in which existential and therefore religious motivations play a part. We know little of Kierkegaard's contact with the doctors. Nietzsche's conception of himself in the context of his illness is fairly informative (reported in my *Nietzsche*, pp. 93–9). In the psychiatric literature see Gaupp, 'Ein cyclothymer Psychiater über seine seelischen Krankheits- zeiten', *Z. Neur.*, vol. 166, p. 705.

# CHAPTER VIII

# THE TOTALITY OF THE MEANINGFUL CONNECTIONS

## (CHARACTEROLOGY—CHARAKTEROLOGIE)

### § 1. DEFINING THE CONCEPT

It is always of first importance in psychopathology that we should make unequivocal use of well-defined concepts. No concept, however, has to carry so many meanings or is put to such multiple use as the concept of personality or character.

### (a) *What personality really is*

We see the personality in the particular way an individual expresses himself, in the way he moves, how he experiences and reacts to situations, how he loves, grows jealous, how he conducts his life in general, what needs he has, what are his longings and aims, what are his ideals and how he shapes them, what values guide him and what he does, what he creates and how he acts. In short, personality is the term we give to the *individually differing and characteristic totality of meaningful connections* in any one psychic life. Within this we now have to to make a number of distinctions:

1. *Personality does not include everything meaningful.* For example, the way in which a sudden sense-perception attracts attention is a matter for general understanding and without relevance to personality, so too with the fascinating power of anything new, etc. Nor do we include in the personality any of those psychic connections which we look at *in isolation* and which *do not carry any meaning on* into the total context but are handled as separate fragments though we may well look at them from within, for their own sake. We just say that all such events have something impersonal about them, even though we understand their meaning. Where the psychic life consists exclusively of such fragments, as in fully developed psychoses, we do not speak of personality at all (though we may still notice something essentially individual in the background of the acute events, showing in the perplexity and the unexpectedly clear judgments).

The psyche, so far as we take it in general as *consciousness and experience,* is not the individual personality but simply the universality of every psychic existence. Personality or character first come into being through the complex unity of content in any one individual.

2. *A totality of meaningful connections does not always mean personality.* For example, an idiot may run away from some terrifying object. We under-

stand this and form some over-all picture of the meaningful connections in his psychic life, yet we hardly conceive of him as a personality. For an individual to be a personality he must have some *feeling of himself*, some *sense of the self as an individual*. We do not mean by this the abstract self-awareness which accompanies all psychic events in identical fashion but a sense of self that is aware of its own particular self in all its historical identity. This is *personality-awareness* as opposed to mere sense of identity. There is no personality without self-awareness. Characterology ends at the lower levels of psychic life, where the self-aware personality also ends. Animal characterology, whether of types or individuals (as with chimpanzees) is of a fundamentally different order. It is an analogous understanding of different types and modes of behaviour of which the creatures themselves are quite unaware.

3. *Not every individual variation is to be ascribed to personality*, and not those individual variations of the psycho-physical apparatus which form the substrate of the personality. Capacity for performance, memory-power, fatiguability, learning ability, etc., every such basic characteristic of the psycho-physical mechanisms, talents and intelligence, in short, all the working-tools of personality which condition its development but are not the personality itself, have to be kept rigidly separate if we want to differentiate within the personality the aspects that have no understandable meaning and the meaningful connections themselves. The close connection between intelligence and personality, even if it is of a reciprocal nature, should not lead us to regard them both as one. Intelligence is a working-tool and we test, measure and assess its power according to its performance. Personality is a connection in the self, aware of itself. The former is passive material, the latter is personal activity moulding this material according to the personal interests, aims and moods. The former is a precondition which makes personality possible in the first place and permits it to develop. The latter is a force which puts the tools to work and if they were not so used they would only deteriorate. The concept of dementia or mental defect as generally current relates to destruction of intelligence *and* personality.

Summarising we can say: personality is constituted from psychic events and manifestations in so far as these point beyond themselves to a single, fully understandable context, which is experienced as such by an individual who is clearly conscious of his own particular self.

## (b) How personality comes into being

So far in our remarks personality or character has been conceived as something which is as it is. It has been there from birth onwards and essentially does not change but only reveals itself, it becomes aware of itself but does not produce itself. This however is only one aspect, which may mislead. Personality is just as much a *development with its consequences*, and attains *reality in the world* through every kind of situation and through the opportunities and objectives that spring therefrom. Personality has an historical basis

and is a *self-creation* of man in time. It is not merely the expression of something that has always been as it is, manifesting itself in time. In this sense
personality only shows itself in the life-history, in as much as this takes in
the whole course of the individual's life with all its possibilities and decisions.

Thinking about personality therefore is full of ambiguities as with all
psychology of meaningful connection. In so far as it affirms *that something is
so*, it turns into knowledge; in so far as it throws light on *what can be*, it works
as a call to freedom.

*(c) The understandable personality and its opposite:*

As our knowledge of meaning grows we are forced up against the non-
understandable. At any given moment the totality of meaningful connections
is grounded in the non-understandable. From the external point of view, the
non-understandable is the *reality of the world* which advances on each individual and determines his life from birth through what it gives or withholds,
demands or lets pass. From the inward point of view it is the biologically
given *Anlage* on the one hand and on the other it is the *freedom* of the individual
as potential 'Existence itself'. This latter is not an object for knowledge nor can
it be investigated, and as psychologists and psychopathologists we only catch
a glimpse of the individual, in so far as he becomes an object for our investigation. The non-understandable element, which is the carrier into actuality of
everything understandable, we try to grasp as something biological.

1. The meaningful connections, instinctual activities, emotional drives,
reactions, acts, aims and ideals always call for the additional construct of an
*Anlage* which manifests itself in these actual conscious psychic events and
their expression. We also call this Anlage personality. By so doing we mean
to convey the extra-conscious disposition that underlies the totality of the
meaningful connections. This will indicate that, although the personality-
Anlage is wholly understandable in its manifest connections, we cannot understand it in its actual existence as a whole, and as such it has to be explained, for
example, by the laws of heredity and grasped as a constitutional entity.

2. That underlying factor of personality which we call its *freedom* is not
an object but a limiting factor in personality research. We may say that one
individual is a 'personality' and that another is not. Such statements are
philosophical assessments and not empirical findings. They are meant to convey that the *truth of Existence itself* seems present in the person. Philosophically we may be able to throw some light on what are then the possibilities
but we can gain no empirical knowledge of their actuality. From the ideas of
Existence itself we can build ideals which philosophically we at once dismiss
as false. By the expression 'personality' we are perhaps conceiving some ideal
of maximum unity as a maximum wealth of particulars in the individual, and
he approximates to this ideal unity all the time as he adapts to the actual
circumstances of his life. Consistent thought and action, coherence, and
reliability are all attributes of this ideal personality. Personality is then

evaluated in terms of the consistent thinker, of the individual with a resolute and consistent will, or an artistic style of life. So we come to speak of different types of ideal personality, for example the sage, saint or hero. But none of these concepts of personality concern us here.

Not only from the philosophical point of view but also in the interests of research we should be fully aware of the limits set to our investigations when we are confronted with the human individual. There are no prohibitions on research, it is true, and we must try to grasp whatever we can in fact grasp, confirm, examine and investigate. But we shall come to grief in our enquiry and go astray whenever we think we know too much or consider we can know the whole or the fundamentals. Where science is baffled radically, investigators may then know that they are entering an area where they no longer confront mankind as scientists but as mere fellow-men. The individual as 'Existence itself' is more than the totality of his meaningful connections and more than the sum of his biological Anlage. All our attempts to define the concept of personality or character have something in common. Personality is always something *inconclusive* and points on to *something else*. In subject-matter the psychology of meaningful connections remains mid-way between all the modes of the non-understandable, yet this only becomes manifest in fact through its operations. Accordingly, the personality which we understand points in the first place to the non-understandable from which it has arisen, that is the *constitution* and all kinds of biological determinants, and in the second place points to the non-understandable which the ever-changing personality both manifests and serves, that is *Existence itself*, the transcendental source and eternal goal of man. In personality we do not see any final Being-as-such, an end in itself. Empirically it can be at times the totality of what is understandable but always in such a way that something remains in the person whereby what is empirically extremely improbable always remains possible. At any moment freedom can have birth and give everything a different meaning. The personality as understood is not what an individual actually is but an empirical and inconclusive phenomenon. What an individual really is himself is his very Existence in the face of Transcendence, and neither of these are ever a subject for scientific enquiry. Existence itself cannot be grasped as personality but it reveals itself in different personalities, which in themselves can never be final.

## § 2. METHODS OF PERSONALITY-ANALYSIS

Analysis of personality has been practised throughout the years by psychologists, others who study mankind, philosophers and psychiatrists, all making use of similar concepts and similar methods.[1] These various efforts at personality-study differ from the biographical approach to personality in that they

[1] Analysis of personality (characterology) is an ancient pursuit: e.g. Theophrastus, *Characters*. Cp. also Bruno, *Das literarische Porträt der Griechen* (Berlin, 1896). Kant, *Anthropologie*. J. Bahnsen, *Beiträge zur Charakterologie* (Leipzig, 1867), 2 vols. (He is the author of the term

try to find out something *typical* that can be given a general formulation. The biographer on the other hand is confronted with the unending task of comprehending a concrete personality and here personality-study may help him to a certain extent. The business of personality-study then is to discriminate the types, the schemata which, in contrast to the concrete personality, stand out plain and clear no matter how they ramify, and it makes use of these, wherever possible, to give some conceptual form to the whole vast range of personality formation in human beings.

Each personality has an infinite reality and potentiality. At any given moment it is the form taken by its own historical contents, a form that has been shaped by fate, calling, function and effective participation in the actual cultural heritage. Thus man in his concrete and complex unity becomes subject-matter for the humanities and social sciences and is not even exhaustible by them. Our conceptual psychological analysis can only offer relatively crude means of orientation. We will now present the methods of such analysis:

## (a) *Awareness of the possibilities of verbal description*

Language provides enormous resources on which to draw for the characterisation of human nature. Klages counted four thousand words in German that denote something psychic and concern aspects of personality, and he is certainly right in pointing out how the infinitely fine nuances of these various terms have got lost in the ordinary usage of the words and have to be rescued deliberately. Whereas the psychologist finds difficulty in securing sufficient terms for dealing with psychic mechanisms, he is here embarrassed with abundance and has difficulty in finding those differentiations of personality which can be taken as really fundamental and profound. No constructed system of personality characteristics is possible which will be comprehensive and generally valid. We can only work through the available analyses and appropriate to ourselves the language of poets and thinkers and in this way achieve some psychological grasp through direct understanding. Only so shall we learn to formulate what we have grasped and these efforts will help us to be flexible, cautious and free of bias. We can make ourselves aware of the way in which language, although in fact it works without any system, is itself permeated by an inexhaustible host of potential systematisations. Language usually holds an unnoticed sway in every psychiatric description—whether meagre or full—and ranges through all the dimensions of social, ethical and aesthetic assessments, quantitative assessments too, as well as the concepts of

'charakterologie'.) Klages, *Prinzipien der Charakterologie* (Leipzig, 1910); 7th and 8th edns., 1936, with the title *Grundlagen der Charakterkunde*. Cp. also p. 262 with its references to the psychology of meaning and p. 221 with references to the study of physiognomy and the theory of expression. There is an extensive and varied literature on this, degenerating into triviality, credulity, quackery and mere enthusiasm, which has increased in quantity since 1920. So far we have no clear, unambiguous science of characterology—or scientific study of personality. There is no method but a conglomeration of all sorts of interests besides scientific ones. Paul Helwig, *Charakterologie* (Leipzig, 1936), gives a good critical review.

the psychology of expression and physiognomy. To be aware of language is a continual reminder of the infiniteness of human nature.

The art of characterisation and personality analysis cannot be methodologically defined nor learnt but it depends on this mastery of language and therefore, at any given time, on the current cultural trends. It will change with general values and modes of thought and in particular with the range of possible human experience.

(b) *The concepts of personality-study are those of the psychology of meaningful connection*

We might say that all psychology of meaningful connection is personality-study, in so far as it concerns itself solely with the connection of what is meaningful in terms of the whole man and tries to grasp the particular quality of an individual.

According to the basic schema that prevails automatically, the meaningful elements are grounded in certain constant '*properties*'. The personality is then conceived as a sum of these properties or as a meaningful connection between them. Properties constitute the lasting foundation. Particular attitudes are thought to arise from a combination of such properties, and there develops an unending play of properties in combination. This sort of language may be unavoidable but as a conceptual foundation for personality-study it is misleading. It robs the personality of movement and, even more important, it removes the dialectic of opposites in everything meaningful.

Suppose we wanted to understand complete personalities as a *combination of properties* and therefore would like to know which properties we should understand as predetermined opposites, which properties were to be understood as linked with which and which were mutually exclusive, we should be landed with some remarkable experiences and learn that our aim was impossible. In every psychology of meaningful connection each contrasting pole is equally understandable and correspondingly the opposites are bound directly to each other. All living that is meaningful functions in opposites. The matter of our understanding dies, as it were, once it has been unilaterally and exclusively fixated at the one pole only. The power of living lies in uniting the opposites, in overcoming them through integration and not in a limited unilateralism. Courage lies in the overcoming of fear and he who has nothing to fear is no longer courageous.

As a result of this basic relationship of the contrasting poles, all the ideal types of 'properties' and personalities that have been constructed tend to fall into *pairs of opposites*. Whereas empirical personality-study of the individual in his unceasing development may at any time confirm Goethe's saying, 'he is no closely wrought ingenious book but a man with his contradictions', the theoretical constructs, on which empirical research depends, are wholly characterised by such contrasting poles. This means however that these constructs are not actual personality-types but constructs of ideal types whereby at times we are helped to understand certain connections. They concern perspectives of understanding, not material being. Such personality constructs, therefore, as have been achieved remain inconclusive so far as human reality is concerned. They are not final diagnoses of a man's quality but a challenge to everyone who would understand others as well as himself to look to the freedom of the potential self. A quality that is absolute in the sense of being finally established always denotes we have reached the limits of our understanding. The quality of a man can never be stated with absolute certainty as to the future and, so far as the actual manifestation has gone, can only be fixed in retrospect by ignoring the play of chance and free decision. Personalities are never whole and conclusive. If they were, they would be without life and potentiality, one-sided and stultified, grown into an automaton.

Thinking about personality therefore returns us via the 'ad hoc' assumptions about 'properties' to the fusion of these in meaningful movement. The turning of qualitative being into something with properties will however always remain a basic shortcoming of personality-study.

## (c) Typology as a method

If we think of a property as something lasting, understandable in its manifestations, in modes of reaction and expression and the general behaviour of the individual, we are in process of developing a type. We form the property and all its consequences into a construct and viewing it as a whole recognise it as something obviously connected. If we then make one or several such properties the basis of a comprehensive totality and proceed to apply it to the person as a whole, noticing the meaningful connection between this and what the individual experiences and does, we are in the process of designing a personality-type.

Such types remain *ideal types* even if we have conceived them from our scrutiny of real people. Their general nature is revealed through the individual, it is not arrived at by deduction or abstraction, but duly perceived by omitting everything that does not belong. They do not come into being as statistical averages but remain purely formal. They only occur in reality as approximate forms, as classical borderline cases. Their truth rests on the inner connectedness of the meaningful whole; their reality, except in the rare borderline case, rests on the fragmentary emergence of the type which is limited in reality by other factors, not to be understood in terms of the type, which cannot therefore exert sole influence.

Every type is of universal application. But individuals lend themselves more or less readily to various types. The types are mutually related in such a way that contrasting types do not exclude each other in the actual individual but are bound directly to each other.

Thus the whole meaning of types makes it impossible for any one individual to be sufficiently characterised by any single type. What corresponds more or less to a type in the concrete individual is always only one aspect of his nature. This is indeed clarified by the attempt at classification but it still does not suffice to describe the man as a whole.

'Type' carries quite another meaning when the term is used to convey a *real type* as against an ideal type. The reality of the type then rests on something that is not understandable, a biological source, a constitutional factor. As a result the type can only be established by making correlations of frequency and can only be partly understood.

Intermediate between the ideal and the real type lie *descriptions of character* based on experience. These have acquired a certain validity for the time being though the principles on which they rest are not really clear.

## § 3. ATTEMPTS AT BASIC CLASSIFICATION OF CHARACTER

Faced with the various classifications of personality we get an impression of endlessness. Almost every fresh contributor thinks he has grasped the essentials of human nature. He sets out his schema rather dogmatically and at first tends to convince uncritical readers. But there is a considerable difference in the various classifications according to the writer's cultural level, the vividness of his observations and in particular the depth of his metaphysics with which are linked his initial presuppositions about human nature. To represent all that has been thought in this field would need some historical account of the various human types which those who study personality have created. In every age certain forms intrude into the current philosophy as essential forms of human life, usually as ideal figures of good and bad, examples of contrasting ideals. We shall only remind the reader here of the enormous literature which embodies such ways of thought, and set out below what seems to be of general importance in all this:

### (a) Single, individual forms

In the first place we have what constitutes the unfailing foundation of all personality-study, that is, the vivid perception of individual forms, which imprint themselves unforgettably on the memory and live on in our imagination. Figures from poetry, historical figures whose biographies are known, living people we have met, are all indispensable for us to keep in mind. This wealth of inner vision, which is there long before concepts arise but is remarkably fruitful, is a precondition for any thinking about personality and every psychopathologist needs to widen and deepen this vision constantly.

Scientific knowledge enters with the tendency to conceptualise and introduce some systematic order, along with the tendency to methodical comparison of ideas and experience. Systematic classifications are of several kinds: *ideal types*, general systems of *personality-structure*, and the setting up of *real types*.

## (b) Ideal types

Typologies which are systems of ideal types outline the personality possibilities in a vast number of *polarities*: self-assertion and submissiveness, happy and sad, extravert and introvert, etc. This schema of opposites appears without exception in all typologies of personality.

The intention is to give pairs of opposites as precisely as possible, define their meaning and distinguish them and keep them apart from human reality. Most important of all, the opposing pairs are not allowed to flow together and be submerged in one contrasting unity.[1] To be ideal, a typology of personality would first have to make a systematic classification of all the possible polarities once they had been precisely defined, a mathematics, as it were, of the meaningful; after this was done it could go on to limitless empirical analysis.

The simple schema of opposites becomes more refined if the meaningful 'properties' ramify out into other dimensions from a single polarity. For example, polarities have been conceived where both poles have a positive value, e.g. frugality and generosity, and there are deviations from both poles, e.g. meanness and prodigality. Or in some systems, a Mean is conceived lying between two extremes, something moderate, genuine and life-enhancing. This in turn is either conceived of as undialectical, an unequivocal quantity avoiding the extreme, or dialectical, i.e. a comprehensive unity with inner tensions and including the extremes within itself as constant possibilities for deviation.

It becomes clear that in all these constructs of ideal types, the types that seek to be comprehensive and make a synthesis cannot be accurately described at any time, while the single type-polarities are unambiguous and clear. But this lack of ambiguity is bought at a price, namely that the single type has to be a deficiency-type and the single, well-defined characteristic acquires a negative value, run aground as it were, and what has become the manifest characteristic is nothing else but a human failing.

## (c) Personality-structure in general

*Klages* made the most effective attempt to bring some order into personality-structure. His study of personality outstrips all the previous efforts. He differentiated between purely formal characteristics of personality, which he termed the *personality-structure*, and what he called the *personality-qualities*, including the instincts, drives and interests.

Within the *personality-structure* three distinctions are drawn:

1. The *tempo* of emotional excitability, i.e. the duration of the emotional wave, the strength of the reactivity. These constitute differences of 'temperament' and there are fluctuations between phlegmatic and sanguine.

---

[1] Psychiatric attempts to create a personality-classification suffer I think from creating *only one* pair of opposites, which then have to contain much heterogeneous material and become confusing although the central theory may be quite clear. Jung, C. G. *Psychologische Typen* (Zürich, Rascher, 1921); Kretschmer, E. *Körperbau u. Charakter* (Berlin, 1921).

TOTALITY OF MEANINGFUL CONNECTIONS 437

2. The predominant *prevailing mood*. This fluctuates between melancholic and euphoric, between dyskolos and eukolos.

3. The *formal properties of volition*. There are fluctuations here between strength and weakness of will. Strength of will appears as an active force in all forms of energy and spontaneous action and as a passive strength in perseverance, tenacity, resistance and, reactively, in obstinacy and stubbornness.

Klages then proceeds to contrast these three structural forms with the *personality-quality*, its substance or essential content as it were. This he terms the system of *mainsprings* (the personality in the narrower sense as against temperament, prevailing mood and formal disposition of the will-power). This is the personality proper. It contains a polarity. Instincts are confronted by the will, conscious goals and purposes are set against the gratifications groped for by the instincts and, alongside the qualities of the world that are merely felt, there are consciously recognised and judged values. On the one hand there are contents, the material out of which the personality is forged, and on the other hand is the will which gives these contents form, inhibits, fosters or suppresses them but cannot add anything to them. The will, from the way it is experienced, always implies an element of control, self-maintenance, awareness and activity. But in all the instinctual drives there is an element of simple permissiveness, self-surrender, unawareness and passivity. On the side of the will and the drive to self-maintenance we find reason (realism, discrimination, sense of duty, conscience) and egoism (acquisitiveness, ambition, caution, craft). On the side of instinctual life and self-surrender we find enthusiasm (drive for knowledge, love of truth, thirst for beauty, love) and the passions (greed, lust for power, sexual drive, revenge).[1]

Klages also most skilfully constructed a number of ideal personality-types lying outside this personality-structure. They are more concrete and truer to life than the theoretical structure which is simply an aid to reasoning when one is trying to classify. The great variety of ideal types is due to the many perspectives according to which man as a whole can be understood. Klages started from basic mood and sensibility, from the tempo and inner tensions of psychic life, from will-power and the mainsprings of the drives and their specific hierarchy.

In contrast to all this, as a last perspective, Klages takes the mode of operation whereby an individual becomes aware of his own self through *reflection*. The personality develops passively out of a given *Anlage* and over against this is the personality that develops reflectively, through the work an individual does on himself and through his own inner activity.

But every analysis of personality halts at the point where man reaches inner superiority over himself and can properly be himself. The individual, who

[1] My exposition does not represent Klages' teaching exactly. He rested everything on his metaphysics, according to which the Will (the spirit) enters life from without as a destroying force, as an absolute devil coming in to the full self-sufficiency of life. 'Personality' only exists in the transitional periods when life is not completely destroyed but in process of being destroyed. Klages' position here is a matter of faith and so cannot be disputed.

becomes matter for his own study without letting this drop to the level of being mere datum or falling himself prey to the devastating effects of reflection, can never be characterised in terms of psychological description.

Once the study of personality starts to pigeonhole people into pure types, it comes to grief. In the first place an individual can never be exhausted by any one type, since this only serves to delineate one aspect of him. In the second place every complete schema of types must be relative, only one out of many possibilities. Thirdly, personality is always part of its own situation which has a host of possibilities that can never be known absolutely. The personality is always in development and can never be sealed off. Speaking scientifically and humanly, with living people we cannot draw a line as it were and balance the accounts, so as to discover what a person really is. To circumscribe a personality-disorder (psychopathy) with the 'diagnosis' of a type, is doing violence to the situation and falsifies it. But in simple human terms, to classify and track down someone's personality implies a categorisation which, if we look at it closely, is insulting and makes any further communication impossible. We should not forget this point when we are trying to throw light on matters by conceptualising the human personality.

## (d) Real types

These arise from the restriction which reality imposes. They take advantage of the ideal constructs of what is understandable but as soon as empirical observation enforces the confusing unity of the understandable and its opposite, they abandon the constructs. The weakness of the real types which have been formulated so far is that their reality-basis is in doubt. They compromise between meaningful constructs and theoretical developments from isolated biological observations. They are satisfying in a few classical cases, giving illustrative 'clinical pictures' but since they are inadequate or not applicable in the great mass of cases, they lack universality. There is no systematic classification of them as would befit their origin in given reality. They can only be enumerated. Thus *Kretschmer* devised three personality types, each moving between two poles, between excitable and sluggish (schizothyme), gay and serious (cyclothyme) and explosive and phlegmatic (viscous). The master-concept into which fall these three sets of polarities, fails because one can only enumerate the concrete sources for these meaningful observations. The true significance here is that underlying these real types there is a biological reality which one day we may be able to grasp (cp. the chapter on constitution). Such a reality as this is quite different from the phenomenon, since in the last resort the phenomenon can be there without the reality as we conceive it. For instance, Luxenburger only accepts schizoid personality-disorders (psychopaths) as such when there is evidence of some blood-relationship with a schizophrenic. There are also schizoid personality-disorders (psychopaths) where this hereditary position does not apply. 'Kretschmer's types if seen in biological proximity to schizophrenics, manic-depressives or hereditary epileptics can only be regarded as genetypically related to these hereditary illnesses.'

## § 4. NORMAL AND ABNORMAL PERSONALITIES

There is no simple answer to the question when and why personalities are abnormal. We have to bear in mind that, speaking generally, 'abnormal' is not a matter of statement but an evaluation. The facts themselves give rise to this evaluation where the personality is considered as the totality of the meaningful connections. Personality characteristics vary according to the *degree of unity* or the amount of scatter in the meaningful elements in a given individual. The more scattered and disconnected these elements are the more abnormal the individual. Alternatively we observe that everything meaningful in the given unity achieves a certain *equilibrium and harmony* which together form a whole, then the more disharmony there is and the less equilibrium the more abnormal the individual (déséquilibré). Or we pay attention to the *polarities and their synthesis* in meaningful living and then the more one-sided the expression is the more abnormal we find it. These, however, are all extremely general points of view, so that we never find the norm fully expressed in any single individual.

The systematic principles indicated in the above paragraph are only to help in the actual perception and representation of exceptional personalities. They are not the source from which such perception and representation derive. Valuable results are obtained in psychopathology through types created by the intuitions of those who investigate and give us impressive and unforgettable delineations of personality that we can recognise. These personality-types are potentially innumerable and they are real types, designed with the help of a number of ideal types. We can only enumerate them, group them and use them as illustrative examples. This is a matter for special psychiatry, and we will comment briefly as follows:

We distinguish *two kinds of real types:* 1. Abnormal personalities, that simply represent dispositions which deviate from average and appear as *extreme variations* of human nature. 2. Personalities that are genuinely ill, where a change has taken place in their previous *Anlage* as a result of some additional *process*.

## I. VARIATIONS OF HUMAN NATURE[1]

Variations of human nature that deviate from the average cannot be called sick as such. Nor do we usually call the least common variations particularly abnormal. In practice we more often investigate those which come within the orbit of clinics and consulting rooms. 'Personality-disorder' (psychopathic personality) is the term which we use in this connection for all those 'who

[1] Attention should be drawn to the oldest and most basic of psychiatric contributions: J. L. A. Koch, *Die psychopathischen Minderwertigkeiten* (Ravensburg, 1891–3). Then to Kurt Schneider, *Die psychopathischen Persönlichkeiten*, 4th edn. (Vienna, 1940). Here there is clear orientation, unprejudiced views and ready access to the entire literature.

suffer from their abnormality or whose abnormality makes society suffer' (Kurt Schneider).

Classification according to the basic concept which characterises the group gives us the following: 1. *Variants of basic personality-disposition* which Klages differentiated according to the 'personality-structure'. 2. Variations of a supposed biological substratum which has been termed *'psychic energy'*. 3. Variants induced by the basic dialectic of all the meaningful elements, the dialectic of *self-reflection* (self-reflective personality-types).

## (a) Variations in the basic personality-dispositions

1. *Basic dispositions of temperament*.[1] An abnormally excitable temperament (*sanguine*) reacts quickly and in lively fashion to every kind of influence, it lights up immediately but excitement dies down equally fast. The individual leads a restless life, and likes extremes. We get a picture of vivacious exuberance or of an irritable, troubled hastiness, a restless psyche with a tendency to extremes. The opposite pole is then a *phlegmatic* temperament. Nothing moves this individual out of his peaceful placidity. He hardly reacts at all and when he does, he does so very slowly with prolonged after-effects.

An abnormally cheerful (*euphoric*) individual bubbles over happily. He is blissfully light-hearted about everything that happens to him and is contented and confident. The happy mood brings a certain excitement with it, including motor-excitement. A *depressive* on the other hand takes everything hard, his mood is always clouded, he sees the worst of everything and tends to keep quiet and immobile.

2. *Basic will-power*.[2] Basic powers of will differ greatly from one man to another, independently of drive or content. *Weak-willed* individuals make any effort of will with much difficulty. They tend to let everything slide. Those who have *no will-power at all*, the drifters, simply echo any influence that impinges on them. They cannot resist and follow wherever they are led by opportunity or other people for better or worse. They may make a show of momentary energy but never stick at anything unless an unchanging environment keeps them to it. Otherwise they follow every fresh impulse evoked by a world that constantly transforms them. They change colour with their environment. *Strong-willed* individuals bring unusual energy and perseverance to all that they do. Their activity pushes everything else aside with a relentless assertiveness. It is as if they could not shake anyone's hand without crushing it, or take up a cause without realising it.

3. *Basic dispositions of feeling and drive*. An individual's nature is most decisively determined by the complexity or the poverty of his drives. Abnormal variations in the quality of the personality proper, of the whole system of instinctual and emotional dispositions, are more profoundly important for the

---

[1] Kretschmer gives an admirable portrait, *Körperbau u. Charakter*, 2nd edn. (1936), pp. 118–35.
[2] Birnbaum, *Die krankhafte Willensschwäche* (Wiesbaden, 1911). E. Grassel, *Die Willensschwäche* (Leipzig, 1937).

nature of the personality than all the other variations in structure, temperament and will-power. There is a more definite cleavage here between people with different dispositions than anywhere else. The most frequently investigated of these well-marked personality-variants is that of *'moral insanity'* (Kurt Schneider's 'affectionless' or 'unfeeling' psychopath). This term has been used to describe personalities who come at the end of a series of transitional states and exhibit the characteristics of the 'born criminal' to an extreme or rare degree.[1] They strike us as strange creatures, highly exceptional in many ways: their destructive drives are unaccompanied by any sensitivity for what is right, they are insensible to the love of family or friends, they show a natural cruelty alongside isolated displays of feeling that seem strange in the context (e.g. a love of flowers), they have no social impulses, dislike work, are indifferent to others' and their own future, enjoy crime as such and their self-assurance and belief in their own powers is unshakeable. They are completely ineducable and impervious to influence.

Another such type is the *fanatic* who devotes himself wholly to a single cause and is blind to everything else. He does this so unconditionally that he will unconsciously risk his whole existence on its behalf. Credulous belief, the exaggeration of some isolated purpose out of all context is a special interest of their existence. They are driven, harried people who get a specific and agonising pleasure from their identification with some solitary cause. Kurt Schneider differentiates the *'combative fanatic'* (aggressive fanatic) from the *'damped-down or more reserved fanatic'*. The former will assert their rights or their supposed rights and are 'querulants'. The latter merely tend to demonstrate and nurse their convictions. They are the born sectarians, cranks and representatives of esoteric doctrines for which they live with an inner self-assurance and proud contempt for everyone else.[2]

*(b) Variations in psychic energy (the neurasthenic and the psychasthenic)*

We speak of neurasthenic and psychasthenic syndromes. They may be characterised perhaps as follows:

1. *The neurasthenic syndrome*[3] is defined by 'irritable weakness'. There is on the one hand exceptional irritability and sensitivity, a painful sensibility and abnormal responsiveness to stimuli of all kinds. On the other hand we find abnormally quick fatiguability and slow recuperation. Fatigue is subjectively

---

[1] Longard, *Arch. Psychiatr.* (D), vol. 43. F. Scholz, *Die moralische Anästhesie* (Leipzig, 1904). Dubitscher, *Z. Neur.*, vol. 154 (1936), p. 422. Binswanger, *Über den moralischen Schwachsinn mit besonderer Berücksichtung der kindlichen Altersrufen* (Berlin, 1905).

[2] Kolle, 'Über Querulanten', *Arch. Psychiatr.* (D), vol. 95 (1931), p. 24. Stertz, 'Verschrobene Fanatiker', *Berl. klin. Wschr.*, vol. 1 (1919). Grohmann, *Die Vegeterieransiedlung in Ascona* (Halle, 1904). 'Ein soziales Sondergebilde auf psychopathischer Grundlage', *Psychiatr.-neur. Wschr.*, vol. 1 (1904). Kreuser, 'Über Sonderlinge', *Psychiatr.-neur. Wschr.*, vol. 1 (1913–14).

[3] Beard, *Die Nervenschwäche* (D), (Leipzig, 1883). Möbius, *Zur Lehre von der Nervosität. Neurol. Beiträge. Heft. 2* (Leipzig, 1894). Krafft-Ebing, *Nervosität u. neurasthenische Zustände* (Vienna, 1899). Müller, *Handbuch der Neurasthenie* (Leipzig, 1893). Binswanger, *Die Neurasthenie* (Jena, 1896). Bumke's *Handbuch*, vol. 5.

strongly felt. There are innumerable discomforts and pains, a dull feeling in the head, everything seems affected and the patient feels battered with intense feelings of fatigue and weakness which turn into lasting phenomena. This syndrome covers all those phenomena that are known as sequelae of fatigue, of exhaustion, overwork and excessive effort but no more than these, and provided such phenomena appear after the slightest stimuli or effort or remain as permanent accompaniments through life.

2. The *psychasthenic syndrome*[1] is less easily detected. The phenomena are many and varied and are held together by the theoretical concept of a 'diminution of psychic energy'. The diminution shows itself by a general low level of psychic resistance to experience. The individual prefers to withdraw from his fellows and not be exposed to situations in which his abnormally strong 'complexes' rob him of presence of mind, memory and poise. Self-confidence deserts him. Compulsive thoughts arrest consciousness or chase through it and he is tormented by unfounded fears. Indecision, doubts, phobias, make activity impossible. A host of abnormal psychic and emotional states are scrutinised and analysed by a compulsion-like self-observation. This results unavoidably in an inclination to do nothing and daydream, and this makes all the symptoms worse. There is occasionally a rush of intoxicating happiness from an impression made by personalities that are idolised but imperfectly understood, or by some quite ordinary landscape which suddenly seems most magnificent, but usually this is paid for by a painful relapse into morbid symptoms. The psyche generally lacks an ability to integrate its life or to work through and manage its various experiences; it fails to build up its personality and make any steady development.

On rare occasions syndromes such as these occur as states of genuine exhaustion or as concomitant phenomena of disease processes. (Some of Janet's cases of psychasthenia are obviously in part schizophrenic.) But they are so closely linked with meaningful contents of the individual life-history that they appear more as personality-variants than syndromes, and as such can be characterised by the diminution of psychic energy and in fact are often linked with some somatic and physiological weakness though they may also occur without this.

Thus one could say that all the variations of personality and temperament may occur as psychasthenia. They may be termed this when there is a prominent element of weakness, a lack of energy and a reduction in effectiveness, when drives are weak and faint, emotion less vivid, the will powerless and performance in any direction grows modest. The best way to describe this type is to make use of the analogy of deficient psychic energy. There is no doubt that something of this sort does exist among the congenital variations.

There are a number of peculiar phenomena which in a mild degree are widespread and can at times also occur as symptoms of phasic and other illness but which we are accustomed to call symptoms of personality-disorder when

[1] Janet, *Les obsessions et la psychasthénie*, 2nd edn. (Paris, 1908).

they are both numerous and troublesome and when there is no manifest illness but something like an illness that dominates the individual's whole life. To these belong compulsive phenomena, the carriers of which are called anankasts (on the basis of the uncertainty of the self, according to Kurt Schneider), also depersonalisation and derealisation, etc., the carriers of which are called psychasthenics.

## (c) Reflective personalities

The personalities we have depicted so far may be understood in terms of a constitution which they have always had. The so-called reflective personality is to be distinguished from these as a personality-formation resulting from awareness of self, from attention directed to one's own nature together with the purposive wish to be 'like this or that'. To this group belong, for example:

1. *Hysterics.* In psychiatry the term hysterical has several connotations: physical symptoms (hysterical stigmata), transient abnormal psychic states with altered consciousness (accidents mentaux) and hysterical personality. It is unfortunate that the same term is given to them all, particularly as hysterical personality is ordinarily used to cover very heterogeneous material. Janet rightly says: 'Hysteria can affect all kinds of people, good and bad. We must not ascribe to the illness personality-traits that would have been there anyhow.' Hysterical personality is common enough but it is not always linked with hysterical mechanisms. Moreover, the types of personality which are called hysterical are very varied.[1] To characterise the type more precisely we have to fall back on *one basic trait:* Far from accepting their given dispositions and life opportunities, hysterical personalities crave to appear, both to themselves and others, as more than they are and to experience more than they are ever capable of. The place of genuine experience and natural expression is usurped by a contrived stage-act, a forced kind of experience. This is not contrived 'consciously' but reflects the ability of the true hysteric to live wholly in his own drama, be caught up entirely for the moment and succeed in seeming genuine. All the other traits can be understandably deduced from this. In the end the hysterical personality loses its central 'core' as it were, and consists simply of a number of different exteriors. One drama follows another. As it can no longer find anything within, it looks for everything without. It wants to experience something extraordinary with its natural drives. It does not rely on the normal processes of life but wants to use these for aims that make the simple drive uncertain or get lost altogether. Through unnecessary and exaggerated expressions it tries to convince itself and others of the existence of some intense experience. It is attracted to anything external that offers strong stimulus, to scandal, gossip, famous personalities, anything impressive, extravagant, or extreme in art or outlook. Hysterical personalities have to ensure their own importance and so play a role and try to make themselves interesting every-

[1] Cp. Kraepelin, for his description in his *Lehrbuch*; also Klages, *Die Probleme der Graphologie*, pp. 81 ff.

where even at the expense of their calling or integrity. If unnoticed for even a brief period, or if they feel they somehow do not belong, they grow unhappy. Such situations immediately make them aware of their inner emptiness. They are therefore extremely jealous if others seem to trespass on their own particular position or sphere of influence. If they cannot otherwise succeed, they will get attention by falling ill and playing the part of a martyr, a sufferer. Under some circumstances they will be reckless with themselves and inflict self-injury; they have a wish to be ill, provided they reap the reward of some corresponding effect on others. In order to heighten life and find new ways of making an effect, they will resort to lying, at first quite consciously but soon this becomes unconscious and they come to believe themselves (pseudologia phantastica)[1]: there are self-accusations, accusations against others of invented sexual assaults, a pretence to strangers that they are important personalities, very rich or of high rank, etc. In all this the patients not only deceive others but themselves as well. They lose awareness of their own reality and their fantasy becomes their reality. But there are certain distinctions to be drawn. In one case we find complete unawareness of falsehood—'I did not know I was lying'. In another case we find parallel awareness 'I was lying but could not help myself'.[2] The more the theatrical aspects develop the more these personalities lose any genuine, personal affect. They become unreliable, are no longer capable of enduring emotional relationships and never reach any real depth. All that is left is a stage for imitative and theatrical performances, the perfect artifice of the hysterical personality.

The nature of hysterical personality has long been known to psychologists with understanding. Shaftesbury used to speak of 'enthusiasm that is as it were second-hand'. Feuerbach describes a 'feigned sensibility which seems to tickle the inner senses compellingly with something that is not really felt but only imagined as felt'. 'In such a state the individual tries to deceive himself and others with a mere grimace of feeling, and as this grows habitual he ends by profoundly poisoning his surest source of truth, his inner feeling. Deception, lying, falsehood, treachery and every-thing that goes with it—these are all seeds of enormous growth in a psyche which is used to falsify its own feeling and, moreover, they very easily suffocate any genuine feeling. This explains why a feigned sensibility can be reconciled not only with a definite coldness but with downright cruelty.'

2. *Hypochondriacs.* It is abnormal for the body as such to play an important part in the individual's concern. The healthy person lives his body and does not think about it. He pays no attention to it. The mass of physical suffering is largely due to psychic reflection rather than any manifest physical illness. Excluding what might be due to a labile physical constitution (asthenia) and what are typical somatic accompaniments of psychic events, we find we are left with a whole field of physical suffering which arises from self-observation and

---

[1] Delbrück, *Die pathologische Lüge* (Stuttgart, 1891). Ilberg, *Z. Neur.*, vol. 15 (1913). Stelzner, 'Zur Psychologie der verbrecherischen Renommisten', *Z. Neur.*, vol. 44 (1919), p. 391.

[2] Wendt, *Allg. Z. Psychiatr.*, vol. 68, p. 482.

worry and which steadily increases as the body becomes more and more the centre of an individual's life. Self-scrutiny, expectation and dread, all disorder the bodily functions, give rise to pain and cause sleeplessness. The fear of being ill and the wish to be ill lead to a constant reflection on the body and together turn the conscious life into a life with a sick body. The person is not physically sick but still he is not simulating. He feels he really is sick, that his body has in fact changed and he suffers like any sick person. The 'invalide imaginaire' is in some peculiar way really ill by reason of his own nature.

3. *The self-insecure personalities* (Schneider, whose description I follow here) or the *sensitive personality* (Kretschmer): In these cases a continuously heightened sensibility is imposed on a reflective awareness of insufficiency. The self-insecure individual finds every experience a disturbing one because he experiences it with heightened sensitivity instead of working through it naturally and giving it some appropriate form. In his own eyes his performance is not sufficient. His position vis-à-vis others always seems to him under question. Actual or merely imagined failure becomes a matter for self-accusation. He will look for the fault in himself and does not forgive himself. When working over his experiences inwardly, he does not repress so much as have an extra battle with himself. He leads a life of inner humiliation and defeat brought about by outside experiences and his interpretation of them. The helpless urge to get some external confirmation of this inner grinding self-depreciation makes him see more or less intentional insults in the behaviour of other people. This may reach the degree of delusion-like ideas (without these becoming delusion proper). He suffers immensely from every external slight for which he once more seeks the real reason in himself. Self-insecurity of this sort leads to over-compensation for feelings of inferiority. Compulsive-like formality, which is rigidly adhered to, strict social observances, lordly gesture, exaggerated displays of assurance, are all masks for the inner bondage. Demanding behaviour covers the actual timidity.

## II. Personality-change Due to a Process

We differentiate abnormal personality-types that are *Anlage*-variants, as described above, from sick personalities in the narrower sense, where the change has been brought on by a process. The fact that most mental illness is accompanied by a marked change in personality has given rise to the statement: mental illness is an illness of personality, but we can see mental patients suffering from false perceptions or even delusions, and yet not showing any noticeable change in their personality at this particular stage. Further, we find acute psychoses that lead to total fragmentation of psychic life into a number of unconnected acts where one can no longer speak of a personality at all, yet one can unexpectedly trace the natural, unchanged personality, temporarily veiled, for which one can have empathy. It shows itself in the patient's perplexity and in the occasional questions and judgments he puts forward.

All the personality-changes brought about by a process have in common the *limitation* or *disintegration* of the personality. The term 'dementia' used in such cases implies disturbance in intelligence, memory, etc., and also a change in personality.

### (a) Dementia due to organic cerebral processes

Certain character traits seem due sometimes to processes of this sort. Thus we find jocularity (Witzelsucht) with certain brain-tumours, 'gallows-humour' in alcoholics, religiosity, habitual lying and pedantic meticulousness in epileptics, and euphoria in multiple sclerotics.

Such traits can be explained partly in the same way and using the same concepts as apply to other changes. The process *removes the acquired inhibitions*, instinctive impulse is translated into action at once without any counter-image or counter-tendency. Once ideas are evoked, they take immediate effect. A paralytic, for example, can easily be made to cry and then laugh by the evocation of opposing ideas ('incontinence of affect').

Disintegration goes furthest in the known organic cerebral processes such as Paralysis (and similarly in severe arterio-sclerosis, Huntington's chorea and other organic cerebral diseases).

### (b) Epileptic dementia

Epileptics who are victims of a progressive process show typical changes in their nature.[1] The slowing down of psychic events (down to the level of the nervous reflexes) shows itself in increasing difficulty of comprehension and the enormous prolongation of reaction-time. To this is added a tendency to perseverate. The affect tends to linger on and stereotypies develop. The loss of spontaneity and activity is accompanied by an elementary, urgent but aimless restlessness. Egocentric touchiness and a craving for constant approbation leads to increasing irritability and explosive reactions. Brutal motor discharges may occur in patients who otherwise are quite inoffensive. There are also descriptions of the so-called 'clinging' patient and attitudes of ingratiating effusiveness. Nervous tension and empty affect complete the picture. The constrictedness of the patients which makes them appear taut, rigid, pedantic and circumstantial can look like conscientiousness, conservatism and solidity etc.

### (c) 'Dementia' in schizophrenia

Among the personalities which are due to a process, those of the schizophrenic group deserve special mention. Many chronic mental hospital patients belong to this group. Variation in personality may range from a very slight alteration in the individual due to a reduction in understandability, to almost

---

[1] K. H. Stauder, *Konstitution und Wesensveränderung der Epileptiker* (Leipzig); Max Eyrich, 'Über Charakter und Charakterveränderung bei Kindlichen und Jugendlichen Epileptikern', *Z. Neur.*, vol. 141 (1932), p. 640.

complete fragmentation of his personality. It is not easy to see any common factor. Earlier psychiatrists tried to characterise something which they called 'affective dementia'. Nowadays we lay additional emphasis on the lack of integration in thinking, feeling and volition, and on the inability to recognise reality as reality and take it properly into account (Bleuler's 'autistic thinking', that is, thinking turned in on itself and on its phantasies with no regard for reality). At the same time, the tools of intelligence remain intact. It is easier to describe the common factor in subjective terms, that is, in terms of the effect on the observer, rather than try to do so objectively. All these personalities have something baffling about them, which baffles our understanding in a peculiar way; there is something queer, cold, inaccessible, rigid and petrified there, even when the patients are quite sensible and can be addressed and even when they are eager to talk about themselves. We may think we can understand dispositions furthest from our own but when faced with such people we feel a gulf which defies description. Also, they do not find those things puzzling which for us are quite unintelligible. They may run away from home for a trivial reason which seems quite adequate for them. They do not draw the obvious consequences from facts and situations, they have no adaptability and show a puzzling angularity and indifference. One such type is the hebephrenic personality, which has been characterised as an hypertrophy and an arrest in development of the awkward traits of adolescence. If we study the nature of these people closely, we find we have to create a large number of types which we shall not distinguish here. The mildest personality change consists in a growth of coldness and stiffness. Patients lose agility, grow much quieter with less initiative.

*How the schizophrenic personality views the change.* Some patients with a mild degree of illness will talk about how their nature has changed. They are 'less excitable', 'their interest is shallower but they talk much more'. They notice that they keep on talking and cannot stop but show no kind of agitation. They sometimes observe that they are staring into the corner for no particular reason and that their general performance is suffering. Some can only say that they feel 'a profound change' has taken place. They feel 'they are not as flexible as before' and not so excitable. Hölderlin has expressed this knowledge of the schizophrenic change in himself in simple and moving words:

> Wo bist du? Wenig lebt ich, doch atmet kalt
> Mein Abend schon. Und stille, den Schatten gleich
> Bin ich schon hier; und schon gesanglos
> Schlummert das schauernde Herz im Busen.

> (Where art thou? So short my life,
> Yet comes my cold evening.
> I am here like the shadows, like them
> I am silent and my shuddering heart
> Has already ceased singing and sleeps in my breast.)

Later on, in the advanced state of his illness, he wrote:

> Das Angenehme dieser Welt hab ich genossen
> Der Jugend Freuden sind wie lang! wie lang! verflossen,
> April und Mai und Julius sind ferne.
> Ich bin nichts mehr, ich lebe nicht mehr gerne.
>
> (I am no longer party to this world's delight,
> The happiness of youth fled long, how long, ago,
> April, May, July I cannot reach,
> Now I no longer live and have no joy.)

# NAME INDEX

# GENERAL INDEX

li

Primitive (*contd.*)
  parallels and analogies, 214
  collective unconscious, 338 f., 361 f.
  'primitive reactions', 390, 533
Prison psychoses, 386 ff., 389 ff., 396, 407
  conversion experience in prison, 388 f.
  'delusion-like fancies' in prison, 409
  day-dreaming in prison, 150
  pseudo-dementia, 220
  —vide: Hysteria, 401 ff.
Private languages, 289
Process, P. and phase; organic and psychic P., 692 ff.
  personality-development or P., 653 ff., 702 ff.
  personality transformation by P., 445 ff.
  limit of understanding, 704 ff.
  P. and neurosis, 704 ff.
  —vide: Development, Personality, Personality-change, Brain-process
Production, cultural p. of patients, 281 ff.
  literary productions of patients, 290 f.
Productivity, fluctuations of P., 216
  morbid P., 284, 287, 294
Prognosis, long and short term, 842 ff.
  —vide: Diagnosis, Cure, Acute
Propulsive 'temperament of development' (Conrad), 660 f.
Protracted recovery, 844
Pseudo-bulbar palsy, 257, 272
Pseudo-dementia, 194, 220, 391 f.
Pseudo-hallucination, 68 ff.
Pseudologia phantastica, 151, 218, 329, 420, 795
Pseudo-understanding, 306
Psychasthenia, psychasthenic, symptom-complex, 216, 441 f.
  'sensitive idea of reference', p. reaction, 409, 640
  p. reaction, 389
  theory of levels, 533
Psyche, psychic, as objectified, 9 f.
  P. as consciousness, 9 f., 137 ff.
  differentiation of p. life, 13 ff.
  expression of P. in body and movement, 253 ff.
  P. and body, 311 ff.
  —vide: Body and psyche, Body
  somatopsychology, 5 f., 222 ff.
  P. between Mind and Body, 311 f.
  —vide: Understanding
  P. and character, 428
  —vide: Character, Personality
  comprehending p. life through opposition of whole and parts, 27 f., 555 ff.
  —vide: Unity (complex), Elements
  P. as Encompassing, 550 ff.
  —vide: Encompassing, 480, 435, 364, Man, Existence itself
  p. energy, variations of, 441 ff.
  dynamic theories, 532 ff.
  association theory, 534 ff.
  p. development from transformation of drives, 324 f.
Psychiatrist, types of P., attitude of P., 806 ff.
  necessity for self-illumination of P., 812 ff.
Psychiatry as an art v. psychopathology as a science, 1 ff.
  history of P., 844 ff.
  German and French, P., 853 f.
  modern P., 854 ff.

Self-revelation, 798 f., 330, 350, 354 ff.
   —vide: Existence, illumination of
Self-sufficiency and dependence, 326
Self-transformation as self-realisation in marginal situations, the therapeutic aim, 330
   —vide: Personality development, Personality-transformation
Self-understanding, 349 f.
   S. of patient in interpretation of his illness, 415 ff.
   misleading pseudo-knowledge, 543 ff., 545 f.
Senile dementia, 218, 686
Senility and old age, 176, 683 f., 686 f., 700 f.
   senile dementia, 218
Sensations, change in intensity and quality, 61 f.
   abnormal accompanying S., 62
   abnormal feeling-S., 112
   subjective bodily S., 227 ff.
Sense-areas, senses, 70 ff.
   hallucinations, 90 f.
   synaesthesias, 74 f.
   simultaneous hallucinations, 129 ff.
   personifications, 129 ff.
   significance of level of attention in false perceptions, 140 f.
   disorders of the sense-organs in production of hallucinations, 169 f., 483 f.
   sense-deficiency, 169
Sense-memory, 66
Sense-perceptions (awareness of body), 88 f.
   hallucinations, 90 ff.
   abnormal feeling sensations, 112
Sensible state, 140 f.
Sensitive, sensitive individual, 445, 327
   'sensitive delusions of reference', 409, 640
   personality and delusions of grandeur and persecution, 411 f., 640
   'sensitive paranoic', 413
'Sensitiver Beziehungswahn'—vide: Sensitive delusion of reference
Sensitivity, reduced S. to pain, 61
Sensory aphasias, 187 ff.
Sex, sexuality, 365 f., 618 f., 623 ff.
   S. and psychosis, 628 ff., 685 f.
Shock, 157
   S.-psychoses, 367 ff., 389 f.
   S.-therapy, 475, 832 f.
Shouting, state of, 124 f., 192, 487, 690
Simulation, 829
   'purposive psychoses', 386 f., 388 ff., 719 f.
   S. and hysteria, 244
Sin, delusions of, 107 f.
Situation, concept of, 325 ff., 10 f.
   marginal S., or frontier-S., 326 f., 330
   social S., 709 ff., 716 ff., 732 ff.
   S. and therapy, 837 ff.
   —vide: Milieu, Environment
Sleep, 144 ff., 232 f.
   S. and hypnosis, 379
   disturbances of S., 233 ff., 87
   sleeplessness, 233 f.
   excessive sleep, 234
   falling asleep and waking, rituals, 234 f., 272
Slowing-down (psychic), 486 f.
Social psychology, 710 ff.
Social psychology and society, 709 ff.

Milton Keynes UK
Ingram Content Group UK Ltd.
UKHW012022041023
429977UK00001B/1